TRAUMATIC APHASIA
ITS SYNDROMES, PSYCHOLOGY AND TREATMENT

JANUA LINGUARUM

STUDIA MEMORIAE NICOLAI VAN WIJK DEDICATA

edenda curat

C. H. VAN SCHOONEVELD

INDIANA UNIVERSITY

SERIES MAIOR

5

1970

MOUTON

THE HAGUE · PARIS

TRAUMATIC APHASIA

ITS SYNDROMES, PSYCHOLOGY AND TREATMENT

by

A. R. LURIA

UNIVERSITY OF MOSCOW

Translated from the Russian

With a Foreword by Macdonald Critchley

1970

MOUTON

THE HAGUE · PARIS

Original title:
Травматическая афазия: клиника, семиотика и восстановительная терапия.
Translated by Douglas Bowden

LIBRARY OF CONGRESS CATALOG CARD NUMBER: 68-17903

Printed in The Netherlands by Mouton & Co., Printers, The Hague.

FOREWORD

by

Macdonald Critchley, C.B.E., M.D., F.R.C.P.,
President, World Federation of Neurology.

Anything which emanates from the pen of Alexander Romanovitch Luria is tantamount to a happening within the aphasiological clique. For the past two decades this author has consistently enriched neurology with his idiosyncratic contributions to the field of higher nervous activity. His work combines in unique fashion all that is most valuable in both Eastern and Western European thought. With Sechenov's ideas as a background inspiration, Luria learned much from his senior colleague Vigotsky, whose premature demise continues to impoverish contemporary thinking. In neurology as in Art, *on est toujours le fils de quelqu'un*, but none the less Luria did not delay his departure from the nest. He has shown himself to be endowed in an unusual degree with intellectual *ingenium* or drive; with an enthusiasm of the Peter Pan variety; and with a cerebral tirelessness which inspires all who are privileged to work alongside him. *Rast ich, so rost ich,* we are told, and this theme has been Luria's life-long driving force. Opportunity ensured a clinical continuum of vexed neuropathological problems which aroused all the peculiar talents of clinical exploration which the good fairies had bestowed upon him. By dint of tenacious and dauntless probing he uncovered the secret mechanism of the faltering efforts of top-level perceptual and communicative activities, utilising to the utmost his own creative thinking. Novel batteries of tests were devised, bringing to the surface faults and failings which the patient had succeeded in concealing from more superficial examiners, who were enmeshed and bogged down in the toils of conventional and less inspired systems of thought.

The secrets of communicative difficulties have for many years intrigued the searching mind of Professor Luria. Being neither a holist nor yet a stubborn localiser, he borrowed what was best from these rival ideologies, and so brought a new look to bear upon problems of aphasia. As a result he was at one and the same time a researcher who both fascinated and yet often goaded contemporary workers. Like Lasègue, he employed at the bedside his very own techniques of investigation . . . "urging, begging, ironical, good-natured, even endearing, permitting the patient to express himself freely, or on other occasions asking him innumerable questions, but never tiring until he was sure to have obtained all possible information". More than any other representative within this field, Luria was a man endowed with fire in his belly, be this a virtue or a handicap. No one who works in this difficult and superficially unpromising terrain can possibly brush aside the contributions of Luria, whether he be in enthusiastic agreement, or in ardent opposition – or whether even he be seated in calculating fashion upon an intellectual fence. Everything he has touched he has adorned, and aphasiology would be a considerably poorer discipline were it not for Luria.

In this present volume on communicative disorders, Luria has limited his pathological material to those cases of aphasia which result from brain-injuries. In so doing, Luria has actually copied the model laid down by Henry Head. Both physicians were influenced by the factor of opportunity and took advantage thereof. Head stressed the peculiar merits of traumatic cases whenever problems of aphasia were under scrutiny. A traumatic lesion is as a rule a cleanly punched-out defect in a cerebrum which is mature and yet not senescent, for in all other respects it is healthy and functionally intact. Accordingly traumatic cases of aphasia are better vehicles for study than those which are due to vascular occlusion, where diffuse arterial thickening or circulatory inadequacies are all too frequent. There exists in such cases an antecedent loss of cerebral virginity, as they say. Moreover, unlike the neoplastic cases, the defect is not of necessity expansive, but is one which may be deemed static or even regressive.

Yet it must be demurred that traumatic cases are somewhat short of the ideal, for the clinical picture is not wholly stable. The opimum research – probably unattainable – would be a definitive study of aphasia based upon cases of cerebral embolism.

To ponder a moment. Aphasia, the touchstone upon which certain rash neurologists are bold enough to test themselves, is a subject of peculiar complexity, frustrating in its obliquity. Some might well look upon it as a chaos of immiscible and conflicting particles. Gowers, master of language as well as of neurology, once laid it down that "the whole subject has afforded abundant scope for word-making; where a large number of new terms have been introduced, most of which are needless, and to some extent injurious, fostering a harmful tendency to divide where it is desirable only to distinguish".

Many physicians who busy themselves with disorders of the nervous system, feel somewhat out of sympathy with those who delve into clinical disorders of expression. The topic, they feel, is unrewarding, impractical, metaphysical, vain. Like Tweedledee in "Alice in the Looking-Glass" they are apt to reject the whole problem of aphasia by saying, "Contrariwise, if it was so, it might be; and if it were so, it would be; and if it isn't, it ain't. That's logic." Indeed, logic it may be, but the aphasiological problems cannot be dismissed as lightly as that.

It has been laid down that there are as many epileptics as there are epilepsies. This aphorism applies still more appositely to patients who have become victimised by defects in self-expression. No two aphasiacs are identical. Biologically speaking this would be impossible. The anonymous coterie of uncommunicating inaccessibles holds no two of a kind. Despite the scores of Russians whose verbalisation is limited to *nyet* and *da*, each monophasic patient represents an autonomous problem, and cannot be strictly compared with the *oui-non,* yes-no, *ja-nein* witnesses who are encountered beyond the borders of the U.S.S.R. To acknowledge this fact implies that a classification of aphasiacs is a more thorny problem than would be imagined at first blush. Some, understandably enough, throw up their hands in despair, and refuse to attempt to classify, preferring to speak merely of "aphasia and its types". Luria, however, boldly promotes his own particular classification.

Time alone will show whether Professor Luria's schemata will survive. If not, then not: the matter is scarcely important. Suffices it to say that this present monograph will for many years cnstitute a conspicuous milestone in aphasiological progress. In writing this foreword it would be tempting to say, with Horace, "*Haec scripsi non otii abundantia sed amoris erga te.*" But more apposite would it be to quote what Sydney Smith once proclaimed ". . . the further he went West the more convinced he felt that the wise men came from the East. . . ."

INTRODUCTION

The present book is the result of observations collected during the Second World War and postwar years when the disorders and subsequent recovery of functions disturbed by brain injuries from fire arms forced themselves upon us as especially acute problems. It does not attempt to cover all aspects of problems which enter into the study of aphasia. Major emphasis is given here to questions of the topical diagnosis of aphasia and to the analysis of particular forms of speech disorders which arise as a result of local brain damage. Consideration of these problems on the basis of war injuries led to answers to important theoretical and practical questions in the field of aphasia.

The basic idea underlying this work is that only by a broad approach to the study of traumatic speech disorders, an approach embracing contemporary knowledge both of psychology and linguistics and knowledge about the structure and physiological functions of the cerebral hemispheres, is it possible to reach conclusions which go beyond the limits of narrow questions of aphasia. The author has attempted to take this approach.

Traumatic Aphasia was first published in 1947 by the Press of the Academy of Medical Sciences, USSR. In 1959 the text has been considerably revised in preparation for the present printing. However, it is obvious that the author was unable to include all new data accumulated in his laboratory as well as in the world literature during the last years. Reading the proofs he could only mention some important works published recently. Two books by the author: *Higher Cortical Functions in Man* (New York, Basic Books, 1966) and *Human Brain and Psychological Processes* (New York, Harper & Row, 1966) can be used as the information of several of his latest works.

The author notes with gratitude the initiative of the publishers, Mouton, who have taken upon themselves the trouble to prepare and print the English edition of this book. He wishes to express his gratitude to Dr. Douglas Bowden for the translation of this book.

Moscow, January, 1967 A. R. Luria

TABLE OF CONTENTS

PART III. REHABILITATION OF PATIENTS WITH TRAUMATIC APHASIA

PART I

GENERAL PROBLEMS AND TOPICAL SYNDROMES OF TRAUMATIC APHASIA

I

THE ORGANIZATION OF BRAIN FUNCTIONS AND PROBLEMS OF APHASIA

A complete understanding of the mechanisms of aphasia and a clear interpretation of the studies in this field can be achieved only if one keeps in mind the theoretical conceptions which have underlain the study of speech disorders in the past. Since these conceptions have determined the positions from which various investigators have conducted their analyses of aphasia, there is every reason to preface the description of our work with a historical survey, though it be only a short one.

The history of the study of aphasia goes back more than a hundred years and consists of a long struggle to achieve a scientific conception of the structure of mental functions and of their localization in the cerebral cortex. It is only natural that at each stage views from which various investigators proceeded were not identical and that progress in this area was intimately bound to the development of their views.

When, in 1861, Broca formulated for the first time the position that destruction of the motor aspect of speech is related to damage of a limited area of the brain he was proceeding from a well defined conception of brain structure and of the localization of functions in the brain cortex. According to this conception, which received support from the anatomical findings of Betz and the physiological investigations of Fritsch and Hitzig, the cortex is a highly differentiated system of areas whose cells possess very specific functions. At this time, when the first anatomico-physiological studies of brain activity were differentiating areas of the cortex which have strictly defined *physiological* (afferent or efferent) functions, clinical investigators were beginning to distinguish areas which appeared to be unique "depots" for complex mental processes and consequently to have definite *psychological* functions. Thus there were described "centers" for the "motor image of the word" (Broca's area) and for the "sensory image of the word" (Wernicke's area). Further, after the works of Charcot in France, Bastian and Broadbent in England, Lichtheim and Kussmaul in Germany, and Henschen in Sweden there were described isolated cortical areas which were "centers" for reading, writing, computation, spatial imagery, and active thought. In the later half of the last century these views were expressed particularly clearly in the publications of K. Kleist, J. Nielsen, and others.

In earlier works, views based on the psychomorphological conception that mental faculties may be considered particular, indivisible functions related to strictly defined groups of cells met with disappointing findings which eventually led them into deep crisis. Theoretically this crisis was related to the fact that the conception of mental processes as isolated indivisible "functions" and "characteristics" rooted in the old "psychology of faculties" very soon ceased to correspond to scientific conceptions of mental processes. Such processes came to be thought of in modern science as a more refined product of complex reflex activity evolving out of the socio-historical conditions of human life. Therefore the idea that it might be possible to relate the highly complex functional systems which underlie such processes as perception, speech, writing, or computation to single limited groups of cells in the cortex rather soon came into conflict with the more modern scientific conceptions. It became clear that such complex forms of reflex activity could in no way be considered direct products of the functioning of isolated cell groups. Thus the conception of mental processes as complex forms of reflex activity forced a fundamental change in ideas regarding the brain mechanisms of this activity.

Doubt regarding the validity of the mechanistic psycho-morphological conception of the "localization" of mental functions was made explicit in the well known positions of principle which were formulated in the modern clinic and which quickly achieved universal recognition. First Hughlings Jackson and later K. Goldstein expressed the idea that the appearance of one or another symptom following damage to a strictly defined area of the brain, gives no basis for assuming the "localization of function". The "localization of symptoms" is of great use to the clinic, but it is reasonable to suggest that the functions disturbed may be based on much broader brain mechanisms. To draw an analogy, the breaking of the pendulum in so simple a mechanism as a clock will make it cease running altogether; but this gives no basis for localizing the "running function" in this broken part! Thus clinicians, with good reason, took the position that the description of the topical site from which a given disorder may be produced must be considered not the end, but only the beginning of the job to determine the function of a given site. The study of focal symptoms should be considered only as one type of material regarding brain mechanisms of disturbed activity.

A final factor which led to the crisis of the psycho-morphological conceptions was related to extreme contradictions among the very facts which had laid the basis for the conceptions of localization just mentioned. Often the foci of damage underlying the disturbance of one or another "function", turned out in practice to be considerably more widespread than would have been predicted theoretically. Even the focus underlying the motor aphasia of the famous patient, whose case served as an example in Broca's first report, turned out, as was shown by Pierre Marie, to extend considerably beyond the limits of "Broca's area". Frequently destruction of the zone designated "center for the motor images of words" was altogether unaccompanied by the expected disorder. (Recently this has been demonstrated by Nissl von Mayendorf and Goldstein who have described motor aphasia in patients with completely intact Broca's areas.) Frequently, damage of completely different cerebral cortex produced apparently identical disturbances, and as a result investigators were forced to describe at least three or four cortical areas, destruction of which led, for instance, to amnesic aphasia, to disturbance of speech comprehension, or to writing disorders. In the end, the clinic was forced to state that the destruction of a single cortical area produced by no means only one strictly defined symptom, but as a rule led to a whole syndrome into which there entered, it would seem, a highly varied combination of disturbances. As examples one needed only point to the sensory aphasia, amnestic aphasia, paraphasia, and agraphia which resulted from injury of the left temporal area, or the disturbed spatial orientation, tactile agnosia and disturbance of logico-grammatical relationships which followed damage to the left parieto-temporo-occipital area.

All this led to the fact that psycho-morphological conceptions of the localization of mental processes in localized areas of the cortex began to lose both their theoretical basis and, to a large extent, even their practical validity. A crisis for these conceptions thus was inevitable.

Criticism of conceptions of strict localization arose very early, even in the years immediately following Broca's first publications, Hughlings Jackson spoke out against such simplified psycho-morphological assumptions. Jackson's views did not receive their due recognition in his time; only more than half a century later did they become guideposts in cortical neurology. While not denying the possibility of localizing certain elementary physiological functions, Jackson expressed the view that attempts to localize complex psychic processes lacked any basis. He insisted that the attempt to account for motor aphasia in terms of the disturbance of "motor images of words" which were presumably localized in a limited cortical area could hardly be considered convincing. In considering motor aphasia he turned attention to the fact that expressive speech is only rarely completely eliminated – that the defect of a function depends on the conditions under which is it carried out, and that usually a patient who is unable to pronounce words voluntarily, to construct sentences and use speech as a means of communication or of expression of his thoughts and desires, is easily able to pronounce various automatic phrases (speech "emboli"), emit various exclamations, and even produce whole sentences if he is in a state of emotional excitement.

This led Jackson to the idea that disturbances of function which arise in various pathological conditions of the brain (including damage to various parts of the brain) must be analyzed in light of the *evolution of mental function,* taking into consideration first of all the *functional level* at which one or another activity becomes disturbed. The fact that the disintegration of activity at a higher ("voluntary") level can be accompanied by the preservation of activity at a lower ("automatic") level led to an essential shift in the treatment of clinical data. It led to a substitution of the conception of genetic levels of functional organization for conceptions of localization of brain activity.

Jackson's conceptions were without a doubt progressive ones. The best neurologists of modern times – Head and Brain in England, Pick, Foerster, and Goldstein in Germany, Alajouanine and Ombredane in France – though they represent various positions, essentially accepted and continued along the lines laid down by Jackson, thus confirming the great scientific significance of the conceptions set forth by that outstanding author.

Despite the advantages of the evolutionary-dynamic conception, however, it had hidden within it considerable dangers. The most fundamental of these lay in the fact that by concentrating all attention on the *level of organization* of various functions this conception in fact discouraged concrete analysis of the topical aspects of various disorders and evaluation in the performance of various functions. By its very nature it diverted consideration of disturbed functions away from the organic substratum and turned clinical case investigations into psychological descriptions of the functional organization of disturbed activity. Not infrequently the brain came to be considered as a single unit not to be analyzed into its various parts.

The danger of the holistic or global point of view, (both of disturbed mental function and of normal brain mechanisms) is manifest in a large number of the investigations carried out in the past fifty years. The lack of concern for neuroanatomy and neurophysiological bases of both normal and disturbed mental function prevented investigators from achieving genuine success in the clinical understanding of focal brain damage. At the very beginning of the twentieth century the dangers involved in a retreat from neurology and neurophysiology became evident in the works of Pierre Marie who, having successfully criticized the conception of strict localization, came himself to the conclusion that true aphasia (which he considered to be Wernicke's aphasia) is not essentially a speech disorder but a disturbance of the intellect and thus not readily accessible to topical analysis. In this assertion he not only improperly differentiated two intimately related processes, viz. thought and speech, but he also closed the door to scientific study of those brain mechanisms which underlie complex forms of mental activity.

Although he set forth valid criticisms of narrow localization theories from a different position, another great neurologist, Kurt Goldstein, actually followed along the same lines to a holistic conception of the brain and mental activity. Extending his view of brain pathology to encompass functional disturbances of the organism as a whole, he eventually had to limit his attention to the most general rules of pathology which he formulated in terms of "Gestalt psychology". Thus in describing disturbances of "abstract behavior" he found no way of relating them to disturbances of brain activity other than by speaking of disturbances of the "totality of brain function" or the narrowing of "dynamic structures". These constructs were not accompanied by concrete suggestions as to the character of disorders which are introduced into various functional systems by damage to specific focal arias.

In Goldstein's work the analytic approach to relatively elementary disorders gave way to an extremely general and global philosophical point of view. In the works of other authors who were dealing with disturbances of more complex processes investigations were carried out which involved attempts at the analysis of brain mechanisms. One need only consider the works of representatives of the so called "noëtic school" (van Woerkom, Bouman and Grünbaum and others) who regarded speech disturbances as the result of damage to "basic mental function" to see that the analysis of pathological changes in mental processes was completely divorced from the investigation of underlying neurophysiological mechanisms. It turned into a purely psychological description of the "disintegration" of complex phenomena. This approach contributed a certain sophistication to the analysis of disturbed forms of psychological activity, it completely side-stepped any study of the concrete brain mechanisms which underlie normal and disturbed mental processes.

It is easy to see that neither the direct psycho-morphological attempts to "localize" mental processes in limited groups of brain cells nor the "noëtic" tendencies to describe levels of organization of psychic processes with no analysis of their brain mechanisms, was capable of further developing this branch of knowledge on a scientific basis.

A scientific approach to the analysis of mental processes and their cerebral organization, while taking into account the level of organization of various functional systems, must not renounce the study of specific brain mechanisms; on the contrary, proposed neurophysiological mechanisms must be subjected to the most careful scientific investigation. Such an approach is by no means to be obtained simply by mechanically combining the two approaches described above. It demands a reexamination of fundamental concepts and renunciation of those false positions assumed by each of the two earlier theoretical systems.

The fundamental positions from which one must construct a scientific theory of brain mechanisms of normal and disturbed mental processes is a conception of psychological processes as highly differentiated functional systems. We shall present here only the broadest outlines of these concepts, leaving more detailed consideration for later.

Even the most simple relationship between organism and environment (even that which we see at the lowest phylogenetic levels) cannot be conceived of as the manifestation of certain "faculties" laid down inside the organism and "localized" in one or another of its parts. The behavior of an organism, beginning with the simplest reactions of living protoplasm, is determined by the specific conditions of its existence in a given environment, by its needs, and by its reactions to stimuli which act upon it. These reactions make possible the best conditions for metabolism by maintaining an "equilibrium" between the organism and its environment. When, in the process of biological development, the environmental conditions in which an organism lives become more complex, its continued existence demands new, more complete forms of orientation to that environment. There arise distance receptors and complex, variable motor mechanisms. At this stage adaptation to the environment comes to be accomplished by means of the distance receptors and those forms of functional apparatus for analysis and synthesis which I. P. Pavlov named "analyzers". It is only natural that at this stage all orienting activity and the active behavior associated with it takes on the character of complex and dynamic functional systems by means of which the organism adapts to nonsteady aspects of the environment. The appearance of temporary connections based on a highly complex dynamic mosaic of excited and inhibited points in the brain cortex constitutes a most important form of analysis and synthesis of external stimuli. It leads to the formation of those complex functional systems which permit the organism to successfully "equilibrate" with its environment.

It is altogether natural that against the background of this conception of the vital activity of organisms the idea of fixed "characteristics" in various brain areas should give way to another more adequate conception of *complex and mobile functional systems* by which the organism becomes adapted to the environment. These functional systems vary greatly depending upon the levels of organization of the activities involved, but they are always based upon the combined activity of the analyzers by means of which the organism orients itself among signals impinging upon it from the external world. It would, of course, be improper from this point of view to conceive of the complex functional systems as "faculties" of limited groups of cells and to "localize" them in definite isolated areas of the brain. "Localization of function" in this case becomes another problem, viz. the problem of the *dynamic distribution of functional systems in central regions of the nervous system* and especially in the cerebral cortex. Instead of conceptions of "centers" for complex psychic processes there arise the concepts of *dynamic structures* or *constellations of cerebral zones,* each of which comprises part of the cortical portion of a given analyzer and preserves its specific function, while participating in its own way in the organization of one or another form of activity.

Everything which we have just said applies in large measure to the complex question of the cerebral organization of *speech processes*. Of all forms of activity, speech is the last that should be attributed to "intrinsic abilities" residing in various regions of the brain. Its sources are not to be found in the depths of the organism, but in the historical conditions out of which emerged the *inter-personal division of labor.* It arose among members of primitive society where the objective necessity for more complex forms of communication first appeared.

Under the conditions of primitive society language began to develop as a means of communication; there, in accordance with laws not yet known to us, *verbal speech* appeared. In the development of verbal speech words gradually became separated from work activities and from signalling gestures; words began to abstract and at the same time to generalize various characteristics of objects. They thus achieved designating and at the same time generalizing-systematizing functions.

In later social history language attained its complex phonetic, lexical, and grammatical structure and gradually became the *objective system of codes* which is well known to contemporary linguistics. Without a knowledge of the history and structure of this system of codes no scientific analysis of the development of speech processes and speech disorders is possible.

The formation of speech processes is related to important changes in the structure of the functional systems of the brain which were spoken of above. With the emergence of what Pavlov considered to be a "second signal system of reality" derived from "abstraction and at the same time generalization of innumerable direct signals", the most complex form of reflex activity, formerly the basis of animal behavior, took on new specific features in man.

The processes of analysis and synthesis of external stimuli, when mediated by speech, acquired new forms. As a result of the changes it is possible to differentiate quickly new signals on the basis of very fine cues. The retention of these cues is greatly changed and mnemonic activity, which becomes reorganized with the appearance of speech, is raised to a new level of stability and flexibility. Modes of orientation to the environment and the formation of reflex connections are essentially altered; instead of the gradual elaboration of new conditioned reflexes which is typical in animals it becomes possible for a connection to be established rapidly by means of its inclusion into one or another thought system formulated in speech. Finally, there emerges a new level of voluntary and conscious behavior which, while predetermined to the same degree as the more elementary forms of reflex activity, differs in the fact that, in this case, behavioral acts are determined by complex systems of connections determined by past experience and evoked by language mechanisms.

All of these facts [1] imply the necessity of a new approach to the organization of psychic activity which we have spoken of above. In particular, it becomes possible to study the functional systems in which the cortical zones underlying speech processes participate. As has been shown by numerous investigations, the higher level of organization of mental activity which arises when the organism's relationship to reality is mediated by the speech process, is of a complex systemic character and cannot be thought of as the result of activity of any one isolated cortical area. This is true even of the most elementary forms of mental process in which speech function plays a role.

Even the simple visual perception of color or shape (and certainly the perception of objects) results from complex activity which involves inspection, comparison

[1] The role of speech in the formation of complex types of activity has been discussed in detail in a series of our works which are reviewed in a special publication, *The Role of Speech in the Regulation of Normal and Abnormal Behavior* (London, Pergamon Press, 1961). Other discussions of this work are to be found in A. R. Luria and F. Y. Judovič, *Speech and the Development of Mental Processes in the Child* (Academy of Pedagogical Sciences of the RSFSR, Moscow, 1956; English edition, London, 1959), and in two volumes of *Problems of Higher Nervous Activity in the Normal and Abnormal Child* (Academy of Pedagogical Sciences of the RSFSR, Vol. 1, 1956, and Vol. 2, 1958) (in Russian).

and naming. As a number of authors have indicated (L. S. Vygotskij, 1934; J. Bruner, 1957) perception is ultimately the inclusion of a color, shape, or object into a *complex system of connections,* by a unique classification or by an act of senseful cognition and thus can by no means be considered an elementary function of some limited area of brain tissue. The same can be said of auditory and kinesthetic perceptual processes. That is to say, *by becoming associated with speech signals even those processes which at lower levels of development may be carried out by relatively limited cortical systems, take on an incomparably more complex pattern of organization,* and come to rest on highly complex interrelationships of various zones functioning jointly. With the development of language cerebral mechanisms lose their localized character and take on altogether new systemic characteristics. These statements relate particularly to the cerebral organization of the *speech processes themselves.*

The social origin of language renders fruitless any attempt to understand the speech process in terms of relatively simple psychological "faculties" which may be "localized" in such special centers as, for example, "centers for the sensory and motor images of words". As we shall see below, even such a relatively simple aspect of speech process as its auditory organization represents the complex result of integrated activity of central mechanisms of auditory and motor (articulatory) analysis. Differentiation of the auditory cues which constitute the signals of a language occurs in the integrated activity of the auditory and articulation systems; as a result of language's phonetic structure it becomes possible to pick out from the flow of speech those distinct and constant elements which also constitute the basis of "auditory speech". This means that even the cerebral organization of the auditory properties of speech cannot be understood as the function of an isolated "center" of auditory speech.

The functional organization of the semantic aspect of speech is even more complicated. At the present time no one thinks that the significance of words can be reduced to simple visual images associated with verbal designations. The significance of a word for a child always rests upon some practical activity. In the course of practical activity abbreviation and differentiation gradually take place leading to that schematized "concept of the object" which a word denominates. By giving the concept a name, language fulfills the function of abstracting necessary cues and introducing it into complex flexible systems. The existence of the lexical and syntactical codes in language makes these systems unusually complex and rich.

On the basis of all this there is no reason to consider the semantic aspect of speech to result from the functioning of some cortical "center" which acts as a "depot" for those images which language denominates. We have every reason to believe that the speech activity associated with abstraction and generalization is a product of highly complex systems of temporary connections which arise in the process of communication with other people. In our present state of knowledge we can only make guesses as to the cortical organization of such systems. It goes without saying that when we go from the more phasic aspects of speech to what linguists refer to as its pragmatic aspect, i.e. its regulatory role in the organization of complex voluntary behavior, the functional systems involved become many times more complex.

The great complexity of speech activity which we have just considered gives no grounds, however, for retreating to descriptions in terms of "higher levels in the structure of mental processes" and refusing to study its underlying brain mechanisms. Nor does it require us to limit ourselves to speaking of "activity of the brain as a whole" as representatives of the noetic school would have us do. Least of all should we speak in terms of spiritual processes which themselves have nothing in common with the brain. Following such a course inevitably leads into the type of dead-end in which even so great a scientist as Sherrington (1935, 1941) found himself in his later years. To separate mental activity from the brain would be to commit a grave mistake against the progressive development of science.

Everything that we know about the development of speech in early childhood, about language in the adult, and about the pathology of speech leads us to consider speech processes as the most complex and specifically human form of reflex activity. This reflex activity has its own neurophysiological basis, its own laws of development, and functional structure. The analysis of brain mechanisms of speech and physiological analysis of what has come to be known in recent years as the problem of "interaction of the two signalling systems" (I. P. Pavlov) should not be allowed to drop along the wayside. On the contrary, it must become a major subject of scientific investigation.

In considering this subject it is necessary to take into account all that is currently known regarding neurophysiology and neuroanatomy. Above all, the study of speech activity must be taken beyond the study of simple language processes, and the study of speech pathology must go beyond the bounds of aphasia. The analysis of brain mechanisms underlying speech and its disorders can follow two closely related lines of development. We have in view the study of both the general and the specific neurodynamic processes underlying speech.

It is known that speech activity (the basis for which lies in the close interaction of the two signalling systems: direct and verbal) obeys the same laws of excitation and inhibition, irradiation and concentration, as any other form of cortical activity. The difference lies only in the fact that verbal processes, which reflect reality by means of relationships fixed in the language, are accomplished by an incomparably more complex system of relations. Thus it is natural that the analysis of psychological characteristics of speech and speech pathology, which were considered by Jackson, Goldstein, Ombredane and others, requires not only a description of the high level of "voluntariness" and "categorization" of speech, but also a clarification of the physiological mechanisms which make the highest forms of verbal structure possible.

A number of investigators, particularly Isserlin (1928-1932), Lotmar (1933), and Ombredane (1951), have approached this problem directly by showing how the processes of word retrieval and word recognition change in different types of aphasia and by analyzing the factors which prevent full use of "voluntary" and "categorical" speech. Although several of these investigators tried to explain their observations in physiological terms a real study of the neurodynamic characteristics of speech processes is still in the early stages of development. An example of this type of investigation is to be found in Ombredane's observations regarding the naming process. In this work, the conclusions are stated in physiological terminology.[2] In the literature one finds only isolated investigations involving the study of neurodynamic processes underlying various forms of verbal activity. Such studies were carried out by I. D. Sapir (1929, 1934), and P. Ja. Gal'perin and R. A. Golubova (1933). They have been in several works of N. N. Traugott (1957, 1958), and A. G. Ivanov-Smolenskij (1952) and his collaborators. Such studies open up an essential path of physiological investigation of the nervous processes, disturbance of which affects the highest forms of speech.

Unfortunately this important approach is not as developed as it should be in the present volume, still there is no doubt that careful study of the pathological changes in neurodynamics which are seen in aphasic patients must eventually lead to the discovery of many mechanisms, disruption of which produces speech disorders.

A second and no less important path of investigation is the study of the partial neurodynamic disturbances which, while not producing a general drop in the level of cerebral activity, may lead to clear cut forms of *systemic pathology*. A wound, hemorrhage, local inflammatory process or tumor which damages the cells of a limited cortical area results in disturbance of neurodynamic processes within the corresponding analyzer (visual, auditory, skin-kinesthetic, motor, etc.). The cortical portions of the damaged analyzer begin to work considerably less effectively than normally. The strength, steadiness, and lability of nervous processes within the limits of a given analyzer may be disturbed, while the functional state of other analyzers remains intact. In connection with such changes, one finds a sharp drop in the ability to differentiate signals, to preserve traces, and to form new connections in the affected analyzer. This is the *primary* result of focal damage.

It must be understood, however, that this primary effect of a lesion is often accompanied by a *secondary* or *systemic effect.* If a given analyzer begins to function poorly, it is inevitable that *all complex functional systems dependent upon the kinds of analysis and synthesis performed by that analyzer will also suffer.* In such cases the pathological process leads not to general, diffuse disturbances but to *selective, systemic disturbances.* It is precisely these systemic forms of disturb-

[2] Ombredane (1951, p. 302) analyzed the time required for patients with amnesic aphasia to produce certain words; his observations led him to the conclusion that "in order to become available for use, the majority of words must be released from inhibitory influences". These inhibitory influences must become the subject of special physiological investigation.

ance which turn out to be so important in cases of focal brain damage; thus they demand special study. Of special interest to us are those cases in which destruction of limited areas of the brain disturbs systems involved in the production of speech. In our investigations we have attempted to analyze the types of speech pathology which result from the disturbance of various systems. By characterizing the primary disturbance produced by focal damage of the cortex and by analyzing its systemic effect, we obtain an analysis of those complex forms of aphasia which arise as a result of disturbances of specific neurodynamic processes.

The approach which we have just described requires a considerable extension of the usual clinical methods of investigation. The basic prerequisite for an effective study of specific forms of speech pathology is consideration of the problem *outside the narrow bounds of aphasia*; one must take into account everything that is presently known about the structure and function of various zones of the cortex.

Investigations of the cytological and neural structure of the brain, of neurophysiology and of higher nervous activity have occupied a whole generation of scientists. The results of this work place us in a much more favorable position for the solution of the speech problem than was open to earlier neurologists. While Broca and Wernicke were forced to create their own hypothesis as to the structure and function of various brain areas, we may, and must, base our investigations on a great body of knowledge regarding the general structure and general functions of various systems. Thus in studying the structure of particular forms of aphasia, we must determine which cortical functions are disturbed in each case.

Today, in the light of the great achievements of numerous anatomical and clinical investigations and, most important of all, following the investigations of Pavlov and his school with regard to the normal and pathological physiology of higher nervous activity, we know considerably more than was ever known before about the structure and function of various cortical systems. We know that the various cortical systems represent central portions of structures responsible for analyzing in fine detail and for synthesizing them into labile dynamic systems. We know a great deal about the fine structure of the cortical portions of the analyzers, about their topical distributions, about their numerous intracortical and vertical connections, and about the specific and nonspecific systems which activate them. Finally, we already have certain ideas concerning the complex functional systems which are accomplished in the brain cortex and which are responsible for those complex and mutable forms of activity which constitute the basis for human behavior. All of this knowledge must be used in a scientific approach to the study of speech disturbances which follow focal brain damage.

How are functional systems of the cortex disturbed by various lesions? What are the direct results of damage to cells within a given focus, and what kinds of secondary systemic disturbances result? What are the distinguishing characteristics of systematic disturbances which arise as the result of focal lesion at various sites? All these questions are of more than clinical interest, for once subjected to careful investigation, they may provide the basis for a better understanding of complex cortical function as a whole.

As indicated earlier we are not in a position to give equally complete answers to all the questions which arise in the study of aphasia. We have had to limit ourselves primarily to particular forms of pathology, but have attempted to consider them in more general neurophysiological terms than is ordinarily done.

For the most part specific pathology of aphasia has been studied on patients with vascular lesions; some cases have involved inflammatory lesions and cerebral tumors. Only in isolated studies have fire-arms served as the basis for study. This circumstance is of special significance in the history of the study of aphasia, since vascular damage more often than not involves the large area of the brain served by one or another branch of a given cerebral artery. Even in the residual phase, a large cerebral area is usually affected. Usually it is observed at a relatively late age and occurs in conjunction with more general changes in cerebral function which attend senile vascular sclerosis.

The study of wounds inflicted by fire-arms offers a number of advantages. As a rule, brain lesions inflicted by fire-arms, e.g. skull fractures and certain noninfected rapidly healing penetrating wounds, provide one the opportunity to observe the effects of quite limited lesions. Also such lesions often occur at an age when the functions of remaining areas are in a much better functional state. The ability to follow the gradual recovery from traumatic injury, from the acute stages through the residual period, is of great advantage when it comes to analyzing the dynamics of the pathological processes involved. Finally, the application of special forms of rehabilitation therapy makes it possible to discover under controlled conditions the ways by which impaired functions are improved and sometimes totally restored.

All of these considerations induced us to make *traumatic aphasia* the object of special investigation. In the following chapters we take up the general characterization of aphasia and an analysis of its basic forms as they relate to the destruction of topical areas. We have devoted a special section to the analysis of the specific disturbances of speech activity which occur in different forms of aphasia. Finally, we have considered in detail the forms of rehabilitation therapy which are appropriate to different types of aphasia and which can become maximally effective only when they have attained thorough scientific verification.

II

APHASIC SYNDROMES AT DIFFERENT STAGES OF THE RECOVERY FROM TRAUMATIC BRAIN INJURY

In early neurological investigations it was firmly established that speech disturbances, aphasias, arise only as the result of damage to certain areas of the left hemisphere. As a rule aphasia does not appear following injury to the right hemisphere or damage of areas lying outside the "speech areas" of the cortex. Thus the early descriptions of aphasic syndromes, which were subsequently made more precise by many authors, attained a distinctly topological character.

The purely topological classification of aphasic symptoms, was however, based only on studies carried out during the *residual state* following brain lesions due to hemorrhage or trauma. In the early period, immediately following trauma the situation is somewhat different.

It is well known, that any acute brain damage, especially brain trauma, produces very gross disturbances of hemo and cerebrospinal fluid dynamics. These disturbances are the result of direct effects of the trauma on the brain tissues and vessels, accompanied by striking of the brain against the skull, plus the development of edema in brain tissues which results from the first two factors. Thus the initial period after injury, just as after acute hemorrhage, can justifiably be considered a period of *general* brain disorder (L. I. Smirnov, 1947).

A very natural question arises, however: is this initial period of traumatic disorder really as "general" as it is often said to be, or do various systems show more or less disturbance from the first moments following local trauma? Is it really impossible during the first week, following injury to note certain correlations between general and local components of cerebral disorder and to distinguish certain *groups of cerebral zones which respond systematically to trauma*? Such a systemic influence of trauma was carefully studied by Monakow in his day. He described the diaschisis phenomenon (systemic shock) which has its onset in the period immediately following acute brain damage. His study was continued by a number of authors, and in the prewar period we succeeded in observing that even acute postoperative edema which persists for five to seven days following brain operations does not affect the functions of all cortical areas equally. Rather it has a distinct regional character and is reflected primarily in disturbances of the system of functions directly dependent upon the damaged zone (B. G. Spirin, 1951).

What is the nature of the speech disturbances which immediately follow damage to various brain areas, and how do they change during subsequent stages in the recovery process? During the second world war at the Institute of Neurology (then the Clinic for Nervous Disorders of the Union Institute for Experimental Medicine) there was organized a systematic long-term study of patients who had suffered traumatic brain injuries. Initial observations were made in the front lines (acute period). These were followed up by observations in Moscow hospitals (acute and subacute periods), and the studies concluded at the Neurosurgical Rehabilitation Hospital in the Urals (residual period). Thanks to this arrangement, we had available by early 1943 detailed material on more than 800 cases of brain trauma inflicted by fire-arms. All cases were studied in detail in the residual stage (two to five months after trauma). A portion of these patients had been under special observation from the very first stages of evacuation.

For purposes of the present analysis we shall exclude cases of damage to the right hemisphere. In such cases there arose quite distinctive forms of speech disturbance which we shall consider separately. For the present we shall restrict ourselves to a detailed analysis of left hemisphere lesions and the associated speech disorders which are of major interest to us.

Even the very first observations revealed a *significant frequency of aphasic disturbances with onset in the initial period after lesions of the left hemisphere*. Of the 394 cases of left hemispheric lesions which we studied,[1] 240 (61%) showed signs of speech impairment in the early period. Such language disorders took various forms. Most often during the first days, and even weeks, they were characterized by total disruption of all forms of speech activity. Patients who had received injuries of the left hemisphere a few hours before examination not only lacked the ability to speak spontaneously or to answer questions, but they could not understand what was said to them. That unity of the meaning and sound of a word which constitutes the special characteristic of any normal speech process was destroyed, and the patient was in no position either to recall the words which designate various objects or to recognize the significance of words spoken to him. Therefore, in the initial period of traumatic aphasia it most often turned out that even the simplest forms of language activity were severely disturbed, so that any communication with the patient became quite difficult.

Speech disorders produced by left hemisphere injuries, however, were not always the same in character. In many cases it was possible even within the first week following injury to observe that a given aspect of the patient's speech was severely disturbed, while others remained relatively intact. Thus in some patients one found pronounced damage to expressive speech functions with almost complete preser-

[1] Subsequently this material was doubled. For the present study, however, we have limited ourselves to the figures obtained in the first summary of the material. In considering them it is necessary to keep in mind that the basic material was collected in a specialized neurosurgical rehabilitation hospital where there was a high percentage of patients with skull and brain injuries and with traumatic aphasia. This selection of material may be reflected in subsequent figures, thus raising the proportion of speech disturbances to total number of brain injuries

vation of comprehenison. (Later patients might note, "It was impossible to talk". "I understood everything, but I couldn't say anything".) In others one saw the ability to pronounce, though perhaps imperfectly, certain isolated words, but comprehension is extremely difficult ("When you talked fast, I didn't understand". "I didn't quite hear what was said".) "When several people started to talk at once I couldn't understand anything". Some patients noted difficulties of articulation during the early period. ("My tongue wouldn't move". "I didn't say that word right".); others noted that the basic difficulty was not in articulation but in finding the right words. "I forgot everything; I couldn't even remember my name". "I couldn't remember my address, even my home address".) All of these disturbances persisted for a certain length of time, from a few hours to many weeks; then, in many cases they gradually disappeared. Usually the recovery of speech function was quite gradual: at first the total block of expressive speech or comprehension and the unity of word and meaning which is basic to language function was reestablished. Difficulties of articulation, word finding, and slight disturbances of phonetic discrimination lasted considerably longer. After two or three months noticeable signs of aphasic disturbances were observed in only 170 (43%) of those patients who had suffered an injury in the left hemisphere.

These observations indicate that speech disturbances quite frequently accompany injury to the left hemisphere, that such disturbances manifest themselves quite clearly in the first stages of traumatic disorder, and that they subsequently give way to a certain degree of recovery.

A. THE SIGNIFICANCE OF DIFFERENT CEREBRAL ZONES IN THE VARIOUS SYNDROMES WHICH APPEAR DURING THE EARLY RECOVERY PERIOD

Since the appearance of speech disorders occurs so frequently during the initial period following left hemispheric injury, it is natural to ask more specifically whether such disorders follow an injury to *any* zone of the left hemisphere, or does the location of the primary lesion play an important role in determining the functional disorders which arise even during the first week following injury? Are injuries of the various cerebral zones more likely to produce certain speech disorders than others?

The observations presented above clearly contradict the idea that systemic disorders do not exist in the initial period – that in the early period the brain is always affected as a whole. If we take disturbances of speech as a guide in the diagnosis of functional brain disorders, we find that specificity of symptoms does exist in the initial stage of recovery.

We have mentioned that lesions of the *right hemisphere* in right-handed patients seldom produce language difficulties (though speech disturbances occur in such cases more frequently than is generally believed). But when speech impairment appears in such cases it is, as a rule, quite different from that of aphasia.[2] This fact alone serves to demonstrate that functional changes – even those revealed by such a delicate indicator as language function – are not expressed to the same degree with injury to various cerebral zones even in the early period of recovery.

Further, examinations within the first few hours or days after trauma to the *left hemisphere* show that, from the very beginning, various zones react to trauma quite differently one from another, i.e., that *the relative frequency of appearance of various speech disorders depends upon the site of the lesion.*

Despite the obvious shortcomings involved in any attempt to localize brain trauma by the site of skull injury, it is worthwhile to present a summary of our observations which correlate the clinical syndromes observed with the external sites of lesions.[3] Figure 1, a summary of all the material examined by us, shows that even in the early period after trauma, injuries of some areas resulted in a considerable number of speech disorders, whereas almost no impairment of speech accompanied injuries of other zones. Thus injuries of the *frontal* and *occipital* poles hardly ever produced speech impairment. When language disorders did occur in such cases, they consisted of certain peculiar difficulties which we shall consider later.

Closely related injuries were those involving the *superior parietal area.* These were accompanied by a number of slight speech disturbances (37% of all cases); in such cases the missile had usually penetrated into other areas of the brain. It is remarkable that these impairments of speech were limited to slight stuttering or complaints such as, "I found some difficulty in speaking", "I couldn't get my tongue to move", "When I wanted to answer, words wouldn't come", etc. They lasted only a short time and left almost no trace in the residual stage of recovery.

The situation is different when one considers certain zones located *nearer to the classical language areas.* These areas occupy an intermediate position in the frequency with which speech disorders follow lesions, these areas occupy an intermediate position.

Injuries here produced speech disorders in 68% of all cases during the initial period, while in the residual stage (two to five months after trauma) speech functions had recovered to such an extent that only 25-50% of cases give evidence of impairment. The first of these areas is the greater portion of cerebral zones known to modern neurophysiology as the "intermediate" or "secondary" zones, or, as they are frequently referred to in modern and anatomico-physiological literature,

[2] They manifest themselves as distinctive difficulties in producing smooth speech, a characteristic type of stumbling, and as disturbances approaching dysarthria. These disturbances have been poorly studied and we shall seldom consider them in this section. We shall consider the aphasic disturbances which may arise as a result of right hemisphere injury later (see Chapter III).

[3] Of course, cases in which shell fragments penetrated to areas far from their point of entry into the skull or cases in which pathological changes were observed in brain tissues far outside of the area of direct injury were excluded from such analysis.

"marginal zones", between the cortical regions of the various analyzers.[4] The chief function of these zones is to integrate the cortical projections of different analyzers and to transform the somato-topical projections represented in the primary zones into functionally organized systems. One should further include here a number of more complex cortical areas which adjoin the classical "speech areas". This group of cortical zones comprises: the premotor area (especially its inferior portion), the anterior temporal areas, the inferior parietal area, the tempero-occipital area, and the parieto-occipital area. These surround the "main speech areas" of classical neurology and make up a group which we shall refer to as "marginal" or "intermediate" areas.

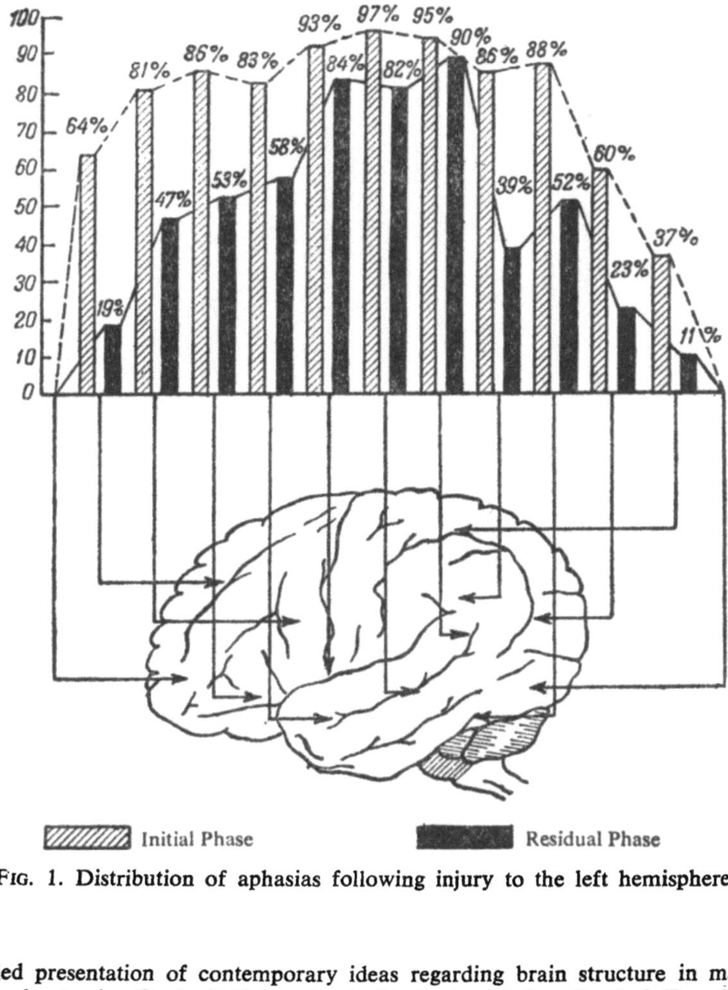

FIG. 1. Distribution of aphasias following injury to the left hemisphere.

[4] A detailed presentation of contemporary ideas regarding brain structure in man is to be found in a chapter by G. A. Poljakov in A. R. Luria, *Higher Cortical Function of Man* (Moscow University Press, 1962); The English Edition: N.Y., Basic Books, 1966.

The third group of zones, those lying on either side of the fissure of Sylvius, constitute a very special category. Injury to these zones almost invariably produces speech disturbances in the early period; exceptions are few. Not only is it characteristic of these zones that injury most frequently leads to speech disorders, but such disorders are extremely severe. A look at the accompanying graphic summary is sufficient to show that in 82-90% of cases involving injury to these zones, servere aphasic disturbances persisted even two to five months after trauma.[5] It is easy to see that we are speaking here of the areas which in classical investigations were considered to be the *principal speech zones*.[6] In all that follows we shall refer to them as such.

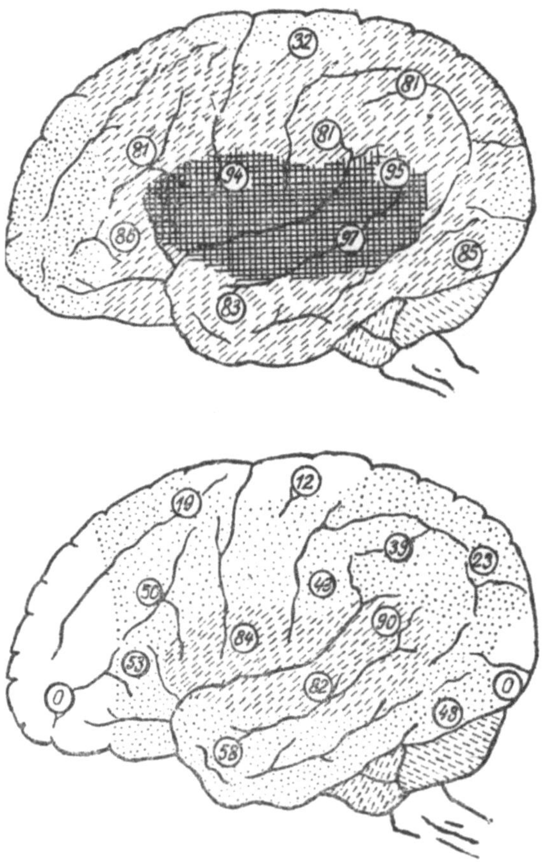

FIG. 2. Frequency of speech disturbances following injuries to different areas of the left hemisphere.

[5] Subsequent analysis of a wider range of material reduced these figures somewhat.

[6] Determination of the principal speech areas on the basis of war injuries was done in France by P. Marie and Ch. Foix, "Les aphasies de la guerre", *Revue Neurologique*, 1917; in England by H. Head, *Aphasia* (1926); and in Germany by K. Kleist (1934) and others.

Analysis of the frequency of speech disturbances following injury to different zones of the left hemisphere led us to the conclusions that *even in the initial period of traumatic brain disorder the disintegration of function by no means results equally from damage to all areas* and that *it is possible, even in the initial period, to determine systems of brain areas which produce different types of speech disorders following trauma.*

The most frequent and severe disturbances were produced by damage to the *principal group of "speech" zones* (fronto-tempero-parietal, posterior temporal, and parieto-temporal). The principal group, which includes zones of complex structure lying at the junction of several large areas, is surrounded by a ring of "marginal" zones. Injury of these marginal areas produces a large number of aphasic disturbances in the initial period. Such disturbances are not, however, so severe and are followed in the residual period by a large percent of total recoveries. Finally, the ring of marginal areas bounded by a group of polar areas which are altogether neutral with regard to speech function. Injury of the latter areas produces only an insignificant number of speech disorders in the initial period; they are usually very slight and almost never persist into the residual period. In Figure 2 we see a schematic representation of the three zones in the left hemisphere and their relationships to speech functions. By combining all our data we obtain Table I, which presents the results of our observations[7] in the most general form. This table shows that while damage to the principal speech areas produced severe disturbance of speech processes, damage to the marginal zones resulted only in temporary block; only in half the cases did the latter disturbances persist. Damage of the polar areas almost never caused speech disorders.

TABLE 1

Aphasic syndromes of different areas at different stages in the period of recovery from traumatic injuries of the left hemisphere

site of lesion	total number of cases	percent of aphasias	
		initial period	residual period
Injuries of the "polar" areas	127	15.0	4.1
Injuries of the "marginal speech areas"	178	80.9	47.2
Injuries of the "primary" speech areas	89	96.7	85.4
Total	394	61	43

[7] Subsequently the number of cases studied was considerably increased; the relations between these figures, however, remained much the same.

B. THE SEVERITY OF APHASIC SYNDROMES AT VARIOUS STAGES OF RECOVERY FROM TRAUMATIC DISORDER

On the basis of the data offerred so far it is only possible to get a general impression of the functional disorders observed in the initial and residual stages of recovery from trauma in various groups of areas of the left hemisphere. For a more detailed picture we must not limit ourselves to such a summary classification but analyze further the syndromes at sequential stages of recovery. So far we have considered aphasic syndromes only in the most general sense; we have spoken of the presence of aphasic symptoms whenever a patient showed signs of impaired complex speech activity or, according to Head's terminology, whenever we observed disturbances of "symbolic formulation and expression". The types and severity of such disturbances were not taken into account. The only cases excluded from this total group were those in which speech impairment did not accompany the elementary or complex disorders (loss of sensitivity, paresis, gnostic disorders), or when speech impairment resulted from dysphonia or stuttering and was clearly unrelated to aphasia.

Such a general classification, however, is of value only as a first approximation. Traumatic aphasia can assume different forms and result from various degrees of brain damage. As a result of brain trauma we may find aphasic syndromes of almost any degree of severity ranging from total aphasia with absolute inability to speak and very poor comprehension to the most subtle and diffuse forms of disturbance which are manifested in some cases only by slight difficulties of articulation, in others by occasional failure to comprehend, and in still others by slight difficulties on naming objects and finding appropriate words.

For the time being we shall put off consideration of the various types of aphasic disorder and take up the question of *severity*. One can arbitrarily separate all cases of aphasia into three basic groups. The first group we shall consider is *total aphasia,* i.e. total block of motor speech or, if we are dealing with sensory-aphasic disturbances, gross disturbance of the ability to attend to and comprehend the speech of others. In this case the pathological process grossly disturbs both the motor and perceptual aspects of speech. We may include in this group those cases in which such disturbances are severe and last at least two or three weeks.

The second group consists of clearcut cases of aphasic disturbance in which the speech disorder does not involve a total block of speech activity, but in which the symptoms of a given type of aphasia are *well expressed.* In cases of damage to the anterior portions of the brain such aphasias take the form of disturbances of articulation which may involve either the inability to "find the correct motor structure of the word" or inability to shift from the articulation of one word to that of another. With damage to the temporal area, such a syndrome may involve a disturbance of discriminative ("phonemic") hearing or the "alienation" of word meanings (great tendency to lose the meanings of words). Injury at other sites may produce clear pictures of disturbance of the semantic (logico-grammatical) code of speech with distinct symptoms of amnesic aphasia or disturbance of the dynamics of verbal thought. Consequently, in this group we have reason to include a number of different types of aphasia the distinctive characteristic of which is a clear cut symptomology and relative severity.[8]

Finally, in the third group we shall include *subtle, slight forms* of aphasic disorder. In some cases one finds a slight loss of the "automatic" character of speech; it becomes less smooth. In other cases there are slight difficulties of articulation which manifest themselves only in the pronunciation of difficult or unusual words. In still other cases disturbance takes the form of a residual amnesic-aphasic syndrome leading to difficulties in the recall of certain rare words or to difficulty in understanding slightly complicated grammatical constructions. A characteristic feature of this group is that the disturbance is not equally apparent at all times; it manifests itself most clearly under conditions of lowered vascular stability (fatigue, affect, etc.). It is well known that the manifestation of disorders due to brain trauma is especially sensitive to such changes.

How is the severity of aphasia related to damage of various zones of the left hemisphere and to the length of the recovery period? The results of our studies are presented in a generalized form in Figure 3. This graphic summary shows that in the initial period which covers the first three or four weeks after trauma, one finds a relatively large number of cases of gross aphasic disturbance with total disruption of speech. These disturbances often lasted from two to six weeks and, if we exclude injuries of the polar areas, they constituted 42% of all cases. Of course this figure compounds two entirely different groups of areas. During the initial period injury of the *principal speech areas* resulted in total disorders in 75% of cases, whereas in the same period damage to the *marginal areas* did not produce such a result in more than 25% of cases. In the latter cases of total disruption, speech function often recovered; whereas with injury of the principal speech areas, there was often no recovery.

This indicates that in the early period of recovery disturbances did not usually reflect a severe irreversible loss of speech, but rather a temporary *block* of speech processes. Such a block arose primarily with injury of the principal speech areas. Though blocks occasionally resulted from injury to the marginal areas, these two groups of areas usualy reacted differently to trauma. With lesions of the principal areas, the speech block disappeared only in about two thirds of all cases; in one third of cases it persisted into the residual period and sometimes lasted indefinitely. Just the opposite was true as regarded marginal area lesions. In these cases total block was always temporary and had to be considered only as a block of the external speech processes.

From this same summary diagram it is apparent that slight forms of aphasic disorder almost never occurred with injury to the principal speech areas. The

[8] These syndromes will be treated in more detail in subsequent chapters (see Chapters V-VIII).

percentage of slight disorders increased only in the residual period after trauma of these areas. Injury of the marginal areas produced slight forms of aphasia in the initial period in 19% of cases, and in the residual period this number increased to 24%, while 19% of cases showed no aphasic symptoms during the initial period and more than 52% showed none in the residual period. It was a common finding that those patients with slight aphasic symptoms in the residual period were ones who had experienced total aphasia in the initial period.

If we submit our data to more detailed analysis by comparing the severity of aphasic syndromes at sequential stages following trauma from focal injuries these

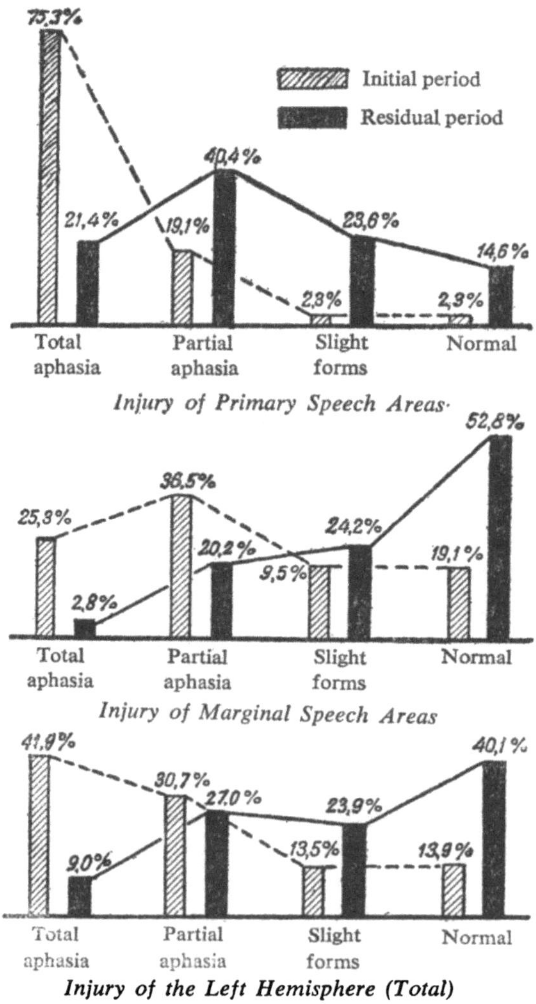

FIG. 3. The severity of aphasic syndromes accompanying injuries to different areas of the left hemisphere.

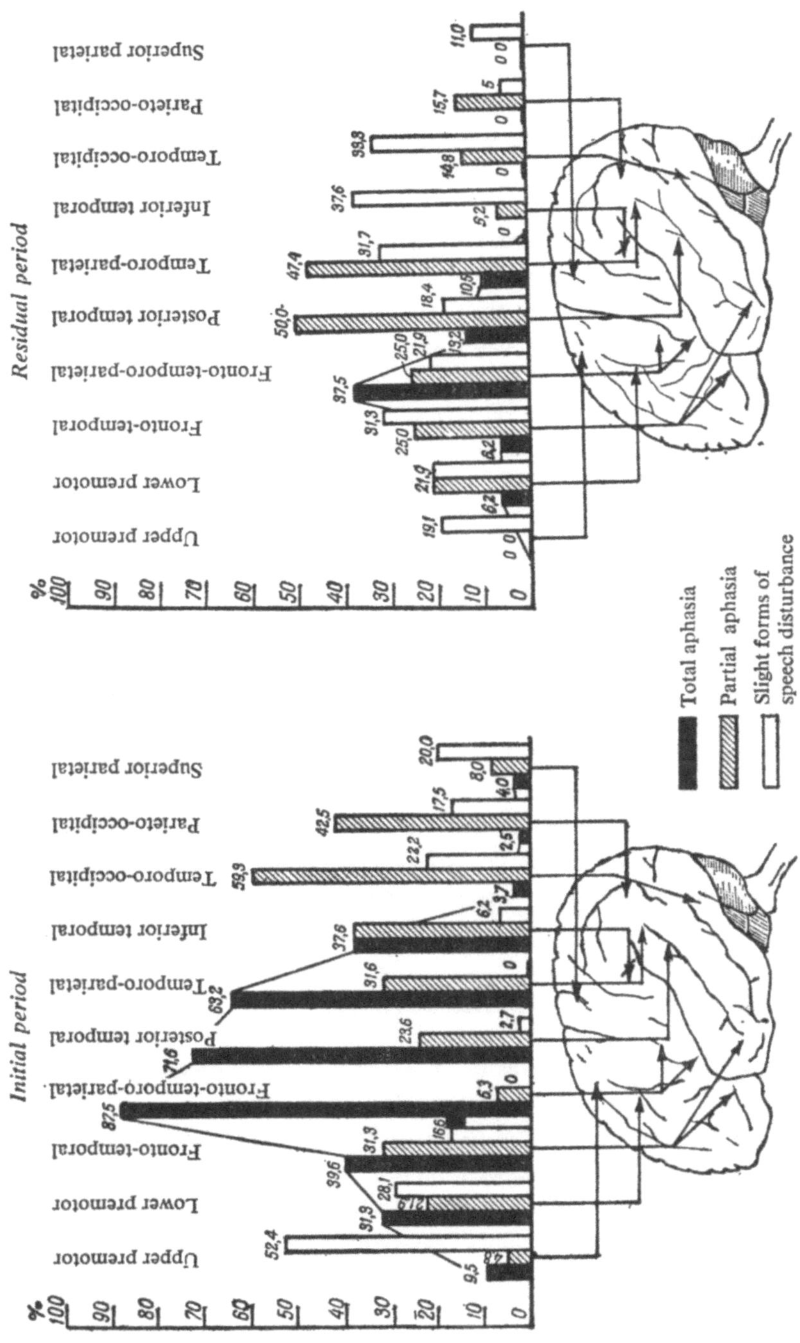

FIG. 4. The severity of aphasic syndromes resulting from injury at different sites.

differences stand out even more clearly. A summary diagram of the results of such analysis are presented in Figure 4.

Gross speech impairment does not result equally from damage to different portions of the principal and marginal areas. From this graphic summary we see that with damage to the anterior parts of the speech area the number of cases of total disruption of speech in the sense mentioned above may reach 80% in the initial period. In the residual state this picture is seen in 38% of cases. Consequently it is possible to say that trauma to this area does not produce a simple block of the speech process. Consideration of the temporal or parieto-temporal area shows that the complete disappearance of active speech occurs in only 63-71% of cases in the initial period; that this type of damage is less severe is evident from the fact that only in 10-12% of cases such total disturbance does extend into the residual period.

Usually the severe, total form of aphasia which extends into the residual period is seen in complicated cases where destruction of brain tissues has proceeded beyond the limits of these areas and involves deeper portions of the brain. Thus the complete disappearance of speech functions involves not simply a speech block, but constitutes a total loss of speech.

An analogous picture, but one less clearly expressed, is observed when one considers cases of injury to the marginal areas. Injury of the anterior portions of these areas results in total aphasia in 31-39% of cases, while damage of the posterior portions (tempero-occipital, parieto-occipital areas) leads to total aphasia and loss of expressive speech in only 2-4% of the cases. In the residual period, the figure for the anterior portions falls to zero.

All this suggests that disturbance of the *motor* aspect of speech which arises in the early period following injury to the anterior parts of the speech zone is related in many cases to *destruction* of the brain areas necessary for expressive speech, while injury of the posterior portions of the speech zone produces primarily a *block* of speech activity.

C. TYPE OF TRAUMA AND THE SEVERITY OF APHASIC SYNDROMES

So far we have considered changes in the severity of the aphasic syndromes during recovery with no reference to the type of lesions involved. Now we must take up this problem and clarify the extent to which the frequency and severity of aphasic syndromes depend upon the *type* of injury.

As a first approximation we shall restrict ourselves to comparing cases of *penetrating wounds* (in which shrapnel or bullets passed through the dura mater to actually penetrate brain tissues) and cases of *nonpenetrating wounds* (in which the missile damaged the scalp and skull, but left the dura mater intact). Despite the fact that a number of features are observed in both cases which may lend them an aura of similarity (e.g. hemorrhage, changes in the circulation of blood and cerebro spinal fluid), we should keep in mind that whereas penetrating wounds are effective primarily due to the *destruction of brain tissues,* nonpenetrating wounds exert their effects by the *temporary inhibition* of function. This difference is accentuated by the gross inflammatory reactions in the meninges and cerebral tissues which often attend penetrating wounds but are absent from wounds of the nonpenetrating type.

What was the effect of these two types of injury on the sequence of functional changes observed during recovery? The answer to this question is to be found in Table 2. There was no significant difference between the numbers of aphasic disturbances arising in the initial period as a result of the two types of injury: penetrating wounds gave aphasic symptoms in 88% of cases, while nonpenetrating wounds gave such symptoms in 75% of cases. Consequently one may assume that *the blocking effect of which we spoke above may be evoked in the initial period both by penetrating and by nonpenetrating injuries, i.e., in the early period the character of the wound does not greatly affect the type of functional defect observed.* A breakdown of these figures considering injuries of the principal and marginal areas separately confirms this conclusion. Both penetrating and nonpenetrating wounds of the *principal speech areas* produce large numbers of aphasias, indicating that the type of trauma does not play a large role here. The difference between the effects of penetrating and nonpenetrating wounds increases somewhat in the case of lesions of the marginal areas, since in 27.1% of cases damage to these zones does not give rise to aphasic symptoms.

The real difference between the functional consequences of penetrating and nonpenetrating wounds appears only in the residual period of recovery.

TABLE 2

Changes in aphasic syndromes during recovery from penetrating and nonpenetrating wounds of the left hemisphere

	Penetrating wounds			Nonpenetrating wounds		
	total number of cases	percent of aphasias		total number of cases	percent of aphasias	
		initial period	residual period		initial period	residual period
All cases of injury to the left hemisphere excluding those of the "polar" areas	203	88.2	67.9	64	75.0	37.5
Injuries of the primary speech areas	73	97.2	93.3	16	93.7	62.6
Injuries of the marginal speech areas	130	83.1	52.3	48	72.9	30.0

Even the over all figures indicate that *recovery from speech defects* is considerably greater in cases of nonpenetrating than of penetrating wounds of the skull. Whereas in the case of penetrating wounds the number of aphasias in the residual period falls from 88% to 68%, in the case of nonpenetrating wounds the *drop is two times larger* – from 75% in the initial period to 38% in the residual period. These figures become even more meaningful if one makes a breakdown according to site of injury. As a rule, penetrating wounds of the principal speech areas are not followed by spontaneous recovery of speech in the residual period, whereas nonpenetrating wounds of these areas are often followed by spontaneous recovery. The number of aphasias resulting from nonpenetrating wounds of the principal speech zones is very high in the initial period, but in the residual stages it drops by a third leaving traces of speech disturbance in only half of the cases. The dynamics of spontaneous recovery from aphasic syndromes following injuries to the marginal zones turn out to be much the same in cases of penetrating wounds as in cases of nonpenetrating wounds; this again supports the idea that the appearance of aphasia following trauma to these areas is usually due to a *blockade of speech function.* All the same, in 52% of cases penetrating wounds of the marginal zones are followed by severe aphasia, while in cases of nonpenetrating wounds such aphasia does not appear more than 30% of the time. Later we shall return to further analysis of this fact.

The data presented thus far have permitted us to establish only the most general ways in which the disturbance and recovery of speech depend upon the type of trauma. Would it not be possible to discover more profound relationships by correlating *type of wound with severity of the aphasic syndrome*? Figures 5 and 6 give the information required for such an analysis. On the basis of summary findings, we have already seen that penetrating wounds produced an extremely high number of severe forms of aphasia. Such disturbances were observed in half of all cases while in cases of nonpenetrating wounds the number did not exceed 16%. With nonpenetrating wounds the number of slight forms of aphasia turned out to be higher in the initial period. These relations changed in the residual period. The difference between the effects of the types of wound was seen more clearly in well expressed (not total) aphasias which predominated in cases of penetrating wounds and the number of symptom free cases which occurred twice as often with nonpenetrating wounds as with penetrating wounds.

As before, this picture becomes especially clear when the consequences of penetrating and nonpenetrating wounds of the principal speech areas and marginal speech areas are considered separately. Penetrating wounds of the principal zones *almost without exception produced permanent, total aphasia,* while nonpenetrating wounds gave a considerably less extreme picture. The latter produced total block of speech only in 50% of cases. The same correlations, though less marked, were seen in the analysis of injuries to the marginal speech zones. There total aphasia was seen in the initial period only after penetrating wounds and almost never arose following nonpenetrating skull injury. Thus, while the type of wound has little significance as regards the presence or absence of speech disturbance in the initial period, it is of essential significance as regards the *severity* of aphasic syndromes: penetrating wounds produced a complete block of speech function more often than did nonpenetrating wounds.

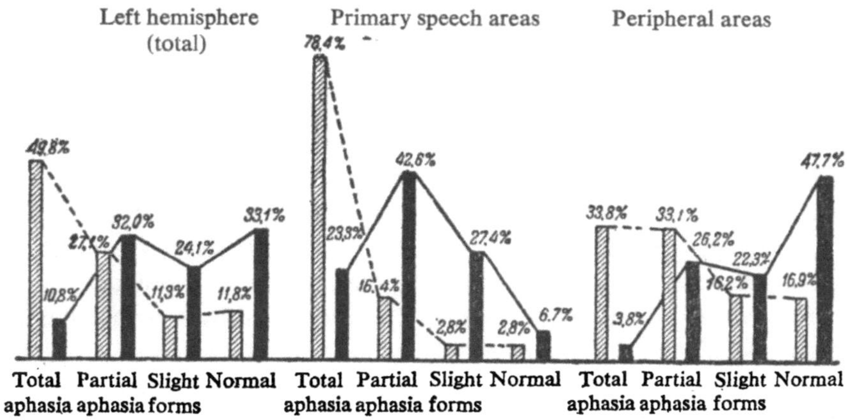

FIG. 5. The severity of aphasic syndromes following penetrating wounds in different areas of the left hemisphere.

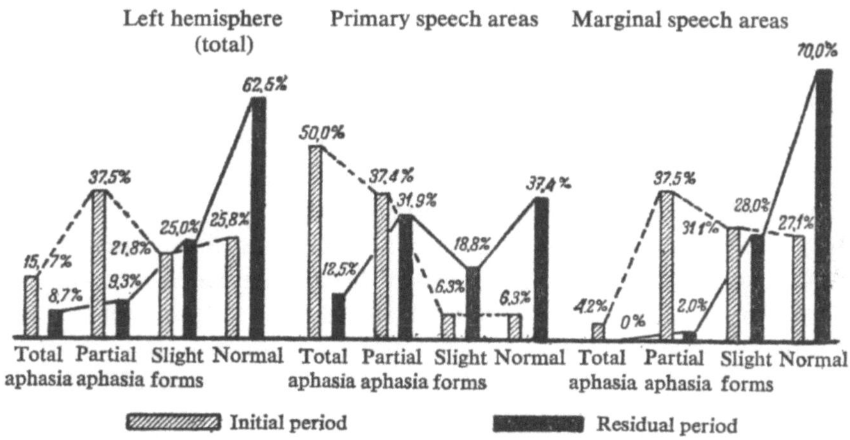

FIG. 6. The severity of aphasic syndromes following nonpenetrating wounds in different areas of the left hemisphere.

A similar picture results when we analyse the *duration* of aphasic disorders after penetrating and nonpenetrating wounds. We had a number of cases in which nonpenetrating wounds of the marginal, or even the principal zones, led only to a transitory total aphasia. Such disturbances lasted from several hours to one or two days after which speech functions were to a certain degree re-established. On the other hand, in cases of penetrating wounds we never found such transitory forms of disorder. This finding introduces another essential difference between the effects of the two forms of injury on brain function during the acute period. It explains why nonpenetrating wounds, which may produce anything from slight contusion of superficial brain tissues to considerable destruction of tissues, can result in clinical pictures having very little in common one with another.

It remains for us to show how the two types of wound affect the changes in aphasic symptoms which occur during the *residual* period. Careful consideration of Figures 5 and 6 will provide the answer. The over all figures show that during the residual period severe aphasic syndromes disappear altogether, while the number of slight speech disturbances and total recoveries increases. This is more true of nonpenetrating wounds, less so of penetrating wounds.

These features stand out quite clearly when one compares injuries to the principal and marginal speech zones. They show a step-like character which reflects the way in which pathological symptoms run their course. The residual period after *penetrating* wounds of the *principal* areas is characterized by a certain stabilization of the aphasic picture. The number of total aphasic disturbances drops here to 23% as the well expressed classical syndroms come to predominate; the number of slight forms is not great, and spontaneous total recovery is limited to isolated cases. *Nonpenetrating* wounds of these same areas give a somewhat different picture in the residual period. It differs in that the number of total aphasias drops even more and that the number of total recoveries grows considerably to 37-40%.

The distribution of aphasic syndromes in the residual period after *penetrating wounds of the marginal zones* approximates the picture which we saw in the residual period following nonpenetrating wounds of the principal zones. Destruction of the marginal zones in a number of cases led to rather permanent aphasic syndromes. Speech was not totally disrupted, but there was a large number of cases sustaining well expressed aphasic disturbances of various types.

Finally, *nonpenetrating wounds of the marginal zones* left no definite aphasic disturbances in the residual period and left slight disturbances only in 28% of cases. In 80% of cases recovery was total. Usually two to four months was sufficient for the reestablishment of speech functions in these cases.

Comparison of the severity of aphasic syndromes observed after penetrating and nonpenetrating wounds of the left hemisphere makes it possible to learn more about the pathological processes which arise in cases of traumatic brain disorder and again shows the distinction which must be made between the *permanent disruption* of functional systems and the *temporary inhibition* of such systems. Special physiological analyses based upon careful study and taking full advantage of modern techniques should clarify the mechanisms of such processes.

D. "FUNCTIONAL" COMPONENTS OF TRAUMATIC APHASIA

The preceding analysis has shown that in the initial period every brain trauma is accompanied by a decrease of functions in the brain areas lying near those zones which have sustained direct injury. Thus the disturbance of cortical function following injury of the left hemisphere turns out to be considerably more widespread and severe than would be expected on the basis of the site of primary destruction. Our analysis would be incomplete, however, if we did not mention one other factor which is of functional significance for speech disorders. During the war neurologists became well acquainted with the syndrome of "reactive postconcussion deafmutism". This disorder has been treated in detail in the Soviet literature by V. A. Gilarovsky, G. V. Geršuni, L. B. Perel'man and others. It characteristically results only from the types of trauma observed during war time; it frequently accompanies typical traumatic aphasias, making them more severe. Considerably less frequently it may lead to pseudoaphasic disturbances and create considerable difficulty for the diagnostician.

Modern warfare, through keeping soldiers under exceptional emotional tension and exposing them to extremely intense sound stimulation, created conditions for the appearance of special forms of "protective inhibition". It commences whenever one or another area undergoes direct trauma. The physiological mechanisms of protective inhibition were studied in detail by the Pavlov school and subjected to further careful investigations by M. K. Petrova, F. M. Majorov, E. A. Asratjan, and others. In some cases it does not proceed beyond a partial reaction in the system damaged. In other cases, especially in those where trauma is inflicted upon personalities with unstable nervous systems, the protective inhibition grows into a special form of "protective reaction". Sensory thresholds rise considerably, the motor systems enter a state of tonic excitation, the damaged function discontinues for an extended period, and the person, in effect, cuts himself off from the traumatizing environment.

The protective inhibitory reaction may assume different forms. In some cases it may lead to protracted catatonia or pseudoparesis which often arise during the recovery from a state of extreme motor excitation. In other cases it may take the form of functional anesthesia or postconcussional deafness with pronounced elevation of thresholds to all types of stimulation. Special observations revealed that these forms of protective reaction may *lead to the complete arrest of functions which have already been disturbed by trauma.* This produces a situation in which subsequently observed functional disorders are not due to the trauma itself, but are the result of *secondary reactions of the personality to trauma.*

Since both barotrauma and extreme intense sound stimulation are very common in modern warfare, such dynamic suspension of function most often assumes the character of reactive postconcussison deafmutism. In these cases mild concussions affecting primarily the auditory system produce temporary deafness, and protective inhibition leads to fixation of this defect for a long period of time. It was shown by G. V. Geršuni that fixation of the defect is accompanied by a rise in the thresholds of all the principal types of sensation and a transfer of function to a "subsensory range". Under these conditions auditory stimuli continue to evoke objectively recordable peripheral and autonomic reactions, but cease to enter consciousness.[9] Observations by a number of authors such as L. B. Perel'man [10] showed that the suspension of function may last for several months if left untreated. On the other hand, under appropriate forms of psychotherapeutic treatment, it may disappear in a few days time.

As a rule reactive postconcussion deafmutism is characterized by long-term suspension of hearing and of speech functions related to hearing. It follows a concussion produced by the shock wave from a bomb explosion; it need not be accompanied by any kind of skull injury or local organic symptoms. This deafmutism differs radically from aphasia in that there is not disruption of speech as a symbolic process, but simply a suspension of phonation and the ability to hear. As a result patients who are unable to hear or speak preserve the ability to communicate in writing. They read without difficulty and write without mistakes.

In some cases reactive postconcussion deafmutism *occurs in conjunction with primary aphasic disturbances*. In such cases it turns the usual forms of traumatic aphasia into complex "mixtures" by supplementing the aphasic symptoms and drastically extending the period required for recovery of speech.

During the war cases of primary aphasia complicated by secondary suspension of speech was reported repeatedly by M. S. Lebedinskij, D. G. Šmelkin and others. We found it most often in the initial period following injury. Any attempt to carry out rehabilitation speech therapy on patients during the first three or four weeks after injury inevitably ran into a certain amount of resistance. Patients avoided making use of even those speech functions which they had left. In some infrequent cases (not more than 5-6% of our patients) the suspension of speech may last for many months and make an otherwise mild aphasia appear extremely severe. Sometimes the disturbance expressed itself in total mutism which might be mistaken for a total motor aphasia; sometimes it assumed the character of verbal stumbling and searching for words, thus simulating an amnesic aphasic syndrome. In all cases the syndrome as a whole reflected the secondary fixation of initial aphasic defects. Sometimes the primary disorders turned out to be unexpectedly minor, and once psychotherapeutic technique had succeeded in removing the secondary suspension of speech functions, it was discovered that the defect in speech activity had already undergone a large degree of recovery. It was apparent that the fixation of the defect had masked the spontaneous reestablishment of function.

[9] G. V. Geršuni et al., "Disorders of sensory and other nervous functions following concussions due to explosions", *Collected Materials on Military Medicine, Academy of Science of the USSR*, II (1945) (in Russian).

[10] L. B. Perel'man, *Reactive Postconcussion Deaf-mutism: Diagnosis and Treatment* (Medgiz, 1943) (in Russian).

Most often the fixation of an initial defect occurs in cases of nonpenetrating skull injuries. But deep penetrating wounds of the left hemisphere may also be accompanied by secondary suspension of speech. This results in well developed mixed syndromes of aphasia and function disorders.

In our files there is a rather large number of mixed cases of traumatic speech disturbances. Two cases should suffice, however, to show the nature of this peculiar type of disorder.

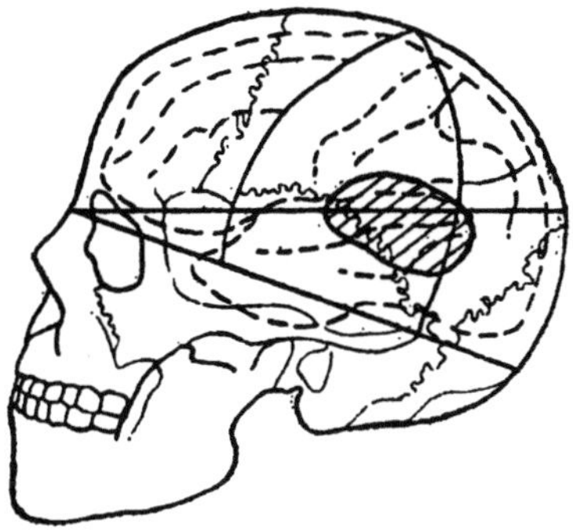

Patient P.: injury diagram (Case 1)

Case 1

On October 27, 1944, Patient P., a 29 year old laboratory technician, was struck by a bomb fragment which produced a wound and a skull fracture in the parieto-temporal area of the left hemisphere. Three days later at operation it was found that dura mater was intact, but under tension and cyanotic; puncture produced no sign of subdural hematoma. Subsequent healing proceeded smoothly under penicillin therapy. The patient did not lose consciousness immediately following injury, but on the third day was beset by confusion which was accompanied by excitement and lasted for four days. The wound produced only a slight right-side hemisyndrome with a decrease both in the strength and sensitivity of the right extremities. Immediately following injury the patient began to show signs of impaired speech comprehension and began to speak with a distinct literal paraphasia. The aphasic symptoms gradually disappeared.

The patient came under our observation three months after injury. In addition to the organic injury, our investigation revealed distinct secondary functional changes. The patient was sufficiently oriented. He gave signs of pronounced instability of vegetative functions, e.g., there were exagerated vascular reactions to all stimulation. Distinct changes of neurodynamic character were noted in sensitivity: although right hemianopsia was absent, there was a definite contracted narrowing of the visual field; there was reduced sensitivity in distal parts of the left extremities as well as somewhat reduced pain and tactile sensitivity in the distal regions of the right side. A more pronounced change was observed in epicritic sensitivity than in protopathic sensitivity.

The mixed character of the disturbances was manifested also in the motor sphere. In addition to a slight weakness of the distal portions of the right extremities, there were much more serious disturbances of a functional type. The patient complained of inability to raise his hand above horizontal, but when his attention was distracted he raised it to a vertical position. His every movement was accompanied by extreme and sustained tension, so that, having raised his arm to a vertical position he seemed unable to let it down. Every voluntary impulse produced spreading tonic tension, so that when trying to stick out his tongue, he strained the entire musculature at the base of the tongue, and in the end proved unable to produce the required movement.

An entirely analogous picture was seen in the patient's speech. Three months following injury there were observed occasional phonetic substitutions, transposition of letters in writing, and verbal amnesia – all typical of residual temporal aphasia. This did not exhaust the types of speech disturbance seen in his case, however, and in fact did not constitute the major type. At this time there was no sign of loss of the meanings of words or of sensory-aphasic phenomena; he showed no defects in reading and only quite infrequent and minor writing defects; he retained all forms of imitative and narrative speech and was able to understand rather complex verbal constructions. In spite of this, the motor speech of the patient was grossly disturbed by a tonic form of stuttering which made it almost impossible for him to speak smoothly. He had a definite dysphasia both in articulation and phonation, so that he was unable to speak in a whisper or sing out loud. These difficulties were evident in all forms of speech regardless of the complexity of the task, and they were intensified by excitement. They were largely removed by psychotherapeutic measures.

This case can be regarded as a mixed disorder involving a relatively slight aphasic disturbance (arising as a result of local confusion in the left parietotemporal area) accompanied by considerable fixation of the defect, thus giving a picture of secondary dysphasia.

The second case differs from the first in that it involves a more radical functional suspension of speech following a penetrating wound of the speech area.

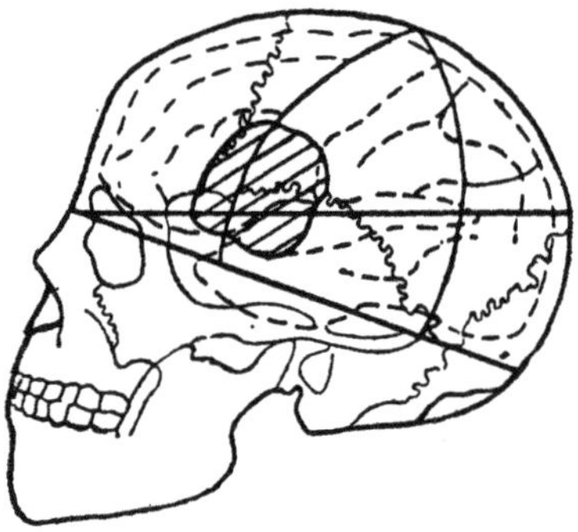

Patient K.: injury diagram (Case 2)

Case 2

On October 17, 1944, Patient K. was struck by a bomb fragment in the left frontotemporal area. The injury resulted in a long loss of consciousness and right side paralysis. An operation was performed on the third day following injury and bone splinters were removed from within the brain tissues.

Immediately after the return of consciousness, a total motor aphasia was observed. Subsequently there were almost no signs of recovery either from the aphasia or from the paralysis. In February 1945, the patient was able, with great difficulty, to stand up and take a few steps; but he remained totally unable to speak. As early as the fifth month after injury it became apparent that the patient's difficulties were partly organic in origin and partly of a secondary reactive nature. He always lay in bed and never gave any sign of attempting either to move or to speak. His rare attempts at expressive speech were marked by poor articulation and lack of active phonation. He usually responded to questions by a shake or nod of the head, though he appeared to understand the speech of others well enough.

The patient came under our observation six months after injury. At that time the wound had healed and by pneumo-encephalography it was shown that the body of the left lateral ventrical had been drawn toward the scar which was located a little higher than the site of scalp injury, i.e. in the sensory-motor area. Hemiparesis of the right side was still evident (most pronounced in the hand) as well as disturbance of all forms of sensitivity, hyper-reflexia (clonus in the right foot without, however, pathological signs), and increased tonus of the right hand. In addition to these findings there were signs of functional disturbance. When the attention of the patient was distracted movement of the right hand increased markedly. Any complex movement of the left hand came to involve a number of unrelated muscle groups and was thus performed only with great difficulty. The same phenomenon was noted in muscles around the mouth: the patient was unable to open his mouth voluntarily, lick his lips, or stick out his tongue. When he attempted to make these movements the muscles at the root of the tongue and in the neck contracted with such force that it was impossible to make the proper movement.

Sensitivity was low on the right side. The same type of glove and stocking loss of sensitivity was seen as in the previous patient, except that in this case it was observed on the left, "healthy" side.

Attempts at phonation invariably produced a general spasm of muscles of the tongue and larynx; attempts to articulate led to perseverative movements of the lips and tongue.

Even very careful observation did not reveal any speech disturbance of a specifically aphasic character. Speech comprehension was preserved, and there was no sign that the patient did not know the meanings of words; only occasionally did he skip or rearrange letters in writing, a typical sign of motor aphasia.

Only by means of psychotherapy was the real nature of the disorder determined. All that was required was repetitive suggestion for this patient, who had sat completely silent for six months, to begin speaking. There was no sign of gross motor-aphasia, agrammatism, or other difficulty to which his previous absence of spontaneous speech could be attributed. What prevented appearance of spontaneous speech was not any kind of aphasic disorder but a disfunctional phenomenon. Despite the penetration wound of the speech zone, the degree of purely aphasic disturbance was so insignificant that the entire disorder could be attributed to the reactive suspension of speech.

We could cite a number other such cases, all of which would differ in detail, but would reflect essentially the same condition.

Damage of the left hemisphere may under certain conditions lead to the disruption of complex speech activity, i.e., to traumatic aphasia. Upon closer consideration, however, this picture turns out to be extremely involved. It is based first upon the disturbance of speech processes which results from injury to one or more cortical areas of the left hemisphere. This disturbance constitutes the nucleus of the aphasic picture which is preserved in the residual period. The second component entering into the picture of traumatic aphasia is the *inhibition* of speech function. Such inhibition is related to changes in cerebrospinal fluid dynamics, cerebral edema, resolving hematomas or reflex vascular changes which accompany trauma. This dynamic component which greatly extends the picture of aphasic disorders is at height during the initial period and most often disappears within three to four weeks. Finally, in some cases, but by no means in all, a third component is superimposed upon traumatic aphasia; this third component differs from the first two in that it has nothing at all in common with aphasia. It is related to reactive (protective) suspension of all forms of speech activity and represents a neurotic reaction to overly intense stimuli.

The suspension of speech functions leads to a sharp rise in the thresholds to all forms of stimulation, and it is accompanied by the suspension of lower levels of motor activity. Such reactions easily assume the character of aphonia (or dysphonia), thus complicating the aphasic picture and often making diagnosis extremely difficult. They are manifested distinctly only in a comparatively small number of cases which, clinically speaking, make up the group of "mixtures". Since they represent a specific phenomenon of military neurology, however, any study of wartime traumatic aphasia which does not take them into account must be considered incomplete.

III

FACTORS WHICH INFLUENCE SPONTANEOUS RECOVERY FROM TRAUMATIC APHASIA

A. THE PROBLEM OF SPONTANEOUS RECOVERY

As we have seen, injuries of the principal speech areas of the left hemisphere often produce clear-cut disturbances of speech processes which later gradually recover. A question arises, however, as to how to explain those few *negative cases* in which *injury of the principal speech zones does not produce speech impairment or cases in which severe aphasic disturbances undergo rapid and complete recovery.* How can one explain the fact that in certain cases one finds *great differences in the dynamics of spontaneous recovery*?

These questions have attracted the attention of a number of investigators. The literature relating to negative cases and rapid recovery of speech functions after severe brain damage runs to tens of volumes. Since it is well established that destroyed nerve cells in the cortex do not regenerate, there are three possible explanations for the conflicting phenomena which we occasionally see.

It may be that in such cases there only appears to be destruction of brain tissue, whereas in reality the injuries only temporarily depress the function of certain areas. This depression, or diaschisis, may spread to a whole system of functionally related zones, when it has passed the disturbed function may recover completely. Such a mechanism might explain cases of rapid recovery after relatively slight injuries.

A second mechanism which may acount for spontaneous recovery of disturbed function is the *adaptive transfer of a given function* from one area of the brain to others, thus compensating for the functional defect sustained as a result of brain damage. Observations recorded by a number of authors show, without a doubt, that in certain cases functions may be taken over by symmetrical areas of the right hemisphere. It is not difficult to show, however, that this functional transfer may be any one of a number of types. It varies from "vicarious" compensation, in which another area of the brain assumes the functions of the damaged area, to more complex *transformations of the function itself.* In the latter case a function comes to be performed by new processes occurring in areas having altogether different functions. Thus it is a universal conclusion among investigators – a conclusion based upon modern study of cortical cytoarchitectonics – that the functions of destroyed brain areas cannot in all cases be directly substituted by other structures. In this regard there are limits to the plasticity of brain function.

It is natural to suspect that, when a function has recovered, the responsible structures will be found either at subcortical levels, e.g. in the subcortical motor nuclei, or in symmetrical areas of the right hemisphere. Proceeding from this assumption a number of investigators have expressed the idea that rapid recovery from aphasic disturbances may be explained either by a transfer of function *downwards* to systems of subcortical motor nuclei of the same hemisphere (this opinion has been repeatedly advanced by a number of French authors), or by a transfer to corresponding zones of the *right hemisphere*. If the latter is true, preservation of the symmetrical cortical areas becomes extremely important.

All of the reasoning advanced so far has taken for granted that zones of the dominant hemisphere always constitute *absolute* "centers", preservation of which is essential for speech function. Might it not be possible, however, to suggest that this necessity is not always absolute – that the degree of *lateralization of complex functions is different in different individuals*? If this suggestion is correct, then cases in which injuries of the speech zones of the left hemisphere produce no aphasic disturbances whatsoever in certain right handed individuals may be explained by the fact that in these cases speech functions were not altogether dependent upon zones of the left hemisphere, but were divided between the *two* hemispheres. Such an explanation differs considerably from our usual ideas. Though it may force us to change some of our habitual conceptions regarding the structure and function of the human brain, it may clarify some of the negative cases which we could hardly explain.

A number of long established facts force us to consider domination by the "leading" hemisphere as most likely. According to the observations by a number of authors which have been summarized by Stier (1911), Ludwig (1932), Nielsen (1944), Zangwill (1960), and others, right-handers who possess various signs of latent left-handedness are considerably more common than is generally believed. Thus left hemispheric dominance is not absolute.

Morphological studies carried out by S. M. Blinkov in the Moscow Brain Institute have shown that the relative sizes of corresponding architectonic fields in the two hemispheres are quite variable. These investigations showed that the "coefficient of assymetry" of cortical areas is especially large in those areas which are phylogenetically youngest. The difference can be as large as 25-30% for areas 22 and 42 (Brodman) but does not exceed 5% for area 41, an old area. Blinkov's data showed that the size of a given area may be larger on the right side for some individuals, larger on the left for others, and approximately equal in the two hemispheres for still others. This plus the fact that in one and the same individual degree of assymmetry is not constant for various areas of approximately equal phylogenetic age, the complexity of the question of cerebral dominance becomes obvious.

Thus both psychological and morphological investigations indicate that there is considerable variability in the degree of dominance of one or the other hemisphere, and that the variability is greatest in the most recently developed cortical structures. Making use of data obtained by careful observation of a very large number of wartime brain injuries, we shall attempt to show what roles they play in the recovery from traumatic aphasia.

B. THE INFLUENCE OF WOUND TYPE ON SPONTANEOUS SPEECH RECOVERY

For the time being we shall not consider those cases in which recovery was achieved by means of long-term systematic rehabilitation therapy, for in such cases radical transformations of speech functions may occur. Rather we shall limit ourselves to the analysis of "negative" cases and cases in which rapid and complete spontaneous recovery was observed. Thus there will be no doubt that all the cases involved *recovery of function* rather than a transformation of function. In order to see the difference between these two means of reestablishing speech functions it is only necessary to compare the slow, strained speech of a rehabilitated aphasic – speech quite similar to that of a foreigner who has just learned a new language – with the smooth speech of a patient who recovered spontaneously and whose language is the same as it was before.

What are the conditions required and how is such spontaneous reestablishment of speech functions accomplished? Is it possible that the absence of aphasic symptoms or the rapid recovery after brain injuries may be explained by the fact that only *slight pathological changes of brain tissues were involved*? The comparison of the recoveries from speech defects after penetrating and nonpenetrating wounds of the left hemisphere which was presented in the preceding chapter provides an unequivocal answer to this question.

From that analysis it was apparent that even in the initial period nonpenetrating wounds were considerably more often accompanied by the absence of speech impairment than were penetrating wounds. This was true both of wounds of the principal speech zones and of injuries of the marginal zones. This difference showed up more clearly in the residual period then in the initial period. During this period penetrating wounds of the principal speech zones of the left hemisphere were seldom completely unassociated with speech disorders, whereas nonpenetrating wounds of the same area showed total recovery of speech function in almost 40% of cases. Consequently the type of wound and the degree of damage sustained by brain tissues is of considerable importance for the spontaneous recovery of functions disturbed by brain injury.

We shall present several examples of rapid and relatively complete spontaneous recovery of speech after nonpenetrating wounds of the speech areas.

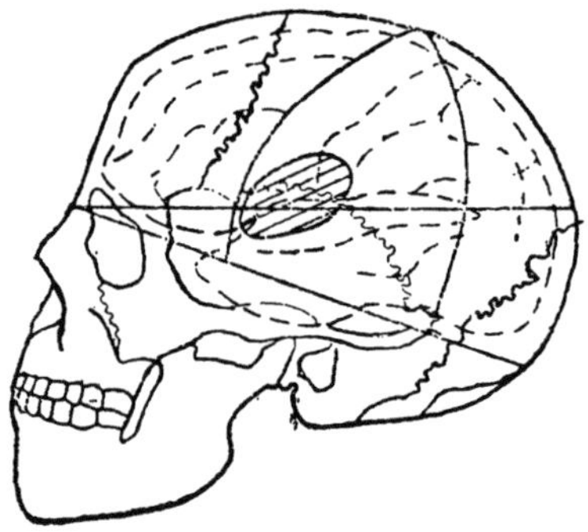

Patient P.: injury diagram (Case 1)

Case 1

On December 21, 1942, Patient P. (case history No. 1395) received a nonpenetrating wound of the fronto-temporal region of the left hemisphere. There was a temporary loss of consciousness and hemisparesis of the right side immediately following the injury. In a short time both movement and sensitivity were re-established, but symptoms of paresis in the area served by the right facial nerve persisted. There was no Babinsky reflex on the right side. For two or three days after injury it was difficult for the patient to talk, but this speech impairment soon passed; four months later his speech was noted to be altogether normal. His only complaint at this time was of a certain lack of continuity of thought.

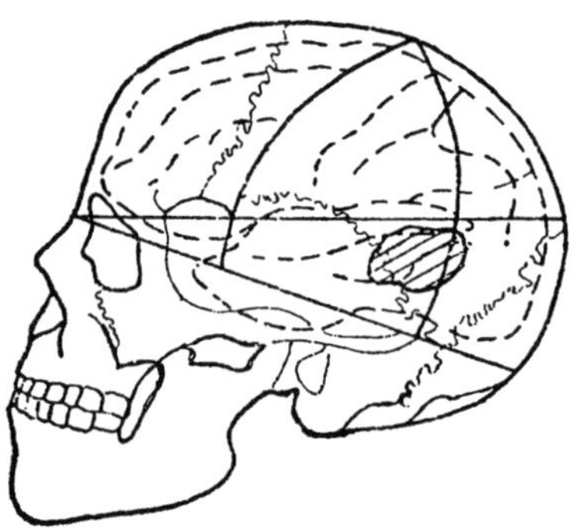

Patient C.: injury diagram (Case 2)

Case 2

On December 13, 1942, Patient C. (case history No. 3187) received a nonpenetrating wound of the left temporal area. Immediately after injury there was a temporary loss of consciousness followed by a longer period of disorientation. There were no signs of paresis; in the residual period slight hypesthesia was noted on the right side. The patient did not speak for five days following injury, although he understood the speech of others. Following this there was rapid recovery of normal speech and after two months there were no signs of speech disturbance except for a very occasional paraphasia (word substitution).

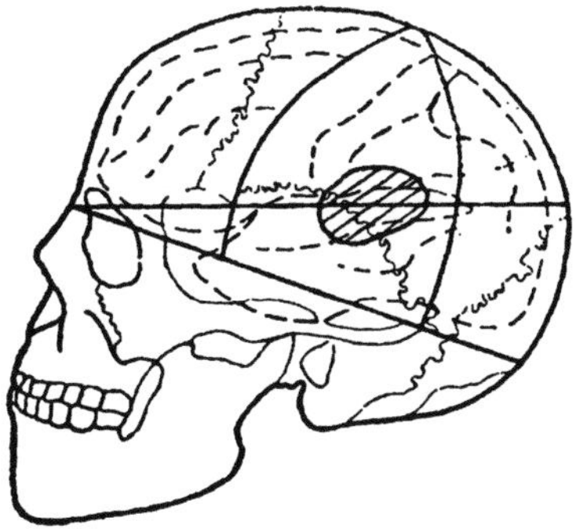

Patient P.: injury diagram (Case 3)

Case 3

On December 15, 1942 Patient P. (case history No. 3357) received a wound of the left temporal area which involved the bone but did not penetrate the dura mater. For several hours following injury the patient was unconscious and showed signs of right hemiparesis. For the first few days after injury he was totally unable to speak, but following an operation to remove bone splinters and bomb fragments, his speech rapidly recovered and in short time was completely normal.

In all of the cases presented above – and this number could be considerably enlarged – nonpenetrating wounds of the skull over the speech areas of the left hemisphere produced temporary disturbances of speech. These disturbances were characterized by a block of speech function, removal of which quickly led to the recovery of normal speech.

C. THE DEPENDENCE OF SPONTANEOUS SPEECH RECOVERY UPON SITE OF INJURY

We have mentioned cases in which nonpenetrating wounds produced temporary blockade of speech functions followed after a short time by complete recovery. There were cases, however, in which *penetrating* wounds of the brain involving hemorrhage, infection, and extensive destruction of brain substance either gave rise to speech disorders which underwent rapid recovery or produced no aphasic signs whatsoever. Some of the cases were shown upon careful examination of the site of lesion to have resulted not from damage to the major speech areas, but from injuries of areas directly *bordering on* the primary areas. Such injuries, which at first glance appeared to be *negative* cases, turned out simply to provide further confirmation for a *topical delimitation* of the speech areas themselves. We shall present several cases which illustrate this point.

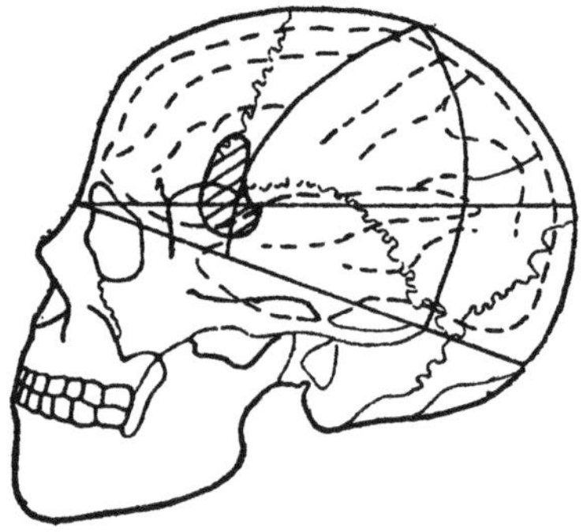

Patient G.: injury diagram (Case 4)

Case 4

Patient G. (case history No. 3276)
The patient was right handed with no signs of left handedness. On January 12, 1943 he suffered a penetrating wound in the fronto-temporal area of the left hemisphere which damaged the dura mater. The injury was followed by loss of consciousness. Gross paralysis was not observed, and no complications arose. Neurologically there were slight signs of a right sided hemisyndrome.

For a period of two weeks after injury the patient had difficulty in speaking ("words wouldn't come"); reading and writing were not disturbed. Two months after injury his speech was perfectly normal; psychological investigation produced no indications of residual aphasic symptoms.

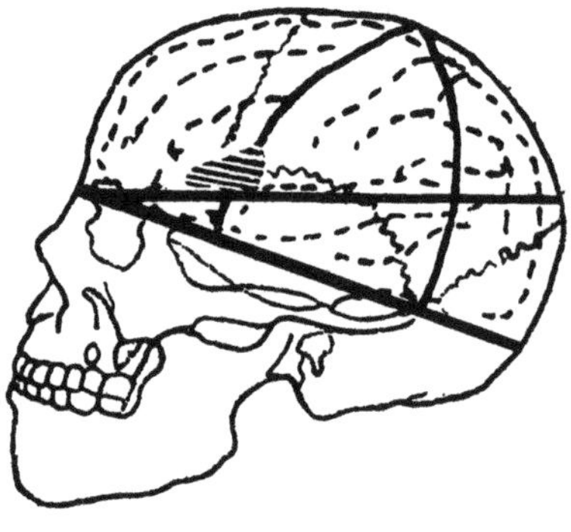

Patient Š.: injury diagram (Case 5)

Case 5

Patient S. (case history No. 3798)
On March 14, 1943 the patient received a penetrating fronto-temporal injury in the left hemisphere which was accompanied by loss of consciousness for two hours. Following injury there were no gross signs of motor or sensory loss. A month and a half after injury there were insignificant signs of a slight residual right sided hemisyndrome. Speech was not lost after injury, and at the time of psychological investigation (two and a half months later) there was no sign of speech disturbance.

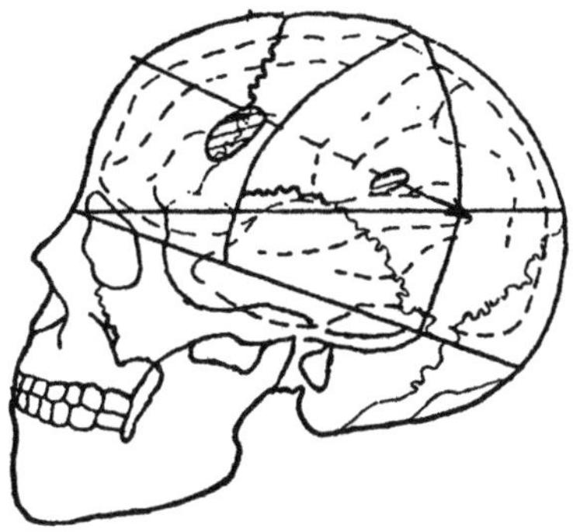

Patient K.: injury diagram (Case 6)

Case 6

Patient K. (case history No. 2827)
The patient was right handed. April 25, 1942 he was injured by a bullet which entered through the lower portion of the left frontal area and emerged from the anterior portion of the lower parietal area. The injury resulted in loss of consciousness for two hours and right hemiparesis and motor aphasia both of which lasted a month before undergoing rapid recovery. Seven weeks after injury an operation was performed to open an absess at the point where the bullet had emerged. This operation also produced no impairment of speech. A thorough examination carried out three months after injury revealed no signs of speech disorder.

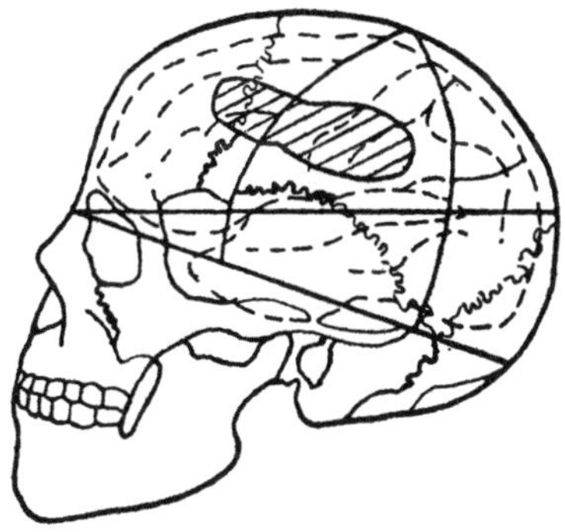

Patient Š.: injury diagram (Case 7)

Case 7

Patient S. (case history No. 3255)
The patient was right handed with no sign of left handedness. January 10, 1943 he suffered a penetrating bullet wound of the left fronto-temporal area with damage in the dura mater and destruction of brain tissue. Several hours after injury he lost consciousness for a long period; after having regained consciousness he noticed a right hemiparesis which was most severe in the hand. This was accompanied by a severe disturbance of speech. For fifteen days he was completely unable to speak and showed poor comprehension. For a longer time he had difficulty in remembering words and experienced some

difficulties in phasic speech, but both of these symptoms soon disappeared. An examination performed two months after injury showed no signs of speech disturbance.

The first two of these cases contributed data useful for delimitation of the *anterior border* of the major speech area, while the latter two contributed to determination of the *superior border.* In all cases injury produced only comparatively short-lived disturbance of speech functions which gave way to rapid and total recovery. Gross destruction of brain tissues in areas bordering on the primary speech zones produced only temporary blockade of speech functions and left behind only slight symptoms. Such examples which at first glance appear to constitute a special group, can thus actually be related to the group of "negative" or "paradoxical" cases.

D. THE DEPENDENCE OF SPEECH RECOVERY UPON THE DEGREE OF DOMINANCE OF THE LEFT HEMISPHERE

After exclusion from the "negative" group of those cases in which absence of aphasic symptoms or occurrence of rapid recovery could be attributed to insufficient depth of damage or to site of injury, there remained a significant group in which indisputable injury of brain substance within the bounds of the primary speech areas of the left hemisphere did not produce speech disturbances or led only to slight forms of aphasia. To these we might also add those cases in which gross damage to the marginal areas produced minor changes in speech with extremely rapid recovery. How are we to explain cases which constitute the core of the "negative" group, i.e. those which contradict our usual conceptions?

It was proposed in the literature long ago that the widespread idea of absolute lateralization of speech function in the left hemisphere is not true. The conception that the right hemisphere may also take part in the organization of speech processes was set forth by Jackson and Bastian in their day, and has received support during the past decade in the writings of Goldstein and Nissl von Mayendorf, Zangwill, Subirana and others. This idea is confirmed by several well known facts. First, total verbal deafness can arise only as a result of symmetrical damage to both temporal lobes (Pötzl, Liepmann, Pappenheim, and others). Also, injury of the dominant left hemisphere may sometimes be slightly compensated for by the remaining intact right hemisphere. It is supported further by the fact that in a number of cases, reported in the literature by Charcot, Monakow, Preobraženskij and others, speech disturbances have occurred in right handers following injury of the right hemisphere. Finally, this conception is confirmed by the fact that in certain cases, gross damage of the speech zones of the left hemisphere in right handers does not lead to aphasic disturbances.

All of these facts support the supposition that in many cases the lateralization of speech function and its dependence upon the *left* hemisphere is not absolute. Actually there is a *whole series of intermediate states* ranging from total and absolute dominance of the left hemisphere to partial or total transfer of the dominant role to the right hemisphere. Thus both the paradoxical appearance of aphasia following the injury of the subdominant right hemisphere in right handers and the absence of, or rapid recovery from, aphasia following injury of the speech zones of the dominant left hemisphere may be explained on the basis of *variation among individuals in the degree of left hemisphere dominance* which is reflected in *variation in the relation of the right hemisphere to speech functions.*

Upon what does this variation in the degree of left hemispheric dominance depend? Is it truly reflected by right and left handedness? On the basis of our observations we must answer the latter question in the negative. It appeared that injuries of equal severity to the speech zones of the left hemisphere in patients who were clearly right handed could lead to disturbances with all degrees of severity and susceptibility to recovery. This fact forced us to seek more fundamental causes for the variability in aphasic symptoms.

One can say that the usual clinical assumption that handedness is a unique indicator of hemispheric dominance is oversimplified. Such a simple view actually has no basis in fact. It is well known that in addition to the obvious sign of handedness one can distinguish a number of more subtle signs. These may show that in certain individuals, whom we would at first glance classify as right handers, the right hemisphere plays at least an equal role with the left. Such signs may be of a morphological character, or they may be purely functional. They have been discussed in the European literature, and especially in the American literature. Thus it is possible to determine *subtle signs of left handedness* in cases where gross observation gives no basis for such a classification.

Here we mention only a few such subtle signs of hemispheric dominance; some of them manifest themselves in anamnesis, while others are revealed only by special experimental tests.

Among the *morphological* signs of latent left handedness are a large left hand, a well developed venous system on the back of the left hand, a wide finger nail on the fifth finger of the left hand, and highly developed expressive musculature on the right side of the face.

The number of *functional signs* of latent left handedness is considerably greater. An individual taught from childhood to use his right hand primarily may always use it for such practiced operations as writing, eating, and manual work; in more primitive functions, however, which he was not taught by others such as actions carried out spontaneously under conditions of high affect (fighting, throwing a handgrenade, etc.) latent left handedness may manifest itself, and the individual may switch to his left hand. Aside from such observations, a detailed interrogation regarding the extent to which the left hand of a given individual can substitute for the right or participate in complex activities with the right hand often reveals irregularities in the dominance of the right hand and turns up individual differences which may have been missed during initial examination.

Another technique for the discovery of latent left handedness involves *special tests.*

Among these are such well known tests as *clasping the hands* (when the fingers of the two hands are intertwined the thumb of a latent left hander comes out on top), *clapping movements* (the left hand of a latent left hander is more active than the right hand), and *tonus tests*, (when the fingers of the two hands are pressed together, those of the right hand beck fack farther than those of the left hand in a left hander).[1] Finally Xaxpuridze, in Tbilisi, has recently described a phenomenon which he refers to as "*sensory asymmetry*." This sign is based upon the fact that a right hander manipulating spheres of equal size estimates the one in the left hand to be larger, while a left hander overestimates the size of the ball in the right hand. The same tendency is observed when two spheres of equal size are presented visually.

These types of test are not limited to functions involving the hand. The procedures include a determination of the *dominant eye*. The patient may be asked to hold a pencil at arm's length and to line it up with a point on the wall three or four meters away. This he must do with both eyes open. If, following this, the pencil appears to shift sharply to the right when he closes his right eye but remains in line when he closes his left eye, the examiner may conclude the presence of right eye dominance. The opposite result signifies lefs eye dominance.

These tests permit us to detect latent signs of hemispheric dominance without depending upon actions involving the hand. Thus one can avoid the use of signs which may prove to be misleading in cases of paresis produced by extensive brain damage.[2]

Simultaneous application of all the methods described above makes it possible to identify cases of latent right hemisphere dominance which would not otherwise be recognized. As a result of this, the number of cases of right hemisphere dominance (or at least of right hemisphere equivalence) rises considerably.

The detection of latent left handedness is not the only approach to a more precise characterization of cerebral dominance. Another line of investigation has developed out of genealogical studies performed by Wilson (1891), Stier (1911), Orton (1937), and a number of others. They believe that, whereas in some cases hemispheric dominance and the accompanying handedness may be the result of learing (as is sugested by cases of identical twins who may show differences in cerebral dominance), in other cases definite genotypic influences have been observed. The fact that in some families there are many left handers while in others there are none can hardly be explained on the basis of upbringing.

If this conception has basis in fact, then we should expect that, along with the overt forms of left handedness, it should be possible to find *latent forms of left handedness* which give no external sign of their presence. Such forms could be identified only by reference to the presence of overt left handedness in other mem-

[1] This last sign was adopted on the basis of a personal communication from Professor Kalman-Šanta (Debrezen).

[2] A new and apparently effective method of detecting hemispheric dominance was introduced in the late forties by the Canadian investigator, Wada. He reports that in cases where there is doubt as to which hemisphere is dominant he injects sodium amytal into the left carotid artery. If the left hemisphere is altogether dominant, injection of sodium amytal produces a transient hemiparesis and aphasia; if the left hemisphere is not dominant Wada observes transient paresis unaccompanied by speech disturbances. Unfortunately this technique appeared in the literature too late to be used in the present study.

bers of the family. The phenotypic absence of left handedness in a number of cases may correspond to the genotype; in other cases it might occur in spite of an underlying latent left handedness. Such latent left handedness might reveal itself if one of the cerebral hemispheres were damaged, for in this case the latent predisposition would have a chance to express itself. The existence of a group of latent left handers could, of course, enlarge the number of cases in which we would expect to see incomplete dominance by the left hemisphere.

Thus one may pose the following question: is it not possible that latent left handedness accounts for cases in which severe damage of the speech zones of the left hemisphere did not produce speech disturbances in right handers or only led to disorders which underwent rapid recovery? Cannot the variation in degree of potential ability of the right hemisphere to substitute for the damaged speech zones account for differences in the *ease* with which speech disturbances gave way to recovery in different patients?

We considered our data from this point of view. Our data indicated that of 420 adult patients, 4.8% were left handed. This is consonant with Stier's finding that the number of left handers in the population does not exceed 4.6% (according to Shaeffer 4.6%, Lombrozo 4.3%, Ogle 6.7%). The number of patients who reported that other members of their families were left handed was also not very large (our knowledge of their genealogy was comparatively limited). According to our observations of a nonselected group of 420 adults, the persons whose families included lefthanders did not exceed 16.2%. The number of cases showing subtle signs of left handedness was of course considerably larger than the number of definite left handers mentioned above.

The next question is whether or not cases of left hemispheric injury which did not produce speech disturbances or gave only short lived impairment included a high concentration of persons with slight signs of left handedness or persons from families of left handers. In order to answer this question we selected a group of 160 patients with penetrating wounds in the primary speech areas and classified them according to severity of aphasic symptoms. This work was begun by us and then continued in our laboratory by E. V. Gurova.[3] The results appear in Table 3.

Table 3 shows that in the initial period, severe forms of aphasia were seen not only in pure right handers but also in righthanders who gave slight signs of left handedness and in individuals with left handers in the family. Slight forms of aphasia, following penetrating injuries in the primary speech areas were seen, however, only in left handers, ambidextrous individuals, or individuals with left handers in their families. Thus not once in 160 cases did a pure right hander show total absence of aphasic disturbance during the initial period following injury; of

[3] This group of patients was subjected to special study by E. V. Gurova. Since this work was carried out in large neurosurgical hospitals and cases were selected which showed either no sign of aphasia or complete recovery in the residual period, the eventual total number of cases studied considerably exceeds the number which enters into our basic statistics.

TABLE 3

*Speech disturbances following injuries of the primary speech areas: signs of slight or latent left handedness and the severity of aphasic symptoms **

Severity of aphasic syndromes / Signs of slight or latent left handedness	Initial period			Residual period		
	severe forms of aphasia	slight forms of aphasia	absence of aphasia	severe forms of aphasia	slight forms of aphasia	absence of aphasia
Number of cases	120	19	21	55	42	63
A. Pure right handers (64 patients)	60 (50)	3 (16)	0	48 (87)	14 (33)	2 (3)
B. Right handers with slight signs of left handedness or with left handers in the family (73 patients)	44 (37)	12 (63)	17 (81)	5 (9)	22 (53)	46 (73)
C. Left handers and ambidextrous patients (23 patients)	15 (13)	4 (21)	4 (19)	2 (4)	6 (14)	15 (24)
Totals	(100)	(100)	(100)	(100)	(100)	(100)
Breakdown of Group B above	(37)	(63)	(81)	(9)	(83)	(73)
a. Right handers with slight signs of left handedness but no left handers in the family (40 patients)	29 (24)	4 (21)	7 (33	5 (9)	14 (33)	21 (33)
b. Right handers without signs of left handedness but with left handedness in the family (18 patients)	5 (4)	4 (21)	9 (43)	0	5 (12)	13 (21)
c. Right handers with slight signs of left handedness and left handers in the family	10 (8)	4 (21)	1 (5)	0	3 (7)	12 (19)

* This table presents the actual number of cases in each group; percentages are presented in parentheses.

the 21 patients with no aphasic symptoms, 17 either showed signs of latent left handedness or were from families with left handers. The remaining four were left handed or ambidexterous. The same preponderance of individuals with slight signs of left handedness was observed among those cases in which injury of the primary speech areas produced a slight, rapidly recovering disturbance. In that group there were only three pure right handers; the vast majority gave signs of either pronounced slight, or latent left handedness.

The role of slight or latent left handedness appears even more clearly when one considers the ultimate development of the disturbances which were produced by injury of the primary speech areas. As the data in Table 3 show, severe aphasia remained during the residual phase in the overwhelming majority of right handed individuals who had no left handers in the family. In only five of 55 cases of severe aphasic disorders were we dealing with individuals showing signs of slight or latent left handedness. On the other hand, of the large group of patients whose aphasic symptoms underwent rapid and total disappearance, despite massive penetrating wounds in the primary speech areas of the left hemisphere, 73% showed signs of slight or latent left handedness, and 24% were left handed or ambidextrous. Only two were pure right handers.

The breakdown of groups in the lower section of Table 3 shows a characteristic tendency for the absence of speech disturbances to occur when injury of the primary speech areas was sustained by patients who gave no signs of left handedness even under careful examination, but whose families included left handers. Of 18 cases studied, half never showed signs of speech disturbance, and the other half lost all signs of disturbance during the residual period.

TABLE 4

Aphasia following injuries to the primary speech areas: hemisphere dominance and severity of aphasic symptoms

Degree of left handedness / Severity of aphasic syndromes	Initial period			Residual period		
	pure right handers	right handers with slight or latent left handedness	left handers and ambidextrous individuals	pure right handers	right handers with slight or latent left handedness	left handers and ambidextrous individuals
Number of cases	64	73	23	64	73	23
Severe forms of aphasia	61 (95)	44 (60)	15 (66)	48 (75)	5 (7)	2 (9)
Slight forms of aphasia	3 (5)	12 (16)	4 (17)	14 (22)	22 (30)	6 (26)
Absence of aphasia	0	17 (29)	4 (17)	2 (3)	46 (63)	15 (65)
Totals	(100)	(100)	(100)	(100)	(100)	(100)

These observations permit us to answer questions regarding differences in the effects of injuries of the primary speech areas depending upon whether the patients are pure right handers, or right handers showing signs of slight or latent left handedness. The data relating specifically to this question are presented in Table 4.

From Table 4 we see that in penetrating wounds of the primary speech areas of the left hemisphere severe aphasia is produced in the initial period in 95% of cases involving pure right handers. In 75% of cases the severe symptoms persist into the residual period.[4] In only two cases was full spontaneous recovery of speech functions observed. On the other hand, if one considers right handers who have slight signs of left handedness or latent left handedness, only 77% showed aphasia in the initial period following penetrating wounds of the primary speech areas. As a rule those disorders which appeared in the initial period were not severe, and within a few months after injury only 7% of cases showed clear residual symptoms. Of the remaining cases two thirds underwent total spontaneous recovery, while in the other third only slight aphasic symptoms remained. Left handed and ambidextrous individuals gave much the same picture as the latter group.

Thus a considerable volume of material leads us to the conclusion that *only in cases of absolute dominance of the left hemisphere do gross lesions of the primary speech areas produce severe lasting aphasic disorders.* In those cases where a "right hander" shows slight signs of left handedness or has left handers in the family, the functional relationship between the two hemispheres is different from that in a pure right hander. The left hemisphere may lack the absolute dominance which we earlier presumed it to have, and injury of the left hemisphere consequently does not produce the disturbances of function which would otherwise be expected. The presence of latent left handedness which is not expressed phenotypically may thus lead to an essential transformation of the interrelationship between the hemispheres following brain injury.

Observations on a wide range of material have led to the conclusion that latent dominance plays a more significant role in brain pathology than might have been suspected at first glance. This does not imply that lateralized functions cease altogether depending upon left, or "leading", hemisphere, but rather that a *whole series of intermediate stages* ranging from absolute dominance by the left hemisphere, through equivalence of the two hemispheres, to dominance by the right hemisphere may be expected to occur. It also means that parts of the right hemisphere which are symmetrical with the speech areas of the left hemisphere may be in large measure capable of assuming the functions of the left hemisphere if it is damaged. Transfer of function to the subdominant hemisphere has been

[4] The lack of correspondence between these figures and those presented earlier is explained by the fact already mentioned that in this group are included specially selected cases of spontaneous speech recovery. Thus, by comparison with the total number of brain injuries, the number of cases with severe residual aphasic symptoms in these statistics is small.

mentioned by many authors, including Wernicke, Goldstein, and Nissl von Mayendorf. The ease with which it occurs appears to depend upon the extent to which various individuals possess the genotypic potential for the right hemisphere to fulfill the complex functions which are usually performed by the left.

We shall present several examples which illustrate the points covered so far. These are cases involving the inconsistent findings of grave damage to the primary speech areas of the left hemisphere resulting in slight clinical symptoms of aphasia.

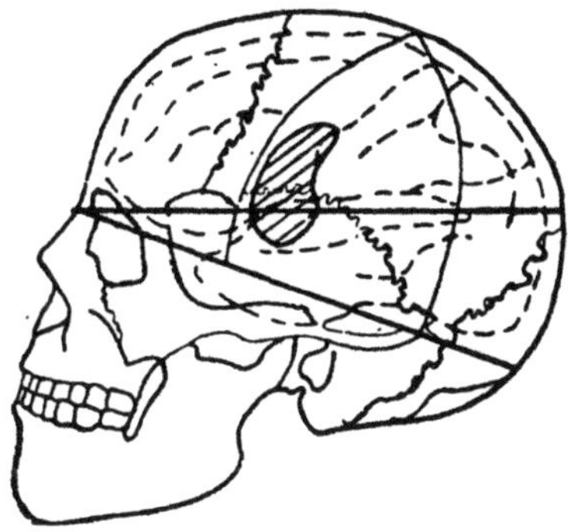

Patient I.: injury diagram (Case 1)

Case 1

Patient I. (case history No. 3656)
On March 5, 1943 this 38 year old man received a penetrating wound from a shell fragment which lodged in the anterior portion of the left Sylvian fissure. He lost consciousness for a short time, but there were no signs of paresis or sensory disturbances. During an operation performed the following day to remove the shell fragments it was noted that the dura mater had been penetrated and that cerebral detritus extruded from the wound. This patient showed no signs of speech disturbance. A careful examination carried out two and a half months after injury turned up no changes either in expressive speech or speech comprehension. The patient was right handed with no signs of left handedness. His father was left handed (information about other members of the family was not obtained).

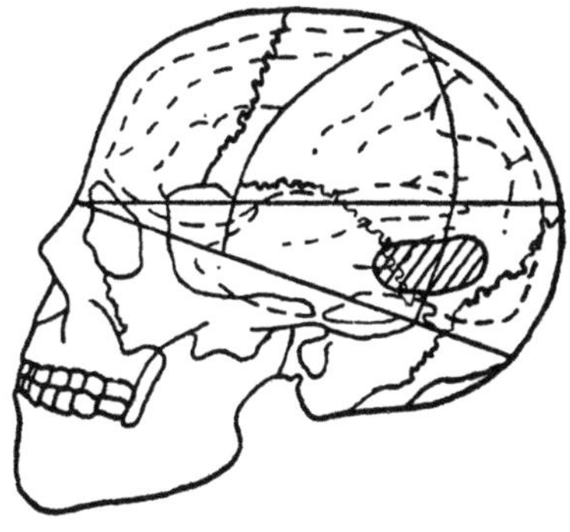

Patient B.: injury diagram (Case 2)

Case 2

Patient B. (case history No. 1715)
On April 3, 1942, this 46 year old man received a penetrating wound from a shell fragment entering the posterior part of the left occipito temporal area. At operation three days later it was discovered that the dura mater had been penetrated and that cerebral detritus extruded from the wound. A neurological analysis produced no signs of functional disorder. Speech was totally intact during both initial and succeeding examinations. Total preservation of mental processes was observed in a careful examination performed three months after injury. The patient was right handed, but there were left handers in his family (son and first cousin).

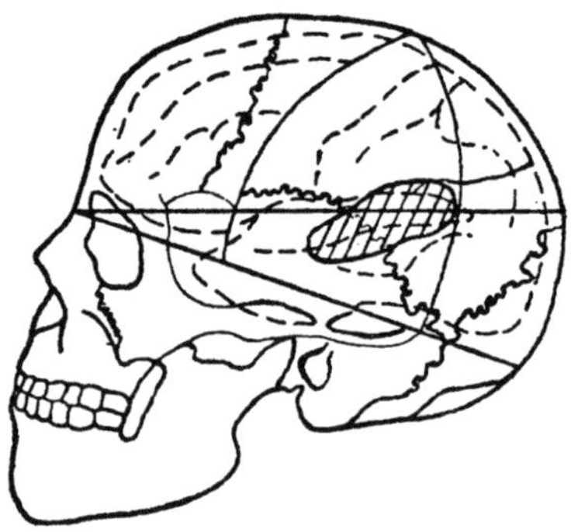

Patient D.: injury diagram (Case 3)

Case 3

Patient D. (case history No. 2890)
On September 1, 1942 the patient received a penetrating wound from a shell fragment in the left temporal area. He was unconscious for some time following injury. Upon operation three weeks later it was discovered that the dura mater had been penetrated. Twenty cc. of purulent exudate were removed from an abscess in the brain tissue and bone splinters were removed. There were signs of mild paresis of the right hand and slight right hemisyndrome with considerable disturbance of motor speech and some disturbance of comprehension (especially evident when the examiner began to speak somewhat more rapidly than normal). Also a writing disorder was observed; letters were misplaced and poorly formed. The speech defects lasted for ten or twelve days and then altogether disappeared. An examination performed three months after injury indicated no signs of speech disturbance; only occasional errors in writing, e.g. substitution of letters similar in sound, and a slight disturbance of verbal memory persisted. The patient was right handed with no signs of left handedness, but in his family there were several cases of left handedness (Fig. 7, left handers in black).

Case 4

Patient B. (case history No. 3262)
On January 9, 1943, this 26 year old man sustained a penetrating injury in the left lower parietal and temporal area. Following injury he lost consciousness for several minutes. At operation five days later bone fragments of considerable size were removed from a depth of 1.5 cm. in the brain tissue. Neither paresis nor reduced sensitivity were

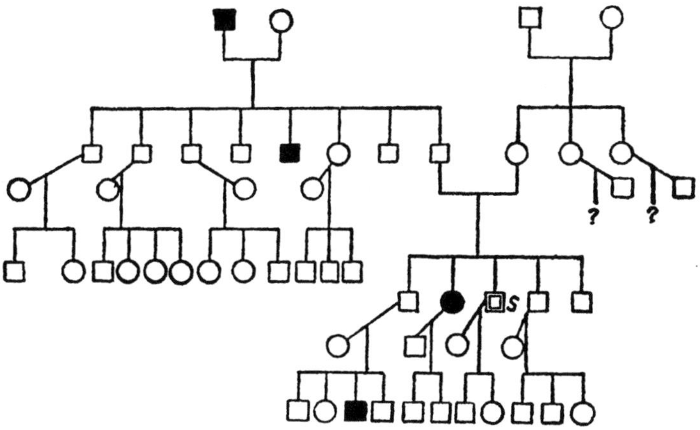

FIG. 6. Genealogy of Patient D. (Case 3)

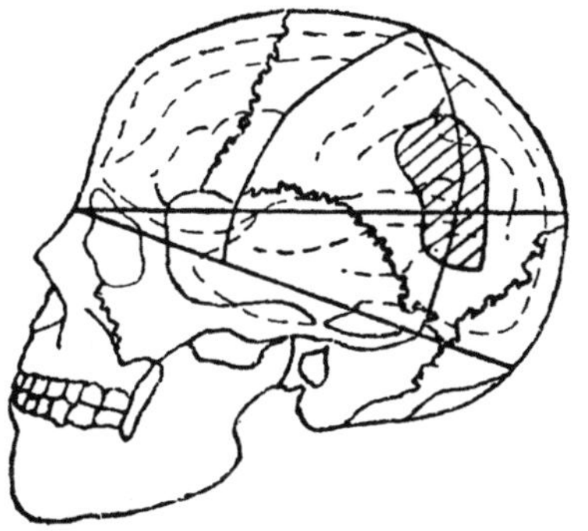

Patient B.: injury diagram (Case 4)

noted, but the patient immediately lost certain speech functions. In particular, he noted a loss of control over of his speech: "I want to speak, but I can't; it always comes out wrong". He was unable to write and experienced considerable difficulty in reading; he was able to name separate letters but could not identify whole words.

These gross signs of speech disturbance persisted for five days and then gradually began to disappear. After a month the patient could talk fairly easily. An examination carried out two months after injury turned up no clear signs of altered speech processes. The only remnants of the previous temporal syndrome were an occasional hesitation in producing words (especially under conditions of excitement) and a slight disturbance of spatial orientation. The patient was right handed, but members of his family were left handed (Fig. 8).

Case 5

Patient T.

On March 15, 1944, this 20 year old man received a penetrating shell fragment wound in the posterior portion of the left temporal and lower parietal area. At operation five days later, it was determined that the dura mater had been punctured and brain substance

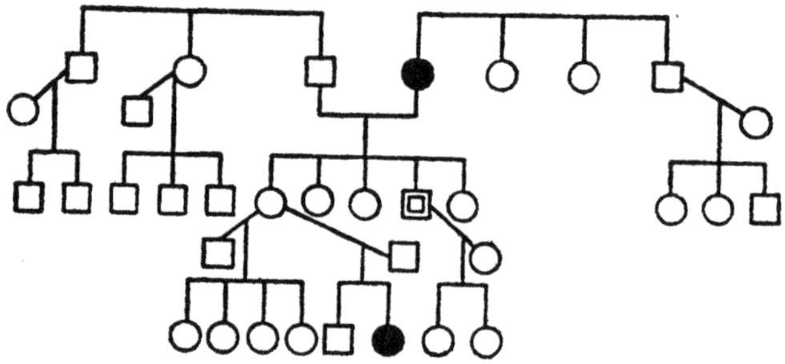

FIG. 8. Genealogy of Patient B. (Case 4)

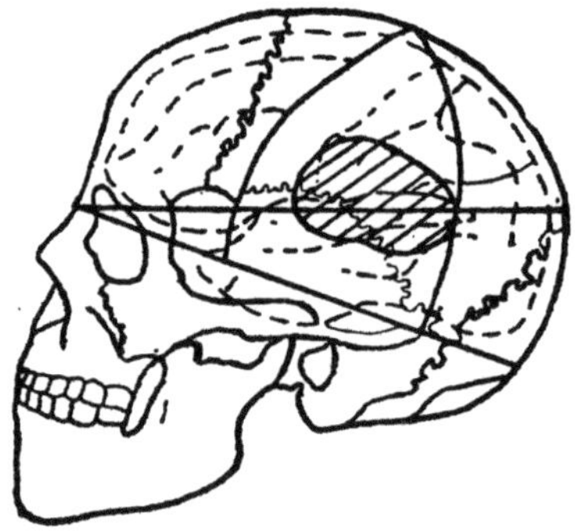

Patient T.: injury diagram (Case 5)

had extruded from the wound. A considerable number of bone splinters were removed from the brain tissues. After the injury, right hemiparesis, hyposensitivity, and hyperreflexia were observed. For two weeks following injury the patient was unable to speak or to understand what was said to him; he could neither read nor write. Many letters lost their meaning; his writing was unintelligible. Gradually all symptoms disappeared and six weeks after injury a careful psychological examination revealed no speech disorder of significance. The patient's speech was smooth and effortless; only occasionally did he experience a certain difficulty in naming things (objectively this was almost imperceptible); speech comprehension, reading, and writing abilities were recovered completely.

The patient had always been right handed with no signs of left handedness, but there were lefthanders in his family (both matrilineal and patrilineal) (Fig. 9).

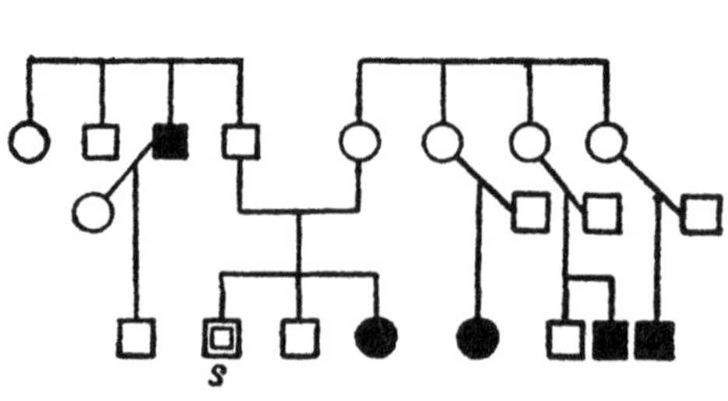

FIG. 9. Genealogy of Patient T. (Case 5)

In all of the cases summarized above, penetration wounds located within the boundaries of the speech zones of the left hemisphere of right handers failed to produce permanent speech disturbances. In every case there were left handers in the family of the individual who was injured.

A second group of cases is made up of nonpenetrating wounds of the same areas which produced virtually imperceptible disturbance in individuals having left handers in the family. Such disorders gave way to complete recovery in the residual period. Here we shall present only one typical example from a whole serie of such cases analyzed in our clinics.

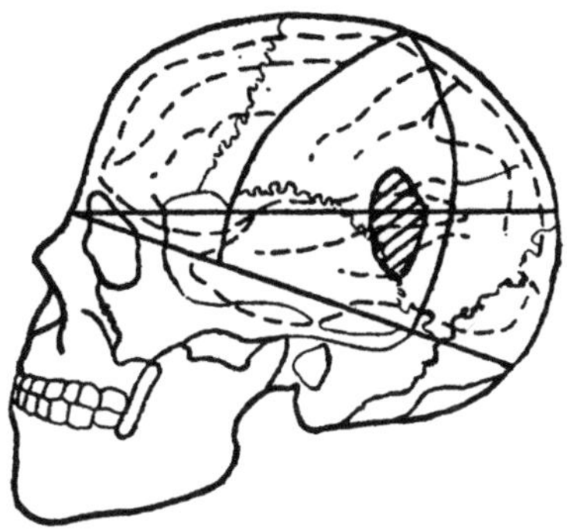

Patient K.: injury diagram (Case 6)

Case 6

Patient K. (case history No. 2682)
On August 10, 1942, this 37 year old man received a shell wound in the left temporal and lower parietal areas. He lost consciousness for two or three hours. Several days later at operation an extensive epidural hematoma was found. The dura mater was intact, and surgical puncture did not reveal any subdural supperation. Immediately after injury there was a notable weakness of the right extremities and disturbance of speech; he did not speak clearly and forgot words; instead of one word he would say another. Within six or seven days these symptoms completely disappeared and the patient began to talk normally. Upon examination two and a half months after injury his speech was altogether intact and only a slight disturbance of phonemic comprehension and occasional dysgraphia gave indication of the previous aphasia.

The patient was right handed, but there were left handers in the family (Fig. 10).

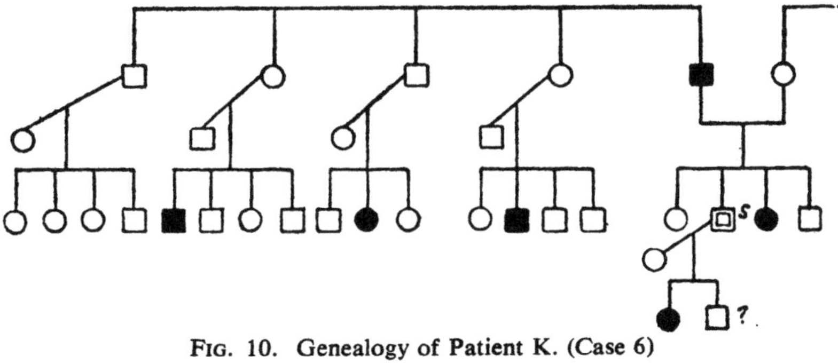

FIG. 10. Genealogy of Patient K. (Case 6)

In all of the cases presented above the only indicant of latent left handedness was the presence of left handedness in the genealogy of the patient. Underlying the phenotypic total right handedness there was a potential for dominance of the right hemisphere, which had never revealed itself in the normal life of the individual.

In a number of cases the latent supremacy of the right hemisphere manifested itself in slight signs of left handedness, and in these cases the functional disturbance could be classified as atypically minor in character. We shall limit ourselves to the presentation of two such cases.

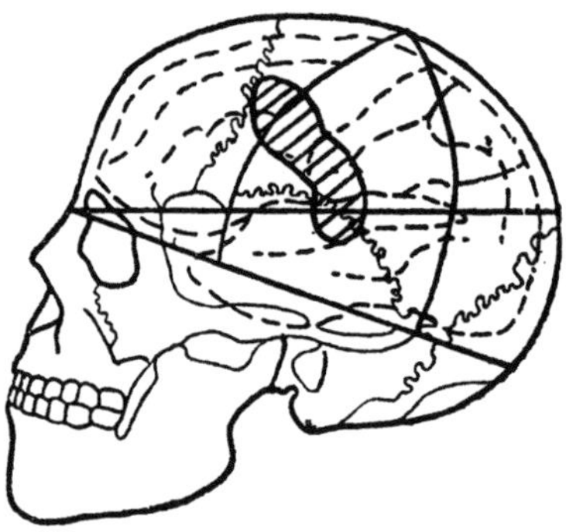

Patient K.: injury diagram (Case 7)

Case 7

Patient K. (case history No. 2822)

On August 10, 1942, this 21 year old man received penetrating bullet wound in the left frontal and temporal areas which involved puncture of the dura mater. He lost consciousness for a short period, but there was no gross loss of sensory or motor functions. For a period of two weeks he spoke poorly, although he easily understood the speech of others. Gradually the disturbance of speech passed and after three months it was impossible to note any sign whatsoever of speech difficulties; all that remained was a very minor defect of phonemic hearing and subjective complaints that he rapidly forgot things which he had heard or read.

The patient was right handed with no left handers in the family; but he himself showed a number of slight signs of left handedness (for instance, the left eye was dominant and when he clasped his hands, the left thumb appeared on top).

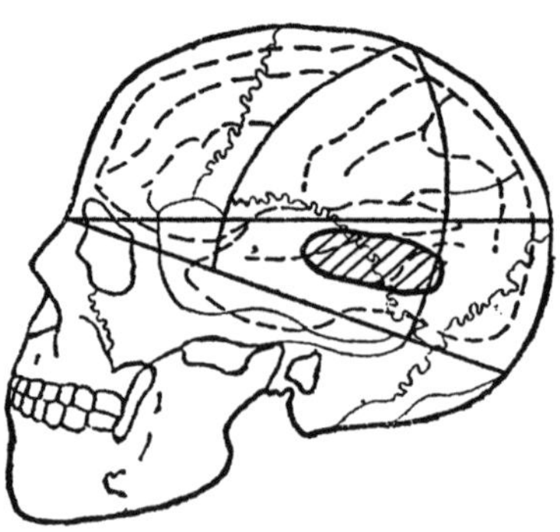

Patient B.: injury diagram (Case 8)

Case 8

Patient B. (case history No. 3644)
On February 18, 1943, this 25 year old man received a penetrating shell fragment wound in the left parieto-temporo-occipital area. The injury was followed by a long period of unconsciousness and right hemiparesis with disturbance of all forms of sensory function most pronounced in the right hand. At operation bone fragments were removed from deep in the temporal lobe. For two weeks, after injury, the patient did not speak at all. Shortly thereafter, however, his speech recovered and all symptoms of aphasia disappeared. All that remained was a severe stuttering which was gradually relieved by intensive rehabilitation therapy.

The patient was right handed with no cases of left handedness in the family. But he himself showed a number of signs of partial left handedness (when clasping his hands, he had the left thumb up; the nail of the fifth finger of the left hand was larger than that of the right hand; he chopped firewood left handedly).

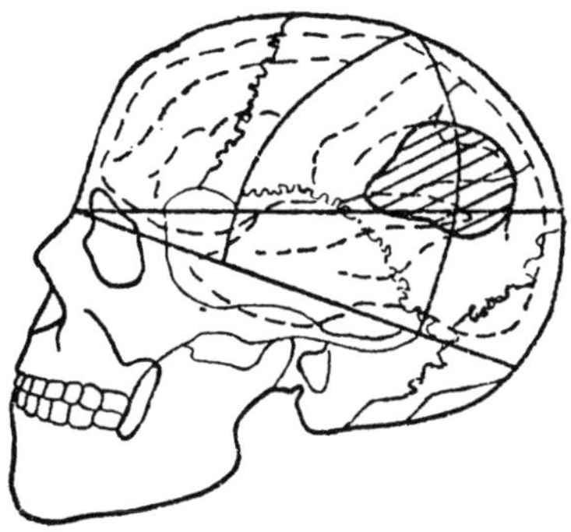

Patient L.: injury diagram (Case 9)

Case 9

Patient L. (case history No. 5005)
On November 2, 1944, this 22 year old man received a penetrating shell fragment wound in the left temporal area accompanied by a large (50cc) subdural hematoma which was drained at operation. After the injury, which was accompanied by a short period of unconsciousness, the patient began to talk poorly. He forgot words and showed many literal paraphasias. The same disturbances observed in speech were also observed in his writing. He poorly understood the speech of others and had the feeling that they were "somehow not speaking Russian". Within a month all of these symptoms completely disappeared, and a careful examination revealed almost no speech defects other than an insignificant difficulty in differentiating similar ("opposition") phonemes and a certain difficulty in comprehending long verbal constructions. By that time neither spontaneous speech nor speech comprehension of the patient differed significantly from normal.

The patient had always been right handed; in his family there were no cases of left handedness. But he himself showed a number of slight signs of left handedness (when he clasped his hands, the left thumb was on top; the nail of his left fifth finger was larger than that of the right; the left eye was dominant).

The idea that slight or latent left handedness can markedly affect the dominance relationship of the hemispheres is supported by cases in which injury of the speech areas of the left hemisphere of right handers does not produce permanent aphasic disturbances. It is supported further by the reverse situation in which injury to the *right* hemisphere produces speech disturbances in a right hander who shows signs of partial left handedness or in a right hander who has left handers in the family.

Such cases of "paradoxical aphasia" have been described in the literature by a number of authors – from Preobraženskij (1893), Senator (1904), Monakow (1914), and Kennedy (1916) to Needles (1942).

Our data show that such cases involved individuals who had slight signs of left handedness. Thus they could be explained in terms of the facts which have already been introduced. We shall present only a few cases to illustrate this situation.

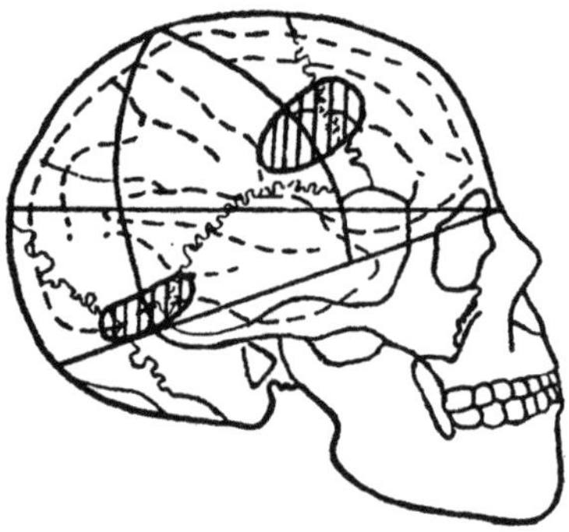

Patient K.: injury diagram (Case 10)

Case 10

Patient K. (case history No. 3090)
On November 17, 1942, this 20 year old man received a penetrating shell fragment wound in the right posterior frontal and right temporo-parieto-occipital area. The injury resulted in a loss of consciousness which lasted for several days. There were slight signs of left hemiparesis. No signs of damage to the left hemisphere were noted. Immediately after recovery of consciousness the patient showed noticeable disturbances of speech which consisted in difficulty pronouncing words and literal dysgraphia. Such disturbances of a distinctly aphasic character persisted for about a month, but after two and a half months only very slight traces of dysgraphia and the amnesic-aphasic disturbance remained.

The patient was right handed, but there were members of his family who were left handed (Fig. 11).

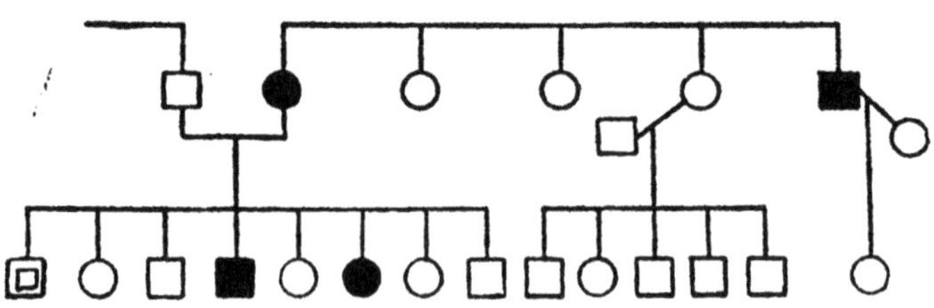

FIG. 11. Genealogy of Patient K. (Case 10)

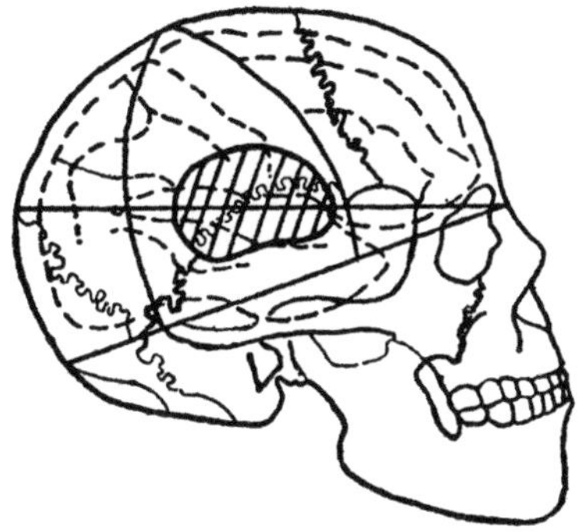

Patient S.: injury diagram (Case 11)

Case 11

Patient S. (case history No. 3661)
On February 23, 1943, this 39 year old man received a penetrating shell fragment wound in the right temporal area which was followed by a long period of unconsciousness. For a short period there were neurological signs of left hemiparesis with hyposensitivity and pathological reflexes on the left side. No signs of injury to the left hemisphere were noted. Immediately after recovery of consciousness, the patient showed symptoms characteristic of aphasia. For instance he was unable to pronounce whole words and had difficulty understanding the speech of others ("I could tell that they were speaking Russian, but I couldn't understand what they said".). Such difficulties were also noted in his handwriting. All of these defects lasted for about two weeks and then gradually disappeared. A detailed examination carried out two and a half months after injury revealed only very slight disturbances of phonemic hearing and residual signs of temporal dysgraphia.

The patient was right handed, but there were a number of left handers in his family (Fig. 12).

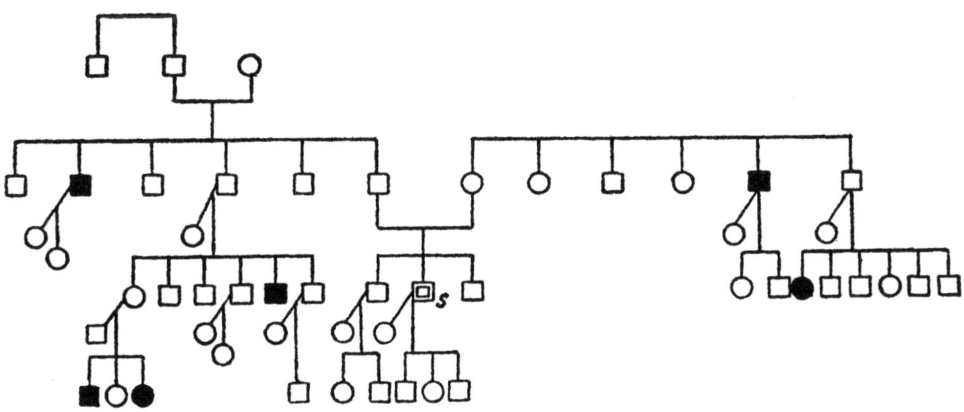

FIG. 12. Genealogy of Patient S. (Case 11)

Case 12

Patient P. (case history No. 3332)
On July 17, 1942, this 33 year old man received a penetrating shell fragment wound in the posterior right parieto-temporal area. An X-ray examination revealed a large metal

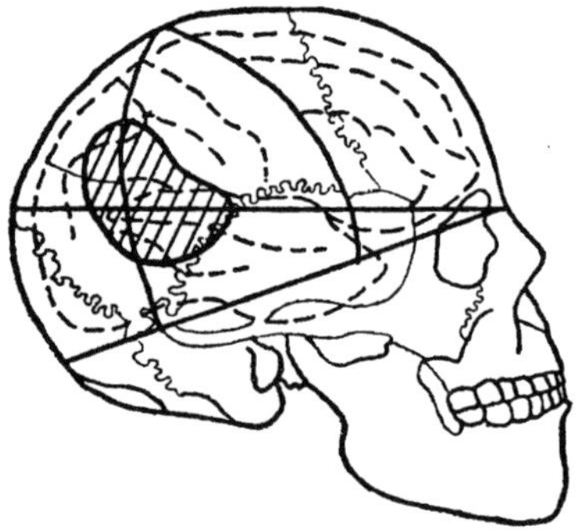

Patient P.: injury diagram (Case 12)

fragment lying two to three centimeters below the cortex. Recovery was impeded by the development of several abcesses.

After injury the patient was unconscious for a long period. A neurological observation revealed signs of damage to the right hemisphere, i.e., a drop in sensitivity on the left side and optico-vestibular disturbances; there were no signs of amnesic aphasia with impaired reading comprehension and agrammatica. These disturbances continued for about five months and again, eight months after injury, an examination revealed a slight temporal lobe syndrome consisting of disturbed spatial orientation, acalculia, and difficulty in organizing thoughts.

The patient was right handed with no signs of left handedness; but at least one member of his family was left handed (brother). (Matrilineal genealogy unknown.)

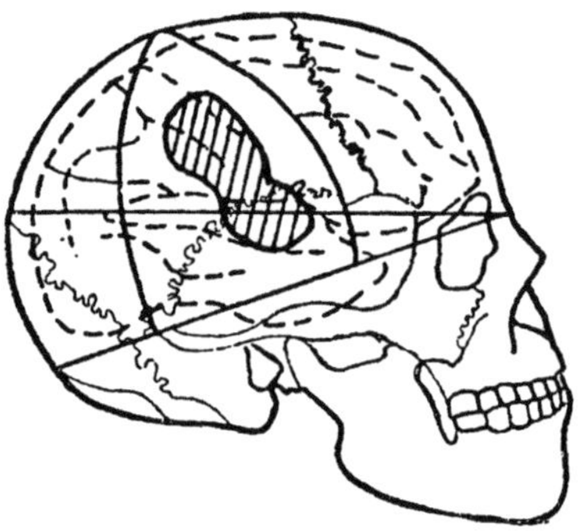

Patient S.: injury diagram (Case 13)

Case 13

Patient S. (case history No. 5005)

On February 7, 1945, this 36 year old man received a penetrating shell fragment wound in the inferior portion of the right sensory-motor area. At operation two days later a number of bone splinters were removed from the brain tissue. The injury produced an immediate and severe aphasic syndrome: the patient was altogether unable to speak, although he understood what others said. Initially there was no paresis, but after he was evacuated by train a left hemiparesis with disturbance of all sensory functions and a left facial nerve paresis were observed. The paresis lasted for about two months but gradually disappeared leaving only a slight weakness of the left hand. The speech disturbances turned out to be considerably more persistent, so that three months later it was still possible to note a distinct syndrome of residual motor aphasia involving a serious impairment of spontaneous speech, a pronounced motor aphasic disturbance of writing, and impaired ability to calculate. Hearing and comprehension were preserved.

There were no signs that the left hemisphere had been damaged. The patient was right handed, but his brother was left handed, and he himself showed a number of signs of partial left handedness (left thumb up when clasping the hands, a wider nail on the fifth finger of the left hand).

In the table accompanying Figure 13 there appear a number of cases in which injury of the right hemisphere resulted in paradoxical aphasia in right handed individuals having signs of slight or latent left handedness.[5]

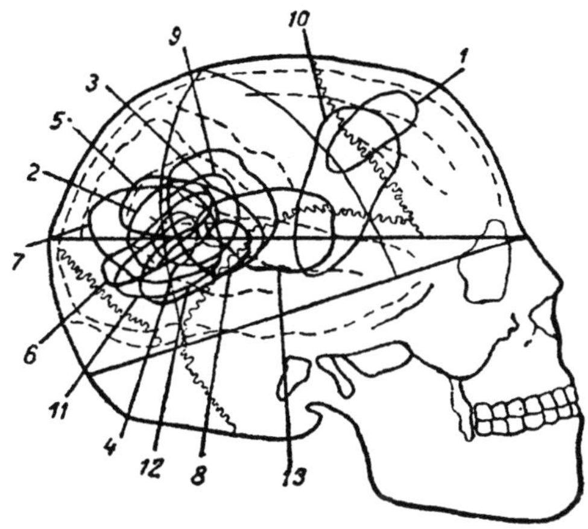

FIG. 13. Schematic diagram of lesions observed in cases of "paradoxical" aphasia following damage to the right hemisphere.

The observations presented above show that latent left handedness not only prevented aphasic disorders or facilitated the recovery from symptoms of aphasia following damage to the speech areas of the left hemisphere; it also can explain the unexpected appearance of aphasic symptoms following injury of the right hemisphere in certain right handed individuals.

Thus in the variations of hemispheric dominance we find an essential factor affecting the severity of speech disturbances that result from injury of the primary speech areas. This factor, which is apparently genetically determined, explains both those paradoxical cases in which massive lesions of the speech areas of the left hemisphere do not produce severe or persistent aphasic symptoms and those cases in which injuries of the right hemisphere of right handers produce speech disorders – a class of cases which up till this time has been difficult to understand.

[5] A part of the cases included in this table were collected by E. V. Gurova.

Cases of "paradoxical" aphasia involving lesions of the right hemisphere

Case No.	Name	Nature and localization of wound	Speech disturbance	Handedness
1	P.	Penetrating shrapnel wound in the right fronto-parietal area; partial left hemiparesis; no pathological signs on the right.	A type of motor aphasia lasting for several weeks and then disappearing.	Right handed with a number of left handers in the family.
2	S.	Penetrating wound in the right parieto-temporal area; slight left hemiparesis; reduced sensitivity on the left; left hemianopsia; right side symptoms absent.	Amnesic aphasia, alexia, and acalculia lasting for one and a half months.	Right handed with no signs of left handedness; mother left handed.
3	K.	Penetrating shrapnel wound in the right temporo-parietal area complicated by an abcess; left hemiparesis with disturbance of all forms of sensation; no right side symptoms.	Severe amnesic aphasia with signs of disturbed writing ability (a type of literal dysgraphia); difficulty in comprehending logico-grammatical constructions; slight visual-gnostic disturbance.	Right handed with no signs of left handedness; paternal aunt and maternal first cousin left handed.
4	Č.	Penetrating wound in posterior parts of the right parieto-temporal area complicated by an abcess; left paresis with disturbance of all forms of sensation; right side signs absent.	Severe disturbances of speech in the form of an atypical aphasia with an unusual aggramatism; reduced speech activity; writing defects (tendency to omit letters); amusia.	Right handed; slight signs of left handedness; brother left handed.
5	M.	Penetrating shrapnel wound in the right parieto-temporal area; persistent left hemiparesis.	Persistent and pronounced speech disorders; only able to pronounce individual words; imperfect comprehension; verbal amnesia; agraphia.	Right handed with slight signs of left handedness (when arms folded, left on top); father left handed.
6	Skv.	Penetrating wound in right parieto-occipital area; left hemianopsia and slight left hemiparesis.	Severe visual agnosia lasting two weeks but disappearing altogether within six weeks.	Right handed; left eye dominant; when arms folded, left on top; sister left handed.
7	Čern.	Penetrating wound in the right parieto-temporo-occipital area with extrusion of brain substance and severe left hemiparesis; right side symptoms absent.	Difficulties in pronunciation and dysgraphia (difficulty in ordering letters when writing) lasting several weeks.	Right handed with a number of signs of left handedness (cuts bread with left hand); many left handers in the family.

Case No.	Name	Nature and localization of wound	Speech disturbance	Handedness
8	Tzynb.	Penetrating shrapnel wound in the right temporo-parietal area; slight left hemiparesis; right side symptoms absent.	Severe residual aphasia with difficulty in repeating words or phrases; loss of meanings of words; slight dysgraphia.	Right handed with slight signs of left handedness (nail of small finger of left hand larger; left eye dominant); father and brother left handed.
9	Les.	Penetrating shrapnel wound in the posterior part of the right parieto-temporal area with shell fragments deep in the right hemisphere; severe left hemiparesis with sensory disturbances; right side symptoms absent.	Severe disturbance of comprehension of logico-grammatical relations and disturbed spatial orientation.	Right handed; slight signs of left handedness (nail of left little finger larger; when arms folded left on top; left eye dominant); sister left handed.
10	Bor.	Penetrating shrapnel wound in the right frontal and parieto-temporal areas without hemiparesis; right side symptoms absent.	Mute for one month but comprehension intact; after a month residual signs of motor aphasia remained with disturbances of reading and writing.	Right handed with slight signs of left handedness (nail on small finger of left hand larger; when arms folded, left up); maternal uncle left handed.
11	Nur.	Penetrating shrapnel wound in posterior parts of right temporal area with slight left hemisyndrome. Right side signs absent.	Mute for two weeks following injury; after four months residual signs of aphasia and disturbance of writing.	Right handed with slight signs of left handedness (left fifth finger nail larger; when arms folded left on top; right eye dominant); mother left handed.
12	Matr.	Penetrating shrapnel wound in posterior parts of the right parieto-temporal area with fragments deep in the hemisphere; left hemisyndrome; reduced sensation and weakness on the left; right side signs absent.	Severe disturbances of speech and writing lasted for two weeks and then gradually disappeared.	Right handed with slight signs of left handedness (left eye dominant).

Finally, the ideas developed above offer an explanation of another fact – the fact that *severe and permanent aphasia seldom follows severe damage to the right hemisphere of left handed individuals*. Having followed through a number of cases not only of traumatic injury, but also of vascular and tumor lesions we have had the opportunity to witness a number of cases in which injury to the right hemisphere produced aphasia in left handers. Only in one extremely severe case of injury to the right hemisphere (perhaps involving the posterior commissural system) did we observe aphasia in a left handed person which lasted for months. Usually the aphasic syndrome appearing in such cases is less severe and less persistent than that seen following damage to comparable areas of the left hemisphere in right handed individuals. This finding can be explained by the fact that in very few cases the phenotypic left handers which we see are "pure" left handers. In contrast to the majority of right handers, most left handers are not from families in which the majority of other members share the same handedness trait. Thus we would be wrong should we expect the effects of right hemisphere injuries in left handers to be the same as the effects of left hemisphere injuries in right handers.

Our account would be incomplete were we not to mention one other essential feature which we consider more a topic for future study than an established fact. Experience shows that just as we have spoken of variation in the degree of dominance of the left hemisphere among members of the patient population, one can speak of *variation in the degree of lateralization of function,* or more precisely, of variation in the degree of dependence of function upon the dominant hemisphere. It is well known that such elementary functions as simple movement, elementary sensation, or sight are directly dependent upon the *contralateral* hemisphere and do not show any selective relationship whatsoever to the dominant hemisphere. In contrast to this, speech depends to a maximum degree upon the dominant hemisphere. Thus disturbances of a purely aphasic character following wounds in the right hemisphere in pure right handers is apparently never seen. Finally, such complex processes as verbal memory and skill occupy some kind of intermediate position as regards dependence upon the dominant hemisphere. This view is based upon the fact that agnostic and apraxic disturbances usually are seen in right handers following damage to the left (dominant) hemisphere. This appears to be so even though one occasionally finds in the literature a case in which injury of the right hemisphere of right handers has produced agnostic-apraxic disturbances.

The varying degree of lateralization of functions may account for a number of cases mentioned above in which injury of the left hemisphere of a right hander with slight signs of left handedness produced no persistent aphasic symptoms, but did produce gnostic disturbances or, as occurred more often, disturbances of complex motor coordination. The possibility that such dissociation of signs may result from the fact that some functions are more intimately related to the dominant hemisphere, while others can more easily be "transferred" to the subdominant, right hemisphere should be investigated further.

IV

TOPICAL SYNDROMES OF TRAUMATIC APHASIA GENERAL PRINCIPLES

So far we have considered questions regarding the pathogenesis of traumatic aphasia and recovery without taking into account the qualitative differences in symptomatology that depend upon what part of the speech area has been damaged. The following analysis will consider special features of the speech disturbances which accompany brain damage at various sites, i.e., the primary syndromes of traumatic aphasia which are associated with lesions of particular brain areas.

A. CONDITIONS UNDER WHICH TOPICAL ANALYSIS WAS CARRIED OUT

It is generally accepted that traumatic injuries, in contrast to vascular and tumor lesions of the brain, do not involve whole vascular beds in the cortex and thus have limited well-defined effects. As a result fire arm injuries constitute very useful material for the analysis of symptoms resulting from local cortical injury. This idea does not altogether hold up under careful examination. As we have already pointed out, the local destruction of brain tissues is accompanied in the initial period by edema, altered hemodynamics, and changes in the cerebrospinal fluid which produce considerably more extensive functional changes than one might expect on the basis of the firearm injury alone.[1]

Thus, during the initial period, whatever permanent losses of function there may be are accompanied by the temporary loss of other functions which are only blocked or inhibited. For this reason traumatic injuries offer real advantages for localization analysis only during the *residual* period.

Even then, however, the analysis of traumatic disorders is not always simple, since the cortical damage is not always well localized. In cases of penetrating wounds by shell fragments, by far the most common type observed during the last war, numerous bits of metal and bone splinters may be left in the brain tissues. These fragments not only produce considerable vascular damage, scar tissues and a source of infection, but quite often they lie far from their point of entry into the

[1] L. I. Smirnov, "Traumatic Brain Injuries", *Questions of Neurosurgery*, 1944; and *The Pathological Anatomy of Traumatic Injuries of the Nervous System* (Press of the Academy of Medical Sciences of the USSR, 1947) (in Russian).

skull. Thus to get a realistic impression of the extent of injury solely on the basis of the external site of damage to the skull can be very difficult. Often one finds extensive simple skull fractures accompanying otherwise highly localized injuries. Hemorrhage and contrecoup may affect other areas of the brain, even in the opposite hemisphere. Add to this complications involving meningoencephalitis, supuration, hydrocephalus, and especially scar formation with consequent distortion of the ventricles and it become clear, that even in the residual period penetrating wounds produced by shell fragments can retain a quite complex character.

Nonpenetrating wounds are more useful than penetrating wounds for localization analysis. They may involve bone damage, but the dura mater remains intact. Sometimes in such cases the inner plate of the skull is broken loose and presses into the dura mater, but it leaves no splinters. The epidural (and sometimes subdural) hematomas arising in these cases are usually relatively limited and leave local foci of softening. The absence of infection leaves this type of wound comparatively localized. To this group also belong *piercing bullet wounds*. Since bullets leave a relatively sterile track through the brain, they are complicated by infection less frequently than are shrapnel wounds. Finally this group includes certain *grazing penetration wounds* in which bone splinters do not penetrate far below the cortical surface and secondary injuries due to repercussion are not involved.

These three groups constitute the basic material for reliable localization analysis, although, even in these cases, scar formation and hydrocephalus may introduce important complications. On the basis of careful study of a large number of cases, however, it is possible to draw certain reliable conclusions regarding the roles of various cortical foci in the genesis of aphasic syndromes.

Analysis of the significance which one or another limited focus may have for the disturbance of a given cortical function depends upon one other condition without which any investigation of the localization of symptoms is futile. In addition to guaranteeing that the site of injury is well established, it is essential to have *a precise conception of the structure of that "function" which is lost as a result of injury and of the structure of the syndrome of functional disturbances* which we see in a given case of brain damage. And since the functions which are disturbed by cortical damage are usually complex functional systems, it is obvious that we must have a clear conception of the *structure of these functional systems* and be able to suggest the *psychological significance of the syndrome* produced by focal brain damage.

In the clinical investigation of functional losses following focal brain damage this important intermediate link is too often omitted and description of the signs observed (e.g. loss of expressive speech or of reading or writing abilities etc.) immediately follows description of the wound site. Such an approach has produced a misleading psycho-morphological conception of the "localization of function". It was justified in early stages of the development of neurology, but with our present state of knowledge of the central organization of mental processes and of the complex structure of functional systems of human activity it has long since become a hindrance to the development of a more accurate understanding of the pathology of complex nervous processes.

It is just such conceptions of the definite localization of "speech function" (or "writing function", or "reading function") in a fixed area of the cerebral cortex that fill the pages of hundreds of investigations related to aphasia. Only in certain of these – following the lead of K. Goldstejn – is the direct localization of complex *"functions"* replace by the localization of *symptoms*. Thus investigators have begun to speak of the localization of various forms of aphasia, alexia, or agraphia in limited cortical areas without going into an analysis of why damage to these areas produces disturbance of such complex functional systems. Such attempts at direct psycho-morphological correlations cannot produce a reliable understanding of the pathology involved.

All complex forms of mental activity, even such activities as observing objects or attending to sounds, are complex functional systems, complex processes based upon the combined activity of various afferent and efferent brain structures. The work of a number of authors shows that such systems develop in the course of ontogenesis. We have already mentioned that even such relatively simple processes as observing objects or attending to sounds are complex reflex acts; they are accomplished by whole functional systems developed in ontogenesis and resting upon a complex "dynamic system" of simultaneously operating areas of the brain cortex. In view of these findings "functions" can no longer be "localized" in isolated areas of the cerebral cortex. This applies in particular to the study of speech processes.

Speech activity, which develops with the mastery of a language in a social setting, must rest upon a dynamic system of the greatest complexity involving the simultaneous functioning of various brain areas. Thus the problem of the neurologist who wishes to study the brain mechanisms of speech processes, must, as we have mentioned above, determine how these complex functional systems derive from the dynamic structure of the cortex and understand the role of each area in these functional systems; but he must not "localize" these highly complex "functions" in separate isolated areas of the brain.

It is easy to see the extent to which this systemic conception of the highly complex forms of nervour activity in man conflict with the mechanistic type of search for "speech centers", "writing centers", or "reading centers". References to such centers give the appearance of scientific explanation, but actually conceal the path to further analysis of underlying mechanisms.

That is why, rather than approach, immediately the actual cortical basis of speech activity, it is necessary to consider the structure of speech processes. This we do on the assumption that only a serious analysis of the functional formations which are lost as the result of brain injuries, an analysis which takes into account contemporary knowledge of the structure and function of cerebral systems, can assure the success of investigations intended to determine the cerebral mechanisms of these disturbances.

We shall consider first the psychological structure of speech activity and then take up the question of just what physiological conditions are necessary for the performance of the speech processes which are disturbed by damage to various areas of the brain. Such an approach should led us to a full analysis of the topical syndromes of traumatic aphasia.

B. THE STRUCTURE OF SPEECH ACTIVITY

Before one can properly investigate the nervous mechanisms underlying speech processes it is necessary to consider speech functions from the point of view of psychology. There was a time when speech was looked upon as the association of images with the conditioned sounds which represent them and the articulatory movements by which they are spoken. According to this conception the mechanisms of speech were thought to lie in the interaction of an idea center (this was sometimes referred to as the "conceptual center" and localized in the parietal area of the cortex), the sound-image center (supposed to lie in the left temporal lobe), and the articulation center (thought to lie in the third gyrus of the left frontal lobe). In any textbook of neurology printed at the end of the last century one can find diagrams of this type. They were based on the work of Kussmaul, Charcot, and others and have survived to the present day without significant changes.

Both the history of language and the psychology of speech, however, suggest that the processes underlying speech activity are considerably more complex than such diagrams would indicate. These simplified schemes must be considerably modified if they are to be made more realistic. The changes required involve equally the inner, cognitive aspect of speech and the more external, expressive aspect.

The idea that various words represent the images of different objects and that speech consists of the associations between such images is an attractive one. There is every reason to believe that speech originated in productive activity and arose first in the form of abbreviated motions which represented certain work activities and pointing gestures by which men communicated with one another. The pointing gesture certainly represented separate objects or actions. But the meaning of the gesture was understandable only in terms of knowledge of the concrete situation in which it was produced; outside a given situation such a gesture had no meaning. Only considerably later, as shown by speech paleontology, did verbal speech develop. Only in the course of a very long historical period was the disassociation of sound and gesture accomplished. During this process a complex verbal code developed by which it was possible not only to represent separate objects, but to abstract action and quality, to categorize objects, to represent their most complex relationships and transmit whole systems of knowledge.

Perhaps the most essential development, occurring during this period which covered many thousands of years was the change in the relation between the verbal *code* and the extraverbal practical *context* to which it relates. We have every reason to believe that in the early stages of language development, the verbalizations which accompanied gestures were by no means so independent as in present day speech. In the beginning they received their significance only from the practical situation in which they were uttered. Also we have reason to believe that in the early stages speech consisted of isolated sound complexes which had very general designative and directive meanings. Investigations of the paleontology of language indicate that, in all likelihood such sound complexes did not have fixed or permanent meanings, but that the meaning arose out of the concrete practical situation.

Even at the first stage of language development, then, it is possible to distinguish two aspects of speech which subsequently constituted the psychological basis of all speech processes: the *nominative* aspect which reduces to the designation of a definite object or concept, and the *predicative* aspect, which consists in the fact that a given designative word or phrase communicates some idea, relates to some concrete activity, and assumes the corresponding meaning. Whereas the first, nominative, aspect of speech was expresed at an early stage by certain very general sounds, which in time came to constitute the first speech *code,* the second, predicative, aspect was generally not expressed and could be obtained only by reference to the concrete "*sympractical context*", i.e., that situation in which the word was uttered. Thus one and the same word used in various situations could take on completely different practical meanings.

The further development of language followed the basic process which we have briefly mentioned. With the development of more complicated forms of collective, productive activity and increasingly complex forms of communication, speech activity became more and more isolated from immediate activities. It came to be a more *independent activity* which man used to abstract the essential cues from the environment, to systematize his experiences, and to communicate them to others. In this way verbal speech turned more and more into a complex system of *phonetic, lexical, and semantic codes* capable of reflecting the most intricate phenomena even in the absence of a concrete practical context. The *sympractical context* which originally constituted an organic constituent of speech became less and less important. This process by which speech was transformed into a new *second signalling system of activity*, social in origin, and bearing the character of a complex code, was fundamental to the historical development of language.

As far as one can judge on the basis of present knowledge of linguistics the further development of language involved two basic changes, each of which contributed a certain improvement to the psychology of the speech process. The first was the development of fixed words which assumed more and more precise meanings and came to reflect deeper and deeper relationships among different phenomena. Words with concrete meanings began to be substituted for diffuse sound complexes. Words came to signify definite attributes and, later, objects or activities. The earlier simple pointing gesture which was incomprehensible out of environmental context gave way to the meaningful elements of a complex system of codes.

The meaning of an element was by no means limited to a single object, however. Linguists from Humboldt to Potebnja, de Saussure and Sapir showed that the meaning of an element involves a certain kind of *generalization*. In the beginning it only singled out an attribute which was common to a number of things. Then it sharpened this attribute and came to relate only to a single category of things. Still later, as prefixes and suffixes accrued to the root of a word, it became the center of an independent system. Each prefix and sufix designated a certain system of relations or a certain class to which the concept represented by the word belonged. In this way the word was worked into a whole system of generalizations. Such linguists as Humboldt and Potebnja have suggested that it is a result of this that man not only reflects the world around him, but also systematizes it.[2]

Thus the entire history of words in human speech has consisted of the development of constantly more refined means of *generalization*. In modern laguage the roots of words are not so much based upon images as upon *concepts or generalizations regarding those things which are represented by words*. In the termoinology of I. P. Pavlov, the second signalling system always possesses two specific features: "abstraction and, at the same time, generalization of innumerable signals". This is a function peculiar to man. Thus in analyzing the sense structure of a word, one must not forget that the word itself represents an abbreviated sum product of the complex activity of man as a social animal. This product is derived from abstraction and generalization and from the specific language codes of a given social system.

The second important aspect of language development was the appearance of means not only for the representation of images or concepts in words, but also for the representation of whole *statements* or thoughts. This we may designate the *predicative* aspect of speech.

The isolated words of which verbal speech consisted in its earliest stages of development were capable of reflecting separate signs or primitive concepts, but they could not express even elementary thoughts. The meaning of a word shifted depending upon the situation and was nonexistent outside certain situations. Whereas words possessed a nominative function from the beginning, the predicative function derived only from the concrete setting in which they were uttered. A

[2] In more recent times the idea of the role of the word in systematizing phenomena of the external world has been emphasized in the works of L. S. Vygotskij (1934, 1956), and J. Bruner (1957).

decisive change occurred when speech went from consisting of individual words to consisting of elementary grammatical sentences, when instead of a single word there arose *a pair or group of words related to one another,* i.e., when the first "syntax" appeared.

The revolution which occurred at this phase in the development of language was truly phenomenal. At the beginning syntax was very primitive and did not go beyond the simple combining of words. But later it was elaborated and came to involve a number of supplementary linguistic principles.[3] Thus verbal speech became capable not only of designating an object, but also of formulating a thought. Verbal speech was still bound up with other forms of expression such as gesture and intonation, but with the development of written language thought came to be expressed altogether by means of language and speech became fully capable of performing the predicative function. Speech became an independent system of codes.

This concept of speech structure naturally renders inadequate the classical ideas regarding basic forms of speech activity and the corresponding conceptions of cerebral localization of speech processes. The fundamental forms of speech defect can not of course be reduced to disturbances of the speech images of words or to the inability to pronounce words. The basic forms of speech disturbance must result from defects in the systems of connections which are concealed behind the word on the one hand and in disintegration of the predicative function of speech on the other. The whole sense of verbal statements resides in this function. Similarly, the cerebral mechanisms which underlie speech processes cannot be attributed to cortical structures which store memory images nor to their associations with "centers of auditory speech" or "centers of articulatory movements".

We are still very far from being able to describe the "functional systems" of excited cortical foci which is the neurophysiological basis of the second signalling system. In seeking the cerebral basis of speech activity we can attempt only the first steps toward an understanding of the cortical structures which permit the analysis and synthesis of external signals by means of language. We are now only beginning to comprehend the function underlying discriminative perception of the significant attributes of things and their systematization into complex systems of generalization.

In order to understand the cerebral basis of speech we must discover the functional organization of cortical processes which allows the codes of language to be used both for the differentiation of significant cues and for the synthesis which makes it possible to take whole categories of cues into consideration at

[3] The history of language as a means of expressing complex interrelations has been especially carefully analyzed for the Japhetic and Paleoasiatic languages by Marr and Meščaninov and for the Russian language by Buslaev and Potebnja. Studies of the Indo-European languages from the point of view of comparative linguistics have been carried out by a large number of authors.

once. These are the functions a person must possess if he is to master the complex nominative aspect of speech.

On the other hand, the predicative aspect of speech is intimately related to the basic motives which direct the activity of the individual. It is tied up with his intentions, with thought. Since a sentence is the manifestation of a thought we cannot restrict ourselves to what was described above. We must seek the other component of these mechanisms in the cortical structures which give rise to unified purposeful activity, i.e., to the storage of a task and conditions which make it possible to turn a long involved statement into an abbreviated pattern of speech which is then transformed into a thought; we must find out how this condensed thought pattern can be reexpanded into a smooth sequential statement (Pick, 1913).

In short, we must understand the mechanism of that shortened *inner speech* which is predicative in function but not sequentially patterned. As L. S. Vygotskij (1934) showed, this mechanism is responsible for the transformation of thoughts into expanded statements and transformation of statements into unitary thoughts. Only a careful analysis of this *dynamic* aspect of speech will permit an understanding of the physiological mechanisms of sequentially structured statements, i.e., an understanding of what Jackson referred to as "propositionizing" and which he considered the fundamental characteristic of active speech.

All of the ideas introduced above concern the organization of the *internal semantic aspect of speech.* During its development the external or vocal structure of speech underwent the same profound changes as internal speech did. In the early history of language development primitive speech sounds only indicated objects which were present at the time they were uttered. They did not represent objects in precise symbols which remained constant from situation to situation. The structure of speech sounds was not differentiated. All that is known about the paleontology of the phonetic aspect of speech forces us to conclude that the initial sound complexes were very diffuse in nature. Certain traces of this stage of development persist in the most primitive languages alive today. Perhaps the closest analogy to such a diffuse organization of vocal speech is to be seen in the primitive sounds which are used in many cultures to express regret, to call domestic animals, etc.

The primitive "prephonemic" stage in the development of the phasic aspect of speech must have given way long ago to the radically different "phonemic" or differentiative stage. When words came to represent different attributes and refer to permanent objects they had to be based upon a definite language code of phonemes – on a system of differentiable sounds. Certain features of sounds were selected out which, in terms of the phonetic code, were to assume a special "signal character". By making these features constant for a given word it attained a constant structure which was not altered by changes in timbre, intensity, or rate of pronunciation. This made it possible to designate a large number of concepts by different combinations of a relatively small number of sounds. Each language came to have its *own special phonemic system*, i.e., its own system of verbal cues which played a leading role in the differentiation of meaning and made possible sound complexes which constituted unchanging, meaningful words.

The history and systematization of this phonemic organization of speech was developed for the first time in the Russian school of phonetics by Baudouin de Courtenay, Trubetzkoy, Ščerba, and R. Jakobson. Later, it was taken up by Sapir, Saussure, and a number of other outstanding linguists. These authors showed that the auditory aspect of speech represents more than the precise acoustic discrimination of sounds. Its essential characteristic is the selection of essential features from the inessential features of speech. Thus it allows the generalization of different sounds into one "phonetic" group and discrimination among sounds which are similar but related to different groups of phonemes. It is this generalized structuring aspect of auditory activity and not in the acuity of hearing that distinguishes the discriminative hearing of man from the non-phonemic hearing of animals.

Phonetic hearing reaches its ultimate in the reading of written speech, for here the most diverse sounds may be represented by a single letter. For instance the letter "d" is the same in different sounding words: "dom" (house), "duma" (thought), "den' " (day), "dikij" (wild); whereas quite similar sounds which are related to different semantic groups may be represented by different letters: "den' " (day) and "ten' " (shadow), or "zub" (tooth) and "sup" (soup).

The phonemic structure of a word is preserved even when it undergoes complex grammatical differentiation. The more involved the complex of sounds constituting a word becomes, the greater the rigidity the phonemes must possess if its meaning is to remain constant.

It is important to note that the phonemic organization of auditory speech presupposes the elaboration of definite *schemata* not only in the *auditory perception* of man, but also in his *articulatory activity*. Physiologically this is a *product of the activity of auditory-articulatory structures.*

Whereas preservation of the constancy of sounds was not necessary in the primitive clicking sounds which expressed a certain affective state or drew attention to some particular object, the change to discriminative representational speech gave the constancy of sounds a decisive significance. A word expressed in a given phonemic code has to remain the same no matter what the timbre, intensity, or rate with which it is spoken. In a complex word this constancy must be maintained no matter what sounds surround a given phoneme. Otherwise the word cannot preserve a specific meaning under diverse circumstances.

This all means that being exposed to a given fully developed language the individual must develop the system of *fine articulatory differentiations* which are necessary for the pronunciation of various discriminable sounds. This coded system of articulatory differentiations must be so generalized and flexible that a given complex of articulatory signs may remain constant under highly diverse conditions of pronunciation. The generalized schemata of articulations which are distinguishable on the basis of fixed phonemic signs could be called *"articulemes"*. These articulemes or differentiated sounds are similar in pronunciation but related to different systems of the language code (for instance lingual-palatal "d", "l", and "n"). They are responsible for the constancy of the meanings of words.

Thus in the organization of the expressive, phasic aspect of speech one discovers the same principle seen in its semantic organization. Here again the basic units of speech are not the isolated verbal elements or the habitual articulatory complexes, but whole *functional systems* which involve the auditory-articulatory structures. They create the systems of sound codes possessing the fixed group of fundamental signs that preserve the constancy of words spoken and heard under variable conditions.

It is altogether understandable that both the disturbance of the vocal aspect of speech and its cerebral localization must be thought of in terms different from those current in classical neurology.

The origin of the impairment of the phasic aspect of speech must be sought in the *disturbance of structures which carry out the combined functions of the auditory-articulatory systems*, i.e. which make possible the complex verbal differentiations necessary for the mastery of the sound code of a language. Receptive speech disturbances result not from the disappearance of individual word images, but from the *disintegration of structured hearing*. This disintegration makes it impossible to separate and retain the sound features which are essential for semantic discrimination. Underlying the disturbance of expressive, articulatory speech is the *destruction of those articulatory* differentiations which are necessary for mastery of the verbal code of the language.

All of the cortical structures necessary for the production of phasic speech constitute a complex system of cerebral zones which permit the development of the auditory-articulatory differentiations necessary for mastery of the phonemic code of language. In attempting to better understand the cerebral mechanisms underlying the external organization of speech sounds it becomes necessary for us not to distinguish various "centers" which would presumably act as depots for individual images, but to specify the systemic mechanisms which would provide for the combined function of separate cortical zones and would make possible the types of analysis and synthesis which are demanded by the complex system of language. This demand holds both for the receptive and expressive aspects of speech and guides our search for the cerebral mechanisms underlying speech activity.

C. THE STRUCTURE OF CORTICAL SYSTEMS

Physiologists have long been aware of the fact that complex forms of behavior must involve the combined activity of numerous *functional systems* which are related to structures widely distributed in the brain. P. K. Anokhin refers to a functional system as the "sum total of all neural excitations resulting in the correct execution of a given act". Analysis of such systems has shown that they are never localized in a single cortical "center", but rather that they require the joint participation of afferent and efferent processes which often involve structures at many levels of the brain and in different parts of the cortex. Together the processes constitute a single, complex, and labile unit of activity.

It was pointed out by Pavlov that even the so called "respiratory center" cannot be conceived of as some kind of circumscribed area in the medulla. This "center" involves a whole group or, to use the expression adopted by A. A. Uxtomskij, a whole "constellation" of neural structures which are sometimes located quite far from one another. If this morphological representation is true of so simple a function as respiration, then it must be even more characteristic of the higher forms of mental activity. The higher psychological functions must be generated by complex functional aggregates of zones which are joined together by temporary connections.

Physiologists (Anokhin, 1935, 1939, 1940, 1942) as well as psychologists (Vygotski, 1934, 1956, 1960), have recognized that the components of a given functional system may change in different stages of its development or as the result of pathological conditions. Thus if we wish to discover the morphological substrate of a complex functional system we must accept from the outset that we are not looking for an isolated "center" fixed once and for all, but that we seek a pattern of neural structures which operate jointly to produce the complex activity in question. It goes without saying that the study of speech activity must be based upon this principle.

The cortical structures which make speech activity possible arose in the course of evolution. It was the birth of language, on the other hand, which brought to life the particular system of simultaneously functioning areas which gives rise to speech. It is important to note that whereas the systems of speech zones appeared in the course of historical development, such systems were based upon cortical structures which had already been provided by previous evolution.

Our task is to present in a nutshell the basic principles of the cortical organization of functional systems. Anatomists interested in brain function long ago rejected nineteenth century conceptions according to which the cortex is composed of isolated cell groups, each of which constitutes the "depot" for a certain type of image or the cortical "center" of a certain faculty. Such conceptions were widely held and reflected the psychology of "faculties" which was current during the second half of the last century. Theory held that all mental experience is derived from the interaction of various faculties. They are represented today only by a few authors such as C. and O. Vogt and K. Kleist. The latter is known for his functional maps of the cerebral cortex in which quite complex psychological functions are attributed to the various cortical areas.

At one time such psychomorphological conceptions played a progressive role in the development of speech physiology, since they drew attention to the cerebral substrate of mental processes. But it is understandable that they should eventualle come into conflict with more advanced knowledge in psychology and physiology. Since they did not point the way to genuine analysis of the cerebral mechanisms of complex functional systems, they became real hindrances to the development of science.

We are still far from a complete scientifically based theory of the functional organization of the human cerebral cortex. We can only refer to some of the findings which have been made during the past half century and which appear to bring us closer to an understanding of the functional organization of the cerebral cortex. These findings can provide the outlines for an adequate theory.

The basic conception which has superceded the principle of narrow localization of complex processes is that of the *dynamic localization of functional systems in the cerebral cortex.* According to this principle, complex functions are not "localized" in particular cortical areas. Instead, their physiological mechanisms are *dynamically dispersed in the cerebral cortex creating systems of zones; each zone plays its own role in the performance of the whole system.* The constellations of zones which work together constitute that "functional mosaic" of the cerebral cortex which was central to Pavlov's theory and which to him represented the dynamic substrate for the most complex cortical functions.

In summing up his many years of work, I. P. Pavlov suggested that the entire cerebral cortex may be conceived of as a central juncture of the separate *analyzers.* He believed that in the cortex signals from the environment are received and subjected to the finest analysis and most complex synthesis. This view coincides with the idea set forth by a number of authors that phylogenetically the brain was superimposed upon the system of distance receptors and became responsible for coordinated function of the different modalities. This principle has found a firm acceptance in the modern literature and has been supported by numerous investigations.

Another widely held principle is that of the *specific (somatotopic or segmental) projection of the peripheral parts of the analyzers to different parts of the cerebral cortex.* Whereas structures of the reticular formation provide diffuse changes in tonus of the whole cortex by a system of nonspecific projections (Magoun et al, 1956; Moruzzi, Jasper, 1949 and others),[4] the receptor systems

[4] A detailed review of the anatomy and physiology of the reticular formation has been published by Rossi and Zanghetti (1957).

are represented by discrete bundles of fibers which carry specific impulses to limited areas of the cerebral cortex. These areas have been well established on the basis of numerous anatomical and physiological investigations. They constitute the "projection areas" of the cerebral cortex or, as Pavlov preferred to call them, the "cortical nuclei of the analyzers".

It is known that the projection area for skin sensation lies in the postcentral gyrus, the area for auditory sensation in Heschl's gyrus, and that for visual sensation along the calcarine fissure of the occipital lobe. It is further well known that in these areas the predominant layer is the fourth or receptive cell layer.

The fact that direct electrical stimulation of the projection areas produces sensations corresponding to the different modalities supports the principle of somatotopic projection from the peripheral receptors. Stimulation of the sensory cortex for instance, produces focal cutaneous sensation (Foerster, Penfield); stimulation along the calcarine fissure and in Heschl's gyrus produce visual and auditory sensations respectively (Pötzl, Hoff, Penfield, Boldrey).

Finally, damage to these areas produces modality-specific loses of sensation. This again illustrated the principle of somatotopic or point-to-point representation of the peripheral receptors in the cortical parts of the various analyzers.

It has been found by a number of investigators that the somatotopic projection has a functional aspect in that the size of the projection area of a given organ depends upon its function. This finding by no means contradicts the principle of somatotopic projection; it simply indicates that the representation of the more important receptor areas must be more specific than that of less important areas. This point is illustrated by Adrian's (1943) discovery of the disproportionately large representations of the snout in pigs and of the lips in sheep, it is further shown by Penfield's famous finding that in man projections from the thumb, forefinger, pharynx, and lips are extremely large.

The principle of specific (somatotopic) projection concerns only the first step in the handling of information which enters the cortex from the peripheral receptors. The second step involves the breakdown of information into thousands of units (corresponding to individual cells of the fourth cortical layer). As a result, it can be restructured in any form. Such a breakdown of incoming information is a necessary step for further synthesis.

Another principle, and one closely related to the specific projection principle, is the *functional organization of information* received by the fourth layer. This *arises through reciprocal adaptation of zones which function conjointly*. It would be extremely unusual for one analyzer to function without involving other systems. As a rule responses to signals from the environment are brought about by the *joint activity of a complex of analyzers*. Even in Sečenov's time it was shown that such a simple function as vision involves coordinated functions of the retina and extra-ocular musculature. Listening, likewise, involves motor as well as auditory activity. Recent work by E. N. Sokolov (1958) has shown that the orienting reflex evoked by the stimulation of any receptor involves a whole system of reactions throughout the body. The fact that every receptor possesses its own proprio-muscular system (Granit, 1956; Kvassov, 1958) is a special instance of this principle. One sees combined functions of many analyzers to an even greater degree in the adaptive behavior of animals and in the complex manipulatory activity of man.

Recent psychological investigations (A. N. Leont'ev, 1958; A. V. Zaporožec, 1959; P. Ja. Gal'perin, 1956, 1957) indicate that the perception of an object, and especially the formation of an image, results from a combination of visual, tactile, and muscular sensations. Initially perception involves comprehensive manipulatory activity; only later does it become abbreviated. This is why the coordinated activity of a group of analyzers (including especially the motor analyzer) is necessary for the formation of any image. This is probably most true of activity involving the second signalling system where analysis and synthesis so often involve several receptors. Thus we see why the coordination of functions of the various analyzers which a child develops in the second half of his first year is so critical for his further mental development. We also see that the combined function of different cerebral areas constitutes one of the most important principles of cerebral activity.

With the work of Flechsig it became accepted that one can differentiate between the primary projection areas, on the one hand, and secondary (projection-association) areas, and tertiary (association) areas on the other. The latter two groups both mature later than the primary projection areas, i.e., myelinization occurs there later. Further, architectonic studies distinguish these areas on the basis of greater development of the superficial "associative" layers. Thus a number of authors have pointed out that they possess all the characteristics necessary for integrating and coordinating the functions of the modality specific areas of the cerebral cortex.

Our knowledge of the secondary and tertiary (association) cortical areas has undergone some fundamental changes in the last few years. Precise histological investigations have shown that the "secondary" and especially the "tertiary" zones cannot possibly be considered purely associative. A number of works have shown that they receive fibers from subcortical structures, just as the primary areas do (Papez, 1944; Poljakov, 1957, 1962 et al.). Also it has been found that they possess the same kinds of cortifugal fibers as the primary projection areas. Pursuing these studies in greater detail, Rose (1950) found that the fibers ascending to the visual association areas do not enter directly from the peripheral receptors nor from the same nuclei of the lateral geniculate which project to the primary visual cortex. Instead, they arise primarily from lateral geniculate nuclei which receive input from other nuclei in the lateral geniculate or from higher structures which transmit impulses of information already integrated in more central areas. Thus Rose suggests calling the fibers entering the primary projection areas "extrinsic" and fibers directed toward the secondary and tertiary zones "intrinsic"; in like manner he speaks of the primary projection areas as "extrinsic areas" and of the secondary and tertiary areas as "intrinsic areas" (Rose, 1950; Pribram, 1958).

Generally speaking, the secondary and tertiary zones of the cerebral cortex appear late in phylogenesis and provide for the most complex forms of integrated function involving different analyzers. Some authors conceive of them as *areas of overlap between the cortical parts of the various analyzers* (Polyakov, 1957). According to this view the intermediate zones were rather poorly developed in early phylogenetic stages and interaction of analyzers was accomplished by the partial superposition of the projection zones. In later stages of phylogenesis the cortical nuclei of the various analyzers became more differentiated. They spread apart, and the intermediate zones formed between them. In the intermediate zones cells from the "scattered periphery" of the analyzers came into contact with cells receiving impulses from fibers of the intrinsic areas. The intrinsic areas participate in the formation of complex labile connections between the analyzers at the subcortical level.

Numerous well known investigations have demonstrated the morphological and functional differences in the two types of intermediate area in man. Whereas the parts lying nearer the primary projection areas possess a structure similar to that of the primary areas, those parts lying further away have a quite different structure. Thus the secondary visual areas 18 and 19, the secondary auditory areas 42 and 22, and the secondary sensory areas 1, 2, (and perhaps 5), are more similar in structure to the primary visual, auditory and sensory areas than are areas 39 and 40 in the parieto-temporo-occipital area or areas 9, 10, 11, and 46 of the frontal lobes. In these latter parts of the intermediate zones the more superficial associative layers of the cortex clearly predominate.

In accordance with the morphological differences between these two groups of areas (the primary areas constituting one group and the combined secondary and tertiary areas making up the other), their functional characteristics are also quite different. Functional differences were noted in the neuronographic studies of Dusser de Barennes (1937, 1941), McCulloch (1941, 1944) and others. They found that when strychnine is applied to a small part of a primary area, e.g. area 17 in the occipital cortex, the spread of excitation is very limited, whereas strychnine applied to a secondary area, e.g. area 18 or 19, leads to changes of potential in a number of structures including the cortical parts of other analyzers.

The same basic principle emerges from more complex studies in which responses of the organism are taken as indicators of function. In experiments where the cortex is stimulated directly, the sensations resulting from stimulation of the primary areas are different from those produced by stimulation of the secondary areas. Stimulation of area 17 (primary visual area), for instance, produces phosphene, a purely visual sensation. On the other hand, stimulation of secondary areas 18 or 19 produces both a visual sensation and the sensations which ordinarily accompany eye movements. Penfield has shown that whereas stimulation of the primary auditory area produces only specific auditory sensations, stimulation of the secondary areas, often leads to complex auditory sensations and acoustico-visual hallucinations. Later we shall consider the results of direct stimulation of the secondary motor areas.

Stimulation of the secondary projection areas of a given analyzer actually brings it into joint function with the other analyzers. It revives traces of the complex temporary connections which have developed as a result of previous integrated activity among the various analyzers. Some authors, e.g. K. Pribram (1957, 1958) suggest that the role of the secondary areas is to program the function of the primary areas on the basis of past experience.

Results altogether consistent with the above are obrained when one observes what occurs following *damage* to the primary and secondary projection areas of the different analyzers. It is well known that total lesions of the primary visual area produce scotoma or total central blindness and that partial damage produces a particular form of "visual asthenia". Lesions of the secondary areas, on the other hand, produce complex impairments of visual synthesis together with abnormal eye movements. It may also lead to various forms of visual agnosia or amnesia, depending upon the degree to which it involves cortical zones of the tactile and auditory analyzers. Later we shall consider analogous auditory and motor disturbances.

We are still far from an adequate physiological explanation of these findings. Yet it is clear that damage to the secondary zones of an analyzer, produces critical disturbances of the systemic forms of acquired activity which develop in the course of ontogenesis. Injury disrupts its integrated functions with other analyzers and destroys the programs stored as the result of previous experience. A brain in which these systems have been disrupted can no longer select out essential signal attributes, inhibit irrelevant attendant impulses, and integrate signal cues into definite systems. In other words, it is unable to carry out the coordination of functions that is necessary for the selective formation of connections and for all forms of adaptation to reality. It is on the basis of this kind of defect that we have come to consider the integrated activity of cortial parts of the various analyzers a basic principle of functional organization of the brain. The integrated activity of these cortical areas is responsible for programming the function of any given analyzer in accordance with temporary connections laid down in past experience.

It remains for us to say something of a *third principle,* an extension of what we have already said. We indicated that the time has passed when mental processes could be considered separate "faculties" or "functions" of "mind". It is now clear that even the highest forms of mental process should be thought of as the *product of complex reflex activity* which possesses both afferent and efferent links. Even such processes as the elicitation of sensory *images* have turned out to be the results of complex human *actions* which were at one time exteriorized as grasping and feeling. In the course of ontogenesis these actions gave way to the examination of objects with the eyes, (an abbreviated form of external activity), and finally to an "image' which although internalized, preserves its motor components and is inseparably related to its verbal denominator.[5]

The adoption of such a conception of mental processes must inevitably introduce significant corrections into previously held conceptions of the cerebral localization of function. As we mentioned earlier, the traditional conceptions of cortical "centers" in which groups of cells possess certain "mental faculties" must give way to the conception of *complex cortical reflex systems,* which carry out the physiological processes underlying complex forms of mental activity.

Modern work in neuronal archintechtonics and neurophysiology give good supporting evidence for the latter conception. The cerebral cortex with its six cell layers can be considered a highly complex reflex organ for two reasons. First we know that each cortical area has fibers entering it and fibers leaving it. Secondly, we know that reflex processes occur in each area. This includes the cortical areas which are parts of the various analyzers where such processes serve to "tune" the analyzers. Corticofugal impulses tune the analyzers by facilitating excitation of certain receptor areas and inhibiting others. It is known that the tuning reflexes may be mediated at different levels. Sometimes they do not involve structures above the medulla or diencephalon; other times they involve a cortical link.

The functions of the cortex are not, however, restricted to this type of reflex processes. They must also include considerably more complex reflex processes in which al parts of the cortex function together. Under certain circumstances it is possible to analyze the behavior of an animal or man into separate partial reflex processes, but *behavior can never be reduced to such processes.* The behavior of a man, like that of an animal, is initiated by the stimulation of afferent systems and always terminates with definite *integrated adaptive reactions of the voluntary musculature.* Any function of the great hemispheres can be broken down into two coordinated systems of activity: one related to the posterior (extero- or proprioceptive) regions and the other to the anterior (motor) regions of the hemispheres.

This is probably seen most clearly in the structure of the sensory-motor areas of the cortex which, according to Penfield (1954) and a number of other authors, constitutes a functional unit. The fact that the posterior-afferent areas are intimately connected with the anterior-effector areas is demonstrated by the fact that stimulation of the areas posterior to the Rolandic fissure can evoke the same movements as are produced by stimulation of the precentral gyrus (Penfield and Boldrey, 1937; Penfield and Rasmussen, 1950). These connections plus the important

[5] The origin of images has been treated in Soviet psychological literature in the works of A. N. Leont'ev (1958), A. V. Zaporožec (1958), and P. Ja. Gal'perin (1956, 1957).

connections of various cortical areas with the subcortical systems are primarily responsible for the integration of cortical functions.

The functional unity of the sensory-motor areas is only one example of the integration of posterior and anterior cortical areas. A second example is the integrated function of a part of the left temporal lobe (Wernicke's area) with the inferoposterior part of the frontal lobe (Broca's area). These areas are united by large U-shaped bundles and are together responsible for audio-articulatory analysis. A third example is the integrated activity of the posterior and anterior oculo-motor centers which are responsible for the fine control of eye movements. Later we shall consider these examples in more detail.

Even these complex acts do not fully explain human behavior, however. As psychologists are well aware, human behavior involves striving to reach goals within a given environmental context. The environment imposes certain *conditions*, and human behavior involves analysis of the conditions and selection of the most appropriate paths by which goals may be reached. In short, it involves complex *analytic-synthetic activity* directed toward the solving of definite problems. Successful actions *are reinforced* thus giving rise to the concept of *back afferentation* or feedback. Through feedback successful actions are separated from all the rest. They become dominant, while irrelevant actions are simultaneously inhibited. On the basis of past experience stored in the form of visual images or verbal associations man orients to problems, creates schemata of possible solutions, – and submits his behavior to them. Of course the various analyzers do not remain autonomous but function continuously in accordance with the overall system of complex structured behavior.

How, in fact, are complex forms of activity carried out? What is the functional organization of neurophysiological mechanisms underlying such activity? We are only beginning to accumulate the scientific knowledge necessary to answer this question. All that we can do is to discuss some of the ideas which have grown out of evidence gathered in the past few years.

The findings of many authors, among them Pribram (1957, 1958) suggest that there are several functional systems in the cortex. Each system is responsible for a certain aspect of complex behavior. One of these systems involves structures in the ventromedial surface of the brain. These areas are projections from nonspecific structures of the midbrain and diencephalon and apparently determine the general dispositions which direct the behavior of animals.

This sytem is distinguished from the dorsolateral surface of the cortex which can be divided into extrinsic and intrinsic parts. It is a highly specialized system which takes part in the central integration of *analytic-synthetic activity*. Thus it is involved in the discrimination of signals and the development of differential responses which are carried out by the various analyzers. We have already spoken of this kind of activity.

There remains one other system which participates in complex forms of activity and which deserves special consideration. According to all indications it is intimately related to functions of the motor analyzer and plays a special role with regard to mental activity.

It is apparent that the effectiveness of any activity is related to the degree to which the traces of successful actions are strengthened and traces of unsuccessful actions inhibited. In other words a major role in the *formulation* of behavior is played by the *feedback* which results from motor action. Feedback makes possible *evaluation* of the effectiveness of an action. It is also necessary for the creation of an image of expected effects and for generating the anticipatory afferentation which directs further behavior. Various authors refer to the function of this system in different terms. Pribram speaks of it as the "economic" aspect of behavior (economic function, utility function, preference behavior); Anokhin (1957) speaks of "acceptor of action". All authors, however, are inclined to relate this highly complex behavioral function to the feedback which arises as the result of a motor act, which signals the completion of the act, and makes possible the regulation of appropriate behavior once it is completed.

We know very little to date regarding the brain mechanisms of the most complex forms of human behavior, the forms of voluntary behavior are regulated by speech and speech-related mechanisms. Only in recent years the psychological development and maturation of these forms of behavior have begun to be investigated.[6] Yet we have every reason to believe that Jackson was correct when he suggested that the cerebral mechanisms of behavior organized at the highest levels are related to the frontal areas of the brain. Not only are the frontal lobes phylogenetically new structures, but in man they undoubtedly play a role in the feedback from systems of connections established by verbal mechanisms and are involved in the regulation of motor processes by the second signalling system. This position, which has been given special attention in our other works (see N. A. Filippyčeva, 1952; A. I. Meščerjakov, 1953; M. P. Ivanova, 1953; Luria, 1962, 1963; Luria and Homskaya, 1966; and others) will be considered further in a later section.

We have presented the principles underlying the relationship between structure and function of the cerebral cortex, i.e. the dynamic systemic distribution of functional systems in the cerebral cortex. These we must keep in mind when we begin to analyze the disturbances of speech activity which result from focal lesions of the brain.

Before proceeding to the discussion of specific forms of disturbance, however, we should take up two other questions. First we should consider the systemic character of disturbances produced by focal lesions; then we should discuss the neurodynamic analysis of symptoms arising in different cases.

[6] We have studied the development of complex forms of voluntary behavior in a number of special investigations most of which are reported in *Problems of Higher Nervous Activity in Normal and Abnormal Children* (Press of the Academy of Pedagogical Sciences, Moscow, Vol. 1, 1956; Vol. 2, 1958). See also A. R. Luria (1959, 1961).

D. PROBLEMS OF CLINICAL ANALYSIS AND THE SYSTEMIC CHARACTER OF DISTURBANCES RESULTING FROM FOCAL LESIONS OF THE BRAIN

No form of mental activity can be thought of as a "function" localized to a limited group of nerve cells. Any form of mental activity, especially speech, is a complex functional system of mechanisms which is dynamically dispersed about the cortex and which must be accomplished by a complex of cortical and adjacent subcortical areas working in coordination with one another. The roles of different areas are not identical; each makes its own contribution to the general "dynamic structure" of cortical zones carrying out a given function. The position we have outlined largely determines the questions which we must consider in studying speech disturbances. It is now accepted that in analyzing the results of brain lesions, one should speak not of the *localization of functions*, but of the *localization of symptoms*. This position which has been so strongly defended by Goldstein was originally formulated by Jackson. According to his conception, a focal lesion of the brain which disturbs a process necessary for the performance of a certain function produces a symptom. In this sense the symptom is correlated with the site of damage, i.e. "localized" to a certain area of the cerebral cortex.

The fact that certain disturbances may be attributed to damage at certain sites cannot be disputed. Indeed were it not for the regularity with which clinical symptoms may be attributed to given sites, neurological and neurosurgical practice would not exist. One problem of the modern clinic is the "localization of symptoms" – the task of description. Beyond this, however, lies a more difficult problem, namely the *qualification of symptoms*. In other words, the clinician must discover the *component functions of different cortical areas,* for disturbance of one of these leads to *corresponding change in a number of functional systems*. Having described the syndromes which arise as a result of local damage to various areas it is necessary to distinguish the *fundamental disturbance* or direct result of a given lesion from its *secondary or systemic effect,* i.e. its effect on functional systems. Only thus can the diagnosis of brain lesions be put on a scientific footing.

As an example of how a functional system can be analyzed we might consider writing activity, since this will concern us in later chapters. The disturbance of writing is a rather common symptom in cases of left hemisphere injury. Only a naive prescientific conception of writing as simply fine coordinated movements of the hand could lead to the idea of "localization" of this act in an isolated cortical "center", e.g., in "Exner's center".

Writing is a complex functional system which originates from analysis of speech sounds, the separation of certain sounds out of the flow of speech and their transformation into constant, generalized phonemes. This first step involving the integrated function of the auditory-articulatory system creates the potentiality for writing. The next step is recognition of these sounds in the various sound contexts in which they appear and analysis of their dependence upon the positions which they occupy in diferent words.[7] Only when these conditions are met is it possible to translate phonemes into "graphemes", to represent the graphemes by motor actions, and to develop the system of smoothly connected movements which are characteristic of handwriting once it has become an automatic activity.

This short and highly simplified analysis of writing activity suffices to show that it is a *highly complex functional system* which must involve a dynamic constellation of areas working together. Each area plays its own role. Occasionally its role is a central one; at other times its function is of more peripheral significance. In ordinary writing, whether it be spontaneous or to dictation, a decisive role is played by the acoustic-articulatory system which breaks down the flow of speech into the phonemes of which it is composed. Another important process is the visuo-spatial analysis and synthesis of the graphemes and the consequent coordination of movements which produce them. No doubt preliminary connections which are established on the basis of internal speech participate in all this. By means of continual feedback they play the role of a collation device or a regulator of coordinated processes.

It is essential to note also that the interrelations of the component functions just mentioned *depend upon the type of writing.* In writing to dictation the stage of acoustic (or acoustic-articulatory) analysis will inevitably emerge as primary, especially if the words are difficult or unfamiliar. On the other hand, in writing down a highly automatized ideogram such as a signature, this stage is of almost no significance. Also, the system of functional components making up a particular writing habit varies depending upon the extent to which it has been practiced. This is true of the dynamic constellation underlying the habit. Thus a child who is just learning to write depends upon altogether different systems of temporary connections than do adults, for whom it has long since become automatic.

In either case, however, writing is a *complex functional system,* which requires the integrated function of a whole complex of cortical areas. Thus it is not surprising that *disturbances of the writing functional system can occur with lesions of several different areas of the left temporal lobe.* They may arise with damage to the posterior temporal area or inferoposterior parts of the frontal lobes. They may also be seen with lesions of the premotor areas, prefrontal areas, or parieto-occipital areas.

Just as writing impairment may arise as the result of damage to a number of different areas, the type of disturbance varies also. The disturbances of component functions such as acoustic and articulatory analysis of sounds, visuo-spatial coordination, or secondary automatization of motor acts which follow damage to certain areas remove various physiological mechanisms necessary for writing. Damage to any such area produces a disturbance of a specific kind. Loss of sound-articulatory

[7] This process has been described in detail elsewhere. See D. B. Èlkonin (1956) and A. R. Luria (1950, 1962).

analysis inevitably leads to incorrect breakdown of the flow of sounds and disturbance of phonemic differentiation. Loss of visuo-spatial coordination results in misshapen letters. Disturbance of the synthesis of motor acts and the related denervation of preliminary movements leads to loss of the kinetic schema of writing. Thus each of these disturbances will inevitably be reflected in a whole series of *symptoms which differ qualitatively* from those produced by the other disturbances. As we shall see below the qualitative differences in syndromes may be quite specific in nature. Thus the systemic character of disturbances *by no means deprives symptoms of their value for topical diagnosis*. The topical significance of symptoms is not seen, however, in the loss of one or another functional system. It is to be discovered by a *qualitative analysis of the syndrome. Careful study of the various symptoms arising in a given case leads to discovery of the component function which has been lost.*

A systemic conception of the structure of "functions" and qualitative analysis of the disturbances which follow focal lesions does more than explain how one and the same "function" may be impaired by lesions at a number of different sites. It also brings us closer to an understanding of the diversity of symptoms which may arise following lesion of a single cortical area.

Clinicians have found that, as a rule, damage to a single cortical area produces a *whole complex of symptoms,* some of which may appear extremely unrelated to each other. For instance a lesion of the posterior part of the first temporal gyrus may lead to verbal deafness (sensory aphasia), agraphia, difficulty in repeating words and sentences, difficulty in finding words, and verbal and literal paraphasias. Similarly damage to the parieto-occipital area may produce such heterogeneous symptoms as a visuo-spatial disturbance, tactile agnosia, acalculia, difficulties in the naming of objects, and difficulties in understanding logico-grammatical constructions.

For decades attempts have been made to explain how such varied symptoms can all arise from lesions of a single area of the cortex. Some authors have attempted to explain this phenomenon on the basis of highly specialized "centers" located close to one another within the damaged area. Such attempts as those of Kleist to find special "centers" for "understanding numbers" or "understanding sentences" and the attempts of Nielssen to find cortical "centers for the perception of animate and inanimate objects" are simply unjustifiable resurrections of the false psychomorphological conceptions originally propounded by Gall.

A systemic conception of functions, and the qualitative analysis of topical syndromes which it implies, leads to altogether different conclusions. There is no doubt that every part of the cortex possesses its *own special function* in the overall picture of cerebral activity and that this function is impaired when the area is damaged. Such specific physiological functions include those of visual, auditory, tactile, or motor analysis and synthesis, integrative functions among the various analyzers, and those functions involving feedback from a motor act. Analysis of the functions related to particular areas is still in its infancy. Future clinical investigations and studies in electrophysiology wil undoubtedly provide the answers.

Although we still know little about the specific functions of different cortical areas and about the complex functional systems which underlie mental activity, what we do know is sufficient to indicate the paths of analysis which are most apt to be productive in the topical study of syndromes made up of diverse symptoms.

Forty years ago Goldstein (1925) introduced the idea that the clinical analysis of a lesion may be considered finished when it is possible, first, to state the *basic disturbance* (Grundstörung) which results directly from the lesion and, secondly, to account for all *secondary symptoms* in terms of the basic disturbance plus the compensatory reorganization of functions accomplished by remaining areas of the brain. Although one may not agree with Goldstejn's (1910, 1926, 1927, 1934, 1947) particular interpretation of the term "basic disturbance" and the conception of aphasia to which it led, there is no arguing with the principle that determination of the basic disturbance and its systemic consequences should have an important place in modern clinical diagnosis. Analyses to determine the direct physiological results of lesions in different cortical areas (we could equally well say, "in the cortical parts of the various analyzers") and analyses of the accompanying changes in functional systems should be the fundamental principle of clinical investigation. Such analyses may also lead to a better understanding of the apparently unrelated phenomena which accompany focal cortical lesions.

Of course, determination of the "basic disturbance" accompanying a given lesion can only be carried out successfully if one has sufficient knowledge regarding the role which it plays in the analysis and synthesis of signals reaching the organism and in the regulation of various types of behavior. Thus the determination of "basic disturbances" must remain incomplete for some time to come. Only careful study of the symptoms which arise as a result of focal brain lesions and physiological investigations involving the stimulation and extirpation of various areas will provide the solution to this problem. Nevertheless, we already know enough about the physiological functions of some areas and about the structure of the complex functional systems in which they participate to throw some light on the syndromes which arise when they are damaged.

If, as we pointed out above, damage to the postero-superior parts of the left temporal area disrupts normal activity in the system of structures responsible for acoustic analysis and synthesis, then it cannot but produce a disturbance of auditory speech (phonemic hearing). In doing this it must affect all forms of activity in which phonemic hearing and the connections related to it play a role. With the disturbance of structured hearing it is impossible to maintain precise and differentiated speech, to find necessary words, or to perform the sound analysis and synthesis necessary for writing. When this basic disturbance is present, secondary symptoms inevitably develop as indirect or compensatory effects. Literal and verbal paraphasias and disturbances in the grammatical structure of speech appear, but such functions as object recognition, orientation in space, and calculation involving elementary written numbers remain unimpaired. Damage to the left parieto-occipital area on the other hand produces different effects which are related to the visuo-spatial analyzer. It disturbs functional systems which cannot operate without simultaneous spatial synthesis (coordination), but it leaves totally unharmed those systems which depend upon other forms of synthesis, e.g., temporal or acoustic integration, and which thus do not involve the damaged system.[8]

Analysis of the primary and secondary (systemic) disturbances resulting from focal lesions not only explains the syndromes arising in such cases, but it also turns out to have *important implications for the study of normal functional systems*. This will become more apparent in subsequent chapters.

This account of principles to be observed in the study of symptoms arising as the result of focal cortical lesions would be incomplete were we not to mention one other point, which unfortunately is not adequately developed in the present volume, *viz.* the neurodynamic analysis of brain lesions.

From the time of Broca clinical investigations have consisted of the correlation of different psychological disturbances with certain focal lesions of the cerebral cortex and it has been common to speak in terms of "loss" of functions. Yet only rarely is a function *completely lost* as the result of a limited lesion. More often a function is merely *impaired*. It may continue to appear but only under certain circumstances; it loses its smoothness and coordination with other functions; sometimes it may simply be weakened. This is why Jackson, whose views were almost a hundred years ahead of their time, spoke not of the loss but of the "disintegration" or "dissolution" of function, of the reorganization of a function, of its descending to a more primitive level.

For many decades simplified conceptions of the structure of functional systems were accepted; the basis for a scientific conception of brain function had not been created. Although the concept of "disintegration" was succesfully employed by such authors as Goldstein and Pötzl, it did not acquire a firm scientific basis and its physiological significance was not clear. Only through the work of I. P. Pavlov and subsequent neurophysiological investigations based upon his ideas did the study of functional defects and focal cortical damage become more precise. The concepts used to define such defects began to take on real pathophysiological significance. It became posible to understand the fact that the partial destruction of cells in an area of the cortex, by changing the circulation of blood and cerebrospinal fluid, gives rise to altered processes. It became apparent that a pathological shift in neurodynamics may express itself in the diminished effectiveness of neural processes, in the instability of neural mechanisms, and sometimes even in considerable impairment of the lability of such processes. It was found that the earliest and most

[8] For a detailed analysis of this subject see "Two types of synthetic activity of the cerebral cortex" (A. R. Luria, 1963).

subtle signs of neurodynamic disturbance are the weakening of internal (active) inhibitory processes and the strengthening of external (unconditional) inhibition. As a result brain does not form stable differentiated systems and the range of possible activities is correspondingly narrowed. It became apparent that the weakness of a neural process leads to pathological disturbance of the systemic functional pattern of which it is a part. Diffuse irradiation of excitation or inhibition takes place instead of the fine interaction of these processes which is necessary for complex differentiated cortical function. It was found to be the pathological basis of perseveration phenomena which were for many decades considered to be psychological in nature, but which are actually quite open to physiological analysis. Finally, it became clear that disturbance of the dynamics of neural processes inevitably leads to a very important phenomenon, *viz* the loss of systemic cerebral activity and defective interaction of the two signalling systems. Pavlov turned his attention to the latter effect in the last years of his life, and only more recently has it begun to be studied with the attention it deserves.

New findings regarding the basic neurodynamic changes which occur as the result of brain injury permit a new approach to a number of the facts investigated by different authors who have studied aphasia (See Isserlin, 1929-1932; Goldstein, 1947; Ombredane, 1951, and others). It is now possible to take a physiological approach in the study of processes underlying the symptoms which we observe. It is possible to analyze physiologically the mechanisms which accentuate symptoms under conditions of fatigue and according to which functions are reorganized during recovery, etc.

In the following pages we shall not see this method applied to the degree it should be, but there is no doubt that the neurodynamic analysis of syndromes will turn out to contribute to the greatest success in the clinical interpretation of focal brain injuries.

E. APHASIC SYNDROMES AND THE RELATIONSHIP BETWEEN "PRIMARY" AND "MARGINAL" SPEECH AREAS

On the basis of our analysis of the frequency and severity of aphasic syndromes we distinguished two groups of speech areas which we tentatively referred to as "primary speech areas" and "marginal areas". The frequency and severity of disturbances were completely different, depending upon which type of area was involved. How are we to interpret this statistically determined relationship in terms of the principles set forth above? *Are only the primary areas directly related to the organization of speech processes so that only damage to these areas can lead to speech disorders?* If so, then the border areas may have no relation whatsoever to the organization of speech processes and damage to them only produces "symptoms by virtue of proximity", i.e. by the spread of damage to involve the primary areas themselves. Alternatively, the relationship between these two groups of areas may be a more profound one in which *each of the marginal areas plays its own particular role in the organization* of speech processes.

The first answer suggested above implies that the brain mechanisms of speech rest upon independent "speech centers" which are sharply delimited from the remainder of the cerebral cortex. The second answer offers the possibility of a systemic structure of complex brain functions involving the integrated participation of different cerebral areas.

The principles which we set forth above regarding the psychological structure of speech processes and functional systems of the cerebral cortex make it possible to give a conclusive answer to this question. Every aspect of speech activity rests upon some organization of afferent or motor processes. Thus it is understandable that the "secondary" cortical areas, the areas which make possible the fine differentiation of functions of the various analyzers, must participate in the cerebral organization of speech activity. Without them speech cannot develop. With the historical evolution of language they underwent certain modifications and their coordination with one another created the cortical functional systems which subsequently became the "basic speech areas".

On close investigation the primary speech areas have turned out to be those cortical areas whose functions are related to the kinds of analysis and synthesis most important for speech or those areas where the cortical parts of different analyzers overlap. The marginal areas have turned out to be not simply zones which happed to lie contiguous to the "speech centers". These areas do not enter directly into the system of speech areas, but are responsible for the secondary integration of certain sensory or motor processes and thus contribute various physiological components necessary for normal speech. Thus when a lesion of a primary speech area is observed, we may expect to see gross and complex aphasic symptoms, whereas with lesions of the marginal areas, more subtle and limited impairment of speech processes is to be expected.

The position we have outlined marks an essential shift from the conceptions which have characterized the study of aphasia up to the present time. *We do not follow the usual course of attributing the slight speech pathology observed in conjunction with lesions of the marginal areas to partial involvement of the primary speech areas themselves. Instead we attempt to understand complex aphasic syndromes by studying the partial disturbances which arise with lesions limited to the marginal areas. These lesions give us the opportunity to identify the different physiological components of more complex aphasic syndromes.*

Thus our analysis will be considerably different from the usual approach of classical neurology. It will begin with a consideration of the *weakly expressed individual signs* of speech disturbance which arise folowing damage to the areas which we have referred to as "marginal zones". Only after the pathology of these areas has become more clear shall we attempt to analyze the more complex and severe form of aphasia. For us the study of marginal zone lesions will not be simply an investigation of the symptoms arising from "lesions to neighboring areas", but rather *a methodological step towards unravelling more complex forms of aphasia into their constituent parts*. This approach only becomes feasible when one goes from studying vascular lesions to the study of traumatic injuries and tumor cases. We believe that it is the only approach which will ultimately permit the analysis of extremely complex aphasic disturbances and that classical studies of aphasia would have achieved considerably greater success had they involved this approach.

V

PATHOLOGY OF TEMPORAL LOBE SYSTEMS AND THE SYNDROME OF ACOUSTIC APHASIA

We shall begin our analysis of the topical syndromes of aphasia with the analysis of sensory aphasia. This has been a familiar syndrome since the time of Wernicke, but, even to the present day, it has not received adequate explanation.

Symptoms of sensory aphasia are generally a sufficient basis for diagnosing damage to the posterior parts of the left superior temporal gyrus. They include an inability to recognize the speech of others, a loss of precise and grammatically structured speech without difficulty in articulation, and frequently inability to repeat words or sentences spoken by others, to name objects, or to write. Often the speech of patients with this syndrome is characterized by severe paraphasias.

But while the sensory aphasia syndrome is quite familiar, the physiological mechanisms underlying the changes involved are far from being understood. Is temporal aphasia a disturbance of *hearing* as was thought by Wernicke? Or is it an impairment of *understanding* and even of thought as Marie believed? What is the basic disturbance that accounts for all the different symptoms in temporal aphasia? And finally, how is one to understand the physiological mechanisms which underlie this disturbance? All of these questions have remained unanswered for many decades. Only now, thanks to achievements in the study of linguistics and the physiology of higher nervous activity is it possible to introduce some clarity into the discussion of this syndrome.

A. THE ACOUSTIC ANALYZER AND ITS FUNCTIONS

When, in 1874, Wernicke described for the first time the syndrome of sensory aphasia, the mechanisms of this disturbance appeared clear. Wernicke believed that the postero-superior portion of the left temporal area is the termination point for fibers conducting the auditory excitation upon which speech is based. Sensory aphasia was thought by him to be a partial deafness ("Sprachsexte" disturbance) which led inevitably to disturbance of the sound images of words.

Further investigation however, did not confirm this initial hypothesis. It turned out that acuity did not change significantly in sensory aphasia and that the patient was quite capable of discriminating pure tones falling in the frequency range of speech sounds. The temporal lobe patient was able to react to tones quite promptly, but did not recognize spoken words. The idea naturally arose that sensory aphasia is not a hearing disturbance but a disturbance of speech memory (Charcot) or even a general intellectual disorder (P. Marie).

Which of these suggestions was correct? In Wernicke's time science could only offer limited data regarding the physiology of the cerebral cortex. A few cortical stimulation studies had been carried out three years before the work of Wernicke. Such work had allowed Fritsch and Hitzig to describe the "motor centers" of the cerebral cortex for the first time. It was only natural that the first conceptions of sensory centers in the temporal area were conditioned by these findings.

In recent decades, however, the knowledge of cortical physiology has been enriched by findings which have fundamentally altered the old conceptions. Following the modern physiological studies the idea became untenable that the cerebral cortex is a place where peripheral fibers end and where the excitations which they conduct become "mental".

The cerebral cortex has come more and more to be thought of as a central unit associated with complex reflex activity, as a junction of the cortical ends of the analyzers which break down the excitation conducted from the periphery into a tremendous number of fractional elements to integrate and synthesize this fractionated mosaic into certain dynamic structures, reinforcing the excitation of some elements and inhibiting others.

The basic characteristics and functions of the analyzers were traced out by the Pavlov school. The primary feature of analyzer function is the reinforcement of certain perceived stimuli so that they become vitally significant as stimulus-signals for adaptive actions. The "signal" characteristics of a stimulus come to be perceived more intensely, i.e. the level of excitability of nervous elements receiving them rises, while sensitivity to undifferentiable non-signal characteristics falls off, and the elements which perceive them become inhibited.

So far we do not have a good electrophysiological conception of this process. Perhaps this will come about with the development of microelectrode techniques, which make it possible to record action potentials from small groups of cells and even from single cells. Nevertheless, the facts obtained so far (G. V. Geršuni 1955, 1957) indicate that, as a result of analytic functions of the cerebral cortex, sensitivity to signal stimuli can increase many hundreds of times.

The function of each analyzer, and primarily of its cortical part, concerns not only the extraction (by analysis) of the signal cues of stimuli. It is related also to the grouping or synthesis of the different attributes of stimuli into whole complexes or systems. Modern physiology showed conclusively that the brain is capable of reacting to a stimulus complex as a whole, no matter whether the components occur simultaneously or sequentially. The brain discriminates with precision, raising excitability to one signal complex and lowering excitability to a different, nonreinforced complex.

On the basis of such work the sensory cortex has come to be thought of as an organ of analysis and synthesis, a complex cerebral "syntho-analyzer". The study of the cortical organs of analysis and synthesis constitutes a major achievement of modern science. Its real significance, however, is understood only when all of these facts are considered in a broad biological context.

The stimulus attributes which are selectively perceived are not fixed once and for all. The selective process is not immutable and, even more important, it is not tied to permanent characteristics of the stimulus. If it were, one would expect, for instance, that a physically more intense stimulus would always be perceived more distinctly than a less intense stimulus. The factors which determine which stimuli or stimulus attributes are perceived with maximal distinctness is governed by *conditions which are not part of the stimuli themselves*. Broadly speaking, such factors comprise the *conditions of life* and ecology of the organism. *The stimuli which are most precisely discriminated are those which have been reinforced and thus have attained signal quality relating to vital activity of the organism.*

In some cases a signal stimulus is so constant a part of the organism's surroundings that it habitually elicits a system of natural adaptive reflexes. It is known, for instance, that for the cat a slight scratching sound is an extremely effective signal stimulus. Other more intense sounds which are of no particular significance to the cat produce weaker responses. Many of the observations of contemporary authors, including Lorenz', have to do with natural (orienting and alimentary) reflexes to constant environmental stimuli. In other cases the signal value of a stimulus is brought about by changing ecological conditions and the reactions result from the formation of temporary neural connections, i.e. conditioned reflexes. In either case, the significance of a stimulus attribute is a function of objective environmental conditions. Its significance determines the function of cortical parts of the analyzers.

Since the various cortical areas make up the central portions of the analyzers it is clear that their basic functions are not limited to control of the general acuity of the different sense modalities. Instead, they are concerned with the *complex selective function* which is performed by these syntho-analyzers. They extract the most significant cues, and damage to them results not in changes in the acuity of perception but in alteration of its analytical-synthetic character. One finds an inability to separate certain patterns of signals while simultaneously inhibiting other patterns.

This clinical finding corresponds exactly to what I. P. Pavlov discovered in experiments on animals. He found that a dog with partial or total extirpation of the auditory cortex was still able to react to individual tones but was unable to select certain signal sounds, raise the level of excitability to these sounds, and inhibit or lower the level of excitability to other, non-signal sounds. In other words, it was impossible to develop fine discriminations among different sounds, although the sensitivity to the sounds *per se* remained as before. The dog with partial destruction of the auditory cortex could still develop differential reactions to auditory stimuli which differed sharply from one another, but it was unable to develop differentiations among sounds which were quite simular to one another or to discriminate complex sound patterns. The latter include features or sequences of tones, which must be analyzed and compared with each other as whole complexes.

Cortical damage, in this case lesions of the auditory cortex, result not in a general decrease in acuity of auditory sensation but in *loss of the functional selectivity of the auditory analyzer*. The disturbance of selectivity deprives the animal of the ability to react appropriately to patterns of sound signals, even though they may be a constant part of the animal's environment.

B. THE HEARING OF SPEECH

How do speech sounds differ from ordinary sounds, and how does the hearing of speech differ from the hearing of nonverbal sounds? Thanks to the findings of modern linguistics, we can now give a much more precise answer to this question than was possible several decades ago. A decisive role has been played in this field by the Russian phonological school (Baudouin de Courtenay, Troubetzkoy, Ščerba, Polivanov, R. Jakobson).

Two complementary features distinguish speech sounds from non-speech sounds. They are always complex sounds produced by the organs of phonation and articulation. These organs include the vocal chords, the oral and nasal resonators, the tongue, soft palate, lips, and teeth, and according to recent findings, the epiglottis.[1] Secondly, and this is a definitive characteristic, they are always formed according to the rules of a given system which has its own particular phonetic structure. The authors mentioned above have shown that, in terms of the phonetic structure of a language, different sound attributes have different values or meanings.

In a given language certain attributes of acoustic stimuli have no significance. For instance it is possible to say the word "dočka" (daughter) in a high or a low voice, a voice of any timbre, fast or slowly, and with any kind of intonation; changing these attributes of the sound does not deprive the word of its meaning. Thus one can say that the tone, timbre, rate, and intonation with which a word is spoken are of no significance for understanding its meaning.

On the other hand, there are other atttributes or features which are significant for the meaning and understanding of words. Physiologists refer to these as signal attributes or distinctive features. In the Russian language, for instance, such fea-

[1] These recent findings were obtained by N. I. Žinkin at the Institute of Psychology, in Moscow by means of an x-ray movie camera and are extraordinarily interesting. (See N. I. Žinkin, *Speech Mechanisms*, published by the Press of the Academy of Pedagogical Sciences, Moscow, 1959; English version: The Hague, Mouton & Co., 1968).

tures include whether a sound is voiced or unvoiced, soft or hard, accented or unaccented. If one substitutes the unvoiced "t" for the voiced "d" in the word "dočka" (daughter), it becomes "točka" (dot), an altogether different word. Similarly the meaning of the word "zalo" (hall) is totally different from that of "salo" (lard), and the meaning of "god" (year) is not the same as that of "kod" (code) or "kot" (cat). One need only change the accent to the first syllable of the word "muká" (flour) to get "múka" (torture).

These sound features which determine the meaning of a word may be justifiably referred to as *signal, semantically distinctive,* or *phonemic*. They are fundamental to language. The speech sounds of which these distinctive features are attributes must be considered the *basic units of spoken language*. In modern linguistics they are referred to as "phonemes".

It is an important fact that the phonemic features which are distinctive for one language and thus constitute signal attributes may lack significance in another language and carry no meaning whatsoever. Thus, while voiced and unvoiced sounds are of decisive significance for distinguishing the meanings of words in Russian, they have no signal value at all in the Chuvash language. The difference between hardness and softness which is another of the distinctive features in Russian (the difference between "pyl" spoken with a hard "l" and a soft "l" is the difference between "ardour" and "dust"). This feature has no significance in German, English, or French. On the other hand the duration of a sound plays no distinctive role in Russian, while in German it is a distinctive feature and changes in the duration of a vowel can alter the meaning of a word, e.g. lengthening the vowel changes the word "Statt" into "Staat" or "satt" into "Saat". Analogously one finds that opened and closed vowels are differentiated in the French language, e.g. French "le, les, lait ou laid". The degree of abruptness is significant in the Georgian language, e.g. Georgian "puri" (bread), as opposed to "p'uri" (buffalo cow); "kari" means door, while "k'ari" means wind. In certain African languages and in Vietnamese a change in the tonality of pronunciation can drastically alter the meaning of a word.

The discovery of the place of distinctive features in language brings us a step closer to answering our original questions regarding speech hearing. The first thing to be noted is that the hearing of speech always involves auditory activity which is complex in two respects.

Speech hearing involves first of all the *analysis and synthesis of complex patterned sound stimuli,* extraction of signals from a current of sounds. *This abstraction and reinforcement of the phonemic cues* characteristic of a given language and the inhibition of extraneous features is the primary function of discriminative speech hearing. A second and no less essential function is the *systematization or generalization of these cues,* the synthesis and transformation of cues into the constant units of a given language – phonemes. This latter process is clearly involved in hearing and understanding the spoken language, but it is seen most clearly in writing. The generalization of cues is considerably complicated by the fact that the actual sound of a phoneme depends upon the sounds which precede and follow it in a given word. In the forms "kota", "kotu", "o kote", and "kotik" the phonetic character of the sound "t" changes.[2] Before the vowels "a" and "u" it is hard, whereas before "e" and "i" it is soft and even approaches the sound "tz" or "ts". The essential condition for understanding (or writing) these words, however, is preservation of the constant phoneme "t" and its differentiation from the closely similar phonemes "d", "c", etc.

The constancy of phonemes is an essential characteristic of both expressive and receptive speech. It is based upon the distinctive features of the language, on the selection of these cues from non-constant, non-signal attributes, and on the generalization of variants of a given phoneme to include a constant well-defined group of sounds. Thus when one speaks of speech hearing as "articulate hearing" one has in mind the breaking down of continuous speech into constant phonemic units and the systematization of speech sounds on the basis of the phonemic structure of the language. Without this, genuine speech hearing is impossible.

What we have just said raises a question which is basic to the theme of this book, viz. whether or not it is possible for a person to *hear* speech which is uttered in a foreign language unfamiliar to him. Obviously a person who attends to speech in a language which is unfamiliar to him hears it; but at the same time there is no doubt that his hearing is not complete. Not only his "comprehension", but his "hearing" is profoundly defective. He hears speech in a strange language but without differentiation, since he is not in a position to separate the necessary (unknown to him) phonemic cues, to systematize the speech sounds into constant phonemes.

If the unfamiliar language belongs to another family of languages, e.g. to a tonal language such as Vietnamese, Chinese, or one of the African languages, or to a family of languages with an altogether different phonemic system such as Georgian or Abkhazian, then a person perceives the speech as an undifferentiated flow of sounds from which it is difficult even to single out "clusters" of sounds which seem to go together. If the language is somewhat closer to the sound system of a language which he knows, a person will translate the phonemic system to which he is listening into his own system to give a kind of "trans-phonematization". This makes itself obvious if he attempts to repeat or write down a word which is spoken to him.

The following examples show to what extent the precision of speech perception depends upon directed hearing based on the phonemic system of a language as opposed to the absolute auditory acuity of the listener.

A person who speaks English is quite capable of distinguishing the sounds "w" and "v" which differ from one another only by the character of the space between the lips, or "th" and "s" which differ only in the degree of resonance. He can distinguish them because these are sounds which act as cues in the English language. They are important

[2] In the literature this has been referred to as a morpheme.

for the *differentiation of meaning*. Thus the words "wine" and "vine" may sound quite similar, but they have altogether different meanings. In Russian language, on the other hand, the distinction between these sounds is not significant, and a Russian has great difficulty in catching the difference between the two sounds even though he may hear quite well. Analogously, the features of hardness and softness which are important for the differentiation of meanings in the Russian language, i.e., which distinguish such letters as "е" and "э", "и" and "ы", "л" and "ль", sound altogether different to the Russian. Whereas the hardness or softness of the "l" makes the difference between "hear" and "dust" ["pyl" (hard "l") and "pyl" (soft "l") respectively] to the Russian, this distinction has no significance whatsoever in the French, German, or English languages. Thus a person who has grown up with the phonetic system of one of these languages does not perceive the fine differences between the two sounds.

The extreme to which a language can come to depend on variations of one feature is to be seen in the Kabardian language, one of the Caucasian group. It has only one system of vowels which differ from one another only in resonance. Thus the distinctions between such vowels as "u", "a", and "o" are not generally recognized by speakers of this language. Yet the differences among a number of sibilant and whistling sounds which are uncommon to the Indo-European group of languages are easily distinguished by speakers of the Kabardian tongue. Again, in the Japanese and Chinese languages differences of intonation which are so slight as to be indistinguishable to the European ear have important phonemic significance. One and the same word pronounced with different intonations can have three different meanings, e.g. the Japanese "ka sa" (hat), "kasa" (syphilis), and "ka sa" (volume). Still, people who catch these differences do not differentiate between the sounds "r" and "l". Thus they may pronounce "Miller" as "Mireru" or "Sebastopol" as "Sebastoporu" or even "Luria" as "Ruria".

The difference in phonemic systems is responsible for some of the difficulties seen among Chinese learning to speak Russian. The difference between "l" and "r" which is so easy for a Russian to recognize is difficult for a Chinese and he does not hear them as discriminable features – as different forms or articulation. As a result, it is easy for him to confuse the two in speaking, and he has a tendency either to use the familiar Chinese phoneme "l" in place of both sounds or to pronounce, write, and understand the two in a random fashion. In my experience there was a case in which a Chinese student, unable to distinguish the words "paradise" ("raj") and "'barking" ("laj"), responded to the exclamation, "What a paradise we have here!!" with a rather puzzled, "what barking?"

These and comparable examples based on the phonemic systems of the Georgian, Chinese, Chuvash, and other languages, which we have discussed in detail elsewhere, all indicate the extent to which hearing is influenced by familiarity with a specific language.

The distinguishing characteristic of human hearing, and particularly of speech hearing, lies not in special acuity or in the range of frequencies which can be heard. There are many animals endowed with greater auditory acuity and capable of hearing a wider range of frequencies than man. Instead, the difference is that human hearing represents a complex system of differentiations which are organized and generalized according to the phonemic system of a given language. Certain sound features are separated out as specific information carrying cues, phonemes.

Having said that speech hearing represents a complex process of auditory analysis and synthesis based upon the phonemic system of the language we have emphasized its complexity, but we have not given a complete account of the physiological processes involved. In order to give a fuller account we must introduce one other very important characteristic of speech. This will bring us to the most important problems dealing with the cerebral organization of speech hearing.

In contrast to other types of sound analysis, the analysis of speech sounds *is not a purely auditory process*. Both in the development of the phonemic structure of the language and in the analysis of speech sounds *articulation* plays a decisive role. This, together with the auditory process, is involved in the extraction of phonemic cues from continuous speech – in the segmentation of continuous speech into a series of constant phonemes.

The participation of articulation in acoustic analysis manifests itself most clearly when a person attempts to analyze the sound structure of a difficult or unfamiliar word. He pieces the word together aloud or, in other words, he submits it to articulatory analysis. This process is easily observed, even without benefit of special recording techniques which may be used, e.g. the electromyogram.

At our suggestion an investigation was once carried out in which the experimentor studied the writing abilities of a second grader. In some trials the child was encouraged to pronounce aloud the word which he was to write; in others he was asked to hold his tongue between his teeth or to keep his mouth wide open as he wrote. The results showed that in the latter case acoustic analysis was not at its best. The number of errors related to inadequate acoustic analysis increased by a factor of six (Nazarova, 1952) when the child did not articulate the word as he wrote it.

All this shows that speech hearing is *a complete systemic function which is based upon the coordinated activity of auditory and articulatory structures of the cortex.*

It has been shown that the speech articulations and phonemic signs which characterize a person's language determine not only how he hears speech, but also the way he hears music. This was demonstrated quite clearly in experiments carried out at Moscow University by A. N. Leont'ev (1957, 1958). Subjects were asked to compare two tones telling which was higher and which lower. Actually the tones were identical except that one was presented with the formant characteristics of the sound "u", while the other was presented with the formant characteristics of "i". A considerable number of subjects (non-musicians) estimated the first tone to be lower than the second; sometimes their estimations of pitch of the two tones were surprisingly different. In order to get such subjects to evaluate them correctly it was necessary to remove the tones from the phonemic system and involve them in another effector system. Thus the subjects were instructed to sing the sounds using the same formant for each. Under these conditions, analysis was freed from the influence of the phonemic structure of speech and it was possible for subjects to recognize the tones as identical.

It is especially interesting that when this experiment was performed with subjects whose native languages utilize *tonality* as a distinctive feature (Vietnamese and Africans), evalution of the pitches of the two tones was made correctly under all conditions. The presence of formants which were not characteristic of their native languages had no effect.

Thus we see another characteristic of auditory speech. If we are to find its underlying mechanisms we must search all the more for the coordinated functions among structures involved in acoustic and articulatory analysis. We must take a new approach to the study of the mechanisms responsible for auditory speech and its pathology.

C. CEREBRAL MECHANISMS OF ACOUSTIC SPEECH. THE FUNDAMENTAL DISTURBANCE IN TEMPORAL APHASIA

Present knowledge regarding the fine structure of the temporal cortex indicates that there is a distinct difference between that which constitutes the central cortical part of the auditory analyzer and the surrounding "secondary" auditory zones, i.e., between intrinsic and extrinsic parts of the auditory analyzer.

The intrinsic area is located in the gyrus of Heschl (Brodmann's area 41) and its structure is characteristic of all the other primary projection areas. The predominant layer is the fourth or receptor layer which has a characteristic somatotopic projection. Some authors, Pfeiffer and others, indicate that the inner part of Heschl's gyrus constitutes the projection area for cochlear fibers which conduct the excitation evoked by high tones, while the outer part received fibers conducting responses to low tones.

In contrast to this the secondary areas of the cortical part of the acoustic analyzer occupy more lateral areas of the temporal lobe. They are found primarily within the limits of the first and, perhaps, second temporal gyri, corresponding to Brodmann's areas 22 and 21. This is the zone which was referred to by Campbell as the "acoustico-psychic zone". Characteristic of the cytoarchitectonics of this area is the predominance of cells in the second and third layers. Recent investigations (Walker, 1938; Papez, 1944; Mettler, 1947; Jasper, Ajmon-Marsan, and Stroll, 1952; Pribram, 1958) have shown that this area is intimately related to nuclei of the thalamus and, through it, with other areas of the cerebral cortex. The essential point is that this area has well developed connections with the anterior speech area. These connections make the two structures components of one functional system.

The anatomical structure and relations of the primary and secondary parts of the temporal area are related to quite different functions. In the literature there are a very few cases in which Heschl's gyrus has been damaged bilaterally. In all such cases (Monakow, Henschen, Morel, Dandy) a central deafness was observed. In a limited number of experiments, direct electrical stimulation of Heschl's gyrus during brain operations (Penfield and Rasmussen, 1950) produced unstructured auditory sensations. A totally different picture appeared when electrical stimulation was applied to the convex areas of the temporal lobe or when these areas were destroyed. Experiments involving stimulation of these areas carried out by Pötzl,

Hoff, Foerster, Penfield and others evoked complex auditory hallucinations. For instance, patients spoke of hearing music, or voices. In short, stimulation of these areas evoked sensations. Damage of the secondary (and especially of the posterior third of the first temporal gyrus of the left hemisphere) produced a type of sensory aphasia which is of special interest to us and which we shall consider in greater detail.

Numerous investigations have failed to show that damage to the lateral parts of the left temporal lobe is accompanied by a diminished auditory acuity to any part of the tone scale. On the other hand they have given convincing evidence of *severe impairment of the analytic-synthetic function of the auditory cortex.*

As early as 1947, N. N. Traugott showed that in children suffering from sensory alalia reflexes may be conditioned to pure sounds, but it is very difficult if not impossible to condition discriminative reactions to any kind of complex sound stimuli. The conditioning of visual and kinesthetic discriminations of these children was not impaired. The greatest difficulties arose in attempting to condition discriminations between two complexes of tones (chords) or between two series of tones presented in different sequences, e.g. ABCD and ACBD. This work was replicated by Kaïdanova in the same laboratory.

Several years subsequent to the work by Traugott experiments involving the conditioning of auditory discriminations were carried over to the study of patients with sensory aphasia by S. V. Babenkova (1954) and L. G. Kabeljanskaja (1955, 1957), collaborators of E. V. Šmidt at the Institute of Neurology in Moscow. In this study patients with left temporal lobe lesions and symptoms of sensory aphasia were required to make different motor responses to discriminative stimuli. Responses to isolated sounds were quite easily conditioned and there was no difficulty whatsoever in conditioning rather fine discriminations among visual stimuli. But the conditioning of precise differentiation among tones which were similar to one another was noticeably impaired and the discriminations achieved were unstable. It was impossible to condition discriminations between complex auditory stimuli such as complex sounds or series of tones presented in different sequences even after many presentations. Interestingly enough all of these results were obtained from patients with lesions in the posterior parts of the *superior* temporal gyrus of the left hemisphere and with syndromes of sensory aphasia and not from patients with lesions in the lower parts of the left temporal cortex. The latter gave a picture of so called "transcortical" aphasia. Figure 14 shows the results of Kabeljanskaja's experiments.

While the experiments described above involved the conditioning of voluntary motor responses, analogous results have been obtained in experiments where involuntary reactions were recorded. N. A. Sukhovskaja, working in the same laboratory at the Institute of Neurology in Moscow, used changes in sensitivity of the retina as the conditioned response.[3]

[3] Sensitivity of the retina was established by determining the minimal area which had to be

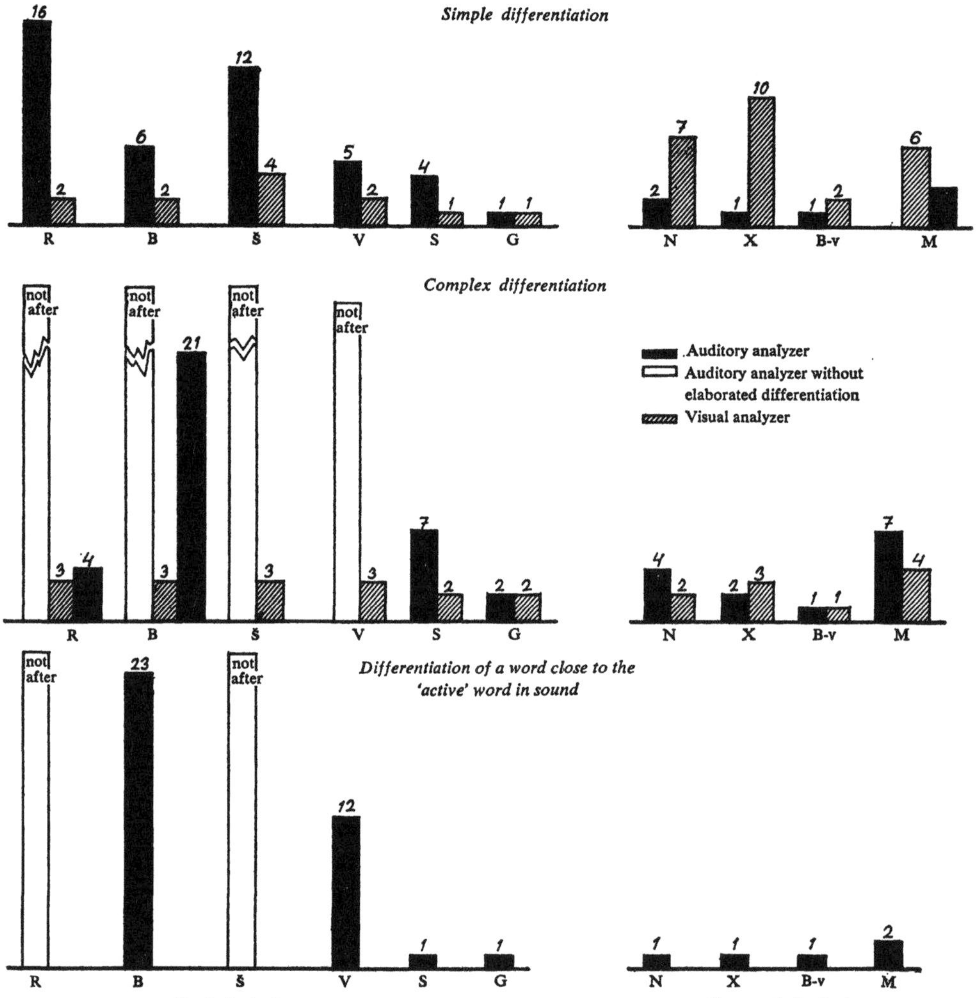

FIG. 14. Impairment in the elaboration of conditioned reflexes and discrimination of auditory and visual stimuli in patients with temporal lobe lesions (from A. G. Kabeljanskaja).

Applying this technique to the study of a group of patients with lesions of the left temporal area and symptoms of sensory aphasia, she obtained results quite similar to those just described. It turned out to be very easy to condition simple responses and differential responses to nonauditory stimuli in patients with lesions

---

stimulated in order to perceive a flash. According to observations made by P. G. Snyakin (Institute of Neurology) the number of active elements in the retina is not constant but varies as a function of certain definite factors. Thus "modulation of retinal sensitivity" may be evoked either by a light stimulus or by a conditioned stimulus which has been paired with the light.

of the superior temporal gyrus. Responses to simple auditory stimuli were also not difficult to condition. But discrimination between two sound complexes, especially sequential complexes, was virtually impossible to obtain. Just as in the experiments mentioned above, reliable discrimination could not be conditioned even with a large number of presentations. Also, just as was found in the first study, this effect was not seen in patients with lesions of the lower parts of the left temporal area and symptoms of "transcortical aphasia".

Such findings help us characterize the basic disturbance observed in lesions of the postero-superior parts of the left temporal area (Wernicke's zone) and the sensory aphasia which arises in such cases. Sensory aphasia must be considered a *disturbance of complex discriminative hearing.* But it is not a simple change in auditory acuity; it is a change in *analytic-synthetic activity.* Any other disturbances of speech comprehension and special "intellectual function" must derive ultimately from this disturbance.

The defect in analytic-synthetic activity of the auditory cortex which arises as the result of damage to the "secondary" areas gives us ample reason to consider the *basic symptom* to be the *disturbance of phonemic audition,* or *speech hearing.* As we indicated earlier, phonemic audition is the same as discriminative hearing in general, except that it is selective audition organized according to the phonemic structure of a given language and is carried out through the coordinated functions of the cortical structures associated with hearing and articulation. Both are based upon the analytic-synthetic function of the temporal (auditory) cortex.

The secondary cortical areas of the auditory analyzer which are most closely connected with articulatory areas lie in the postero-superior part of the temporal lobe. Might we expect that damage to this area could occur without disturbing phonemic hearing? Numerous observations of both tumor cases [4] and firearm injuries of the left temporal area have indicated to us that when the postero-superior region is damaged, preservation of speech hearing is out of the question. Lesions in this area produce a sensory aphasia which is *always associated with impairment of discriminative phonemic audition.*

The experimental technique which brought us to this conclusion is very simple. It is known that the phonemes of a language constitute well differentiated systems of sounds (Troubetzkoy, R. Jakobson). Among the different groups of phonemes one finds some so called "disjunctive phonemes" which differ from each other by a number of distinctive features, e.g. "b" and "r", or "s" and "m". Other differ from one another only by a single feature; for instance one may be voiced, whereas the other is not. This is the difference between the phonemes "b" and "p", "d" and "t", or "z" and "s". Phonemes in pairs of the latter type stand in opposition to one another and are referred to as "oppositional" or "correlative" phonemes. In

[4] A detailed study of the syndromes which arise in cases of left temporal lobe tumors is included in an unpublished monograph by the author, "Studes in Aphasia, part 1: Temporal Aphasia" (Dissertation, Moscow, 1941).

recent years several authors (R. Jakobson, 1956, and others) have used new electro-acoustic techniques to determine with utmost care the oppositional phonemes characteristic of different languages.

It is obvious that the differentiation of disjunctive phonemes does not demand such fine auditory processes as differentiation between oppositional phonemes, since disjunctive phonemes differ from one another by a number of features. Thus one of the methods used in evaluating the degree to which phonemic speech is preserved is to test the differentiation of disjunctive and oppositional phonemes.

We can outline several simple and clinically useful techniques for investigating the degree to which differentiations of various degrees of complexity are disturbed. With a patient whose active speech is intact it is possible simply to give several disjunctive phonemes, of the type "b", "s", "m", "r", or several oppositional phonemes of the type "b", and "p", "d" and "t", "z" and "s", and ask him to *repeat* them. If one wishes to test for finer differentiation the phonemes are presented in pairs which the patient is to repeat ("r-b", "m-s"; or "b-p", "d-t" and "t-d", "z-s" and "s-z"). An even more sensitive test is to present phonemes in *threes* (disjunctive phonemes: "b-r-m", "b-r-k"; oppositional phonemes: "b-p-b", "p-b-p").

If the patient has difficulty in repeating these sounds, or if the investigator has reason to suspect an inertness of motor speech (motor perseveration) the same tests may be carried out in different way. Instead of being asked to repeat the sounds, the patient is asked to *write* them down. The shift from speaking to writing sounds may remove the perseverative effect and reveal defects of sensory differentiation more clearly.

If both of the above methods fail the investigator may attempt to *condition* different reflexes to the different sounds. For instance, in testing the discrimination of disjunctive phonemes he may instruct the patient to raise his hand when he hears "r" but keep it in place when he hears "s". A differential conditioned reflex is considered to have been elaborated if the hand is consistently raised in response to "r" and if this reflex is absent following the presentations of "s". The same procedure is repeated using oppositional phonemes. In this case one of the phonemes, "b" for instance, receives positive reinforcement, while the other, "p", is inhibited. Differentiation is considered established once the patient confidently raises his hand in response to "b" but withholds the response when the phoneme "p" is presented.

For finer analysis this technique can be extended by substituting phoneme *complexes* for individual phonemes. In this case the patient is instructed, for example, to raise his hand in response to "b-p" but not to respond to any other combination – "p-p", "b-b" or "p-b". (Of course if the patient does not comprehend verbal instructions the examiner may move his arm for him or hold it still in order to reinforce the appropriate sounds or pairs of phonemes.) Just as with the previous method, the establishment of a differential response is evaluated by the development of a stable reaction to one sound complex and no reaction to other complexes.

One advantage of this last technique is that it permits one to determine both the *stability* of the discrimination and the *rate* at which it is established. In order further to check the stability of the discrimination it is possible to change the rate at which stimuli are presented, introduce extraneous stimuli, or repeat the same experiment after a four or five minute pause. What is most important is to introduce greater and greater complexity, for instance, to pronounce different phonemes at one pitch or the same phoneme at different pitches. All this not only allows one to ascertain whether impairment is present or not; it also submits whatever impairment may exist to *neurodynamic analysis*.

Application of the techniques described above produced quite clearcut results in the study of patients with focal brain damage. Whereas patients with lesions not involving the left temporal areas had no difficulty whatsoever in performing these tasks, patients with lesions of the postero-superior temporal area had considerable difficulty.

In the most severe cases patients had difficulty in repeating disjunctive phonemes as well as in developing differential reactions to them. As a rule, however, patients were able to repeat disjunctive phonemes. Their performance became poor only if the tests were prolonged; with extended testing they sometimes showed fatigue effects earlier than normal. Severe and, often, overwhelming difficulties arose in tests which involved the *repetition of oppositional phonemes* or the *conditioning of differential reflexes to oppositional phonemes.*

Our observations of patients with tumors or firearm wounds in this area indicated that the great majority were unable to repeat correlative phonemes. For instance they were unable to clearly distinguish "ba-pa" from "pa-ba" or "da-ta" from "ta-da" or "ta-ta". In some cases patients would indicate that these pairs were somehow different from one another, but they could not say exactly what the difference was. Occasionally patients were able to repeat the pairs correctly for a short time, but very soon they ceased being able to do so. The instability of functioning of the auditory analyzer and the rapidity with which it became tired made practice useless. The discriminative responses which appeared were unstable and extended practice did not strengthen them; rather it produced greater fatigue and eventual loss of the ability to repeat the phoneme pairs correcly.

Comparable results were obtained in experiments where differential motor responses were conditioned to oppositional phonemes. Such results were especially clear when pairs of phonemes were used. Usually patients with lesions outside the temporal areas rapidly formed conditioned differential responses to the phonemic cues, and these systems of reflexes were quite stable. The patients *always* responded to the sound "b", for instance, by raising their hands and withheld the response to "p". (The pitch with which the phonemes were pronounced had no effect on the response.) Patients with lesions of the *left temporal area,* on the other hand, were either totally incapable of forming such differential reactions, or the differentiations established were highly unstable. Sometimes if the "b" was pronounced at a high pitch and "p" at a low pitch these patients could distinguish the two, i.e., they would raise their hands only in response to "b". It was easy to show, however, that in these cases pitch had become a signal feature and that the original phonemic cue had lost its signal character; for these patients came to raise their hands in response to any phoneme pronounced at a high pitch and to withhold the response to low pitched phonemes. Also, when "b" and "p" were pronounced at the same pitch, these patients were unable to discriminate between them.

The impairment of phonemic hearing as an aphasic symptom is of topical significance; the degree of disturbance reflects the degree to which the lesion involves a certain cortical area. It is important to note that disturbance of phonemic hearing is usually the *earliest symptom* observed in cases involving tumors of the left temporal area. Impairment of phonemic hearing may occur long before more severe signs of speech disturbance and more obvious neurological symptoms appear. It is not seen, as a rule, with tumors involving other cortical areas. This is true even when the more anterior and inferior parts of the temporal lobe itself are affected. Besides being the first symptom to appear in cases where lesions involve the left postero-superior temporal area, impairment of phonemic hearing is the most stable symptom and the *last to disappear* in the recovery period.

In the large volume of data collected in our study of war injuries, impaired phonemic hearing turned out to be of *great significance for topical diagnosis.* Figure 15 gives a graphic summary of observations made on about 400 cases involving lesions in the left hemisphere. It is apparent from this figure that disturbances of phonemic hearing were seen only in cases where the lesion involved the posterior part of the temporal lobe or adjacent areas. They were seldom observed to accompany lesions at other sites. Injuries in the right hemisphere,

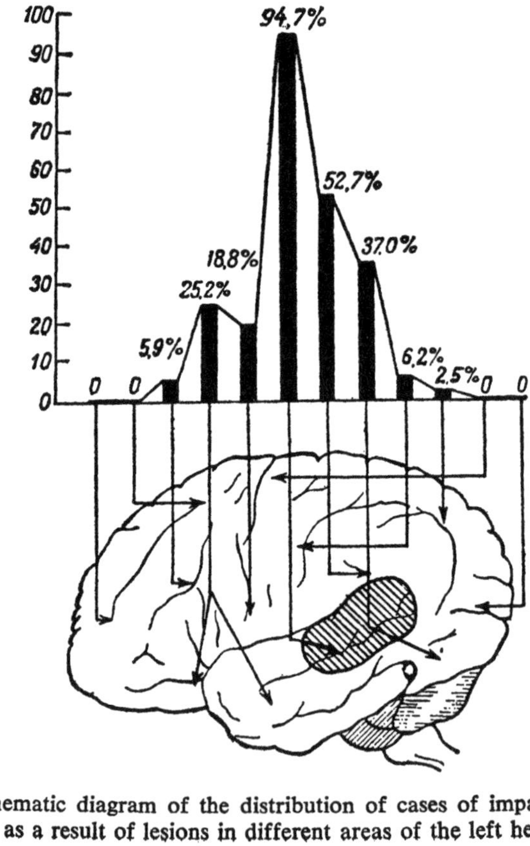

FIG. 15. Schematic diagram of the distribution of cases of impaired phonemic hearing as a result of lesions in different areas of the left hemisphere.

which are not included in this figure, virtually never resulted in phonemic hearing disturbances; previous studies of brain pathology have laid the groundwork for the conception of functional structure of the left temporal lobe to which these findings bring us.

The temporal area as a whole is like other cortical areas (the visual and motor areas) in that it has a complex hierarchical structure. Heschl's gyrus is the basic part of the temporal auditory system. It represents the primary auditory projection area, the "portal" or "entry" for complex auditory perceptions. Here one finds the same kind of precise somatotopic structure which occurs in the precentral gyrus or in the visual projection area of the occipital lobe. According to evidence obtained by Pfeiffer, the fibers which convey impulses in response to high tones project to the central part of Heschl's gyrus, while fibers responding the low tones project to the more lateral part.

Just as in the motor and visual systems, one finds secondary areas which supplement the primary auditory system. The secondary cortical parts of the auditory analyzer are well connected with the other analyzers by association fibers and constitute the "areas of overlap" between analyzers. They take part in complex functions. The division of the auditory cortex into primary and secondary areas gives it a definite *functional organization.* The lateral surfaces of the left temporal lobe (Brodmann's areas 42 and 22) play a role in the auditory analyzer which is analogous to that played by the premotor cortex and post central areas in the motor analyzer or that of Brodmann's areas 18 and 19 in the visual analyzer. According to all that is presently known, these areas permit the secondary organization of auditory perception, i.e. integration of auditory analysis and synthesis into a single functional system with the articulatory process. Thus they are involved in the transformation of simple hearing into the kind of auditory perception, which is organized according to the phonetic system of a particular language. Apparently the function of these areas is to extract the essential cues from continuous speech and to generalize variants of these cues into constant "phonemes", the basic units of human speech. It is natural that, while damage to Heschl's gyrus leads to a central hearing deficit, damage to more lateral parts of the left temporal lobe leads to defects of auditory analysis. The impairment of auditory analysis is reflected in certain kinds of *agnostic disturbances* in which the elementary auditory system remains intact, but the complex system of auditory analysis and synthesis involved in auditory speech is greatly disturbed. One of the most important disturbances which may occur is disintegration of the system of selective speech sounds which plays a programming role in auditory perception. Ultimately this may lead to loss of the functional systems of complex auditory speech; in such cases a primary defect appears which is characteristic of lesions of the postero-superior parts of the left temporal lobe.[5]

[5] We have intentionally omitted here discussion of other functional disturbances related to auditory experience. A number of special studies which we shall consider elsewhere reveal the

D. SYNDROMES OF TEMPORAL (ACOUSTIC) APHASIA

In man the cortical organization of auditory processes is so intimately related to the phonetic system of language that is it virtually impossible for it to be disturbed without profoundly altering all forms of speech activity. Thus it is not surprising that a large proportion of all acoustic-gnostic disturbances is made up of different forms of *acoustic aphasia.*

Table 5 shows that in the overwhelming majority of cases damage to the postero-superior areas of the left temporal lobe produced severe aphasic disturbances. In 82% of cases such disturbances persisted into the residual period.

TABLE 5

Severity and duration of aphasic syndromes following lesions of the left temporal lobe

Site of injury in temporal area	Total number of cases	Initial period			Residual period		
		severe forms (%)	slight forms (%)	total (%)	severe forms (%)	slight forms (%)	total (%)
posterior	38	95	3	98	63	18	81
inferior	27	63	22	85	15	33	48
anterior	48	66	17	83	31	31	62

Injuries in the anterior and postero-inferior temporal areas resulted in significantly fewer aphasic syndromes in the initial period, and of those which appeared, a smaller proportion was severe in nature. A considerably smaller percent of the syndromes observed persisted into the residual period (anterior areas: 63%, postero-inferior areas: 48%). If one considers only those cases in which severe symptoms continued into the residual period, these figures become even smaller (anterior areas: 31%, postero-inferior areas: 15%). Despite the fact that one cannot usually determine the exact sites of lesions in cases of traumatic injury, the accumulation of a large number of cases makes it possible to determine which area

functional structure of the temporal area in its full complexity. There is some evidence to indicate that the anterior parts of the left temporal lobe, while unrelated to phonemic hearing, are intimately related to the integrated auditory perception of rhythmic melody. Similarly it appears that the postero-inferior parts of the temporal lobe lack any connection with phonemic hearing; they are probably related to further integration of auditory perception. These findings require further discussion and will be taken up in more detail later.

is most likely to be responsible for a given syndrome. In this study we were able to present enough cases to make the data obtained relatively reliable.[6]

The data presented in Table 5 correspond exactly to the distribution of cases of disturbed phonemic hearing shown in Figure 15. The greatest proportion of disturbances accompany lesions in the postero-superior part of the left temporal area and there is a considerable drop in the number of such disturbances with lesions in the anterior and inferior parts of the temporal lobe. This suggests a close relationship between the impairment of phonemic hearing and the temporal aphasic syndrome. It indicates that the basic disturbance associated with damage to the left temporal lobe is the impairment of auditory analysis and synthesis and the disintegration of phonemic hearing.

Still the question arises as to what are the *secondary or systemic disturbances* which may develop as a result of this basic defect, and what kind of a *syndrome* is most likely to appear as a result of the primary and secondary disturbances? Careful neuro-psychological analysis of temporal aphasia has made it possible for us to answer this question; thus we shall consider it in somewhat more detail.

In most severe cases and in the earliest stages of left temporal lobe injury the functional disturbances may at first glance appear to be so massive as to make it virtually impossible to distinguish the major symptoms. Even in the initial period, however, these patients are seldom totally unable to speak. When they attempt to say something it is apparent that they are still able to articulate individual sounds, but their speech is garbled and it is difficult to understand what they say. Often only a few introductory phrases or interjections, such as "listen a second", "that's it", or "well now, how would you say . . ." remain. Though limited in content, these expressions may be pronounced with normal intonation. Attempts to go on from these phrases to statements of greater content are seldom successful, however, and the patient, exhausted by unsuccessful attempts, commonly ends up wringing his hands and exclaiming, "Well . . . I can't . . . It won't . . ."

Even the names for things which might be expected to be most permanently a part of one's memory are often inaccessible to these patients. Patients in this group may be unable to remember their own names or addresses and may be hospitalized for long periods of time listed as "name unknown".

Generally the patient with a temporal lesion is capable of carrying out simple instructions such as "Open your mouth", "show your tongue". Careful observation often reveals, however, that the apparent comprehension of verbal instructions is actually more a result of guessing than of genuine speech comprehension. Thus it is advisable to go through the tests several times, repeatedly instructing the patient to point to his nose, eye, or ear. Often as a result of the fatigue of auditory analysis these words will cease to signify anything to the patient and he will begin to point

[6] We have done autopsy studies of tumor cases in order to check the pathology associated with different syndromes (Unpublished). See A. R. Luria, *Studies in Aphasia*, part 1, *Temporal Aphasia* (Dissertation, Moscow, 1941).

out the different organs at random. Disturbances of comprehension stand out even more clearly when the patient is asked questions which have nothing to do with the immediate surroundings or context.

The nature of this complex syndrome becomes apparent when it is submitted to sequential analysis. We ordinarily begin such analysis with an investigation of the *acoustic*, or *phasic* aspect of speech.

If we ask the patient to repeat individual speech sounds after us, we find the same kind of impairment of phonemic hearing that we described earlier as characteristic of patients with temporal aphasia. The repetition of simple syllables is often accompanied by substitution of oppositional phonemes. Sometimes if the patient is asked to delay repeating a syllable for ten or fifteen seconds the differentiated trace of the auditory engram disappears altogether and the patient is unable to repeat it, no matter how simple a combination of sounds it may have been. If the syllable presented is more complex, e.g. if it contains two consonants adjacent to one another, the patient may not even be able to perceive it.

Perseveration often sets in very early; sometimes it is observed from the beginning. The patient, having repeated one syllable, continues to repeat it no matter what syllable is subsequently presented to him. Such stagnation of nervous processes is characteristic of cases involving functional disturbances of the auditory analyzer.

The repetition of words turns out to be as difficult for these patients as the repetition of individual speech sounds. Only occasionally, when the words presented are phonemically simple or very familiar, are patients able to perform this task correctly. Even when a patient is able to repeat certain words, however, the disturbed neurodynamics of the auditory analyzer become readily apparent when the examiner changes from one word to another and the patient fails to repeat it correctly. He either continues to respond with the previous word or to incorporate part of the previous word into the new one. Thus, one sees such paraphasic responses as "kartoška" instead of "katuška" after repetition of the word "karandaš", or "roga" instead of "ruka" after the word "noga". Another common finding is that the patient distorts the word which he is to repeat, so the "kolxoz" is repeated "kolz", "gols", or "glos". Similarly the word "jumor", becomes "umar" or "umer", and the word "inej" is pronounced "imja" or "imej", etc. (the latter examples are taken from observations of Ė. S. Bejn). The more the patient attempts to pronounce a given word correctly, i.e., the more he attempts to analyze it acoustically, the greater his helplessness becomes. Another common observation is that a patient may presented a word and respond with words which are in some way related to it; such substitutions are spoken of clinically as "verbal paraphasias". They occur when unsuccessful attempts to reproduce the original word lead to inhibition of the necessary sound structure and substitution of the trace of another word. The other word has some connection with the word sought and they are both members of a certain common "cluster of associations". Examples of such verbal paraphasias are substitution of the word "karandašik" (a small pencil) for "mal'čik" (a boy), "kupit'" (to buy) instead of "vspomnit'" (to remember), "glaza" (eyes) instead of "očki" (glasses), etc. There is every reason to believe that, whereas literal paraphasias should be considered secondary (compensatory) symptoms.

The *disturbance of writing*, which is one of the basic symptoms of sensory aphasia, is analogous to the verbal disturbances just described in that it is closely related to loss of the sound structure of words. It is similar to the disturbance of repetitive verbal speech except that the defects related to auditory analysis and synthesis manifest themselves much more clearly when the words are written down.

The act of copying (more precisely, the act of visual copying) is ordinarily preserved in these cases, as are such *habitual acts as writing one's signature* or writing one's name and address. These forms of writing often do not require sound analysis and can be reproduced on the basis of kinesthetic stereotypes. We once had occasion to see a patient with a severe sensory aphasia who was able to write down several common words if he wrote them *quickly*. If he attempted to write the words *slowly*, however, he had no success whatsoever, since in this case his writing had to be mediated by sound analysis of the words; he could not take advantage of the motor stereotype. In this, as in *writing to dictation* or *writing spontaneously*, the patient had overwhelming difficulties associated with the defect of auditory analysis and synthesis of words.

In the most severe cases and often in the acute period following injury to the left temporal area, patients are totally unable to differentiate the phonemes making up a given word or to keep phonemes in the proper sequence. Their difficulties stand out most clearly when the words to be written are phonetically complex, e.g. words in which two consonants occur adjacent to one another. In less severe cases the disturbance manifests itself in the substitution of oppositional phonemes for one another, so that the word "zima" may be written "sima", "ogurec" may be written "okules" etc.

Occacionally a patients's attempts to write reveal the defect in auditory analysis at its extreme. Figure 16 shows some examples of such writing. Our earlier attempts to test orally the degree of difficulty which this sensory aphasic patient had in the auditory analysis of words did not reveal the disturbance with such precision as did the writing test. For instance it was difficult for us to note exactly how he answered a given question, how many letters were in each word, which phonemes followed which etc. Sometimes in the oral test he would attempt to produce a complete word by pronouncing the different sounds separately; the sounds might be separated by long pauses or even conjunctions. These forms of auditory analysis present overwhelming difficulty for the sensory aphasic, not because they represent "abstract forms of activity", but because the voluntary production of the sounds comprising words is extremely difficult for a patient whose auditory analyzer has been damaged.

Analogous signs are also observed if one investigates the reading ability of patients with temporal lobe lesions. In children who have just learned to read such

Dictated	Kaša	Gora	Griby	Zdorov'e
Written	Taša	Karaa	Kribi	Storov'e

Patient C. with left temporal lobe lesion (7 class education)

Ogurec	Djatel	Kombajn	Krovat'
okurec	tjatel	Gambaen	Kpobaint'

Patient O. with left temporal lobe lesion (7 class education)

Sobaka	"List'ja šuršat"
forara	lizda šolsad

Patient N. with left temporal lobe lesion (10 class education)

Komnata	"Krugom plamja"
Gonmada	Grukom blame

Patient Z. with left temporal lobe lesion (7 class education)

FIG. 16. Samples of writing by a patient with sensory aphasia (Facsimiles are replaced by printed words for better understanding of the mistakes).

impairment may be virtually complete. In adults, however, it may take a less severe form, so that reading is less affected than the ability to write. The adult sensory aphasic may only notice some difficulty when it is necessary for him to identify an unfamiliar word on the basis of its phonemic structure. In the most severe cases, such reading-by-letter may be completely disrupted, while the direct visual, "ideogrammatic", recognition of familiar words remains relatively intact.

An interesting exception to this rule is found if one considers the reading and writing of numbers, for these functions do not require auditory mediation and remain perfectly preserved in such patients. Usually the ability to make written computations is retained, while the abilities to compute orally or to do computation silently are lost, because of the instability of the verbal signals upon which they depend.

We have frequently observed that patients with left temporal lobe lesions and sensory aphasias read and recognize the meanings of words presented to them, even though they might pronounce the same words incorrectly or even be unable to pronounce them. As an example we might cite a case in which a patient could easily read aloud his own name, "Levskomu", ("to Levskij") as it appeared on an enveloppe, but was incapable of reading just the first syllable, "Lev", by itself.

These findings will be considered in greater detail in another chapter.[7] They indicate that the ability of these patients to read is based upon direct visual recognition or "ideogrammatic" recognition. Thus they avoid the disturbed function of auditory word analysis. Clearly the disturbance of systemic phonemic hearing which we have described must result in that *disassociation of the sounds and meanings of words* which is basic to the sensory aphasic syndrome.

A striking symptom seen in sensory aphasia is a kind of "word blindness". A word which sometimes is heard as "kolos", sometimes as "golos", and sometimes as "kols", or "glos", loses its meaning and ceases to be understood. Similarly a word originally heard as "med" may come to be heard as "mit", "mjat", or "mat" and is rendered incomprehensible. Thus a word loses its precise meaning and comes to be perceived as an indefinite and variable collection of sounds. The patient can no longer repeat, recognize, or recall it, and begins to look upon his language as a foreign and incomprehensible flow of undifferentiable sounds. It is this very symptom which gives rise to the general name "sensory aphasia". It has been the basis for cases in which soldiers wounded in the left temporal lobe and unable to understand the speech of their comrades have thought themselves to be enemy spies; only the understanding of their fellow troops saved them from a tragic end.

A case in which a patients's native language sounds foreign to him often turns out to be a consequence of acoustico-gnostic disturbances, i.e., the dissociation of sound and meaning mentioned above. The forgetting of a word is reflected both in the spontaneous speech of the patient, and also in his attempts to remember the names of different objects. The latter, incidentally, is not characteristic of other forms of aphasia. As a general rule, the forgetting of words in these cases differs from that seen in aphasias due to parietal lobe lesions (see Chapter 7) in that here it results from disturbance of their sound structure. These patients are unable to analyze the phonemic structure of the words they hear; verbal prompting usually does not help them.

In addition to dissociation of the sounds and meanings of words, the *semantic aspect* of speech is profoundly disturbed in the patient with temporal aphasia. It is not surprising that with the general inconstancy of phonemes and phonemic sequences the parts of the word which conveys its basic meaning becomes distorted, so that it loses its significance altogether. Thus the patient no longer possesses large numbers of words, and the few which he retains convey little meaning. This is why in the acute period such patients only utter such transitional phrases as "well . . . so, how do you . . . that means that . . ." etc. For a long time their speech is limited to these transitional expressions, interjections, and introductory phrases which lack any real meaning. One such patient, in trying to describe

[7] See Chapter 13.

the situation in which he was wounded, said, "It get's me . . . and that's all . . . it was like – boom! – I don't know . . . I mean . . . I still don't know . . . when I'm here – I can't . . . I can't . . . right now I just can't . . . maybe . . . no, it just won't . . . Before, I could . . . ha ha ha! Good! But right now I just can't." Although intonation and gesticulation to some extent conveyed the meaning which this patient wanted to express, his speech was altogether lacking in substantive words. On the basis of this kind of direct communication, it became clear that he had been wounded, lost consciousness, did not remember anything for a long time, and was beginning to improve; it was apparent that before the injury he had been a very good speaker.

When such a patient under therapy has partially recovered his speech and begins to recall the words he wants, the confusion and instability of words and meanings become more apparent. One sees typical literal and, more often, verbal paraphasias, e.g. replacement of the desired word by a word which sounds like it or by one which is related to it in some kind of associative complex. The confusion and inconstancy of verbal meanings affects not only the expressive speech, but also the receptive speech of the patient. The involvement of receptive speech is seen in the fact that, while he may have lost the ability to reproduce a certain word, he retains the system of semantic associations of which it was a part. Thus if he is asked to tell what a shoulder is, he may be totally unable to repeat the word "shoulder" or to explain its meaning directly; but by pointing to the arm or elbow, he reproduces approximately the "semantic sphere" of the word. Loss of the meanings of words in other situations is based upon exactly the same defect. It is characteristic of these patients that they comprehend the phraseological relations and grammatical attributes of words, such as suffixes and inflection, much better than they remember the semantic content. Thus their ability to catch logico-grammatical relations, especially those conveyed by the tonality and inflection of speech, proves to be much better preserved than might be concluded on the basis of a cursory examination.[8]

It remains for us to say a few words about the *thought processes* of patients with sensory aphasia, if only because the treatment of this subject has for so long been hampered by adherence to a vexing number of misconceptions.

The position of P. Marie who holds that sensory aphasia is not so much a disturbance of speech as a disturbance of thought (a particular form of dementia) is unacceptable. If we disregard the complete lack of justification for his dissociating thought from speech, the weakest point in this author's argument is its sharp contradiction with the facts.

A number of authors (the best recent examples being È. S. Bejn, 1947, and Ombredane, 1951) have shown that the primary defect in sensory aphasia is the

[8] Analysis of the meanings of words and intellectual operations available to patients suffering from temporal aphasia has been a subject of special investigation. See È. S. Bejn, *A Psychological Analysis of Sensory Aphasia* (Dissertation 1947).

disturbance of analysis and synthesis in the auditory analyzer. As a rule, those abstract concepts which originally arose on the basis of language but which with further development largely ceased to require verbal involvement, are preserved. In experiments carried out by È. S. Bejn this has been supported by a number of findings indicating that patients are capable of employing quite complex concepts if they can avoid the auditory difficulties involved in grasping the corresponding words. Evidence that aphasics in this group are able to perform written calculations, to the extent that they do not involve purely verbal steps, supports this position. Among our patients there was one bookkeeper with a clear-cut sensory aphasic syndrome who forgot words and confused the names of his fellow workers. All the same, at the end of the year he was able to make up his office's annual financial report.

The disturbance of those forms of logical thought which depend upon verbal considerations and verbal conclusions is altogether understandable, but it gives no basis for assuming that *intellectual* defects are primary to sensory aphasia. We have every reason to believe that the basic defect in temporal aphasia is the disturbance of auditory analysis and synthesis which leads to the loss of phonemic hearing and, as a secondary result, to the disturbance of all functions which are dependent upon this physiological function.

At this point we would do well to introduce some examples of traumatic aphasia involving the temporal lobe. We shall first present cases involving mild forms of aphasia which occurred as the result of partial injury to the left temporal lobe and then compare them with cases of more severe temporal aphasic syndromes.

In the first two cases slight symptoms of acoustic aphasia followed focal injuries limited to areas lying just anterior or just posterior to the primary auditory speech areas.

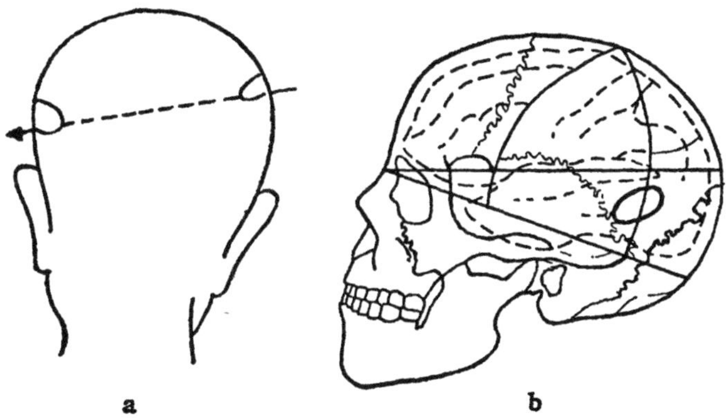

a b

Patient Voev.: injury diagram (Case 1)

Case 1

On December 21, 1943 patient Voev., age 19, was wounded by a bullet which entered the skull in the lower left temporal area near its occipital border; the shell emerged from the right parietal area. The patient was unconscious for a long period of time. From the beginning there were no severe neurological signs. The borders of the visual fields were not well defined, but this defect was not sufficiently severe to merit classification as a scotoma.

Immediately after injury the patient noted considerable difficulty in conversation. He was able to understand the speech of others well enough, but could not retain what he had heard: "Everything immediately flew away". As a result he was unable to follow a few easy words; he was unable to recall less common words, and was completely unable to name objects. He could not write: "The words, fell to pieces". This picture remained the same for about a month and then, as healing of the wound progressed favorably, these functions were gradually recovered.

Three and a half months after injury the patient was given a thorough examination. At this time no neurological losses whatsoever were observed. His spontaneous speech was normal except that he occasionally had to search for words. He easily understood complex logico-grammatical constructions and had no articulation difficulties. His only complaints had to do with the fact that he easily forgot words and occasionally had difficulty to understand them. Sometimes words appeared to him to have an unexpected meaning, or he did not know what they meant. This uncertainty and instability of verbal images interfered with his speech and thought by depriving it of its usual rapidity and smoothness, and often left him with a feeling of confusion and "absurdity". The patient noted that he was completely incapable of writing connected text: "What I get are individual absurd sentences which, taken together, don't mean anything".

A thorough investigation revealed certain disturbances, especially of auditory speech. Phonemic hearing was slightly impaired. Sometimes the patient repeated pairs of oppositional phonemes without clearly differentiating them. He easily recognized common words, but less familiar words appeared strange to him and he was frequently unable to recall their meaning immediately. He also had a certain degree of difficulty in naming objects, e.g., he occasionally misplaced the accent of words, substituted one word for another, or instead of saying, "Mother is older than her sisters", said "Mother is better than her sisters". The patient wrote well, but sometimes made spelling errors. His visual memory was normal. After a few repetitions he was able to draw ten abstract geometrical figures which he had seen, yet, after ten verbal repetions of a list of ten words, he was still unable to repeat them himself (Fig. 17). He was also unable to repeat sentences and invariably responded to the request to do so by saying that he was unable to remember them.

This mild syndrome of aphasic disturbances became greatly intensified whenever the patient was excited. When he became agitated his speech immediately lost all substantive words and was composed of the phrases typical of patients with sensory aphasia. The following is a sample of this kind of speech: "I told him ... that's enough ... when this ... when this is all over ... maybe this won't end ... They say not to climb up there ... and just get out of here ... and that's not right .... this helps ...", etc. When he was in this condition he was unable to pronounce certain words or to repeat phrases and his ability to comprehend what was said to him was considerably impaired.

This case is characteristic of lesions located in the border area between the temporal and occipital areas in that it presents a definite but mild syndrome of auditory speech disturbances. The primary symptom was a characteristic *instability* of the auditory images of words. This condition becomes more severe when a shift in affective state results in disturbance of the vascular equilibrium of the cortex and temporal area systems become disfunctional.

The next example shows the picture seen when the area damaged is that lying just anterior to the primary temporal speech area.

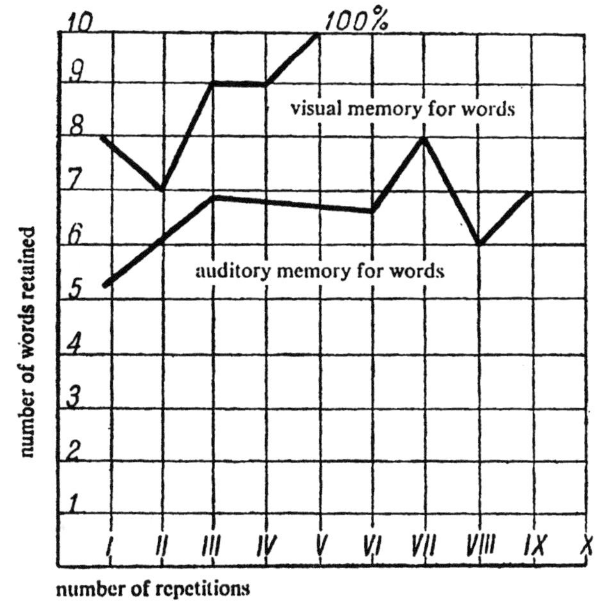

FIG. 17. Patient Voev.: memory curves for word lists.

Case 2

On December 2, 1941, patient Rom., age 22 (case history No. 1419) received a penetrating shrapnel wound of the right premotor area. A large part of the missile passed through the entire brain and came to rest in the central part of the left temporal lobe.

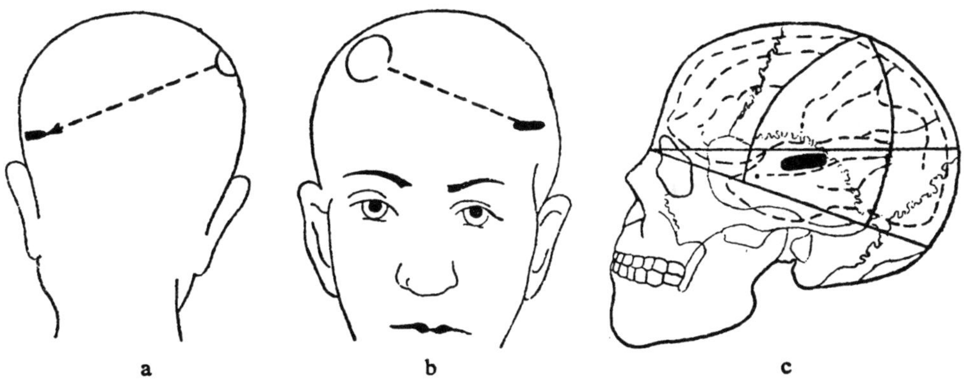

Patient Rom.: injury diagram (Case 2)

On the basis of X-rays it was determined that it lay in the area just anterior to the zone of Wernicke (Fig. 18). The patient was unconscious for a long period of time after injury; he showed a right hemiparesis which was especially prominent in the hand. The injury also produced severe disturbances of both sensory and motor aspects of speech. (The patient did not adequately comprehend the speech of others, forgot words, and was unable to pronounce them for a long time). His writing was seriously impaired. Gradually the paresis disappeared leaving only a very slight weakness in the right hand and hyperactive reflexes on the right. Severe speech disturbances continued for about one and a half month and then gradually disappeared.

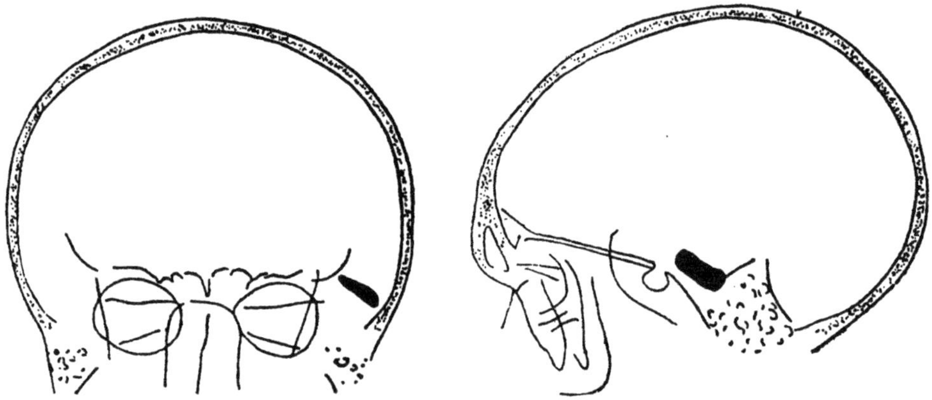

FIG. 18. Skull x-rays of Patient Rom. (Case 2).

When the patient was given a careful examination three months after injury he showed only slight residual signs of the righ hemisyndrome and a mild disturbance of complex coordinated movements. He had great difficulty in differentiating between different rhythms and perceived them poorly (this symptom will be considered further below). Spontaneous speech was relatively intact, and he understood the speech of others well enough. Against this background, however, clear signs of an auditory speech disorder were evident. The patient did not always distinguish clearly between similar phonemes; in some cases he had difficulty recognizing words; with several repetitions and changes in the instruction to point to his nose, eye, and ear he relatively quickly ceased to perceive the meanings of the words and began to confuse them. He was unable to represent to himself the phonemic components of words and had great difficulty when attempting to answer questions regarding the number of letters in the word "dom" (house), "most" (bridge), etc. His writing was severely impaired. Sometimes he would leave one or two letters out of a word; other times he would transpose letters making typical phonemic errors. It was very difficult for him to relate narrative material; he complained that he was unable to hold any kind of long phrase or quote in his memory. Intellectual functions unrelated to auditory speech, computation for example, were unaffected. After rehabilitation therapy the patient was released from the hospital with a slight residual disturbance of phonemic hearing, impaired abiliy to discriminate different rhythms, and a slight disturbance of the auditory analysis of words and written material.

The two cases presented above involve lesions of areas adjacent to the primary temporal speech areas. The same kinds of mild symptoms may also be seen in cases of nonpenetrating wounds which produce local contusions of the left temporal lobe. They differ from the previous cases primarily by the fact that the symptoms disappear more rapidly. We shall present one case which is typical of this group.

Case 3

On July 11, 1943, patient Budk., age 18 (case history No. 4056) received a shrapnel wound in the left temporal area. The skull itself was not damaged. As a result of contusion he lost consciousness for half an hour and was deaf in the left ear for a period of two days; no severe neurological symptoms were observed. Following the injury there

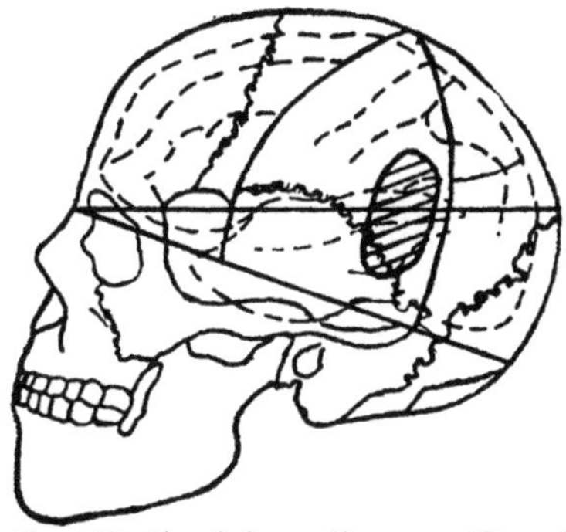

Patient Budk.: injury diagram (Case 3)

was a noticeable disturbance of speech processes. The patient did not always comprehend the speech of others; sometimes common words sounded unfamiliar to him, "as though they were not spoken in Russian". Sometimes it was necessary to ask the patient several times what word he was trying to say before he pronounced it clearly enough to be understood. He also had active speech difficulties; he often confused words and was unable to express his thoughts. These disturbances lasted a few days. Upon examination two weeks after injury his speech had recovered well, his memory for spoken phrases was good, and only a slight but persistent disturbance of phonemic hearing gave indication of the focal lesion. In this case the subsequent rapid and complete recovery of all functions may be ascribed both to the nature of the wound and to characteristics of the patient himself. His genealogy was such as to suggest the presence of latent left handedness.

All of the cases presented so far show that wounds of the left temporal lobe which primarily produce contusions with no widespread destruction of brain tissues, can evoke mild forms of the temporal aphasic syndrome. In some cases these may persist for a long time; in others they may undergo rapid recovery. More severe damage to the left temporal lobe, the postero-superior part in particular, usually produces pronounced and long-lasting aphasias. We shall present two cases belonging to this group.[9]

Case 4

On July 21, 1942, patient Burs., age 30, (case history No. 2218) received a penetrating shrapnel wound of the posterior portion of the left temporal area. Later this injury was complicated by the development of an abcess at the wound site. The patient was in deep coma following injury; when he recovered consciousness a transient right hemiparesis and more persistent right hemianopsia were noted. From the time of injury the patient was unable to understand the speech of others; when more than one person spoke at a time or someone spoke to him from a distance the words seemed to blend into one another and what he heard was undifferentiable noise.

Spontaneous speech was difficult for him because of in inconstancy of verbal images and because he often could not find the words he wanted; instability of the phonemic com-

[9] These patients were given detailed psychological examinations by Ė. S. Bejn, who also directed their rehabilitation therapy.

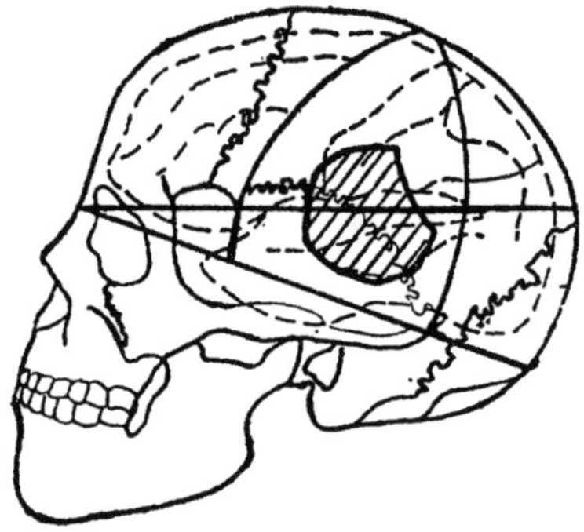

Patient Burs.: injury diagram (Case 4)

ponents of words prevented him from communicating. He showed clear signs of an amnesic disturbance which gave his speech a halting quality. He was unable to remember his address or the names of relatives, and even his own name sometimes sounded so strange to him that he was unable to recognize it. He was completely unable to write.

A detailed examination of the patient was initiated a month after injury. At that time there were no signs of sensory deficits or pathological reflexes; only the right hemianopsia remained. He had no motor speech difficulties, but his spontaneous speech was marked by constant searching for the correct sound images of words; he would repeatedly pronounce aloud the word he wanted until he found the pronunciation which sounded correct. His intonation was expressive, but his speech contained very few substantive words. Literal and verbal paraphasias were very common ("My head is ba . . . bad. They had to do an . . . this . . . offe . . . my head . . . they . . . operation . . . it was bad . . . it hurt . . . they had to . . . I myself . . . this . . . ka . . . ha . . . heart . . . out – in the Far East . . . I was there . . . From the first they took . . . us triko . . . tracto . . . tractor . . . drivers . . ." etc.) Perception of sounds was clearly impaired. The patient repeated and wrote down pairs of oppositional phonemes incorrectly ("bapa" was pronounced "baba" or "papa", etc.) and it was clear that he was unaware of the errors which he made. It was virtually impossible for him to repeat complex words, much less whole phrase, since he did not perceive the individual sounds of which they were composed ("futljar" (box) became "ful . . . fulton . . . fulatrij . . ."; "karandaš" (pencil) became "gragaš . . . dra . . . . . . tarakaš . . .", etc.). Writing to dictation was equally severely impaired. Only with great difficulty was the patient able to find the correct names of objects, and the process by which he sought words showed that the difficulty was in finding the sound components. Thus when he tried to pronounce the word "nogot" (finger nail) he uttered the following: "neyk . . . neyko . . . nyet . . . oboždi (no . . . wait) . . . tzokol (base) . . . nakal . . . lokol . . . nakol". Similarly, when he tried to say the word "futljar" (box) he uttered the following: "how do you . . . oh yes . . . fljurt . . . fli . . . fljar . . ." When the examiner prompted him with the syllable "fu" he continued, "fljurt . . . fut . . . fut . . . ne fljar (not "fljar") . . . flar . . . fljur . . ." With further prompting from the examiner, "futlja . . ." he continued again, "fuglja . . . filtra . . . fljurta . . ." Word comprehension was also severely impaired and, while he was able, at the beginning, to point correctly to his nose, eye, and ear, after a few times he became confused and asked, "nos . . . nos . . . nas (nose . . . nose . . . us) . . . what is that?" Of course the meanings of less familiar words were even less accessible to him. When asked the meanings of such words, he would try repeatedly to figure them out. Thus being unable to recognize the word "lososina" (salmon meat) he attempted over and over to recall its meaning and, in the process, confused it with other words which are similar in sound: "osina (aspen tree) ... liso ... lisosina ... lisosina ... What is it? I don't know." The patient was better able to understand whole sentences; usually he was able to catch fragments and the general context which permitted him to understand their general meaning. Often he was able to do this so successfully that his disability was inapparent, but if one then presented sentences which were more complex he fell into a state of helpless confusion which clearly revealed his difficulty. Thought processes which depended upon speech mechanisms were naturally disturbed by the inconstancy and confusion of verbal meanings. Intellectual operations other than overt speech, e.g. written calculation, were performed with minimal difficulty, but if they were made so complex as to demand incorporation into a verbal plan, they became insolvable.

Writing was definitely disturbed; in the initial period after injury the patient was unable to write even the simplest letters, syllables, or words as they were dictated to him. On the other hand he was fully capable of copying written material.[10] He was able to write numbers which were dictated to him more accurately than other words, although even in this case, loss of the meanings of the words representing digits was occasionally revealed when he would substitute one number for another. Initially his reading ability was limited to the recognition of very common words (visual ideograms). Eventually he was able to read better than he could write.

After four months of rehabilitation therapy the patient was released from the hospital with his symptoms greatly reduced.

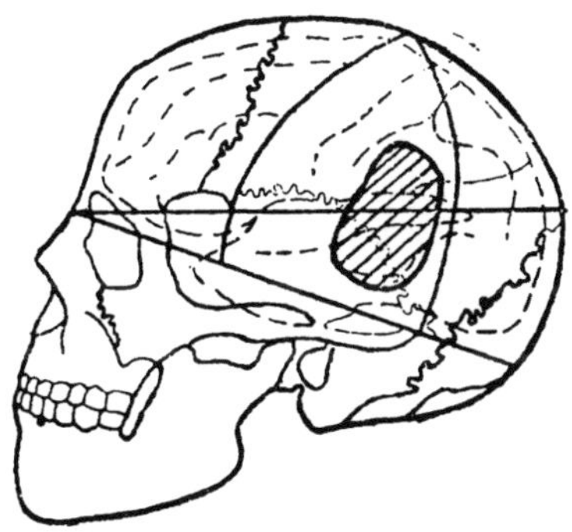

Patient Zvor.: injury diagram (Case 5)

Case 5

In May, 1942, patient Zvor., age 24, (case history No. 1991) received a penetrating shrapnel wound in the posterior part of the left temporal area. He was unconscious for a long time after injury and suffered from a severe right spastic hemiparesis which was most pronounced in the arm. He also had pathological reflexes of the right and a right hemianopsia. From the time of injury he had a total aphasia; he could neither talk nor understand the speech of others. He was treated at several different hospitals "name unknown" and came under our observation two months after injury. It first became possible to communicate with the patient one month later. Up until that time his speech was unintelligible, he continually confused word sounds, and, pointing to his arm, leg, or tongue would say: "Trudno ... trudno (it's hard ... I want to ... and I don't know". His spontaneous speech was made up of fragments of phrases and words, some of which had meaning and others of which were nonsense: "Ja ranen ... ranen (I'm wounded ...

[10] For a discussion of this phenomenon, see Chapters 13 and 16, Part 4.

wounded) ... projd ... front (front) ... brop ... davlo ... ne mogu (I can't) ... tak (so) ... flonde ... raka (brandy) ... fu ... i nu evo (and, well, his ...)". The patient was unable to give his own name and was only able to show where he had come from by pointing out the place on a map. His phonemic hearing was severely disturbed; he could not discriminate between correlative phonemes and, as a result, was unable to repeat phrases or name objects. Speech comprehension was disturbed as a consequence of a severe word deafness; when he was asked to point out his nose he repeated the word "nose" several times and then said confusedly, "I don't know". Writing was severely disturbed; he was unable to write down a single letter dictated to him. Only later did his ability to write recover, and it was accompanied by considerable difficulty in the sound analysis of words.[11] He was unable to do simple calculations orally, although with pencil and paper he was able to calculate relatively well; functions involving spatial analysis were retained.

The patient improved considerably with rehabilitation therapy. He still showed signs of defective phonemic hearing, but he could understand the speech of other relatively well and had no difficulty in writing or expressing his own thoughts orally.

The two cases just presented show clearly the syndromes of temporal, acoustic aphasia. Underlying this syndrome is a phonemic hearing disorder as a result of which the subjective sound of a word ceases to be fixed and constant, the precise meaning of a word is easily lost, and all that remains of its meaning is the general "semantic sphere" to which it belongs. Oral speech becomes impossible, since it is deprived of substantive words and is interrupted by numerous paraphasias. Writing ability is severely disturbed.

The study of a mass of wartime traumatic injuries made it possible for us to observe this syndrome in a rather large number of cases involving lesions of the superior parts of the left temporal lobe (primarily in the posterior area). Figure 19 and the corresponding table summarize these data.

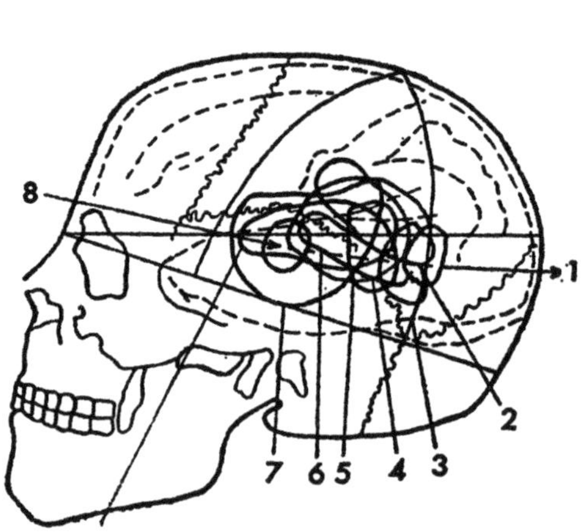

FIG. 19. Schematic diagram of lesions in cases of temporal (acoustic) aphasia.

[11] Samples of the writing of this patient are presented in Chapter 13.

Lesions observed in cases of temporal (acoustic) aphasia

Case No.	Name	Nature and localisation of wound	Speech disturbance
1	Pavl.	Penetrating shrapnel wound in superior part of left temporal area; right hemianopia.	Severe sensory aphasia with impairment of phonemic hearing, loss of the meanings of words, inability to name objects, literal and verbal paraphasias, and writing disturbance.
2	Gird.	Penetrating wound by a bullet which entered the anterior part of the left temporal area and emerged from the posterior part of the same area; persistent right hemiparesis with sensory disturbances and right hemianopia.	Residual severe sensory aphasia with disturbance of phonemic hearing, loss of the meanings of words, considerable difficulty in naming objects, and writing defect.
3	Tar.	Penetrating shrapnel wound in superior part of left temporal area; transitory hemiparesis with sensory disturbance; right hemianopia.	Signs of sensory aphasia with impairment of phonemic hearing, loss of the meanings of some words, literal paraphasias, and severe writing disturbance.
4	Vlas.	Penetrating shrapnel wound in left temporal area; severe right hemiparesis.	Signs of sensory aphasia with disturbance of phonemic hearing, loss of the meanings of words, difficulty in naming objects, literal and verbal paraphasias, and writing disorder.
5	Bash.	Penetrating shrapnel wound in the left temporal area; transitory right hemiparesis.	Severe signs of sensory aphasia with disturbance of phonemic hearing, loss of the manings of words, difficulty in naming objects literal and verbal paraphasias, and severe writing disorder.
6	Nik.	Superficial penetrating wound in the left temporal area; right hemiparesis.	Residual signs of sensory aphasia with disturbance of phonemic hearing, difficulties in the auditory analysis of sounds, and signs of temporal dysgraphia.
7	Osip.	Penetrating shrapnel wound in the left parieto-temporal area; transitory right hemiparesis; right hemianopia.	Severe sensory aphasia with disturbance of phonemic hearing, loss of the meanings of words, extreme difficulty in naming objects, literal and verbal paraphasias, and difficulties of auditory analysis; severe writing disorder.
8	Chus.	Direct shrapnel injury in the left temporal area with massive damage to cerebral structures; severe right hemiparesis.	Severe sensory aphasia with a clear disturbance of phonemic hearing, total loss of the meanings of words, "verbal salad", and total writing disability.

The clinical picture described thus far does not cover all of the symptoms which may be seen as the result of temporal lobe lesions. If *inferior parts* of the left temporal lobe are damaged, the syndrome is different.

So far we know little about the cortical structures which make up the postero-inferior part of the left temporal lobe. All the evidence collected to date indicates that the posterior part of Brodmann's area 21 and the adjacent part of area 37 are no less complex in structure than the area considered above. According to S. M. Blinkov these constitute the newest part of the temporal area. Judging from its structure, which is characterized by a rather diffuse distribution of cells and predominance of association fibers, it belongs to the more complex group of structures.

There is probably some basis for the idea that area 37 plays an important role in the coordination of functions between the auditory and visual analyzers. Penfield has given great attention to analysis of the temporal systems and has suggested that they are important for the *preservation and re-excitation of memory traces.* His findings support the position outlined above.[12]

The best data regarding the function of these areas come to us from clinical cases involving tumors or otogenic abcesses which sometimes came to involve the posterior part of the second temporal gyrus. Such cases have been studied by Niessl von Mayendorf, Luciani and Sepilli, Monakow, Kleist, and others. They involve a characteristic disturbance of *auditory memory*, thus giving rise to a special form of "amnesic aphasia" which has taken its place in the neurosurgical and oto-neurological clinics.

Patients with tumors or otogenic abcesses involving the inferior left temporal area usually do not show severe sensory disorders initially; their difficulties are more closely related to disturbances of auditory memory. Although writing ability and the comprehension of speech are preserved for a longer time in these patients, they are unable to remember a long sentence or to reproduce certain words; they may have serious difficulty in naming objects. Initially their intellectual faculties remain relatively intact, and their verbal thought processes are only marred by the great instability of their speech processes.

At first glance this "acoustic-amnesic" syndrome[13] appears to exist independently of any other form of disorder; but on more careful observation it is found to be

[12] We are unable here to give a detailed account of Penfield's hypothesis in this regard. It has been discussed in a number of publications (Penfield, 1952, 1954, 1959 *et al.*). Attempts to relate memory function directly to the temporal lobe seem to us to be somewhat premature, and at the present time not very convincing. Such conjecture will require considerably more physiological and psychologcial analysis before it can be accepted with confidence. Most significant, it seems to us, is the general finding that in man (who possesses auditory speech) memory, as a highly verbal function, is related to the temporal areas of the brain.

[13] During last years a careful study of the disturbance of acoustic verbal memory was carried out by Dr. M. Klimkovskij in his dissertation *Disturbances of verbal acoustic memory with lesions of the left temporal lobe* (Moscow, 1966).

intimately related to more general temporal disturbances, in particular to the sensory aphasic disorders observed in cases of damage to superior parts of the left temporal area.

Kabeljanskaja, Sukhovskaja, and Markova have observed that in some of these patients auditory analysis and synthesis may remain relatively intact. Phonemic hearing is often not severely disturbed. In more severe cases or by the use of more sensitive tests on less severe cases it is possible to demonstrate a slight auditory impairment which sometimes makes relatively common words sound strange or foreign to these patients. They do not show striking signs of sensory aphasia, but when the acoustic "load" is great certain words lose meaning for them. This form of acoustic aphasia does not involve words representing objects as often as it does terms which are uncommon in every day speech. The forgetting of words which occurs in these patients may appear to be an isolated symptom, but occasionally it can be quite clearly shown to be based upon a defect in auditory memory, i.e., it turns out that prompting by the investigator is of no help to the patient. This confirms the fact that an acoustico-gnostic disturbance underlies the overt memory difficulty. Finally, there is one other observation characteristic of these patients. In some cases a word will preserve its precise phonemic structure for the patient, but he will gradually forget its meaning; it comes to sound like a new word, and he is unable to recognize it.

All of the above findings bring this group of cases closer to the general group of temporal aphasias. They simply show that the "alienation" of word meanings may arise at different stages in the auditory recognition of words, and that the sound structure of words, which presupposes a unity of sound and meaning, must be studied more thoroughly. At present the correct interpretation of this syndrome is unclear. Some authors (Bejn) see it as a stage in the recovery from sensory aphasia; while others (Šmidt, et al) believe that it should be considered a separate syndrome. The latter refer to it as the syndrome of "transcortical temporal aphasia" and suggest that it arises from a complex disturbance of an associative system.

Our observations of traumatic brain injuries incurred on the battlefield confirmed the fact that the type of syndrome just described may arise as the result of injury in the inferior part of the left temporal area. It was characteristic of these cases that in the initial period following injury there was no severe disruption of speech hearing accompanied by the usual total agraphia and inability to communicate verbally.

Usually during the early post-traumatic period these patients had difficulty in understanding the speech of others, but this symptom rapidly disappeared leaving behind no severe impairment of phonemic hearing, reading, or writing. Ordinarily the only persistent disturbance affected the organization of internal processes related to auditory memory.

We shall present two cases illustrating this group of disorders.

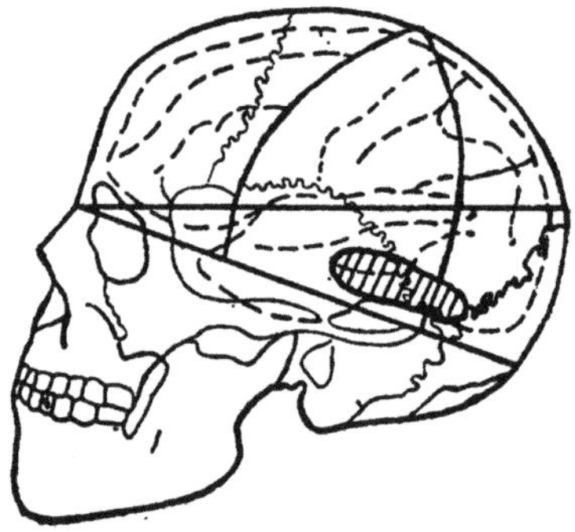

Patient Kash.: injury diagram (Case 6)

Case 6

On February 11, 1942, patient Kaš., age 25 (case history No. 1629) received a penetrating shrapnel wound in the lower left temporo-occipital area. The injury was not accompanied by any serious motor or sensory deficits, but there was a noticeable right hemianopsia. Immediately following injury he did not speak and did not understand the speech of others: ("I could hear, but I couldn't imagine what the words meant".) Speech comprehension recovered somewhat within a month, but it was still necessary to repeat every sentense several times before the patient understood it. He would perceive the first word but was unable to remember the remaining words and the sentence as a whole was lost. There were analogous disturbances in his active speech. He could pronounce individual words but was unable to form whole sentences, since he was unable to embrace all of the component words at once; ("I would say one word but forget what was to come next, or I would say the next and forget what word went before, and I could not connect words into sentences"). When the patient came to our attention (three months after injury) the impairment of phonemic hearing was hardly noticeable. His spontaneous speech was frequently interrupted by word searching which resulted from the fact that he was unable to retain whole sentences. Paraphasias were not observed. By the end of a three month stay, the lability of phonemic hearing had completely disappeared. The patient was able to pronounce individual words without difficulty, but there remained a rather severe impairment of the ability to repeat long phrases; even after seven or eight attempts he was unable to repeat a long sentence presented to him orally. This symptom contrasted sharply with his excellent memory for individual words and made considerably more difficult any kinds of intellectual functions which might be performed orally or silently. The patient was released from the hospital with his speech well recovered, but with a definite impairment of the ability to remember long statements.

Case 7

On September 29, 1942, patient Pol. (case history No. 3312) received a penetrating shrapnel wound in the infero-posterior part of the left temporal lobe at its occipital border. He was unconscious for a long period of time following the injury but showed no signs of motor or sensory deficits. There was a pronounced right hemianopia. Motor speech was not disturbed and the patient usually comprehended the speech of others; occasionally he did not understand long sentences and complained that he was unable to keep in mind the sequence of components in such sentences. He had difficulty in recalling certain words and frequently was unable to name various objects. When he was asked who had wounded him he substituted "a Finn" for the forgotten word "German". From the beginning he had no difficulty in writing, but he was unable to compose

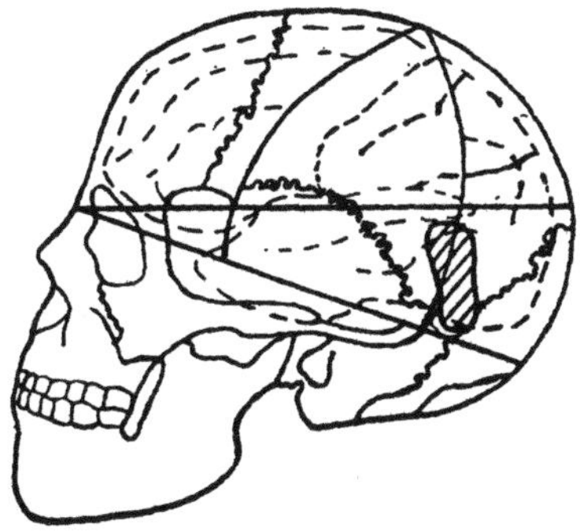

Patient Pol.: injury diagram (Case 7)

sentences. When he was admitted to the hospital two and a half months after injury he was perfectly capable of understanding common words, although he had forgotten the meanings of many less familiar words. Phonemic hearing was preserved; he wrote without error. There were virtually no signs of word deafness. He had difficulty in committing to memory any material of a sequential nature if it was presented in verbal form; he also had difficulty in carrying out a list of instructions in the required order. This symptom was all the more interesting in view of the complete preservation of his ability to remember individual words. The deficits of auditory memory described above prevented the patient from performing any type of intellectual operation involving verbal functions. After three months he was released from the hospital. His condition had improved considerably, but he still had difficulty in remembering the sequence of verbal items presented orally.

The impression that two different syndromes accompany lesions to different parts of the left temporal lobe appears to be based on fact. Clinical analysis indicates that the two syndromes are distinguishable not only by the frequency with which they occur but also by the level at which the integration of auditory processes is disturbed.

Careful analysis shows also that the sites of lesions giving rise to the two syn-

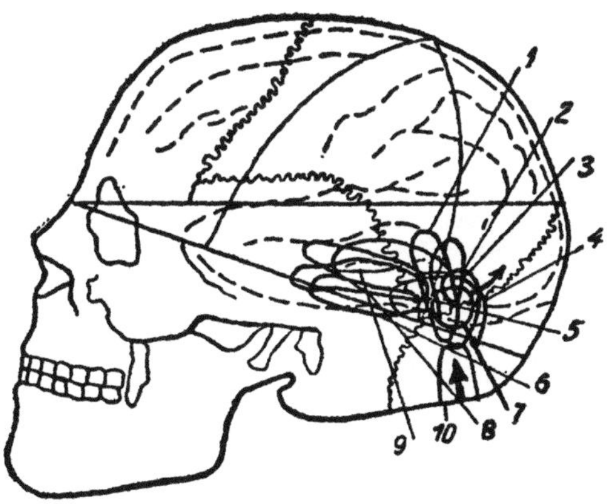

FIG. 20. Schematic diagram of lesions in cases of the temporal acoustico-mnestic syndrome.

Lesions observed in cases of acoustico-mnestic aphasia

Case No.	Name	Nature and localization of wound	Speech disturbance
1	Petr.	Penetrating shrapnel wound in the left temporo-occipital area; right hemianopia.	Signs of acoustic-mnestic aphasia, negligible disturbance of phonemic hearing; difficulty in remembering long sentences; speech pure with no sign of paraphasia; writing intact.
2	Gus.	Penetrating shrapnel wound in the left temporo-occipital area; hearing impaired in the left ear; noticeable ataxia; nystagmus.	Slight signs of acoustico-mnestic aphasia with negligible disturbance of phonemic hearing, preservation of articulation, and slight temporal dysgraphia.
3	Siz.	Penetrating shrapnel wound in the left lower temporo-parieto-occipital area; right hemianopia.	Severe acoustico-mnestic aphasia with loss of word meanings; phonemic hearing preserved; literal paraphasia absent; writing intact.
4	Volk.	Penetrating shrapnel wound in the left lower temporal area; vestibular disturbances; visual field defect on the right.	Residual signs of acoustico-mnestic aphasia; considerable difficulty in retaining sequential material; phonemic hearing intact; writing intact; connected speech unchanged.
5	Mor.	Direct penetrating wound in the left temporo-occipital area; residual right hemiparesis and visual field defect on the right.	Clear signs of acoustico-mnestic disturbance (difficulty in naming objects, loss of the meanings of words difficulty in remembering sequential verbal material); phonemic hearing undisturbed; literal paraphasia absent; writing intact.
6	Red.	Penetrating shrapnel wound in the left lower temporal area; no severe neurological symptoms.	Residual signs of temporal aphasia; definite disturbance of phonemic hearing and loss of the meanings of some words; residual dysgraphia.
7	Khrom.	Penetrating shrapnel wound in the left temporo-occipital area with disturbance of reading and right visual field defect.	Residual signs of temporal aphasia; certain difficulties in remembering long sentences; phonemic hearing preserved, but the sequence of sounds not retained; speech and writing intact.
8	Karp.	Shrapnel wound in the left mastoid process with contusion of the temporal lobe.	Slight signs of temporal aphasia; difficulty in remembering verbal sequences and loss of word meanings; phonemic hearing undisturbed; speech connected and expressive; writing intact.
9	Pod.	Direct shrapnel wound in lower parts of the left temporal area; metal fragments imbedded deep in brain structures; slight right visual field defect.	Residual signs of acoustico-mnestic aphasia with slight impairment of phonemic hearing, obvious difficulty in finding words, but rare difficulty in understanding the meanings of words; writing intact.

dromes are different. A comparison of Figure 19 with the combined lesions shown in Figure 20 is sufficient to show this difference. Figure 20 presents cases in which damage to the infero-posterior border of the left temporal lobe produced the second form of temporal aphasia described above. It indicates that these areas are probably directly related to the higher integration of auditory speech processes.

We have taken for consideration those syndromes of temporal aphasia which are directly associated with damage to the cortical part of the auditory analyzer and for which the physiological mechanisms are most clear. Other clinical syndromes which are referred to as "transcortical aphasia" or "visual aphasia" and which arise as the result of lesions in the temporal or temporo-occipital areas have not been mentioned here. The physiological basis of such syndromes will be given special consideration in another place.

VI

THE PATHOLOGY OF AFFERENT SYSTEMS AND THE SYNDROME OF "AFFERENT (APRAXIC) MOTOR APHASIA"

We have considered disturbances of the external, auditory aspect of speech which occur as the result of damage to cortical parts of the auditory analyzer located in the left temporal area. Now we shall turn to a consideration of the brain mechanisms underlying the *motor aspect of speech*; we shall take up the analysis of focal lesions which give rise to *expressive, or motor aphasia.*

Motor aphasia, the first form of aphasia to be met in the clinic, was first described almost a hundred years ago. Despite this, however, recent physiological findings require that we substantially alter our approach to the study of brain mechanisms underlying the motor act and revise our conceptions of what causes disturbances of the motor aspect of speech.

A. THE AFFERENT ORGANIZATION OF MOTOR ACTIONS AND DISTURBANCES OF MOVEMENT

At one time it seemed to be a well established neurophysiological fact that motor activity is related primarily to efferent structures of the nervous system, e.g., the anterior horns of the spinal gray matter and the cortical motor areas. Studies in recent decades, however, have forced significant changes in this viewpoint. Investigations carried out by I. P. Pavlov and his collaborators (Krasnogorskij, 1911; Miller and Konorskij, 1936; Skipin, 1951; and others) have shown that the central cortical structures associated with the organization of movements should be considered to make up a special *motor analyzer*. The only difference between this analyzer and those associated with exteroceptive analysis lies in the fact that its function is related to the analysis and synthesis of proprioceptive and kinesthetic impulses rather than impulses arising in exteroreceptors. Such impulses arise in the muscular structures and are transmitted to the central parts of the analyzer. By facilitation (raising the excitability level of some complexes of active elements) and inhibiton (lowering the excitability level of others) the same processes of analysis and synthesis are performed as occur in the cortical parts of other analyzers. We are also indebted to Pavlov for another no less important conception. According to his findings the cortical part of the motor analyzer is by no means restricted to the precentral gyrus. It is true that this cortical area may be looked upon as the special "exit route" of impulses arising in the cerebral cortex, but according to his conception, the motor analyzer itself is made up of a large number of associated but widely distributed structures lying both anterior and posterior to the precentral gyrus.[1]

Our present conceptions regarding the role of afferent structures in carrying out movements are based upon a large series of investigations performed by Soviet physiologists in recent decades. Early experiments by L. A. Orbeli and Kunstman showed that deafferentation abolishes the control of limb movements. P. K. Anokhin (1935, 1955) came to the same conclusion on the basis of experiments demonstrating that after deafferentation an extremity loses its characteristic forms of movement; subsequently its movements are restricted to those which are organized at a lower level as part of a system which is still intact, e.g. the respiratory system. Another investigator who has done no less for the theory regarding organization of movements is N. A. Bernštejn (1935, 1947). He has shown that the number of degrees of freedom of movement in most joints of the extremities is so great that it is in principle impossible that they be controlled by efferent impulses alone. A decisive link in the control mechanism underlying variable voluntary movements is the afferent part of the reflectory arc. When we consider the fact that the afferent limb transmits impulses back from the moving muscles and joints themselves, our former conception of the reflex arc gives way to the conception of a "reflex circle" or a "closed reflex ring". Modern concepts of cybernetics confirm conclusively the importance of feedback for the structure of any regulatory mechanism and again, bring our attention to the role which the afferent systems play in patterning of motor activity. These concepts have forced us to take a new approach to questions dealing with the cerebral organization of motor processes.

Contemporary views regarding the motor area of the cerebral cortex differ considerably from those held earlier. More and more frequently one finds in the literature the view that the sensorimotor area of the cortex, where the precentral and postcentral gyri unite, is essentially a *single structure*, or that it acts as part of a more complex functional system. (Cf. Phillips, 1966.)

Penfield and Rasmussen (1950) have found that motor reactions may be produced by stimulating either the precentral or postcentral area directly. In their experiments it appeared that the parts of the postcentral gyrus which were most clearly associated with carrying out motor acts were those related to hand movements and those related to the articulation and phonation apparatus (Fig. 21). Two important anatomical findings support the view that structures other than the precentral and postcentral gyri participate in the organization of movement. First, there are well developed connections between the precentral and post-

[1] We have reviewed this conception of the motor analyzer in another place. See A. R. Luria, "The Motor Analyzer and the Cortical Organization of Movement" in: *Human Brain and Psychological Processes* (Moscow, 1963); English edition, N.Y., Harper & Row, 1966.

central gyri, many of which pass through the thalamus; secondly, according to the (1938-1948), Woolsey (1952 *et al.*) only a relatively small proportion of fibers making up the pyramidal tract actually arise from Betz cells in the motor cortex.

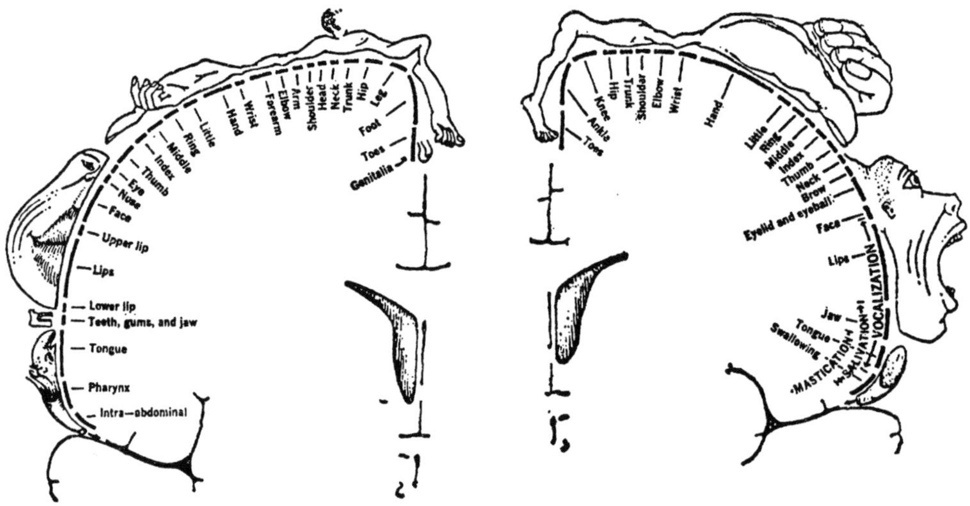

Fig. 21. Somatotopic representation of motor and sensory processes in the precentral and postcentral gyri (Penfield and Rasmussen).

What kind of role might postcentral cortical structures play in the formation of motor activity? We have accumulated some data relevant to this question from cases involving focal lesions of the postcentral areas. Clinical observations have clearly indicated that the "sensory" areas (tactile and kinesthetic) and the complex secondary areas adjacent to them play an important role in the organization of motor processes. Early neurological investigations showed that the cerebral mechanisms of complex coordinated actions do not reside altogether in the precentral motor cortex but are associated with functions of the postcentral structures. The latter appear to suppress irrelevant impulses and thus permit expression of the correct synergic systems. Damage to these areas can produce quite diverse motor disturbances. In some cases one observes a "pseudo-paresis" in which a limb retains its original strength but, having lost all sensation, cannot be controlled. In other cases these motor disorders take the form of ataxias and other disturbances of coordination which are well known to the clinic. Finally, in the most complex cases, one sees a loss of the motor components of complex activities. All of these disturbances lead to the loss of differentiated motor impulses, to the loss of the ability to shift the extremities rapidly and smoothly into a desired position. Patients lose the ability to carry out differentiated movements.

The postcentral gyrus is not the only afferent structure of the cerebral cortex which may play a role in increasing the precision of motor action. A number of investigations have shown that damage to more complex secondary areas located in the inferior portion of the parietal lobe may also affect motor activity. These areas are involved in the integration of exteroceptive and proprioceptive impulses into spatial schemata, and damage to them can produce "mnestic" (ideational) forms of apraxia. It is characteristic for patients with such lesions to substitute one movement for another, so that it becomes impossible to carry out any kind of complicated sequence of motor acts. They do not possess the variety of spatial and proprioceptive schemata which are necessary for movements oriented toward external objects.

Special electromyographic studies of patients with lesions of the postcentral cortical areas have added more precision to our clinical observations and have taken us a step closer to the physiological analysis of movement. In an investigation carried out in our laboratory by I. Zambran (1948) it was shown that, whereas in normal subjects the acts of grasping and opening the hand involve a high degree of coordination of agonists and antagonists, in patients with lesions of the postcentral area the picture is considerably different. Impulses lose their selectivity and come to activate muscles which are not related to the desired movement. In Figure 22 we present a sample electromyogram showing the degree to which impulses may be misdirected to various muscle groups in cases of postcentral cortical lesions.

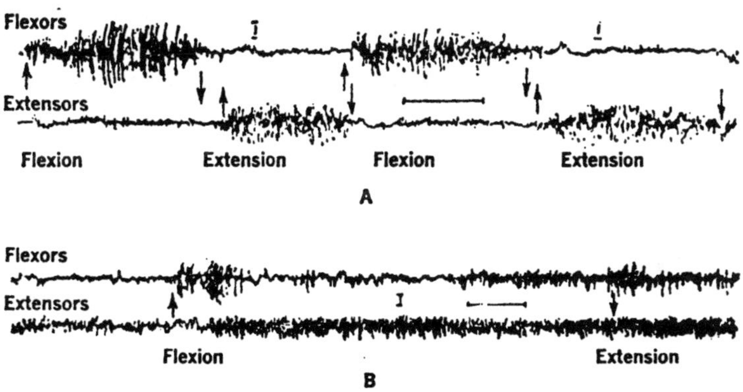

FIG. 22. Electromyograms showing flexion and extension of the hand by a normal subject and by patients with lesions of the postcentral area. A: normal; B: a case involving a tumor in the postcentral area — a. before operation; b. after operation; c. after operation. (From I. I. Zambran).

On the basis of the above evidence we are forced to conclude that *the postcentral parts of the cortex play an important role in the organization of motor acts*. By making more precise the direction of impulses from other analyzers to specific muscle groups, they play a programming role in the organization of motor impulses.[2]

[2] Pribram (1958), in particular, has pointed out such a programming function and its relationship to the secondary afferent areas of the cortex (the intrinsic dorsolateral areas).

Under various conditions the pattern of afferent impulses necessary to evoke a given movement is not always the same. Depending upon the situation and the type of movement, it may originate from different sources and be mediated at different levels. Thus the afferent synthesis necessary for the coordination of locomotion, i.e., for the patterning of movement in space, occurs at a level which involves the objective perception of points in space. This function is performed by structures associated with vision and kinesthesis. They are the afferent structures which give rise to the patterns of excitation leading to appropriate movements. Patterns of activity organized at the "object manipulation level" on the other hand, require an altogether different type of motor coordination than that required for locomotion. Here the spatial patterns involved are of considerably less significance. The coordinations which this type of activity involves are more complex and variable, because it is possible to accomplish a certain change in the environment by any one of a number of muscular action patterns. The substitution of one action for another does not, in this case, change the significance of the organization of the manipulatory act. It involves the complex integration of visual, vestibular, and kinesthetic impulses, perhaps, but this function is subordinated to higher processes associated with the most complex areas of the inferior temporal cortex which integrate the activity of the different analyzers. Finally, there is the system of still more complex movements which are related to all the forms of symbolic gesture and speech. This system is organized at a higher level than manipulatory activity. It makes new demands upon the afferent systems. The structures associated with this type of activity (meaningful activity mediated by the second signalling system), have a special relationship to afferent structures of the auditory analyzer. Speech movements require the neural organization of delicately patterned articulatory impulses which give rise to the utterance of words. These articulatory impulses can easily be substituted for one another in the sense that a given meaning may be communicated by any one of a number of different verbal constructions. But any given word in such a construction requires a specific pattern of articulatory impulses which give rise to a precise phonemic verbal speech pattern. It is natural to expect that a system for coding acoustico-semantic units into their kinesthetic equivalents should be an essential prerequisite for such afferent integrations.

All the ideas which we have outlined so far force us to recognize the importance of the postcentral cortical areas for the organization of motor processes.[3] Recent evidence regarding the anatomy of the cerebral cortex provides further basis for these conclusions.

The postcentral cortical areas comprise the postcentral gyrus (areas 3,1, and 2 of Brodmann), caudal parts of the parietal lobe (areas 5 and 7) and the anterior part of area 40. These areas developed largely as an outgrowth of that single sensory-motor area

[3] Many of these ideas have been developed in detail by N. A. Bernštejn in his book *The Structure of Movement* (Moscow, Medgiz, 1947).

in lower mammals which is associated with the integration of sensory and motor functions. In man this area has expanded and differentiated into several areas which are distinguishable from one another on the basis of their cytoarchitecture and their connections with other areas. From these characteristics it is possible to draw certain conclusions regarding their different functions. We have every reason to believe that areas 3 and 1 make up the primary sensory projection area and are, in this sense, analogous to area 4 of the motor system. The most outstanding characteristic of areas 3 and 1 is the predominance of the granular layer of afferent cells; there is an extremely well developed complex of projection fibers and stellate cells (Ramon y Cajal, G.I. Poljakov). Areas 2 and 5, typical examples of secondary areas (intrinsic areas), differ considerably from 1 and 3. Analogous to posterior parts of the premotor cortex, which preserve certain characteristics of the pimary motor cortex in area 4, these areas preserve the well developed granular layer seen in the primary sensory area. The greater development, however, of the second, third, and superficial part of the fourth layers, the "association" layers) in these areas compels us to think of them as playing an integrative role in cortical function. The neurons in these areas usally have short axons and are correspondingly arranged in associative complexes. This, plus the fact that these areas have been shown to receive a rich supply of vertical fibers from secondary thalamic nuclei (n. medialis dorsalis, n. centromedianum, n. anterior medialis), indicates that they should be considered secondary areas or, according to the terminology of G.I. Poljakov, "projection-association areas". The predominance of the association layers is characteristic also of area 7 and, to some extent, of the anterior parts or area 40, which represent the secondary cortical areas of greater complexity. These "projection-association" areas are associated with the organization of particular sensory-motor functions.

All of the evidence cited above causes us to expect that the postcentral cortical structures are an important part of the motor analyzer and that they are of great significance in the formulation of movements. The major difference between their function and that of the anterior premotor systems (which will be discussed further in the following chapter) is simply that they are involved in the *spatial* organization of complex coordinated actions, whereas the premotor areas play a role in the *serial* organization of motor actions (Lashley, 1937). The secondary postcentral areas are associated with programming that pattern of impulses directed to various muscle groups, which makes possible complex movements. It is inevitable that the afferent role which these areas play in making movements more precise should be reflected in a higher degree of topical specificity than is seen in the anterior, premotor areas.[4]

All of the views summarized so far are supported by the kinds of clinical findings associated with damage to postcentral cortical structures. If a wound directly involves the postcentral gyrus it naturally gives rise to disturbances of all forms of sensation, including deep sensation. More often than not it is accompanied by a clearcut motor disturbance, sometimes a particular form of "afferent paresis".

If an injury is located caudally, only partially involving the sensory projection area, but involving a major part of the secondary postcentral area, the resulting

[4] This fact is considered in more detail in Chapter 7.

paresis may be quite mild. The primary disorder seen in this case is either a cortical ataxia or the kind of disturbance of coordination which Foerster described in such detail and which resembles the syndrome referred to in classical neurological literature as "sensory apraxia" (see Monakow, 1914, p. 496). Patients with such injuries usually do not use the affected hand, even though it retains its strength and the movements which it makes are about as fast as normal. Ordinarily only fine selective movements are lost. The patient is unable to move his fingers individually or to place his hand in a desired position. He can only make rather undifferentiated movements ("shovel-hand"). Impulses destined for particular muscles of the fingers or hand sometimes arrive at the muscles for which they are intended and other times activate altogether different muscle groups. Sometimes they activate both agonists and antagonists diffusely, thus resulting in no movement at all; this may create the false impression that muscle power has been reduced. The misdirected transmission of impulses results in severe cortical ataxia and dysmetria which disrupts the schemata of coordinated movements and leads to the execution of movements which are inappropriate to the task at hand. These disturbances usually appear in the hand contralateral to the damaged cortical hemisphere and are most clearly expressed in cases where the dominant, left hemisphere is involved. When the lesion occurs in the left hemisphere, the ipsilateral hand may also be affected. The disturbance observed in either case is clearly afferent in nature (cf. Foerster, 1936).

Afferent disturbances of movement are not always associated with severe sensory disorders. If they involve higher levels of afferentation they do not disturb the acuity of sensation, but seriously affect the cutaneous-kinesthetic analysis and synthesis of impulses. The result is a loss of complex kinesthetic schemata which inevitably leads to the disturbance of coordinated movements. In this case, however, one does not observe paresis or ataxia, but rather faulty execution of the kinds of complex motor acts involved in manipulatory activity. Of course in these cases the disturbance of afferentation at a complex level is not limited to the contralateral limb. Loss of the afferent integrative function abolishes the ability to carry out complex movements with either hand. As we said earlier, such disturbances are observed most often in cases involving damage to the postcentral and inferior parietal areas of the *left*, dominant, hemisphere. The patient is unable to place his hand in a desired position. Thus when he is asked, for example, to extend his thumb and fifth finger or to make threatening or beckoning movements with his hand, he is unable to do so immediately and begins to search helplessly for the desired movements. He does not sense the correct position, and makes helpless, sometimes awkward, corrections of his first attempts. Only after repeated attempts and with great effort does he finally produce the necessary movement.

Such a "positional apraxia" reflects severe disturbances of the cortical organization of synergic muscle actions and often is a relatively isolated symptom; it may be unaccompanied by visuo-spatial or manipulatory apraxia. The technique for studying these disturbances will be described later. It is important to note that all of the disturbances which accompany these lesions differ radically from those observed in cases of premotor area lesions. As we shall see later, damage to that area affects the *temporal (dynamic) organization* of movements; there is a loss of smoothly changing kinesthetic patterns, loss of the smoothness of movements, and loss of the automaticity of sequential motor activity. In the present case, on the other hand, cortical damage is reflected in disturbances of the *proprioceptive and structural organization of movements*. Here there are no significant changes in the speed or smoothness of movement. Disturbance of the proprioceptive organization of movements leads to a characteristic *ataxia or positional apraxia*. This is the defect in function of the motor analyzer which arises as the result of lesions to the postcentral systems. We must keep this disturbance in mind when we analyze the different types of motor aphasia which result from such lesions.

B. THE SYNDROME OF AFFERENT (APRAXIC) MOTOR APHASIA

The syndrome of motor aphasia has been known for more than a hundred years; in fact, if one takes into account the work of Mark Dax, it has been known even longer. Yet neither the structure of this syndrome nor the precise cortical area associated with it have been definitely established. For this reason K. Goldstein, (1948) in a comprehensive review of his work, referred to "peripheral motor aphasia" as one of the most confusing problems of neurology. Whereas at one time motor aphasia, or "aphemia", was regarded as "forgetting of the motor images of words" and distinguished from dysarthria, recent investigations have severely shaken this position. As early as 1906 Marie set forth the idea that Wernicke's aphasia is a "true aphasia", whereas Broca's syndrome must be considered aphasia complicated by dysarthria. He saw the latter as a purely motor disturbance. Although this conception was not widely accepted in the form in which Marie presented it, the results of studies carried out by a number of different investigators tended to confirm it. Liepmann, Monakow, Nissl von Mayendorf, Nielsen, and others pointed out the apraxic nature of different forms of motor aphasia. Alajouanine, Ombredane, and Durant (1939), and later Ombredane (1951), on the basis of specially designed experimental investigations, described the phenomenon of "phonetic disintegration". They held that motor aphasia is a complex clinical entity which can be shown to possess paretic, dystonic, and apraxic components, any one of which can produce a severe articulatory disorder. More recently E. Bay (1957) has come to a similar conclusion on the basis of special studies involving the glossogram. This kind of evidence has made it necessary to turn away from more simple conceptions of motor aphasia and to begin to analyze the factors which produce motor speech disturbances; these studies indicate that the different components of motor-aphasias may vary in severity, independently of one another.

Numerous authors, in discussing the significance of different forms of motor aphasia in locating cortical lesions have commented on the complexity and lack of homogeneity of the different syndromes. Marie, who was the first to challenge the classical conception of motor aphasia, showed that the brain lesion in Broca's famous patient was not limited to the posterior parts of the third frontal gyrus; it extended considerably further posteriorly. Other cases have been described in which damage limited to Broca's area in right handers was not accompanied by aphasia in any form (Monakow, Goldstein). Finally, a number of authors (Nissl von Mayendorf, Monakow, Liepmann) have described cases in which motor aphasia resulted from lesions in areas bordering the lower part of the Rolandic fissure (Rolandic operculum). Such aphasias are associated with apraxia of the oral, lingual, and pharyngeal musculature. The idea that motor aphasia is a particular type of apraxia was developed in detail in the works of Liepmann and, to some extent, in the works of Monakow and others.

We have good reason to consider seriously the works of these authors and to accept the idea that motor aphasia presents a complex picture which may be broken down into a number of variations. Some forms are associated with disturbance of the *afferent organization of movements* and in particular with the afferent disturbance of movements of the speech apparatus. These are the types of motor aphasia which arise as the result of damage to the Rolandic-operculum and inferior parts of the left postcentral area. The results of those lesions in the postcentral area which we have described in general terms in the preceding pages are by no means restricted to difficulties in control of hand and finger movements. A number of such patients show analogous signs of *apraxic disturbances of the tongue and speech apparatus.*

Apraxic disturbances of the speech apparatus may be demonstrated by very simple tests. In severe cases (most commonly the result of lesions in the middle inferior parts of the postcentral area) even such a simple task as extending the tongue is impossible. Instead of putting out his tongue the patient goes through a whole series of helpless attempts of a clearly apraxic nature. In less severe cases this simple movement may be possible, but an instruction to touch the tongue to the upper lip may produce, again, only helpless uncoordinated attempts.[5] Sometimes the disturbances are even more subtle. For instance, the patient may be capable of passing all tests when he is relaxed; under more strained conditions, however, he experiences considerable difficulty. If he finds it difficult to touch his tongue to his upper lip, he may try to use his fingers to bring it into correct position, or he may use a mirror so as to be able to control his tongue movements visually.

This difficulty in performing motor acts according to instructions lies midway between the gross disorders described earlier and one last group of difficulties which may arise as the result of disturbance of the afferent systems. The last group is made up of patients who are able to carry out all of the instructions described

[5] Techniques for examining oral movements are presented in a later chapter (see Chapter 11).

above, but who are unable to perform any kind of symbolic movement of the tongue and lips. They are unable to demonstrate the movements involved in kissing, spitting, or clicking the tongue. This "symbolic" apraxia concludes the list of oral apraxias which are seen in cases where afferent systems of the posterior cortical areas are damaged.

We still do not have adequate knowledge about the localization of lesions which produce the kinds of syndromes described above or about the disturbances of afferent systems which underlie these syndromes. There is some reason to believe, however, that such syndromes are seen most clearly in cases involving lower parts of the postcentral area of the left hemisphere. Confirmation of this impression must await special investigation.

The idea that complex motor speech disturbances can all be reduced to disorders of oral movement is untenable. It is important to note that *the loss of precise oral movements removes an essential physiological prerequisite for accurate verbal expression*, and thus creates all the conditions necessary for the appearance of a special type of *"afferent motor aphasia"*.

"Afferent motor aphasia" is no novelty to the neurological literature. As early as 1900, Liepmann indicated that motor aphasia may sometimes be interpreted as an "apraxia of the speech musculature". A number of authors including Goldstein, Nissl von Mayendorf, Nielsen, Pötzl and Leonhardt have referred to the syndrome of "apraxic aphasia"; and Pötzl, in particular, has suggested that there exists a special "pseudo-motor aphasia" which may arise as the result of parietal lesions.

We studied this second form of motor aphasia on a number of patients who received brain injuries during the war. Disturbances of articulation were by no means seen in all cases involving damage to the postcentral systems. Thus we can say that there is a great degree of topical differentiation in this area. Table 6 shows that, in the initial period following injury to superior parts of the parietal lobe, only 40% of al cases showed signs of speech impairment; of these only one-third of these fell in the group showing severe symptoms, and symptoms persisted into the residual period in less than half of them. In cases involving injury to inferior parts of the parietal lobe, on the other hand, the number showing speech impairment in the initial period reached 95%, of which 75% remained in the residual period. In this group the overwhelming majority of disorders was severe. These figures show that clear forms of apraxic aphasia did not always follow left parietal lobe injury. They also help us to identify a mechanism which constituted an important component of a number of motor aphasias.

On the basis of careful examination it was possible to describe rather clearly the characteristics of "apraxic" aphasias. If it had been true that the disturbances were limited to the impairment of very simple sensory afferentation, then the motor speech disorders should all have been of an elementary nature. We would have observed a certain ataxia of the lingual musculature, imprecise articulation, and, in cases of bilateral injury, disturbances bordering on dysarthria. In some cases

TABLE 6

Severity and duration of aphasic syndromes with lesions in the left postcentral area

Site of injury in postcentral area	Total number of cases	Initial period			Residual period		
		severe forms (%)	slight forms (%)	total (%)	severe forms (%)	slight forms (%)	total (%)
Superior	32	16	25	41	0	19	19
Inferior	40	88	5	93	48	28	76

these were, indeed, the symptoms seen. But more often, parietal injuries resulted not in simple dysarthria but in disturbance of the selective schemata of articulation and a nearly pure aphasic syndrome.

In cases involving relatively small lesions, one may see simply an impairment of differentiated speech. The patient's speech becomes awkward and slow; he must often go through several attempts before he is able to find the correct position of the tongue for the word he wants to pronounce. In the most severe cases, the articulation difficulty may be so great that the patient is unable to utter a single sound. In less severe cases, pronunciation of consonants is more severely impaired than the pronunciation of vowels. Only after extensive retraining involving special techniques is such a patient able to relearn to articulate speech sounds.

The disturbances of articulatory processes seen in these cases differ sharply from those seen in cases involving lesions of the premotor systems (to be discussed below), and from the types of dysarthria which arise as the result of subcortical lesions. They differ also from the disturbances seen in the pseudo-bulbar syndrome which may arise as the result of bilateral cortical injuries. These disorders differ from those seen in premotor lesions in that the articulation difficulty is unaccompanied by any sign that the dynamics of speech processes have been disturbed. Here the disturbance of expressive speech consists in difficulty finding the necessary articulatory movements; this difficulty affects the pronunciation of individual sounds and sound sequences which go to make up words and phrases. Once the movements necessary for a given sound have been found, however, it is pronounced with none of the distortions which characterize the pronunciation of patients with premotor lesions. On the contrary, the attempts of these patients to produce particular sounds are highly variable. They produce a large number of inappropriate sound combinations with random substitution of individual sound components. Each attempt gives rise to a new complex of sounds. Thus the basic disturbance can be looked upon as a *positional apraxia of the speech organs and search for the articulatory movements appropriate for different sounds.* It is not a de-automatization of continuous speech or increased inertness of articulatory activity. With training the patient can relearn the tongue and lip positions necessary for producing different sounds and this difficulty disappears. He may continue for some time, however, to substitute one sound for another when the positions of the speech organs for the two sounds are similar, e.g., he may say "l" instead of "n" or "d", or he may say "m" instead of "b", or may say "s" instead of "t".

The disturbance of differentiations among similar articulatory positions is one of the most characteristic symptoms of this form of motor aphasia. Thus patients with afferent motor aphasia have special difficulties in articulating the sounds they want, i.e., in differentiating them from other sounds. Often such a patient will attempt to distinguish the articulatory positions for different sounds by feeling his own tongue and lips with his fingers as he pronounces them; he attempts to memorize the positions which produce appropriate sounds. Very often he will begin to use a mirror so as to be able to see the positions of his lips and tongue. He attempts to use these visual images for mastering the desired articulations. Discovery of the appropriate positions of lips and tongue turns out to be the primary obstacle to recovery of speech by such patients. Thus even in the latest phases of recovery, when they have adequately compensated for the basic disturbance, their speech is strained due to the high degree of voluntary effort required for articulating the desired sounds.

The form of "afferent (apraxic) aphasia" which we have been describing also differs in several respects from the usual syndrome of dysarthria. In cases of dysarthria the disturbance affects all types of fine movement which involve the tongue and vocal cords; the result is a characteristic slurring of speech. In the kind of motor aphasia which we have described, however, the disturbance is a selective one; it involves only the generalized schemata by which sounds are articulated. Thus a series of tests may indicate that such a patient is capable of producing some sounds relatively clearly, whereas he is incapable of producing others. In his attempts to articulate the latter sounds, he produces various incorrect sounds at random. Related to this is the fact that a patient with apraxia of the vocal apparatus can benefit from the use of visual and visuo-kinesthetic cues or even from verbal explanations of the way in which different sounds are articulated.

In addition to the characteristics already mentioned, this form of aphasia differs from dysarthria and "efferent motor aphasia" (to be described in the following chapter) by its special dynamics and its characteristic form of recovery. As we shall see, the articulation of different sounds poses no particular difficulty to patients with the kind of efferent motor aphasia which arises following lesions to the premotor and frontal systems. Their difficulties arise in the transition from articulation of individual sounds to the pronunciation of words and phrases, or in the transition from repeating words spoken by the examiner to spontaneous speech. These difficulties are altogether different from those seen in cases of "afferent motor aphasia". The difficulty in the latter lies almost completely in mastering the schemata of articulatory movements for different sounds. Thus, a given individual sound may be articulated differently depending upon the syllable in which it occurs. In general it makes little difference to these patients whether they are articulating individual sounds or syllables; similarly, they have no more difficulty with spontaneous speech than with repetitive speech. As a result, once they have regained the ability to pronounce individual sounds, they encounter no particular difficulty in the recovery of all other forms of speech.

It would be a mistake, however, to conclude that all the disturbances observed in cases of afferent motor aphasia result directly from the loss of articulatory processes. Disturbance of the generalized articulatory schemata is so fundamental a change that the appearance of secondary disturbances is inevitable. Although all systems of speech activity may be altered to some extent, the major disorders involve auditory analysis, auditory synthesis, and writing. The fact that the patient is unable to find rapidly the articulatory positions for different sounds deprives his speech of a basic essential, and it markedly disturbs those conscious acoustic speech processes which occur so easily for the normal individual. When speech sounds cease to be generalized into discrete "articulemes", they can no longer be differentiated out of the flow of continuous speech. They cease to be differentiated from other sounds and are not retained. As a result the patient is often unable to indicate what sounds constitute a given word. The individual sounds which make up a given syllable may be articulated differently depending upon the other sounds in the syllable. Thus a single articuleme may have several "variants", e.g., in Russian, the hard "t" in the syllable "to" is articulated considerably differently from the soft "t" in "te". This further complicates the basic difficulty which the patient has in determining the categories to which different sounds belong. Once he has relearned one variant of the articulation of a given sound, he is still incapable of recognizing its other variants and either fails to pronounce it in some syllables or replaces it with another sound which is articulated similarly.

It is understandable that the loss of generalized articulatory schemata should lead to pronounced *writing* disturbances. The patient commonly has difficulty in writing the letters which represent sounds he is unable to articulate. Sometimes he refuses to write anything; other times he attempts to comply with instructions but makes letter substitutions, e.g. he may write "b" as "m", and "d" as "l" or "n". This sort of literal error is the predominant kind of mistake seen in the writing of such a patient. It is important to note that the skipping and reversal of letters, and the perseveration so characteristic of patients with efferent motor aphasia, are seldom seen in the writing of patients with afferent motor aphasia.

Even after a patient has learned to use tactile and visual images to articulate various sounds (and this in itself takes a long time), these images by no means immediately become generalized and constant internal schemata. He may be able to speak only when he can watch himself in a mirror; he may be able to write only if he speaks the words aloud simultaneously. If "external articulation" is excluded in such a case, the patient's speech is again disturbed. Similarly, S. M. Blinkov at the Moscow Brain Institute found that if he had such a patient hold his tongue between his teeth, so as to preclude external articulation, the patient was completely unable to write.

The loss of articulatory schemata affects the process by which words are synthesized out of individual sounds. Consequently it must be expected to affect *reading* ability also. Having lost the ability to categorize the letters which he reads into variants of particular articulemes, such a patient experiences great difficulty in combining separate sounds into whole words, e.g., in transforming the sequence of sounds "s-t-e-n-a" into the word "stena" (wall). Thus he is often unable to read certain words. Underlying this difficulty is the same disturbance discussed above, and the patient who reads the sound "n" as "l" or "d" can, of course, not understand words in which "n" appears. As we shall see below (Chapter 9), this defect may sometimes prove to be so severe that the patient is totally unable to read, even to himself.

It is interesting that the defects of articulatory schemata described above can lead to secondary disturbances in receptive speech and thus, to unreliability in the *comprehension* of words and sentences.

Our observations indicate that the syndrome described above does not appear with equal frequency or severity following damage to different parts of the postcentral (afferent) areas of the left hemisphere. In lesions which involve the *superior and middle parts* of the postcentral area, apraxia may be absent altogether or may affect only the hand. In these cases, the patient has no articulation difficulties or he may experience temporary difficulties during the initial period following injury. He may indicate that for a short time after he was wounded it was difficult for him to talk. Such disturbances are usually transient in nature and do not affect the patient's reading or writing abilities. We shall present only one example of such mild speech impairment. This case involves almost no aphasic symptoms and is only included here only in order to show the role which the nonspecific parts of the postcentral "marginal" areas can play in the regulation of speech processes.

Case 1

On March 2, 1942, patient Sav., age 25 (case history No. 2224), received a grazing bullet wound in the left parietal area; he was unconscious for a short time after the injury. At operation it was found that the parietal bone had been fractured and splinters from the inner plate were imbedded in the brain tissues. A subdural hematoma had developed at the site of injury. Right hemiparesis and a disturbance of sensation on the right side were observed. Simultaneously it was noted that the patient's speech was impaired in that he was unable to articulate words which he wished to speak. There was no noticeable writing disability. Five months following injury, movement of the extremeties had recovered but deep pressure sensation remained reduced. The patient's

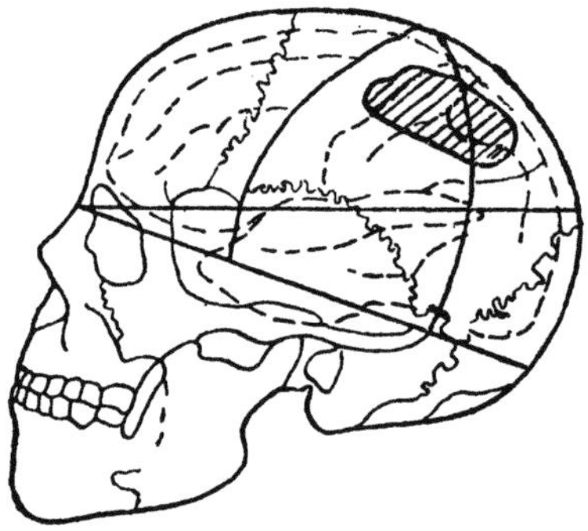

Patient Sav.: injury diagram (Case 1)

movements were somewhat awkward and he had difficulty in controlling movements of his fingers. These disturbances were seen in both hands, but were more pronounced on the right. At this time there were still noticeable signs of lingual ataxia, e.g., the patient was not immediately able to touch his upper lip with the tip of his tongue. Speech comprehension and the grammatical structure of speech were totally preserved, but there remained a certain hesitancy and lack of clarity in his pronunciation. In pronouncing complicated words he often slurred syllables. His pronunciation of individual sounds was imprecise.

Speech disturbances of this type are slightly apraxic in character. They do not have a profound effect on the organization of speech activity and appear to come and go. As a rule they arise as the result of lesions of the superior and middle parts of the postcentral area. Figure 23 and the accompanying table present a number of cases similar to the one described above.

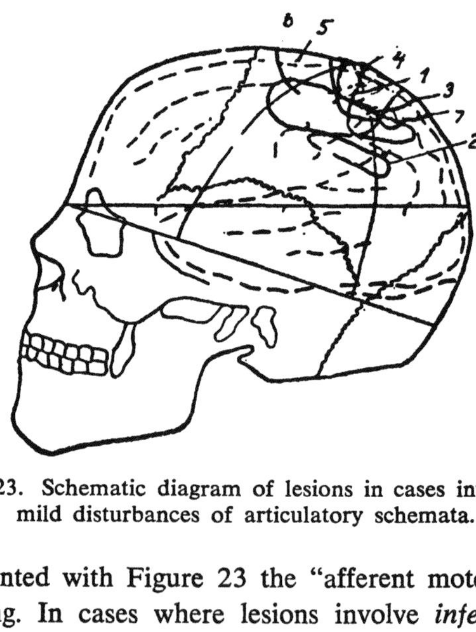

FIG. 23. Schematic diagram of lesions in cases involving mild disturbances of articulatory schemata.

In the cases presented with Figure 23 the "afferent motor aphasia" syndrome was not very striking. In cases where lesions involve *inferior parts* of the left

Lesions observed in mild cases of afferent motor aphasia

Case No.	Name	Nature and site of injury	Speech disturbance
1	Bark.	Direct penetrating wound in upper part of the post-central area; right hemiparesis with sensory disturbance.	For a month following injury, distinct apraxia of organs of speech with corresponding speech defects (he "mangled words" and was unable to pronounce desired sounds); after six months, speech recovered relatively well.
2	Gor.	Penetrating shrapnel wound in left lower parietal and occipital areas with loss of brain tissue; right hemiplegia with impairment of all forms of sensation.	After injury, severe motor aphasia with difficulty in finding the articulations of desired sounds, confusion of sounds with similar articulatory patterns, and substitution of letters in writing.
3	Kon.	Direct penetrating wound in upper parts of left parietal area; slight right hemiparesis with sensory disturbance.	For some time after injury the patient's "tongue was disconnected"; it was difficult to pronounce words distinctly; after three months speech relatively intact with very slight residual signs of lingua apraxia.
4	Bal.	Direct shrapnel wound in left postcentral area with damage to brain tissues; right spastic hemiparesis.	For a long period of time, speech characterized by stumbling due to slight lingual apraxia.
5	Burk.	Superficial penetrating wound in upper part of parietal area with damage to left postcentral area; paraparesis of lower extremeties.	For a long time following injury, motor aphasia with difficulty in articulation of sounds; subsequent indistinct pronunciation of complex words; no signs of denervation.
6	Gus.	Direct penetrating wound in upper parts of parietal area with slight signs of right hemiparesis and sensory disturbance.	For some time after injury, severe motor aphasia with articulatory difficulties; seven months after injury, noticeable disturbance of articulation of speech sounds; residual signs of apraxia of pose.

postcentral area (usually including both the sensory motor area and anterior parts of the inferior parietal area), this syndrome appears in a considerably more severe form. Generally the positional apraxia seen in these patients is quite pronounced in the hand; apraxia of the vocal apparatus is usually well expressed, however, and is sometimes associated with reduced deep sensation in the tongue. Often in the early stages following injury such apraxic disturbances are so severe that the patient is incapable of voluntarily executing the movements involved in inspiration, expiration, kissing, etc. At subsequent stages functions like these may recover, especially in case the patient is retrained. The only residual signs of disturbance may be a difficulty in finding the internal articulatory schemata necessary for the pronunciation of complicated sounds, e.g., sounds which can be produced only when there is precise coordination of vocalization with a particular positioning of the tongue, lips, and soft palate. In the final stages of recovery even these symptoms may be greatly reduced in severity, but this usually requires a long period of retraining. Ultimately, the only defect may be the absence of those internal generalized schemata which were mentioned above. These apraxic phenomena constitute an important component of many forms of motor aphasia. The high frequency with which motor aphasias involve complex symptoms can easily be understood when one considers, first, that the inferior parts of the post-central area are intimately involved in functional systems with the speech areas and, secondly, that they lie precisely between the inferior parietal area (Brodmann's area 40) and the sensory-motor areas.

Here we shall present several examples of such "afferent motor aphasia".

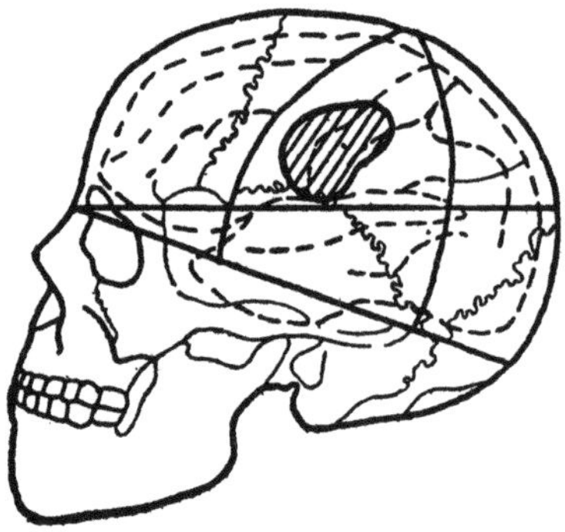

Patient Prus.: injury diagram (Case 2)

Case 2

Patient Prus., age 32 (case history No. 3865), received a penetrating shrapnel wound of inferior parts of the left parietal area which involved the Rolandic operculum as well. Bone splinters were imbedded in the brain tissues to a depth of two or three centimeters. There was no loss of consciousness following the injury, but weakness and reduced sensitivity were observed in the right hand. The patient walked for a distance of 100 meters after being wounded before he became aware of the fact that he could not talk. Speech comprehension was not impaired. His speech recovered gradually, but remained significantly impaired for a long time; often he had difficulty in finding the correct articulatory movements for certain words. He also read poorly, substituting sounds, so as to produce words other than the ones desired. Writing was difficult; he did not know how to place the letters, and his hand curled up in such a way that it was impossible to write clearly. Deep sensation was impaired in the right arm and lip. The patient felt that the right side of his mouth was deformed.

Within six months after injury the paresis disappeared completely, but there remained a certain awkwardness in carrying out complex coordinated movements; he had to search continually for the arm positions desired. His speech had improved considerably, but it was still marred by imprecise articulation and frequent searches for the articulatory movements required to produce certain sounds. In writing he often omitted letters; sometimes he transposed letters and failed to differentiate the sound components of words correctly. In reading he complained that he was unable to "catch the right sounds." and to find the corresponding articulatory movements. Thus the residual disturbance appeared to involve only the phasic, articulatory-auditory aspect of speech.

In the case just presented, apraxia of the vocal apparatus was relatively unsevere. More massive lesions of this area produce more pronounced syndromes.

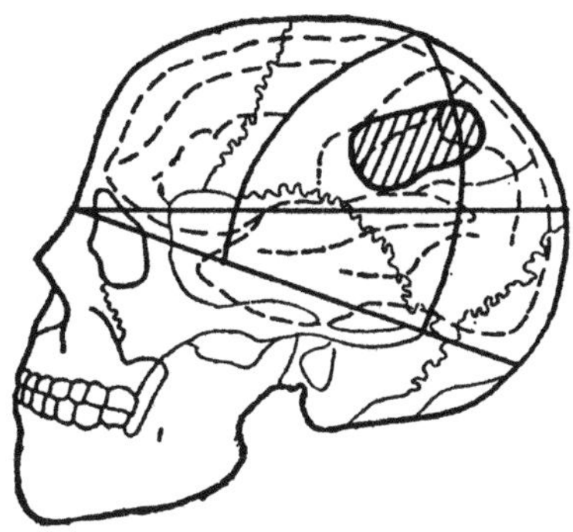

Patient Ljut.: injury diagram (Case 3)

Case 3

In July, 1941, patient Ljut., age 35, received a penetrating shrapnel wound in the middle part of the left parietal area. The injury was complicated by extrusion of brain substance from the wound. The patient lost consciousness, but only for a short time. Right side hemiparesis with impaired sensation were noted. There was a total motor aphasia, but speech comprehension was preserved. A careful examination begun three weeks after injury indicated that the underlying cause of speech impairment was a severe apraxia of the vocal apparatus. The patient was unable to extend his tongue or to touch it to his upper lip; he could not mimic symbolic movements made by the examiner. He was unable to produce voice sounds either by hearing them or by imitating tongue and lip movements of the examiner. Once he had mastered the articulation of a given sound, however, there were no signs of inertness in its pronunciation. Hence the underlying defect was the absence of articulatory schemata and not an inertness in the execution of speech patterns. A writing disability was also observed. Errors resulted from the omission, substitution, or improper ordering of letters.

Systematic rehabilitation therapy was begun relatively soon after the injury with primary emphasis on position of the tongue and lips for the articulation of various phonemes; external visual and kinesthetic cues were used. As a result the apraxia of the speech apparatus began to disappear; the most persistent symptoms were the awkwardness and strained character of articulation. These lasted for several months. As might be expected, once the patient had mastered the articulation of individual sounds, the transition to pronouncing words and speaking phrases and sentences was not difficult for him. His speech was only occasionally agrammatical, and even this defect was overcome by further therapy. As a result of all the above observations this case was classified as belonging to the group of afferent (apraxic) motor aphasias, and its primary symptom was taken to be the disturbance of articulatory schemata.

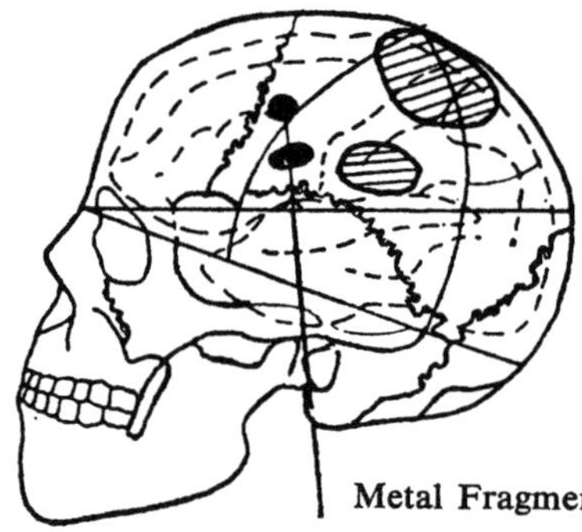

Patient Khol.: injury diagram (Case 4)

Case 4

On August 6, 1944, patient Khol., 18 years of age, received multiple injuries from fragments of an exploding mine. The fragments were localized primarily in the superior and middle postcentral areas of the left parietal region. A month after the injury an operation was performed in which bone fragments were removed from the brain tissues; two fragments were detected by X-ray. The first was 4-5 cm. in diameter and was located in the superior part of the postcentral area; the second was somewhat lower, in the middle area. A long straight fracture extended posteriorly and inferiorly from the first lesion. Embedded in the brain tissues near the midline were two metal fragments. Purulent abcesses were formed and brain tissue extruded from the wound for a period of about three months.

Immediately following the injury the patients lost consciousness and remained unconscious for a long time. There was a very severe hemiparesis, all forms of sensation were impaired, and pathological reflexes were observed on the right side. Gradually leg movements were recovered, but paresis of the upper extremity persisted and was most pronounced in the hand. There were also very persistent aphasic symptoms.

Even a month and a half after injury there was a noticeable disturbance of positional movements of the left, "healthy" hand, and an extremely severe apraxia of the speech apparatus. Neither in response to verbal instructions nor by imitation was the patient able to control his respiratory movements, extend his tongue, or touch with it his upper lip. Under these conditions, of course, he was unable to articulate the various speech sounds. When he came under our observation three months after injury he was unable to pronounce a single sound. Speech comprehension was relatively well preserved, but his reading was limited to the recognition of a few words, common visual ideograms.

Therapy for this patient began with the learning of articulatory positions of the speech apparatus and the development of elementary motor coordination.[6] In the course of therapy both the apraxia of the hand and the severe signs of apraxia of the speech apparatus gradually disappered. Nevertheless, it was a long time before new movements of the tongue and lips could be performed easily. The patient gradually mastered a number of sounds, but the number was limited, and those which he could pronounce required great effort. He was unable to produce the articulations for many sounds and was fully aware of it. In general, once he relearned a sound he had no difficulty in going on to use it in words and phrases, and he had no more difficulty in spontaneous speech than in imitative speech. In contrast to the previous patient, he continued to speak

[6] A more detailed description of the therapy provided this patient is presented below (see Chapter 16).

agrammatically even in the last stages of the therapy. The aggrammatic character of his speech was noticeable, but it was not so severe as to be considered an example of so-called "telegraph style".

The writing of this patient was severely disturbed in the initial period following injury, but it gradually recovered. Peculiar to his writing was the fact that while he could perfectly well tell how many sounds made up a given word, he was often unable to think of the sounds and their corresponding letters. As a result he would frequently write dashes in place of the missing letters. Only after extensive training in the articulation of various sounds, first by imitating lip and tongue movements of the therapist and later by observing the movements of his own speech organs in a mirror, did he become able to articulate sounds and recall the corresponding letters. Not only writing, but also the acoustic analysis of verbal speech remained difficult for him. He often noted that he could not clearly distinguish the sounds making up a given word and sometimes could not remember their sequence in the word. Long and concentrated therapy was necessary to remove this defect and to restore the process by which whole words are synthesized out of individual (auditorily or visually presented) elements.

In the cases presented above severe aphasic syndromes were seen in the presence of pronounced paretic symptoms, indicating that the sensory-motor areas or areas associated with them were pathologically involved. Both the massive disturbances of deep sensation and severe apraxias of the speech apparatus distinguish such cases as belonging to the group of afferent motor aphasias.

Figure 24 presents a summary diagram of sites of injury in cases where the primary symptom was an apraxic disturbance of speech activity. It shows that in many cases of afferent motor aphasia the primary lesion was located in postcentral afferent systems of the left hemisphere.

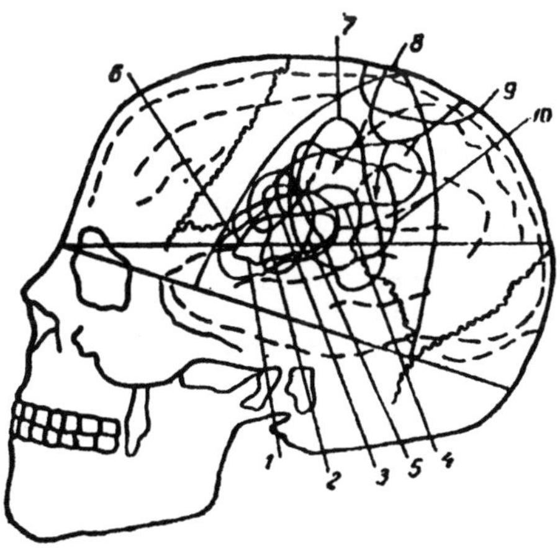

FIG. 24. Schematic diagram of lesions in cases involving severe disturbance of articulatory schemata.

Our discussion of afferent motor aphasia would remain incomplete were we not to mention a final group of disorders which are in many ways similar to those just discussed, but which differ in certain important respects. In some cases these disorders are seen with lesions involving the posterior part of the parietal area farthest from the sensory-motor area; in other cases they may be looked upon simply as stages of recovery from the usual afferent motor aphasia.

In all of the cases described above the disturbance of articulatory schemata was reflected directly in the expressive speech of the patient. Not infrequently, however, one observes cases in which the patient has regained the ability to articulate sounds, but the disturbance of generalized and constant articulatory schemata remains, becoming evident only when he has to deal with sounds at a conscious level. This becomes most apparent in his reading and writing. Attempting to read a certain letter he may search helplessly for the correct articulation by gliding from sound to sound; attempting to write down an orally presented sound, he may repeat it incorrectly and then, in writing it, substitute another similar letter. There can be no doubt that this is primarily an articulatory rather than an auditory defect. The same disturbances appear not only in writing, but in any conscious analysis of the auditory aspect of speech. In attempting to enumerate the sounds of which a par-

Lesions in cases of severe afferent motor aphasia

Case No.	Name		Speech disturbance
1	Dan.	Penetrating shrapnel wound in left postcentral and infero-parietal areas leaving metal fragments imbedded deep in brain tissues: right hemiparesis and sensory deficit most pronounced in the hand.	Severe motor aphasia with disturbances of articulation and oral movements; at first only able to pronounce vowels; subsequently able to pronounce consonants and simple words.
2	Gorb.	Penetrating shrapnel wound in inferior parts of sensori-motor and postcentral areas; right hemiparesis with disturbance of all forms of sensation.	Severe motor aphasia with disturbance of articulation, but without loss of attempts to communicate verbally and without tendency to perseverate.
3	Kor.	Direct penetrating wound in lower middle part of sensori-motor area; right hemiparesis with sensory impairment.	Severe motor aphasia with apraxia of of the organs of speech, and difficulties in articulation; writing defect of a literal type; no sign of perseveration.
4	Lat.	Direct shrapnel wound in left postcentral area with right hemiparesis and sensory deficit.	Severe motor aphasia with apraxia of the speech apparatus, articulatory difficulty, and writing defect; recovery accomplished on the basis of visual analysis of articulatory pose.
5	Pr.	Direct penetrating shrapnel wound in lower parts of left sensori-motor and postcentral areas; subsequent brain abscess; right hemiplegia with sensory deficit.	Motor aphasia with articulatory difficulty in the pronunciation of syllables and words, but with preservation of attempts to communicate verbally and no perseveration of difficulties.

Case No.	Name		Speech disturbance
6	Nas.	Penetrating shrapnel wound in lower parts of sensori-motor and postcentral areas, abscess and scarring of brain tissue; right hemiparesis with sensory loss.	Severe motor aphasia with disturbance of oral movements, articulation difficulties, and corresponding disturbances of both imitative and spontaneous speech; writing disorder with obvious articulatory substitutions; speech recovered on the basis of visual analysis of articulatory positions.
7	Gur.	Superficial penetrating wound in posterior parts of left parietal area; persistent right hemiparesis with sensory loss.	Clear aphasic syndrome with unreliable recognition of articulated sounds; tendency, in writing, to confuse letters representing sounds similar to one another in articulation; elements of semantic aphasia.
8	Khol.	Direct penetrating wound in upper parts of sensori-motor and postcentral areas, multiple metal fragments remaining imbedded in brain tissues; persistent right hemiparesis with sensory loss.	Severe motor aphasia with profound impairment of oral movements; initially, complete lack of ability to pronounce sounds or to write; speech gradually recovered on the basis of visual perception of articulatory movements; later, difficulty in recognizing letters representing series of sounds; noticeable lag of vocal speech behind writing.
9	Sukh.	Direct penetrating shrapnel wound in left parietal area near the midline, damage to brain tissues, deeply imbedded fragments; right hemiparesis with sensory disturbances.	Persistent motor aphasia with severe lingual apraxia and articulatory difficulty; no tendency to perseverate; writing disorder.
10	Ščep.	Direct shrapnel wound in lower parts of left postcentral area; paresis of right hand with severe sensory deficit.	Persistent motor aphasia with disturbance of control of movements of the speech apparatus; considerable articulatory difficulty.

ticular word is composed or to articulate a word more precisely the patient, again, often slides from one articulation to another and may have to use a mirror, so that he can analyze visually the position of his speech organs. If he changes this position or is asked to think silently, however, he loses the ability to analyze "internally" the phonemic constituents of the word; as a result his ability to read or write it is lost. All of these findings indicate that even after the recovery of external speech the role of internal articulatory schemata in speech recognition processes may still be severely disturbed. We shall present only one example of such a syndrome.

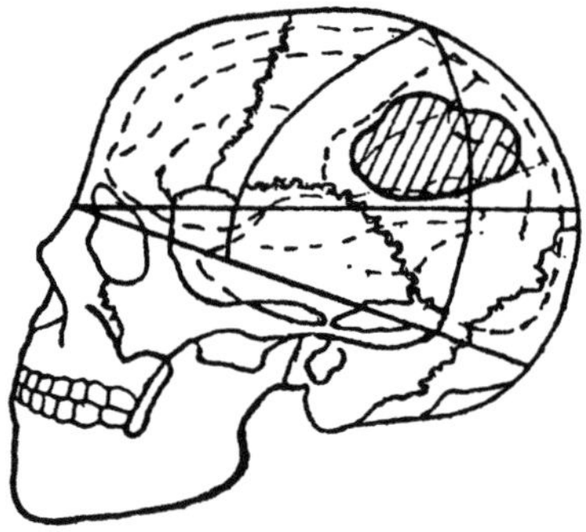

Patient Gur.: injury diagram (Case 5)

Case 5

Patient Gur., age 18, had finished seven years of school. On October 25, 1944, patient Gur., age 18, was wounded by a bullet which entered the middle part of the post-central or parietal area and emerged from the postero-inferior part of the parietal area. At operation the following day bone splinters were removed from the wound. Subsequently the injury was complicated by extrusion of brain tissue, necrosis of the part exposed, and local encephalitis.

Immediately following the injury a right hemiparesis with impairment of all forms of sensation was observed. This was accompanied by a total motor aphasia; speech comprehension was retained to a certain degree. Within three months the motor aphasia disappeared; the patient was able to talk, although he tended to express himself in single words or incomplete sentences. He had noticeable difficulty in understanding complex logico-grammatical constructions (we shall not give a detailed analysis of this symptom at the present time).

At the time our investigation began the patient was no longer having difficulty in the articulation of particular sounds. But if one changed the task so that a word became the object of conscious analysis, i.e., asked the patient to name the sounds which composed it, the instability of articulatory schemata became very apparent. Thus, in attempting to tell what sounds make up the word "kot" (cat), he would "feel out" the letters one at a time: "k . . . o . . . r . . . no, o . . . p-o . . . t . . . no, s . . . s . . .," or, defining the sound composition of the word "sup" (soup), would say, "s . . . u . . . a . . . a . . . no, u . . ., the third is m . . . m . . . p . . . m . . .," and then stop in perplexity. In these cases as in many others the patient, in trying to pronounce certain letters, would drift into the articulation of other leters which were different in sound but similar in articulation, e.g., "m" and "b", "t' and "n", etc.

An analogous disturbance characterized the patient's reading. The presentation of a letter to be read elicited a series of articulatory attempts among which were heard sounds with articulatory positions similar to that of the given sound. Thus he read the written letter "p" as: "f . . . f . . . p . . . f . . . pu . . . p . . ."; the letter "t" he read, "n . . . n . . . s . . . l . . . l . . .". As might be expected, he had difficulty spelling in out the letters of words presented to him in written form. "Sito" (sieve), for instance was spelled "s . . . s-a . . . l . . . l-o . . . s-a-l-o (fat) . . . no, s. . . s-i . . . l . . . l . . . s-i-l-o"; or the word "guba" (lip) was spelled "g-u-m-a", a typical mistake for this patient. Because of the diffuseness of internal articulatory schemata he was incapable of reading to himself except insofar as the words to be read were familiar enough to be recognized as ideograms.

The same diffuseness of articulatory schemata revealed itself in the patient's writing.

He often substituted letters for one another; the letters substituted were not necessarily similar in sound, but were similar in the sense that the articulatory position of the speech apparatus in pronouncing the two sounds was approximately the same. The writing defect was the most serious disturbance observed in the late stage of recovery. Figure 25 presents several examples of the kind of "articulatory substitution" which he made, e.g., "khalat" (smock) became "khadat" or "khanat", etc. Here one can see quite clearly the disturbance of internal articulatory schemata which characterized this patient's speech processes.[7]

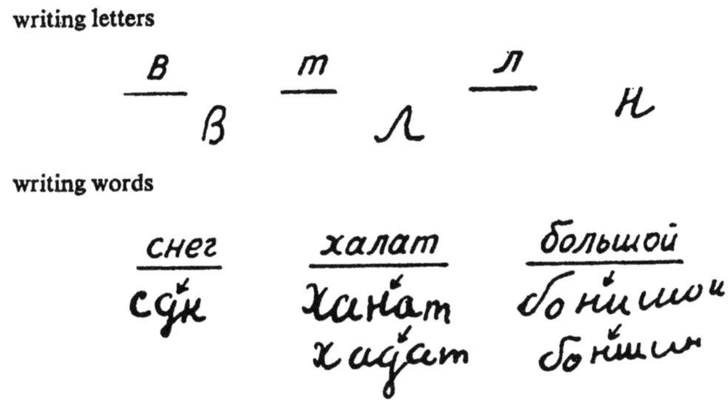

Transliteration:

(v)	(t)	(l)
(v)	(l)	(n)

(sneg)	(khalat)	(bolshoi)
(sdk)	(khanat)	(bonishoi)
	(khadat)	(bonshin)

Patient Gur. Lesion of left postcentral area. Afferent motor aphasia.

FIG. 25. Articulatory substitutions in the writing of patient Gur. (to dictation).

We have presented a series of cases of afferent motor aphasia beginning with the mildest and "purest" disturbances of afferent motor processes and proceeding to more severe appraxias of the speech apparatus, which are often complicated by various secondary symptoms. The common feature of all these cases was that the speech defect was related to loss of afferent motor schemata and not to disturbance of the dynamics of expressive speech. In some cases the impairment of speech appeared as a specific kind of speech dysphasia, in others it took the form of a more severe apraxic functional disintegration. The difference between the first and second types corresponded to a difference in the sites of injury. The milder disturbances usually occurred with lesions of the more superior parts of the left postcentral area, while the more severe and more complicated syndromes resulted

[7] The internal mechanisms of reading and writing will be considered in greater detail later (see Chapter 13).

from lesions of the more inferior areas bordering on the Rolandic operculum and involving other systems of speech areas. In all cases, however, the fundamental defect had to do with the afferent aspect of motor speech processes.

In some cases the apraxic disturbance of expressive speech may constitute the basis for a particular simple form of "afferent motor aphasia", while in others it is just one component, though surely the fundamental one, of a motor-aphasic disturbance of much greater complexity. In either case analysis of the expressive speech defect in terms of modern theories regarding the structure and function of different cortical areas permits us to think of "motor aphasia" as a considerably more complex disturbance than was possible when the study of aphasia was in its infancy.

VII

PATHOLOGY OF THE PREMOTOR SYSTEMS AND SYNDROMES OF "EFFERENT (KINETIC) MOTOR APHASIA"

The formation of movements is by no means completed by the central and post-central afferent systems; it would be truer to say that this is where the organization of movement begins. Equally important to the motor analyzer are areas lying in more anterior cortical areas, *viz.* the premotor areas and parts of the frontal cortex. These areas contribute to the organization of movement by making possible the analysis and synthesis of motor acts. No discussion of the motor analyzer would be complete without taking them into account. It is impossible to understand the mechanisms of aphasia if one omits consideration of the forms of speech pathology which may arise as the result of lesions in these areas. Thus, we shall consider the physiology and pathology of these systems in some detail.

A. THE DYNAMIC ORGANIZATION OF MOVEMENTS AND PATHOLOGY OF THE PREMOTOR AREAS

Almost a hundred years ago the great Russian physiologist I. M. Sečenov, in commenting upon the cerebral organization of mental processes, noted that brain activities can be divided into two types of processes – we would say two forms of synthetic activity. One type of process is related to the integration of simultaneous sensations to produce the unified perception of a *spatial array*; the other type has to do with impressions which arrive in *temporal sequence*. As Sečenov himself indicated, an example of the first type of process is the perception of a spatial object which derives from the complex interaction of excitations arising in the retina and cutaneous receptors. Examples of the second type of process are the perception of musical melody or the generation of a series of rhythmic motions. These two types of synthesis require the function of different structures with different working parameters.

Almost three quarters of a century after Sečenov, Lashley (1937) returned to the problem of spatial (simultaneous) and temporal (successive) cortical functions. Having stated that the two types of function are in principle, incompatible, or more precisely, that both parameters cannot be governed by one and the same complex of nerve cells, he suggested that spatial synthesis is based upon visual, cutaneous, and muscle sensation, while temporal synthesis is based upon the auditory and motor organization of activity. He associated spatial integration with the posterior cortical areas, while sequential integration was attributed to the more anterior areas.

The conception of two types of synthesis carried out by the visuo-spatial and audio-motor analyzers respectively is very important to understand the brain function.[1] We shall give special attention to those anterior cortical areas which have been shown to be directly involved in the organization of sequential activity. We shall consider both the normal structure and function of these areas, as well as the disturbances which arise when they are damaged.

About fifty years ago Hughlings Jackson suggested that the entire anterior part of the cerebral cortex is related to the organization of motor activity at its highest level. Subsequent investigations have altogether confirmed his view. A large body of material accumulated by physiologists and morphologists indicates that the cortical structures involved in the formation of motor behavior are not limited to the precentral pyramidal cell area. Just anterior to the precentral gyrus lies an area which by morphology and physiological function is directly associated with the organization of motor processes. This area, referred to by Campbell as the "intermediate motor zone", has come to be called the "premotor zone" (Brodmann's areas 6 and 8). It is quite different from other areas both in the nature of its connections and in its function.[2]

Cytoarchitectural investigations have shown the structure of the premotor areas to be similar to that of the other motor areas with the exception that here the pyramidal cells of the fifth (efferent) layer are smaller and more sparsely distributed; also the third (association) layer is better developed than in the precentral gyrus. These characteristics make the premotor area well fitted for integrating and organizing impulses generated in the primary motor area.

The same role is further suggested by the great variety of connections which the premotor area has with other areas. Of special significance are the rich vertical connections of this so-called "extrapyramidal motor area" with thalamic nuclei and with the basal ganglia. These tracts have attracted increasing attention recently (see the works of Lassek, 1939-1948; Magoun et al, 1949, 1952; Penfield and Jasper, 1954). It is now well established that the premotor area has intimate connections both with the primary motor cortex and with subcortical structures (thalamus and striopallidal system). In Figures 26 and 27 diagrams are presented showing the various connections of the premotor area. The significance of these different tracts will be discussed later.

[1] We have discussed this problem in detail elsewhere. See A. R. Luria, "Two Forms of Synthetic Function Performed by the Cerebral Cortex" in: *Human Brain and Psychological Processes* (Moscow, 1962); The English edition, New York, Harper & Row, 1966.

[2] A special summary of anatomical, physiological, and clinical studies of the premotor areas (excepting the work of Fulton) was published in a review by P. Bucy in 1944, *The Precentral Motor Cortex.*

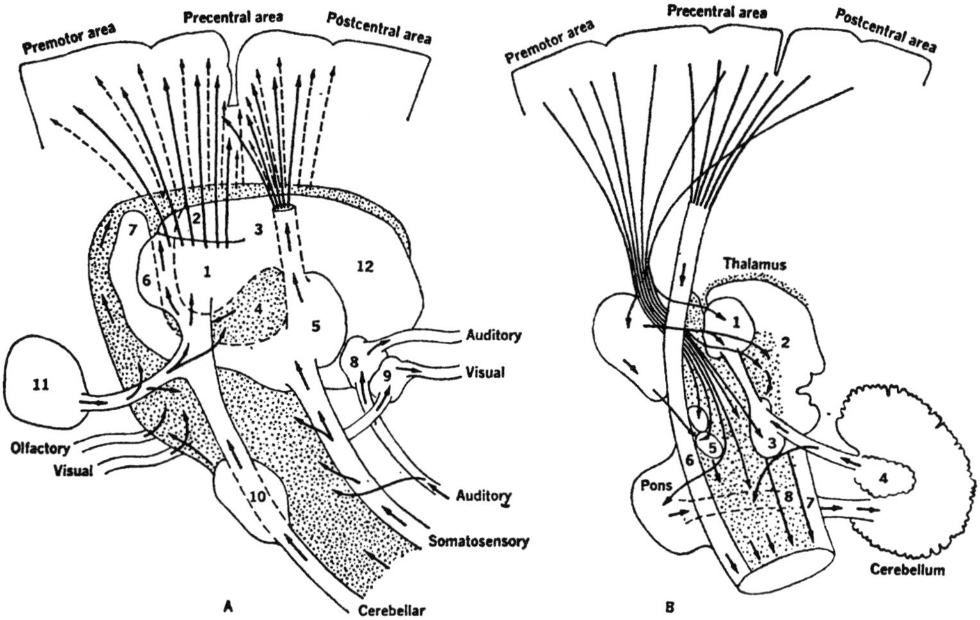

FIG. 26 and 27. Ascending and descending connections of the sensorimotor and premotor cortical areas (Penfield and Jasper, 1954).

The functions suggested by the anatomical characteristics of the premotor area have been revealed more directly by experiments involving direct electrical stimulation, by observations regarding the motor disturbances which arise as the result of premotor lesions, and by the analysis of epileptic seizures spreading from foci in the premotor area. Direct cortical stimulation has shown to what extent the function of this area differs from that of the primary motor area (Brodmann's area 4). Whereas stimulation of the latter area leads to localized movements of various parts of the body, depending upon the point stimulated, stimulation of the premotor area produces more gross movements involving whole muscle systems. Thus the premotor area has been shown to have a much less somatotopic representation than the primary motor area. A further finding is that stimulation of the premotor area with individual impulses does not lead to correspondingly discrete muscle reactions. In experiments carried out by Wyss in Fulton's laboratory it was found that single electrical impulses applied to the premotor area had no effect; if a series of impulses was applied, however, a long tonic movement was evoked which gradually involved various synergic muscle groups and eventually produced a rudimentary integrated act. These findings are quite consistent with the results of experiments performed by Foerster (1936), Penfield and Boldrey (1937), and Penfield and Jasper (1954). These authors found a special "supplementary motor area" within the premotor region, the stimulation of which evoked complex movements. Such findings confirm the complex synthetic activity of the premotor area.

The integrative function of this area appears most clearly in clinical cases involving chronic irritative lesions such as scars or tumors. In such cases so called "adversive" epileptic seizures have been observed in which the characteristic sequence of movements is conjugate deviation of the eyes to one side, turning of the head and body to the same side, and a grasping movement of the arm and hand. Here, again, the movement involves not a single muscle group, but a whole system of muscle groups working in synergy.

Finally, Dusser de Barennes and McCulloch (1941) and Penfield and Jasper (1954) have shown that stimulation of the premotor zones (zone 6 α, β according to the former; "supplementary motor area" according to the latter) depresses motor responses to stimulation of the primary motor areas. Thus the premotor zone not only integrates motor impulses, but it has also a "denervating" function in that it inhibits superfluous inappropriate excitation.

Another source of information is the study of experimental animals in which the premotor area has been partially destroyed. Experiments by Fulton and his school showed that extirpation of the premotor area, while producing no severe paralysis, inevitably resulted in the impairment of fine skilled movements. Animals from which the premotor cortical area was removed showed no signs of apraxic motor disturbances. This made sense, for one would hardly expect to find an apraxia in which relatively complex innate behavior was retained, while manipulatory movements were lost. The major finding was that all of the animals' movements became slow and awkward; the smoothness of movements was disturbed.

Much more well defined losses have been observed in cases of premotor area lesions in man. The findings of a number of authors, our data included,[3] indicate that damage to the premotor area in humans does not produce paralysis, or apraxia of the ideational or ideomotor types. Even a patient with massive destruction of the premotor area is able to place his hand and fingers in a position requested by the examiner; the pattern of impulses necessary to do this is immediately available to him. He is easily able to place his arm in a particular position in space and has no difficulty in using various objects. Symbolic and constructive activities are equally unaffected.

Motor disturbances only become apparent when one goes from the analysis of simple acts to *complex dynamic coordinations* and serially organized (successive) movements. Here motor disturbances are unmistakable. The primary defect in these cases rests in the patient's inability to master tasks which involve any kind

[3] A. R. Luria, *Higher Cortical Functions in Man* (Moscow University Press, 1962) (English edition, New York, Basic Books, 1966). A. R. Luria, *Human Brain and Psychological Processes* (Moscow, 1963) (English edition, N.Y., Harper and Row, 1966); see also E. G. Skol'nik-Jarros, *Disturbances of Movements with Damage to the Premotor Zone* (1945) in: A. R. Luria and E. D. Homskaya (eds.), *Frontal Lobes and Regulation of Psychological Processes* (Moscow University Press, 1966 [Russian]).

of active motor pattern that must be worked out against a certain dynamic "background". By "motor background" we mean the tonic preparedness of synergic groups of muscles to act, even though they are not taking part in the motor pattern being executed at a given moment. The active motor pattern lacks the appropriate dynamic plasticity. The denervation or discontinuation of efforts once they have been initiated ceases to be accomplished automatically and it becomes necessary to generate special voluntary impulses for this purpose.

Dynamic disturbances are seen most distinctly when patients must carry out serially organized movements. Pathology of the premotor areas results in disruption of the smooth automaticity of motor habits which a person acquires as the result of great practice. Practice transforms a sequence of discrete motor impulses into a smoothly flowing "kinetic melody". Damage to the premotor areas, especially to the left premotor area, leads to loss of the automatic character of motor habits, i.e., it leads to a situation in which a single generalized impulse is insufficient to generate a series of movements. Every individual act comes to require its own special impulse; the possibility of learning motor habits or automatic responses of a higher order is reduced or abolished altogether. Movements lose the smoothness and plasticity which characterize the activity of normal individuals. Having lost the ability to execute serial movements directly, the patient seeks indirect means of producing the component acts individually. In very severe cases smooth movements give way to chains of individual acts, each of which is evoked by a special effort. It is important to note that damage to the premotor area of the dominant hemisphere affects not only the contralateral hand, but also the ipsilateral, or "healthy", hand. Again, it is clear that the premotor area does not possess a simple somatotopic representation of the contralateral extremities.

Loss of the smoothness of complex motor activities is reflected most clearly in tests requiring reciprocal coordination of the two hands or in tests requiring shift of innervation from one finger to another, e.g., when the patient is asked to move his first and second finger, then his first and fifth finger he may have difficulties. Here the task involves not simply one change in finger position, but the execution of a series of different movements.[4]

In addition to this disturbance so typical of patients with premotor lesions, one observes another very important symptom. Not only do serial movements lack continuity, but is is often difficult for the patient to shift from one act in the sequence to another. For example, it is difficult for him to tap his finger in a given rhythmic pattern; if he attempts to increase the rate of tapping, he tends to make perseverative, superfluous movements. The shift from one motion to another is made difficult for him by the persistence of impulses more appropriate to the motion just produced than to the one he wishes to produce. Once he has thoroughly mastered a given rhythm, he may be incapable of shifting to another. With great frustration he may continue to repeat the first rhythm even though he recognizes

[4] The techniques involved in this and further tests are discussed in detail in Chapter 10.

it to be wrong. He is unable to overcome the inertia of the system generating the first motor pattern. This persistence of excitation patterns once they are aroused may be especially strong if the lesion extends anterior to the premotor area or if it involves much of the underlying white matter. We have observed loss of the smoothness of movements and difficulty in shifting from one movement to another in cases involving lesions of subcortical nuclei or destruction of the fiber tracts connecting them with the premotor area. Such symptoms are especially likely to arise in a patient who has undergone surgery of the premotor area which resulted in hemorrhage or postoperative edema. He may easily begin to carry out the required task, e.g., drawing a circle or writing a number, but be unable to shift from the first figure to another. Usually in such a case the unit of repeated activity is not a particular component of the movement, but the movement itself. In Figures 28 and 29 we present two examples of the pathological inertia of motor activity. The first case involved a hemorrhage in the left premotor area as a result of a ventricular puncture; the second involved cerebral edema following an operation on the left premotor area. In the second figure, one sees that the pathological inertia of motor pattern gradually disappeared as the edema subsided.

All of these phenomena appeared in the majority of cases which we observed, and they persisted into the residual period. The most severe symptoms were seen with lesons of the left premotor area; lesions of the right (subdominant) hemisphere resulted in less pronounced disturbances. As a result of our observations we were able to attain a more adequate conception of the functions of the premotor area than was available to us before.

In view of current neurological principles we may look upon the premotor area as an important component of the cortical motor analyzer; it plays a special role in the smooth execution of complex serial movements. According to all available evidence the function of this area consists of the transformation of individual impulses arising in other (afferent) cortical areas into complex dynamic patterns, each component of which is easily denervated once it is completed, thus making way for the succeeding component. Only thus is it possible to generate patterned unitary movements.

In investigating the elaboration of motor habits (or higher automatisms) one is forced to conclude that the basic mechanism underlying such kinetic patterns is the creation of specific dynamic stereotypes. It is apparent that the various individual acts making up a complex movement do not have to be initiated by separate impulses. Instead, they are run off as a *unitary series,* initiated by a single generalized impulse. Such dynamic organization of movements makes it possible to combine separate components of a movement into a single dynamic structure; each link in the chain of activity, is denervated as the next link emerges. Both electrophysiological evidence and clinical observations indicate that creation of the dynamic systems which permit the coordination of sequential motor acts is a specific function of the premotor area.

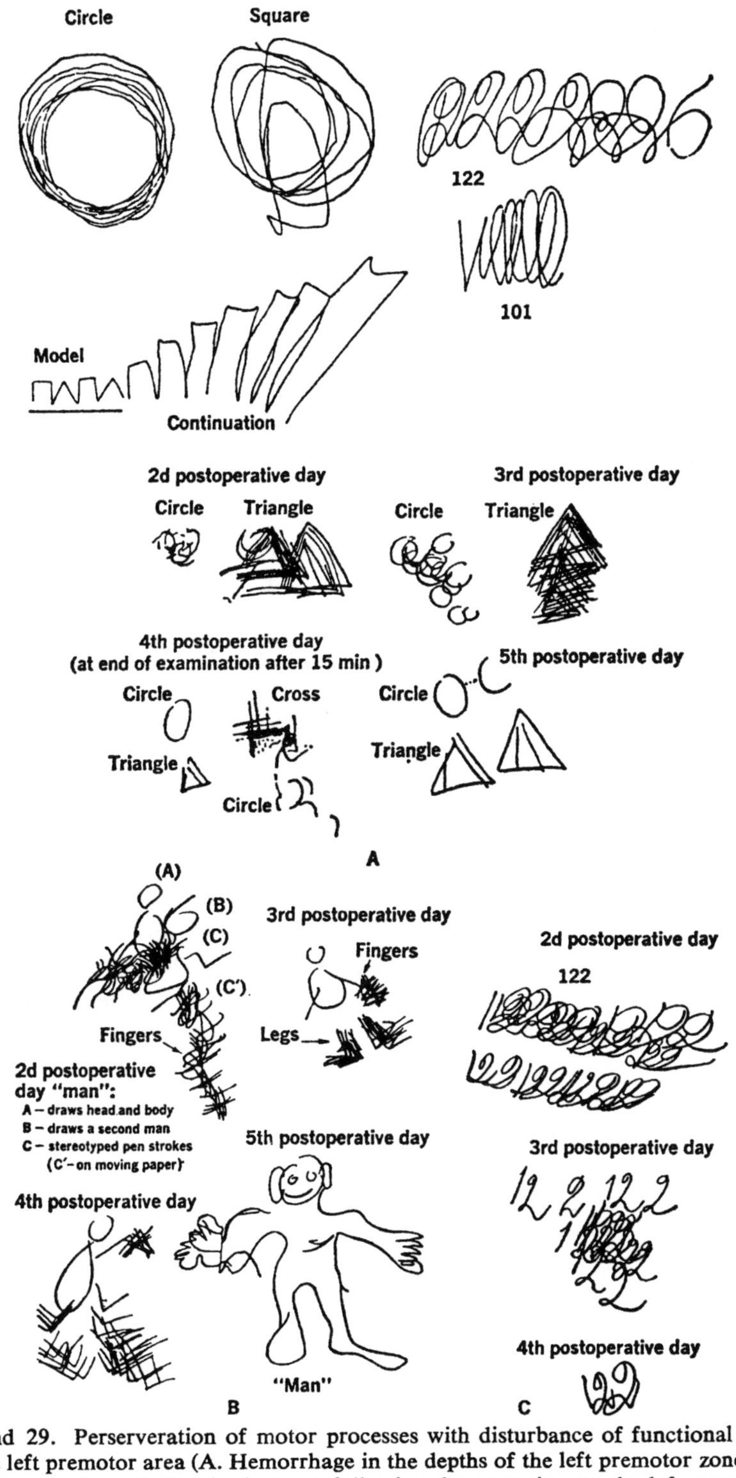

FIG. 28 and 29. Perserveration of motor processes with disturbance of functional systems involving the left premotor area (A. Hemorrhage in the depths of the left premotor zone as a result of ventricular puncture; B. Cerebral edema following the operation on the left premotor zone).

There is, however, a second principle underlying function of the premotor area; that is the principle of segmental representation. It is well known that the principle of segmental, or somatotopic, representation characterizes the primary projection areas of the cerebral cortex. Experiments involving stimulation and extirpation indicate that the organization of the premotor areas is more functional than somatotopic. Even here, however, the principle of somatotopic projection holds to a certain extent.

The Vogts were the first to show that one part of the premotor area (6a α) is largely associated with integrated movements of the trunk, while another (6a β) is primarily concerned with fine movements of the extremities, particularly of the hand. Anterior to this area lies a zone concerned primarily with coordinated eye movements (area 8). Finally, at its lower border, there lies a zone which, according to its morphological, genetic, and functional characteristics, should be considered separately, viz the motor speech area, or Broca's area (Brodmann's area 44).

There is no basis whatsoever for the idea that this area is anything other than a highly specialized part of the premotor area, even though it may be true (as some authors believe) that it appears only in man. Campbell was the first to show that the cytoarchitecture of Broca's area is very similar to that of the rest of the premotor area, or as he referred to it, the "intermediate precentral" area. One sees relatively small pyramidal cells sparsely distributed in the fifth (efferent) layer and the deeper part of the third layer is well developed. The third layer which, apparently, has a secondary integrative (associative) function is even more prominent here than in other parts of the premotor area.

This area differs from other parts of the premotor cortex, however, in two respects. First, it lies directly adjacent to that part of the precentral gyrus associated with movements of the facial musculature, lips, and tongue; thus it is natural to expect that the organizing function of this area may be primarily associated with movements of these areas. Secondly, it possesses a much more fully developed system of afferent connections than more superior parts of the premotor area. It is not only connected with the postcentral (kinesthetic) cortical structures, which are necessary for carrying out finely differentiated movements, but it is also under the influence of a very well developed system of afferent tracts arising in the auditory projection area of the temporal lobe. These latter connections are so great as to make it reasonable to think of Broca's area and the temporal area as constituting a single auditory-articulatory functional system.

Both of these conditions make the inferior part of the premotor area particularly suited for the integration of speech movements. On the basis of this alone we would predict that damage here should produce primarily disturbances of expressive speech. Our consideration of effects of lesions in this area can only be fully productive if we keep in mind the relationship of this area to the rest of the premotor area; in studying its pathology we should attempt to identify its losses analogous to those losses which we observed in cases of premotor area lesions. This task is, of course, complicated by phenomena peculiar to disturbances of speech activity, but it provides the general guidelines for our investigation.

B. SPEECH DISTURBANCES WITH LESIONS OF THE PREMOTOR SYSTEMS

Premotor area lesions which are capable of producing the decomposition of motor processes described above must inevitably also give rise to speech disorders. In studying speech pathology, it is a mistake to consider only lesions of one small part of the premotor area, i.e., Broca's area, and to ignore the kinds of speech disturbances arising as the result of damage to other parts. Sixty years ago Campbell (1905) pointed out, "Broca's area, so-called, is a part of the premotor cortex controlling motor speech". He suggested that the entire premotor cortex takes part in speech activity, and, "although clinical confirmation of this idea is unfortunately lacking", he was convinced that it was true.

Campbell's prediction was absolutely correct. Consequently, we must begin our analysis with a consideration of the speech disturbances which arise as a result of lesions to the premotor area proper, an area which we consider to be one of the "peripheral" speech areas. By analyzing the relatively mild aphasic disturbances which arise in such cases we can expect to discover one of the important prerequisites for organized speech activity in its purest form.

Careful study of a large number of cases reveals, indeed, that damage to premotor areas other than Broca's area often produces speech disorders. As Table 7 shows, speech disturbances are encountered frequently in cases having lesions in the part of the premotor area directly bordering on Broca's area. In the initial period following injury, 83% of such cases exhibited signs of speech disorder; in 56% of cases the disorders persisted for a long period of time (3-5 months). A "motor aphasia" syndrome was clearly seen in a large proportion of these cases.

TABLE 7

Aphasic syndromes with lesions in the left premotor area

Site of injury in premotor area	Total number of cases	Initial period			Residual period		
		severe forms (%)	mild forms (%)	total (%)	severe forms (%)	mild forms (%)	total (%)
Superior	37	30	43	73	0	38	38
Inferior	43	53	30	83	23	33	56

Even lesions in parts of the premotor area quite far from the classical Broca's area, however, did not leave speech as well preserved as one would expect on the basis of narrow localization theories. Wounds involving the upper part of the premotor area gave rise to speech disturbances during the initial period in 73% of cases; in 38% the disorders persisted for more than three to five months. These disturbances were not so frequently classifiable as motor aphasias, however. The majority were so slight as to be easily missed, yet they were of great interest. The fact that a large number of them were very stable indicated that they did not arise simply as the result of secondary involvement of Broca's area by edema or vascular changes, but that they were a consequence of injury to the premotor area itself. This finding was of considerable interest and made further analysis of the premotor syndromes imperative.

What is the nature of speech disturbances arising as the result of damage to the premotor systems? What aspects of speech suffer? What complaints and speech defects does one find?

It appears that damage to the premotor area can produce at least two different syndromes of speech impairment. One arises, as a rule, in cases involving lesions of the upper portion of the premotor area; the other arises as the result of damage to lower areas, including Broca's area. The latter is more specifically a disturbance of speech processes than the former. Despite their differences, the two syndromes actually represent two variants of a single type of psycho-physiological disturbance and may, thus, be considered together.

1. *Speech Impairment Following Lesions of the "Marginal" Parts of the Premotor Areas*

First we shall consider the speech defects which arise following damage to those parts of the premotor area which are not a part of the specialized "speech" area. In such cases one does not observe the classical form of motor aphasia. The pronunciation of individual sounds and even of whole words may remain unaffected. On the other hand, from the very beginning, one observes a *loss of the smoothness of speech* which is simply one aspect of the change in the smoothness of movements which we mentioned earlier. The patient begins to pronounce individual words (in severe cases, individual sounds) haltingly; the transition from one word to another is accompanied by a long pause. This loss of the rapidity and automaticity of speech is a superficial sign, however; a qualitative change underlies it. The unit of innervated action is no longer the *sentence or phrase*, as it is for the normal individual. The patient no longer utters a whole meaningful complex "in a single breath". Instead, the unit becomes the individual *word or syllable*. The patient speaks in a monotone and haltingly. The position of a word in a sentence no longer determines the intonation with which it is spoken. As one of our patients characterized his own speech, "Since the injury . . . I stumble . . . in my speech: like a hobbled . . . horse . . . hops . . .". The loss of automaticity affects not only the patient's spontaneous speech, but also the way in which he repeats sentences or reads aloud.

It would be incorrect, however, to think of these speech disorders as pure disturbances of vocal speech. Investigation has shown that the more general processes underlying expressive speech may be affected, i.e., the processes by which verbal speech is generated and comprehended. Many patients with premotor area lesions are unable to narrate a story spontaneously. The speech of such a patient is simplified grammatically "expansive" sentences so constructed that he has to keep in mind what he has said in order to complete them disappear. He is unable to preserve an "inner set". There is a similar loss of "inverted" grammatical constructions, i.e., a loss of sentences in which the order of words does not correspond to the order of thoughts.[5] His vocal and written speech are characterized by short sentence fragments in which the important words appear directly adjacent to one another. Thus he is able to avoid the necessity for preserving the schemata of inner speech.

Not only expressive speech changes in such a case; as a rule speech comprehension is affected also. At first it may appear that comprehension is simply slowed. In attempting to understand a sentence, the patient may have to hear it or read it through several times; more significant is the fact that he may have to repeat it to himself, either silently or aloud. If a complex sentence is presented once, only certain substantive fragments of it remain in the patient's consciousness, e.g. "Something about a valley . . . something about an evening and mist." The meaning of the sentence as a whole is by no means preserved. Requiring the patient to hold his tongue between his teeth is often sufficient to make him totally incapable of understanding connected speech. In this situation he has to rely completely upon the schemata of inner speech which, in his case, are defective. As a result, it is impossible for him to comprehend complex speech immediately.[6]

Thus, as the result of careful observation, we can say that both speech comprehension and the intellectual processes associated with it suffer the same loss of automaticity as does the expressive speech of the patient. It is obvious that one sees here the loss of dynamic systems that underlies the disturbance of body movements following damage to the premotor area. Instead of resulting from a disturbance of the "inner schemata of movements", however, the speech symptoms result from a disturbance of what psychologists have referred to as "inner speech", *viz.* the abbreviated schema of speech which precedes the speech act itself (Vygotskij,

[5] An example of the first, or "expansive" type of construction would be the sentence, "The mountain, which we climbed, was high". Another, stylistically more complex, would be, "The wide valley, lying between two mountain ridges, submerged in the dense evening mist, spread out before us". An example of inverted sentence construction would be, "The boy was bitten by the dog", or any other passive construction.

[6] The disturbance of comprehension which arises in such forms of aphasia has been investigated in detail by O. P. Kaufman of our laboratory.

1934). As a result of the disturbance of the schema of speech, patients with premotor lesions come to speak haltingly and in very simple terms. In order to understand the speech of others, statements must be presented several times to such a patient. Though the patient is unable to rely upon inner processing of what he hears, repeated presentations may act as a substitute.

Loss of the automaticity of speech underlies the *"mild forms" of aphasia* which arise as the result of premotor area lesions. As we have seen, damage to the upper part of the premotor area may result in a "premotor syndrome" which is limited to loss of the smoothness of speech, or it may take a more generalized form, in which intellectual functions lose their automaticity. With more severe lesions, especially those involving both the premotor cortex and its connections with subcortical structures, the loss of dynamic speech systems may be complicated by a third symptom. The patient with a premotor area lesion may be unable to suppress words once he has uttered them. Thus he may fix on the articulatory motor pattern of the word just spoken and perseverate, rather than switch to the next word and continue. His speech is reduced to a series of attempts to overcome the persistence of words spoken, and it is made all the more difficult by the fact that this obstacle arises out of the speech process itself.

In some cases, especially those in which lesions do not extend beyond the borders of the premotor cortical area, perseveration is seen simply as a tendency to repeat the first or last syllable of the word just uttered before going on to the next word. Sometimes it is limited to the appearance of perseverative trembling of the lips or a labial intention tremor. In severe cases, on the other hand, syllabic perseveration may be so pronounced as to totally disrupt normal speech. Perseveration assumes yet another character, especially when the lesion extends beyond the premotor area to involve a portion of the frontal cortex.[7] Here one may see not only perseveration of words, but even perseveration of sentences. If one has the patient repeat a series of syllables, e.g. "bi-ba-bo", or three words, e.g. "house-table-cat", his difficulty is quite different from that of a patient with a temporal lobe lesion. The latter patient is unable to retain a series of auditory signals in their original order. The patient with a premotor area lesion, on the contrary, is unable to alter the order in which he pronounces the items. He is unable to utter the same items in a different sequence or to substitute any other items for the ones originally presented. The dynamic speech pattern which arises during initial utterance of the series persists, causing him extreme difficulty.

These are the symptoms which make up the syndrome of *efferent motor aphasia*. The basic disorder is *not a loss of the ability to create new speech articulations, but an inability to overcome articulatory patterns once they have been created*. This group of symptoms often arises in conjunction with the other forms of disturbance

[7] The psychophysiological mechanisms of these different types of perseveration are clarified elsewhere. A. R. Luria, "Two Kinds of Perseveration in Massive Injury of the Frontal Lobes", *Brain*, Vol. 88 (1965), pp. 1-10.

which we noted earlier as resulting from damage to the premotor systems. We shall present a series of examples illustrating the premotor aphasic disturbances just described. The first cases show the kinds of symptoms which arise with lesions of the upper and middle portions of the premotor area. They do not lead to severe articulatory disturbances but impair the automaticity of speech and intellectual processes.

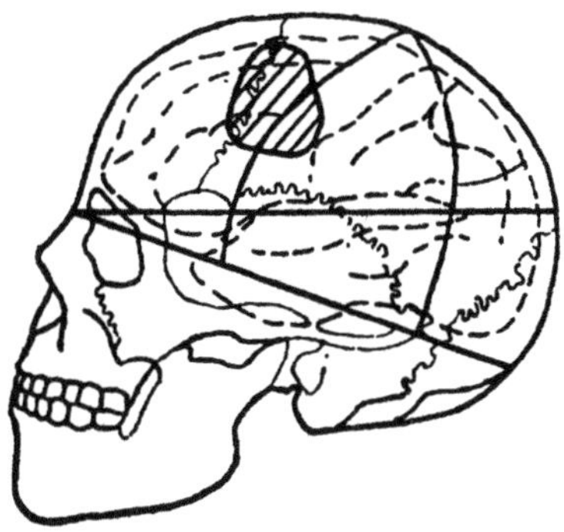

Patient Pavl.: injury diagram (Case 1)

Case 1

On January 20, 1943, patient Pavl., age 46 (case history No. 3501) received a direct penetrating wound in the middle part of the left premotor area. Following the injury he was unconscious for a short period of time. Weakness appeared in the right extremities and persisted for a much longer time. No further complications arose during the recovery period. Two months following injury there were persistent signs of generalized depression. Signs of reduced strength and sensitivity in the right extremities and hyperactive reflexes on the right were observed. From the time of injury the patient noted a clumsiness in the movements of both hands, especially the right hand, and a certain disturbance of speech. As he noted: "My speech was broken up. I would stumble in speaking". An examination two months after injury revealed a disturbance of complex coordinated movements. In tests involving opposite movements of the two hands (e.g. (1) pronation of one hand while clenching the other, (2) reversal of position, so that the first hand clenches while the second pronates) the patient responded slowly and with uncertainty. When he was asked to reverse positions more rapidly, he confused the movements and began to make the same movements with both hands. When asked to alternate between a fist and apposition of the thumb and forefinger to form an "O" he could only repeat stereotyped movements, as though it were impossible for him to denervate, i.e., discontinue, the movements which went before. This awkwardness was seen to some extent in the left hand, but was most pronounced on the right side. Similar loss of automaticity was observed in the patient's speech. His narrative speech lacked expression; it was interrupted by numerous pauses, and was sometimes agrammatical. The sentence structure and intonation were abnormal. He spoke in sentence fragments. "The farmer had ... a hen ... there was gold ... and then ... he killed the hen ... got the gold ... but no gold ...". The patient's spontaneous speech was reduced to little more than a broken series of such phrases interrupted by his searching for words. He had no difficulty in naming objects. He was generally able to repeat statements presented to him, but long sentences were repeated in a broken manner. Sometimes he was unable to retain a long sentence and would repeat only isolated parts of it. He showed similar difficulty in maintaining the serial order of items when solving problems in arithmetic; he easily solved problems involving two steps, but problems involving three steps were extremely difficult for him. Similarly, he had difficulty in carrying out any series of three or more instructions, though he could carry out two instructions easily enough. For instance he could respond correctly to the instruction: "Draw a cross and a circle", but the instruction, "draw two crosses, a triangle, and three dots", was impossible for him. The sequence of steps to be carried out was forgotten, so that he would carry out the initial steps over and over again, with long pauses. The patient had difficulty in understanding the speech of others. Although he might eventually comprehend even the most complex series of instructions, he was unable to master it immediately; thus obtaining the meaning of a statement had to become a conscious process, just as did any complex movement. He had to read a sentence through several times before he caught its meaning. Characteristically, he had to read a sentence aloud in order to understand it. Exclusion of external speech considerably reduced his comprehension of written material. He could write only if he simultaneously spoke the words aloud.

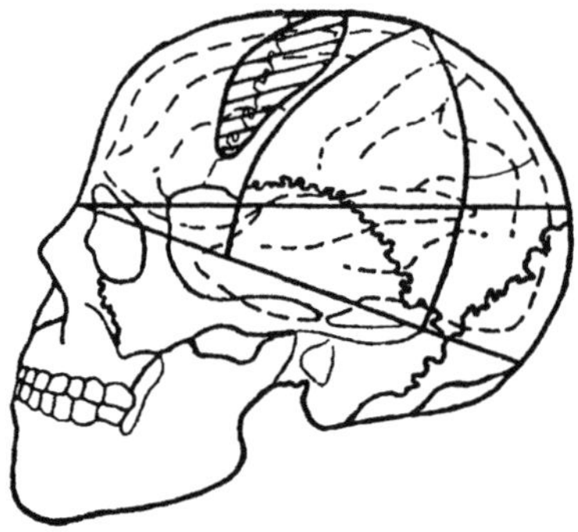

Patient Kar.: injury diagram (Case 2)

Case 2

Early in November, 1942, patient Kar., age 29 (case history No. 1217) received a penetrating shrapnel wound in the left premotor area. In the initial period he suffered a right hemiplegia, reduced patellar and Achilles tendon reflexes, and a total motor aphasia; the latter lasted for a relatively short time. Two months later there was only slight weakness and hyperreflexia on the right. By this time his speech had greatly recovered. At examination four months after injury it was found that individual movements were totally preserved, whereas complex and continuous movements were still severely impaired. The patient was unable to carry out the reciprocal coordination test which requires rapid shift from one position to another (see case above). Series of discrete movements took the place of smooth kinetic patterns. A severe "apraxia of sequential action" (Kleist's "Apraxie der Handlungsfolge"), resulted from attempts to produce any kind of complex movement. Instead of a continuous movement, the patient would produce a series of disconnected motions representing the various sequential elements of which it should be composed. His articulation was not affected in the least, but he spoke very slowly. His speech lacked its normal automaticity and was punctuated by pauses during which he searched for words. Such "amnesic phenomena" did not at all affect the naming of objects. A special effort was required to utter each word, so that the smoothness of speech was altogether lost. "Before I was injured I used to put out a thousand words a minute. I gave speeches; but now I can't. No words; embarrassing." Associated with the loss of speech schemata there was a decrease in the grammatical complexity of the patient's speech. Whole sentences gave way to disconnected speech elements. The patient's memory for past events was totally intact; yet he could not describe his occupation as a welder: "And so . . . an electric arc . . . 3500° C . . . (a smile, embarrassment, pause) . . . that's all . . . it's here . . . the memory . . . about the past . . . how it was . . . but I can't say it . . .". He understood perfectly well the meaning of a selection which he read. For instance, he recounted a story about an eagle that kidnapped a child in order to recover her own fledgling as follows: "In a word, an exchange: they exchanged . . . the eagle gave the little girl back . . . and took the eaglet . . .". But he was only able to understand the story after having read it through several times aloud. When external speech was excluded, he would utter a few unrelated words, and then give up trying. Although he had great difficulty in retelling such a story, he could easily answer questions about it. He was unable to memorize verse even after numerous repetitions, though he might know its content perfectly. The patient's intellectual capacities were preserved, but they were characterized by the same lack of automaticity seen in his speech. Hearing and the articulatory aspects of his speech were not affected.

These two cases illustrate premotor speech disturbances in their purest form. They show that, by eliminating the dynamic schemata of speech, premotor lesions produce a characteristic type of "kinetic" aphasia. At first glance the syndrome which appears may be taken for a very slight and superficial form of speech impairment, but upon closer investigation it becomes obvious that beneath it there lies a gross disruption of all forms of continuous speech (and intellectual activity).[8]

The syndrome of "premotor aphasia" can vary considerably depending upon site of lesion. Injuries at different sites affect different aspects of the functional system with varying degrees of severity. If a penetrating wound is sufficiently deep to affect the cortical organization of the extrapyramidal systems one sees more than a simple loss of the automaticity of speech. In addition there is greater difficulty in the suppression of speech patterns once they have arisen, so that one characteristically observes hyperkinesis and "motor emboli" in the behavior and speech activity of the patient.

Case 3

On July 18, 1943, patient Papk., age 20 (case history No. 4247) received a graze wound of the skull over the left premotor cortical area. The injury resulted in a transitory loss of consciousness, a disturbance of movements in both legs and the right hand, and motor aphasia. During the first month following injury there was a loss of voluntary bladder control, so that while the patient was aware that urine was flowing, he was unable to

[8] We have presented elsewhere a special analysis of the syndrome arising in cases of premotor area lesions. See A. R. Luria, "Psychological Analysis of the Premotor Syndrome" in: A. R. Luria, *Human Brain and Psychological Processes* (New York, Harper and Row, 1966).

stop it. The dura was damaged, and at operation two days following injury bone splinters were removed from the brain tissues. Movements gradually reappeared, and speech began to return. After twenty days the patient was able to pronounce individual words, and a short time later he could produce whole sentences. Only an impairment of narrative speech remained; the phrases which he desired were inaccessible to him, and he spoke very slowly.

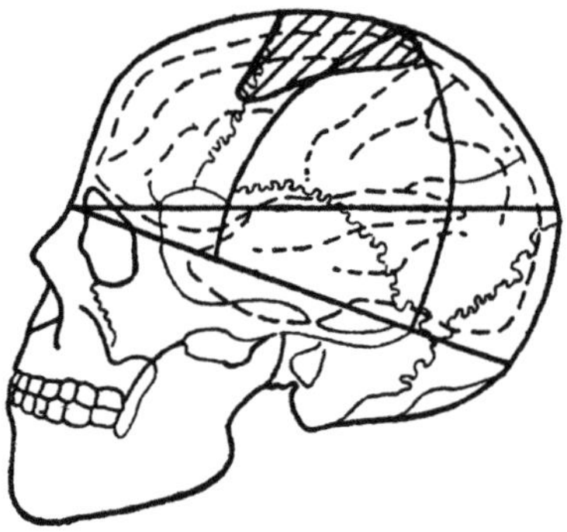

Patient Papk.: injury diagram (Case 3)

A month after injury the patient was transported away from the front. The trip was made in a jolting vehicle, and his condition subsequenly worsened. His speech became considerably worse. Later he reported that during this time his speech had become harsh and guttural, and that he had suffered from a particular kind of stuttering defect, *viz.* having once uttered a word he found that he had a tendency to repeat it, that he was not able to get rid of it.

The patient came under our observation two months after injury. At this time the wound had almost completely healed. A right hemiparesis with clonus of the right foot, hyperreflexia, pathological signs, disturbance of pain and deep sensitivity on the right and a pronounced grasp reflex in the right hand were observed. He easily placed his hand in any desired position and showed no signs of apraxia. In a test of the ability to reproduce kinetic patterns, however, severe difficulty was noted. He performed simple rhythmic tapping tests very slowly; every attempt to tap more rapidly resulted in inappropriate motions which he was unable to suppress. Attempts to carry out more complex patterns of movements were accompanied by great effort and were generally unsuccessful. His speech was grammatically correct, but disconnected; each word required a special effort. Often the patient had to search for words, and this difficulty might be complicated by a tendency to repeat the initial or final syllables of words, giving rise to a certain form of stuttering. He did not have difficulty in naming objects. Speech comprehension and simple intellectual functions were rather well preserved, but they required more time than normal and exclusion of external speech reduced these functions considerably.

Three and a half months after injury the patient experienced further trauma; he suffered a blow to the occipital region of the skull. This was not followed by any important change in neurological status, but he noted that his speech became much worse. The stuttering was intensified and he found that he had difficulty in releasing objects once he had grasped them. "You grab – and you can't open your hand."

Six months following the original injury, the patient again came under our observation. At this time there remained only a slight restriction of movements of distal portions of the right extremities with an accompanying reduction in strength. No sensory deficits or pathological signs were noted except for an occasional Babinsky sign on the right. Encephalography indicated the presence of an extensive scar in the parietal area in a parasagittal plane with retraction acting to deform the body of the left ventricle. Both lateral ventricles and the third ventricle were distented. As before, there was no sign of a positional apraxia; the ability to make symbolic gestures was totally preserved. On the other hand, the disturbance of dynamic motor acivity observed earlier was considerably more severe. Fine finger movements of he left hand were made difficult by synkinesis of all the fingers; the fingers of the right hand were similar disabled. The patient was totally unable to reproduce a tapping pattern, even though it consisted simply of a pair of taps. Once he began tapping with his finger he was unable to stop and produced numerous extra taps, even though he was perfectly aware that he was producing too many. He was even unable to draw two dots or two dashes on paper; he invariably drew a whole series of them as though he were unable to denervate and act once it was initiated. Tests of reciprocal coordination indicated severe kinetic disturbances; the ability to alternate between two acts necessary for such tasks was absent.

Analogous disturbances characterized the patient's speech. Spontaneous speech was just as disconnected as it had been earlier. Against this stable background, however, the tendency to repeat certain words or syllables stood out even more sharply than previously. In general there was a large difference between his spontaneous speech, which was severely disturbed and complicated by word searching, and the smoother speech which he exhibited when repeating sentences, or even literary selections. Whenever the patient was faced with the problem of denervating a certain articulatory pattern, e.g., switching from the series of syllables "bi-ba-bo" to "bo-bi-ba", he failed. Sometimes such difficulties arose in the repetition of sentences, so that once having repeated the sentence, "In the garden behind the high fence there grew some apples", he was unable to repeat the sentence. "In the garden behind the wide gate there stood a well." Instead he would reproduce it, "In the garden ... uh ... behind the high fence ...", "In the garden behind the high gate ...", etc. The tendency to perseverate was most pronounced in the performance of movements. Somewhat less so in oral speech, and almost imperceptible in the patient's writing.

Intellectual functions remained as they had been at the earlier examination, but even here the dynamic disturbances were great. Thus intellectual operations which involved only one step were preserved. The grasp of logical relationships, comprehension of the grammatical structure of meaningful speech, and understanding of numerical relationships remained intact. He had great difficulty, however, whenever it was necessary to carry out a smooth sequence of intellectual operations. Even as simple a task as successive subtractions of seven from hundred turned out to be impossible for him, since he was unable to keep in mind the sequence of operations and thus direct the overall process.

Although this case shows the same symptoms as the previous two, the focus of difficulty is shifted from the disturbance of the inner schema of kinetic patterns to a disturbance of the denervation process. Here there is an element of perseveration which was absent in the preceding cases and which apparently arises as a result of the direct involvement of deeper extrapyramidal structures. Such deep lesions in patients who do not show absolute left hemisphere dominance lead to loss of the automaticity of movements and increased effort, but aphasic symptoms are less prominent, being largely restricted to disturbances of the smoothness of speech.

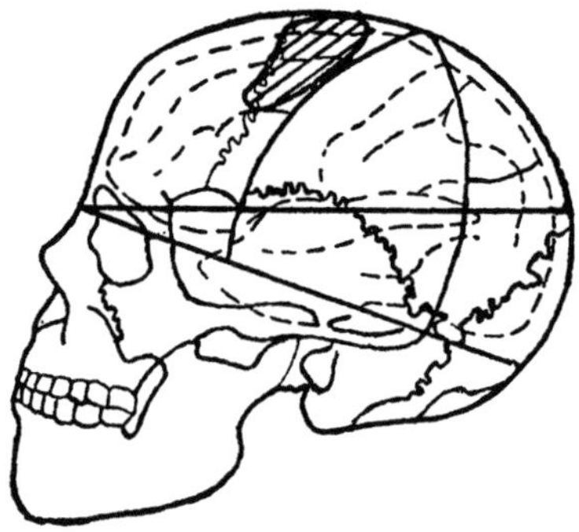

Patient Pitk.: injury diagram (Case 4)

Case 4

On September 1, 1944, patient Pitk., age 28 and left handed, received a penetrating shrapnel wound in upper parts of the left premotor and sensorimotor areas near the midline. At operation several days after injury bone splinters were extracted from the lesion which extended ventrally, anteriorly, and to the left from the site of skull injury through brain tissues. The post-operative condition of the patient was complicated by meningo-encephalitis which, however, responded favorably to therapy. An encephalogram made eight months later revealed porencephaly complicated by a multilocular cyst which extended from the premotor area ventrally to the subcortical motor nuclei.

Immediately following injury, right hemiphlegia and motor aphasia were noted. The aphasia disappeared relatively rapidly: after a month the patient began to pronounce individual words, and after three months he exhibited only a mild form of speech defect of which more will be said below. The paralysis of the right extremities was more persistent. Movements of the leg reappeared within two months, and movements reappeared in the arm after three months, with only the hand excepted. Sensation of the right side of the body was rapidly restored fully but movement was noticeably restricted, especially in the right hand, which remained paralyzed. At this time there appeared a definite grasp reflex which appeared even before an object was placed in the hand. The reflex was insusceptible to voluntary control and could be elicited by the mere approach of an object. This reflex remained even after there had been some recovery of strength in the hand. Eight months after injury any attempt at voluntary movement of the right hand produced initially a forced grasp reflex, only after this had been forcefully overcome was the patient able to carry out the desired motor act. In some cases voluntary control of the hand proved to be impossible. If, for instance, the patient was asked to reproduce a simple rhythm such as paired tapping, he would produce instead a steady series of taps, as though he were incapable of stopping the particular motion involved. Similar rhythmic movements could be performed by the left hand, but they required a considerable degree of conscious effort and never became automatic.

The same effort and loss of automaticity characterized the patient's speech. Although he had been a good speaker before the injury, he began to speak slowly and brokenly with long pauses between words and forced articulation of each word or phrase. Quite often, the utterance of a word would be preceded by a tremor of the lips. His speech was characterized by the perseverative utterance of words from which he was unable to release himself; as a result his attempts to retell a story were interrupted by intervals of forced repetition of individual words.

All the signs of perseveration and loss of automaticity were limited in this case to the motor aspects of the speech process. No signs of loss of the inner grammatical aspect of speech, agraphia, or motor-aphasic disturbance were observed. (Perhaps the absence of motor-aphasic disturbance was related to the fact that the patient was ambidextrous.)

Cases involving a loss of the automaticity of speech processes are typical of lesions of the superior parts of the premotor area, those parts not directly related to speech. The schematic diagram presented in Figure 30 shows the areas in which lesions were observed to produce disturbances of this sort.

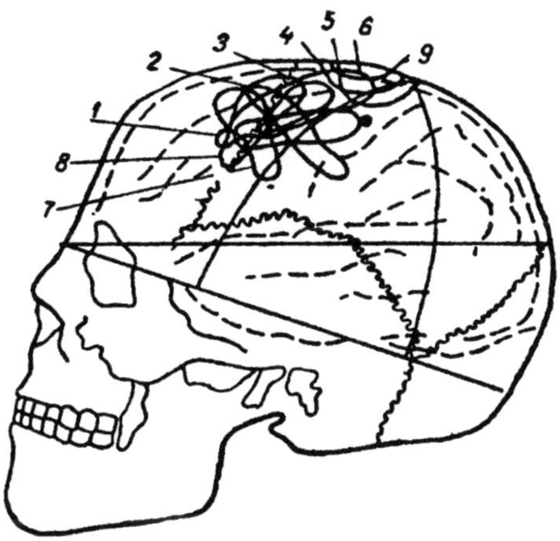

FIG. 30. Schematic diagram of lesions giving rise to premotor speech disturbances.

2. *The Syndrome of "Efferent Motor Aphasia"*

The disturbances described above which most often arise as the result of lesions involving *superior* parts of the premotor area may severely disrupt speech processes, but, still, they can be considered *external* disorders since they do not destroy the speech act itself. In those cases where the lesion extends to involve the *inferior*, specialized, parts of the premotor area the picture may be considerably different. It is not determined simply by the relationship of this strip of cortex to the cortical projection areas from the mouth, lips, tongue and throat, but also by the fact that it has an integral functional relationship with the speech areas which lie more posteriorly. The general loss of motor patterns may be less prominent, but the functional disturbance, preserving all of the features just described to a

Lesions observed in cases of premotor speech disturbances

Case No.	Name	Lesion	Speech disturbance
1	Ak.	Direct penetrating wound in the left premotor area with involvement of the motor area; right hemiparesis; disturbances of coordinated movements of left hand.	No speech for three months after injury; after three months speech lacked all continuity; after a year: slow, broken speech; writing similarly disturbed.
2	Ber.	Nonpenetrating injury of middle part in the left premotor and motor areas; right hemiparesis; severe coordination defect and loss of skilled movements.	Expressive speech disturbed after injury; after three months: broken speech with tendency to perseveration.
3	Šul.	Nonpenetrating wound in the left premotor area with compression fracture and contusion of underlying tissues; clearcut premotor syndrome with disturbance of coordinated movements.	Speech lacked its automaticity for a long time after injury; there were also disturbances of the continuity of thought processes and writing.
4	Lev.	Penetrating shrapnel wound in the left premotor area near the midline; slight right hemiparesis; pronounced premotor syndrome.	Motor aphasia immediately following the injury gave way to halting speech with disturbances of the continuity of thought processes and severe defects of inner speech.
5	Khor.	Penetrating shrapnel wound in superior parts of the premotor and motor areas; right hemiparesis; clear signs of premotor syndrome affecting left arm.	Motor aphasia persisting for a long time after injury; a year after injury speech lacked automaticity; loss of inner speech and pronounced writing defects.
6	Ter.	Nonpenetrating wound in the left premotor area with depressed bone fracture and injury of underlying brain tissue; slight residual right hemiparesis.	Transient motor aphasia following injury giving way to pronounced premotor syndrome and loss of the continuity of speech processes.
7	Op.	Direct penetrating wound in the left premotor area with involvement of brain tissue but no paresis.	Severe disturbance of motor speech for two months following injury; comprehension intact; clear premotor syndrome subsequently with loss of speech continuity and difficulty in making the transitions from one speech unit to another.
8	Žeg.	Nonpenetrating shrapnel wound in the left premotor area with compression fracture; residual right hemiparesis; definite premotor syndrome.	Motor aphasia following injury gave way to halting speech with denervation disturbances.
9	Čern.	Nonpenetrating wound in the premotor area near the midline with no paresis or sensory disturbance; severe premotor syndrome.	Loss of the continuity of speech processes and disturbances of inner speech.

certain degree, is dominated by the disturbance of the inner dynamics of the speech act. Thus there arise those forms of "efferent motor aphasia" which have been familiar to clinicians. The nature of these disturbances becomes more clear, however, in light of the above described functional disturbances which arise following lesions to the premotor zone in general.

The disturbances described above involved two components; loss of the inner structure of the speech act with its complex system of dynamic coordination and an increase in the inertia of neurodynamic processes within the motor analyzer. With lesions of the lower (specialized) parts of the premotor area of the left hemisphere both of these symptoms are present and they involve primarily *speech* processes. Damage to these highly complex and specialized structures leads to disintegration of the *sentences* and *words* in which the dynamic unity of speech and thought consists. We shall consider each of these components separately.

The basic product of that dynamic system which arises through integrated activity of the motor and sensory cortical areas is the *word*. Words results from the dynamic organization of the acoustic-articulatory analyzer which makes it possible to carry out the sequential articulations of which words are composed in unitary kinetic patterns. It is this unity which is lost following lesions of the specialized inferior parts of the premotor area. With disruption of the dynamic schemata of words, the unit of innervation becomes the individual articulatory act, so that whereas the individual articulation may be easily carried out, there is a general decrease in the plasticity of speech and the switching from one articulation to another becomes difficult. As a result the normal articulation of words becomes impossible.

Characteristically there is no impairment of the ability to articulate individual sounds. The patient has little difficulty in finding the lip and tongue positions which are necessary for the pronunciation of single sounds. He fails, however, when he is required to pronounce the same sounds as parts of whole words, i.e. to pronounce sounds in serial combination. In general, the patient loses the inner *schemata of words*; in addition he loses the ability to shift smoothly from one articulatory position to another.

This situation is complicated by one other factor. The articulatory positions for individual sounds depend to a certain extent upon the words in which they appear. They usually acquire certain "positional characteristics"[9] depending on the preceding and succeeding sounds. For the patient who has lost the inner sound schemata of words, however, it becomes extremely difficult to produce the appropriate articulatory positions of a given sound in different contexts. Thus, while such a patient can easily pronounce "pure" sounds individually, he is quite unable to find the articulatory variations appropriate to the sound contexts of different words.

[9] In the Soviet literature, these characteristics have been discussed in greatest detail by D. B. Èlkonin (1956).

In the most severe cases this loss of the dynamic aspect of speech affects not only the patient's oral speech, but also his writing. Quite often he is able to write down individual letters as they are dictated to him; but if syllables or words are dictated it quickly becomes apparent that the writing process is severely disturbed. Because of the loss of the inner schemata of the sound sequences and the inability to shift readily from one letter to another, the patient is unable to write a simple syllable. His attempts are characterized by perseveration of the first letter written, so that instead of a whole word he produces a stereotyped series of letters.

In sum we can say that the severe phenomena of efferent "motor aphasia" result from a *loss of the dynamic aspect of speech activity*. Occasionally these dynamic disturbances are so severe that the patient appears to have a true "apraxia" of the speech apparatus, but further investigation shows that this "apraxia" is either a result of the perseveration just described or, as happens quite frequently, is a reflection of traumatic involvement of afferent structures themselves to produce the symptoms discussed in a preceding chapter (See Chapter 6). The most obvious defect lies in the disturbance of articulatory processes; but this is not the only dynamic disturbance characteristic of efferent motor aphasia. Behind this are concealed more subtle defects which emerge with some clarity when the articulatory difficulties themselves have been overcome and when the patient is again capable of active expressive speech. They are associated with the disturbance of inner speech and with disintegration of the dynamic unity of *propositions*.

These disturbances also lead to defects in the verbal formulation of thought which are among the most severe signs of damage to the anterior parts of the cortical speech area. Hughlings Jackson was the first to state the view that the proposition is the basic unit of living speech and that the primary function of speech is the *formulation of thoughts into propositions*. A proposition always has a *predicative aspect*. It always says something about something. Thus behind every proposition there lies a thought. This thought is embodied in a sentence. For a young child such a sentence may be very short, sometimes limited to a single word, but even this word is, in its own way, an abbreviated proposition with a predicative aspect. As the child becomes older the propositions which he generates may become very involved, but the predicative aspect is always present to carry the meaning of the proposition.

Psychological investigations of speech development, in particular those of L. S. Vygotski, have shown that the transition from thought to external speech is invariably mediated by inner speech. In its global and purely predicative form the formulation in inner speech contains the rudiments of the dynamic schema of a sentence. The transition from inner speech to external speech consists in the unfolding of this preliminary schema, i.e. in its transformation into the structure of an externally conveyable proposition.

The grammatical structure of active speech is based upon generalized dynamic schemata to which linguists refer collectively as "the sense of the language". This sense is very deeply ingrained and may be preserved even in severe forms of dementia. It is these dynamic schemata of propositionizing, however, which suffer most in efferent forms of motor aphasia. Thus R. Jakobson (1956) has justifiably pointed out that whereas various forms of sensory aphasia are reducible to disturbances of the auditory *code* of a language the form of aphasia which we are discussing here involves disturbances of the *dynamic context* of the language.

Here loss of the dynamic schemata of sentences manifests itself in the fact that even when he has regained the ability to pronounce individual words, the patient is incapable of stringing them together according to proper schemata to form smooth grammatically structured sentences. The defect lies in the fact that the linguistic units innervated are not whole sentences but individual words. Its psychological nature, however, goes even deeper. The most important defect is that the word retains only its static nominative, designative function. The dynamic, predicative function of the word is completely destroyed. Thus, the patient can name an object standing before him relatively easily, but he is unable to express verbally any kind of desire or thought about it. The behavior and gestures of such a patient retain their sequential character, but his speech loses its sequentiality. He asks for objects by reaching for them directly; verbally he can do no more than name them.

Sentences disappear altogether from the patient's everyday speech. Inner speech, the "kernel" of the thought and the rudiment of the sentence to be unfolded, suffers most in this patient, and it becomes impossible for him to formulate sentences. Even in attempting to repeat sentences, such a patient is only able to reproduce a few words, usually substantives. His spontaneous speech is transformed into serial naming of objects. Such speech is composed of unrelated nouns; verbs are altogether absent (so-called telegraph style). In the residual period one sees typical difficulties in finding words to express thought and difficulty in the formulation of sentences, while the naming of objects presents no particular problem.

It is natural that the most persistent symptom of this disturbance should be impairment of the verbal expression of thought. Even in the later stages of recovery the patient may be able to repeat a complicated sentence, but he continues to experience significant difficulty when required to formulate his own thoughts in connected speech. His spontaneous discursive speech remains disturbed for a long time and he may continue to complain that he is unable to write connected sentences, that he forgets what he is talking about, and that he is unable to actively formulate the thoughts which he desires to express.

In cases where it is possible to follow the symptoms of speech disturbance from the earliest stage (a few weeks after injury) through the entire recovery period (many months later) one may observe the sequential development of all the symptoms which we have described. One observes the initial loss of expressive speech activity, due to disruption of the dynamic structure of individual words, giving way at later stages to specific agrammatisms, which reflect the loss of the dynamic schemata of sentences and disturbance of verbal thought. Careful analysis of the course of recovery reveals the common basis of symptoms which might otherwise appear to be quite unrelated to one another.

We shall present here only a few typical examples to illustrate this course of development. First we shall consider cases in which massive and deep penetrating wounds have destroyed the inferior part of the premotor area and tracts lying deep under it. Here one observes both a severe disturbance of the dynamic aspect of speech and specific speech denervation difficulties.

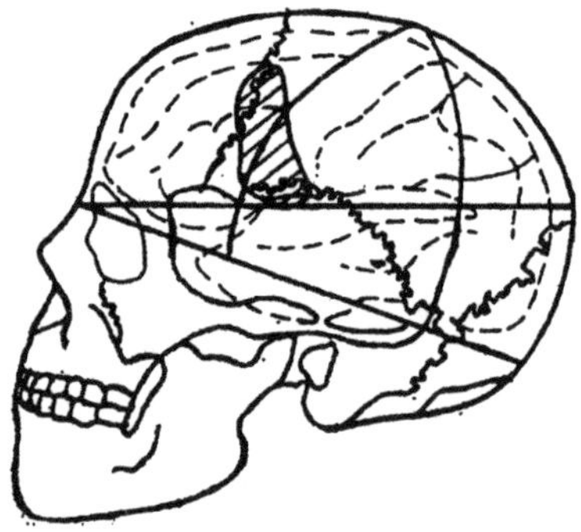

Patient Cap. eight months after injury.

Case 5

On November 3, 1942, patient Cap., age 21 (case history no. 3069) received a bullet injury of the middle portion of the left premotor area partially involving the precentral gyrus. Injury was followed by a long period of unconsciousness, complete right hemiplegia, and motor aphasia. The wound was complicated by an infection and cerebral scar tissues which were removed at operation a month after the injury. There was a considerable increase in tonus on the right accompanied by right ankle clonus and hemiparesis; sensitivity was slightly impaired on the right. Both the hemiparesis and the sensory deficit gradually disappeared and left only a residual disturbance of movement of the distal extremities and pathological sign of pyramidal damage. These symptoms remained during the patients entire hospitalization.

At the time he came under our care three weeks after injury the patient showed symptoms of a severe motor aphasia with partial disturbance of speech comprehension. He was unable to pronounce a single word, and when he needed something he could only point at it helplessly. He was able to understand words spoken individually, but did not comprehend sentences. He could neither read nor write, and he had more difficulty with written instructions than with oral instructions. Thus his speech difficulties during the first weeks after injury took the form of a severe motor aphasia which, at first glance, might appear to involve a "general" disruption of speech.

During the first six weeks, however, certain unifying characteristics of this motor aphasic syndrome became evident. The patient was examined psychologically with great care and showed no detectable signs of spatial apraxia in the "healthy" left hand. He was easily able to follow instructions to place his hands and fingers in given positions and equally easily changed the position of his hands as instructed. Sometimes he could perform more complex tasks (of the type described by Head) involving reversed imitative movement. He showed no signs of disturbance of constructional activity. He was able to reproduce rhythms, although more slowly and somewhat less automatically than normal. Tests of sequential motor activity revealed severe disruption of the *serial organization of movements.* He was unable to change the position of his hand three times in succession in response to a single instruction (strike the table with the fist, open the hand, and place it on the chest). Once he had placed his hand in a given position he was unable to reach the second position and usually repeated the first movement several times. He was unable to draw several lines in succession; here again he made several perseverative attempts (Figure 31).

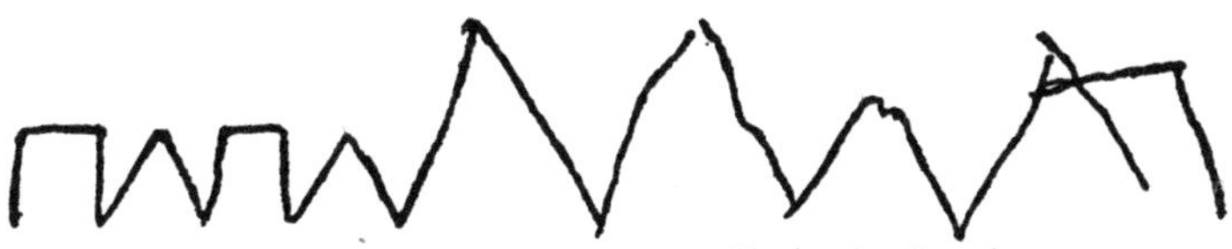

FIG. 31. Drawing test of the ability to shift from one motion to another; Patient Cap. eight months after injury.

Similar but much more pronounced disturbances were noted in the patient's *speech processes.* He was altogether incapable of spontaneous speech or of answering questions orally. The basis for this disturbance, however, was by no means an apraxia of the speech apparatus. He was able to carry out all the normal movements of tongue and lips and pronounced individual consonants and most vowels without difficulty. The pronunciation of each sound, however, was characterized by an abnormal "inertia" of the associated articulatory set. Thus having pronounced the sound "t" the patient was unable to shift to the sound "m" and began to stammer helplessly, "ah . . . well . . . ah . . ." as he attempted to eliminate this perseverative articulatory set. This "inertia" or "persistance of set" turned out to be the major factor preventing utterance of sound sequences. While he was able to pronounce isolated sounds relatively easily, he could not repeat a complex series of sounds. He was able to repeat such pairs of sounds as "pa-ba" or "da-ta", but the repetition of a series of three syllabes e.g., "bi-ba-bo" was impossible for him and gave rise to a stereotyped "ba-ba-ba", even though he tried continuously to escape from this forced repetitive pattern. Comparable difficulties appeared also in the repetition of meaningful sound sequences. The patient was only able to repeat a few one- and two-syllable words before the same kind of persistence of articulatory set and transition difficulties interrupted his speech. His difficulty became most pronounced with words involving three syllables. He repeated "Katja" as "Tjatja", i.e. made typical anticipatory substitutions. "Doroga" (road) was pronounced "do-da" or, after multiple attempts, as "do-ra". Never was he able to reproduce the series of three syllables correctly.

Characteristically the persistance of articulatory set in this patient was not limited to the perseveration of syllables within words. It also prevented him from uttering a second word. Thus having repeated the word "dom" (house) he was unable to repeat a second word "roga" (horn). Instead, he reproduced it as "do-da". In attempting to name objects presented to him the difficulty became more severe, but its nature remained essentially the same. Combinations of two words or elementary sentences were of course impossible for this patient, so that he repeated the phrase, "Daj pit'!!" simply "tit' " (as if "let's drink" were uttered "link" – trans.). Accompanying exclamations, such as "ah . . . ta . . . ah . . ." made it clear that the patient was dissatisfied with his own response, but he was unable to overcome the pattern of articulation which forced itself upon him.

The same difficulties emerged in the patient's *writing,* thus revealing a second important aspect of the basic defect. At the beginning of our detailed investigation (6-8 weeks after injury) the patient was able to write individual letters in response to dictation. He tired rapidly, however, and began to substitute previous letters for the ones dictated. The most severe disturbances arose when he went from letters to syllables and words. The ability to copy was relatively intact, i.e. he was able to copy words letter by letter, but he was completely unable to write simple words to dictation. His attempts to do this revealed that the *inner schemata of words,* the sequential schemata of sounds from which different words were composed, were lacking. Thus he sometimes repeated the

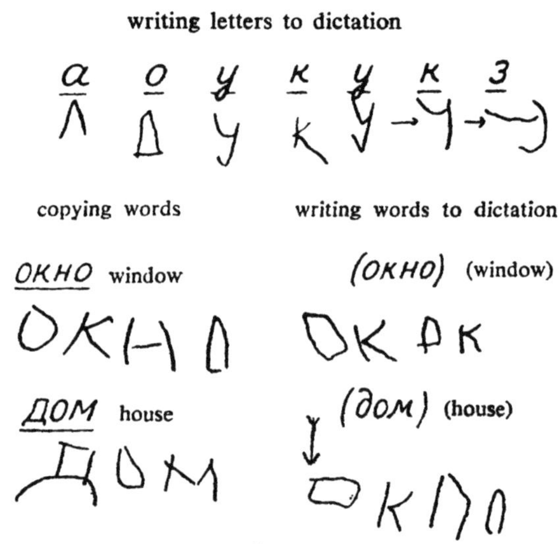

Transliteration

a	o	u	k	u	k	z
l	?	u	k	u	u	u

copying words	writing words to dictation
"Okno" (window)	(dom) (house)
OKNO	OKPO
Dom (house)	("Okno") (window)
DOM	OKOK

Patient Cap.: lesion of the anterior part of the left premotor area.

FIG. 32. Writing of Patient Cap. eight months after injury.

first letter or first syllable of a word several times; sometimes he would substitute conglomerations of incorrect letters for the correct ones. Figure 32 shows several examples of this. The loss of the schemata of words and the persistence of articulatory set affected not only the expressive speech of the patient but also his receptive speech and simple intellectual processes. At the time we studied the patient he had regained the ability to understand individual words; he was also able to point at objects which were named for him. If words were presented in groups, however, the patient soon ran into difficulty. His comprehension became less reliable; the words lost their precise meanings and he had a tendency to point repeatedly to one and the same object. Thus when he was presented a *pair of words,* e.g. pencil-key, comb-pencil, etc., he was almost never able to remember the two objects long enough to point at them both. It was also impossible for him to carry out instructions presented orally. Instead of phrases, he caught only individual unordered words. As a result, he was helpless to carry out the actions expected of him.

The same "narrowing" of the perceptual field to a single element and inability to transform a task into a schema represented in inner speech was also seen in the patient's attempts at *calculation.* He easily recognized the meaning of individual numbers as they were named, i.e. he was able to write them down or show the corresponding number of fingers. But the inability to remember series of numbers prevented him from carrying out any kind of calculation.

This was the clinical picture observed during the first stage of the patient's aphasic syndrome. It is easy to see that it consisted *not so much in the disturbance of articulatory movements as in loss of the dynamic schemata of words and the resulting destruction of the schemata of sequential mental operations.*

The patient underwent extensive retraining, the basic purpose of which was to reestablish the defective schemata of sound sequences and to eliminate the pathological persistence of excitation. This form of therapy shortly led to a stage in which it was possible to see specific disturbances of speech structure which had earlier been masked by the total motor aphasia. Five to eight months after injury, the paresis was restricted to the right hand. Movements of the leg and proximal portions of the arm were regained after special pharmacological therapy. In the left (healthy) hand all forms of manipulatory movements were retained as before, except that they lacked the smooth automaticity of skilled activity. Only with great effort was the patient able to make smooth serial movements.

His speech had recovered considerably. He was able to repeat easy words with no signs of oral apraxia and only showed difficulty when required to repeat very complex combination of sounds. The repetition of series of syllables or series of words, however, created great difficulty. He was unable to repeat three syllables, e.g. "bi-ba-bo"; instead he might respond with a simplified sequence, e.g. "bi-bo-bo". Having spoken the word "bulka" (roll) he was unable to utter the word "bublik" (thick ring-shaped roll) and repeated several times "bulka . . . bulki . . . bulbik . . ." as though he were unable to suppress the first articulatory set once it had been established. The patient was easily able to repeat a series of three words, e.g. "house, cat, table", but if the order of the words was altered, e.g. "house, table, cat", he was unable to overcome the inertia of the sequential pattern first established.

The disturbance of the schemata of words as sequential sound complexes severely affected the ability of the patient to analyze consciously the sequence of sounds in words and his ability to write words to dictation. These symptoms proved to be the most difficult to overcome in the course of retraining.

Six months after injury the patient was unable to analyze the sequences of sounds in simple words, even though he could easily pronounce them. Thus, while he was able

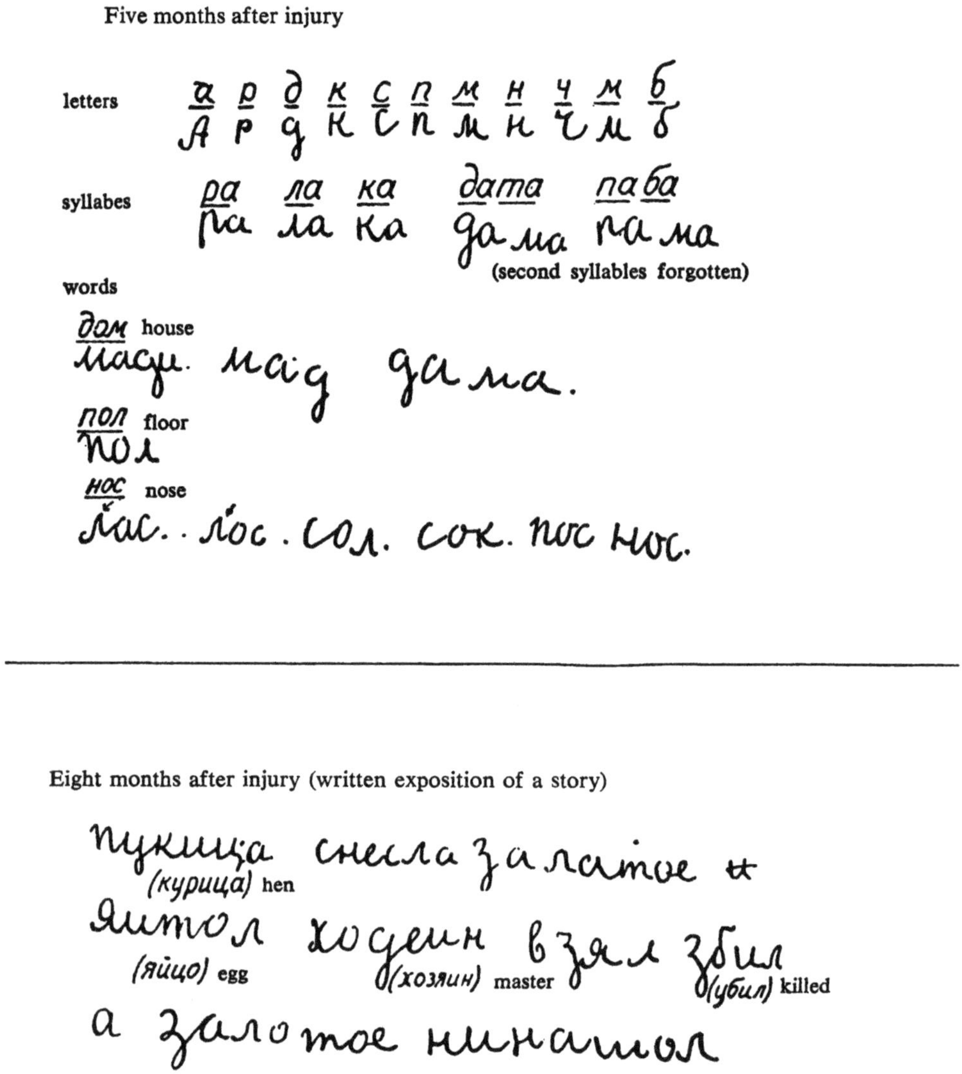

Patient Cap.: lesion in the anterior part of the left premotor area; motor aphasia.

FIG. 33. Writing of Patient Cap. 5-8 months after injury.

to say that the word "kot" (cat) consisted of three letters, he might say that the first letter was "k" the second "t" and the third "o". He had the same difficulty in maintaining the order of constituent sounds when he interpreted the sounds "t-o-k" (current) as "kto" (who), and the sounds "b-r-a-t" (brother) as "rab . . . bar . . . brig" (slave . . . bar . . . brig). Needless to say, at this stage the patient also had great difficulty in writing words. He often omitted letters, so that only skeletons of words remained; he confused the order of letters, or replaced the appropriate letter by perseverative repetition of previous letters (Figures 33, 34). Thus difficulties which had already largely dis-

Transliteration of Fig. 33

Five months after injury

letters	a	r	d	k	s	p	m	n	č	m	b
	A	r	d	k	s	p	m	n	č	m	ɦ

syllables	ra	la	ka	data	paba
	ra	la	ka	dama	pama (second syllables forgotten)

words

dom (house)
mad i   mad   dama

pol (floor)
pol

nos (nose)
las . . .   los . . .   sol   sok   pos   nos

Eight months after injury (written exposition of a story)

pukica	snesla	zalatoe	i
(kurica (hen)	(lay)	(gold)	
jaico	xozjain	vzjal	ubil
(egg)	(master)	(took)	(killed)
a	zalotoe	ninašol	
(but)	(golden)	(not found)	

Patient Cap.: lesion in the anterior part of the left premotor area; motor aphasia.

FIG. 34. Writing of Patient Cap. 5-8 months after injury.

appeared from the patient's oral articulation of words remained in his writing where conscious analysis of the order of constituent elements was required.

Although the articulation of individual words was relatively intact during this period, very severe disturbances persisted in more complex forms of speech, e.g. in sentence structure. Observation of the patient's attempts to repeat simple sentences revealed gross disturbance. The patient would repeat a short sentence as though he were simply enumerating the individual words of which it was composed. He was most likely to enumerate the *nouns*, which have no predicative function. Verbs and, to an even greater extent, adjectives, conjunctions, and pronouns were omitted; so that all that remained of such sentences were their "nominative" (substantive) skeletons. Even sentences consisting of two or three words were repeated agrammatically. Thus a sentence of the type, "Winter is coming", was reproduced as "Winter", or "Winter . . . is coming . . . winter

. . ."; and "The weather was nice yesterday", as, "Was . . . weather . . . sun . . .". The patient was clearly unable to reproduce the grammatical schemata of sentences.

The patient's agrammatism resulting from retention only of the nominative aspects of words emerged most clearly in his narrative speech, which consisted of nouns designating certain major events of the story with no elaboration of sentence structure. This is how, for instance, he related the contents of a certain movie: "Odessa! a swindler! down there . . . to study . . . the sea . . . (a gesture to represent diving) . . . into . . . a diver! Armena (Armenia) . . . (a ship . . . went . . . oh! Batum! a girl . . . ah! Po-li-ceman . . . ah! . . . I know! . . . cashier! . . . money . . . ah! . . . cigarettes . . . I know . . . this guy . . . beer . . . mustache . . . ah . . . money . . . Mikalai ("Nikolaevskie") . . . ah . . . suit . . . di-ver . . . ah . . . a mask . . . a light . . . ah . . . up . . . came . . . the girl . . ." etc. The entire grammatical sentence structure was lost and the patient showed extreme disturbance of the inner schemata of connected speech.

This breakdown of grammatical speech structure into single nominative words is not simply the result of an articulatory difficulty or due to a disturbance of the "conservation of energy" to which many authors have referred in analyzing the phenomenon of "telegraph style". Behind it there lies a disintegration of the dynamic schemata of speech and a severe disturbance of inner speech which leads to loss of the "feeling for language". This is seen in the fact that, even though the patient attempts to correct the defects of his agrammatical sentences, he is unable to do so. Clearly incompatible sentence fragments stand side by side and words are used in their basic "null" form (nouns in the nominative case, verbs in indeterminate forms) as though the patient is not always aware of the inaccuracy of such forms. Another aspect of the problem is seen in the fact that the patient has great difficulty in comprehending complex sentences. He must repeat them several times aloud before their meaning becomes clear to him. If speech is excluded, i.e. if he attempts to understand the meaning of a complex statement without repeating it to himself, comprehension is impossible for him. Apparently, comprehension becomes impossible with loss of the capacity for preliminary processing which the normal person carries out by means of inner speech.

In many ways this case is a typical example of efferent motor aphasia. Here there is no difficulty in finding articulatory positions and no oral apraxic difficulties. There is a disturbance of the schemata of serial movements in general and of speech sequences in particular. Eventually the syndrome is reduced to a residual defect in the dynamic schemata of connected grammatical speech. The ability to articulate individual sounds does not guarantee the ability to pronounce whole words. The mastery of whole words likewise does not necessarily permit the utterance of sentences. In such a patient loss of the articulatory *synthesis of words* may prevent the pronunciation of words and loss of the synthesis of sentences may preclude the recovery of connected speech; for these are the dynamic units of verbal thought. This is the reason why the patient's primary difficulty during the early stages of recovery lies in the pronunciation of sound complexes, and gives rise to literal dysphasias and writing disturbances. This is also why during later stages of recovery such a patient passes through a phase of severe agrammatism which very often takes several months to overcome.

On the basis of the case just described we can now analyze the essential components underlying "efferent" motor aphasia. This form of speech disturbance arising with lesions of the lower, specialized parts of the premotor area, may involve extremely severe disturbances of expressive speech. Sometimes the disturbance of expressive speech may be extremely complex and involve several features which we shall consider below. This is explained by the fact that "Broca's area", receiving inputs both from postcentral and temporal structures, is apparently the final common path for the generation of speech impulses. Thus it possesses a very complex function which is still not fully understood and damage to it, by altering the overall functional system may prevent normal functioning in the structures which send information to it. On the other hand, Broca's area is so small that an injury seldom affects it alone; the adjacent sensory motor area is also usually involved. We have succeeded, however, in picking out those disturbances which arise as the result of direct involvement of the premotor area and thus constitute the essential defect of the underlying efferent motor aphasia. The essential elements of "efferent motor aphasia" are loss of the serial organization of speech which arises as the result of a pathological inertia of individual articulatory impulses shortly following trauma, and the disturbance of inner speech which develops in subsequent stages as the result of motor agrammatism and loss of the predicative significance of words.

We found the difficulty in the transition from one sound, syllable, or word to another which disrupts normal speech activity to be the predominant feature in a large group of cases involving lesions of this area. The diagram in Figure 35 makes it clear that lesions in the anterior parts of the speech area itself rather than lesions in the postcentral part are responsible for the syndrome characteristically referred to as "efferent motor aphasia". A description of the disturbances observed as the result of lesions in the postcentral parts of the speech area will be presented below.

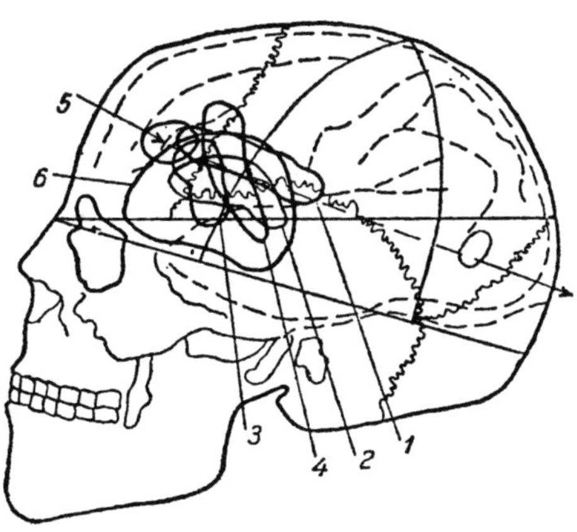

FIG. 35. Schematic diagram of lesions giving rise to efferent motor aphasia.

Lesions observed in cases of efferent motor aphasia

Case No.	Name	Lesion	Speech disturbances
1	Sam.	Superficial penetrating wound in lower parts of the left premotor and sensorimotor areas; severe right hemiparesis.	Motor aphasia with preservation of the ability to pronounce individual sounds; great difficulty in pronouncing complicated syllables and words; pronounced impairment of the ability to denervate speech units; writing defect.
2	Dim.	Direct penetrating wound in lower parts of the left frontal area with extrusion of brain substance and right hemiparesis.	Motor aphasia with preservation of the ability to pronounce individual sounds and, sometimes, short words; severe difficulties in uttering series of syllables, long words, or sentences; a similar writing disturbances; spontaneous speech totally absent.
3	Khv.	Penetrating shrapnel wound in lower parts of the frontal area and border of the temporal area; right hemiparesis.	Severe motor aphasia with preservation of the ability to pronounce individual sounds but great difficulty in pronouncing combinations of syllables or words; similar disorders affecting writing.
4	Čum.	Penetrating shrapnel wound in lower parts of the premotor area involving part of the sensorimotor area; right hemiparesis.	Motor aphasia of moderate severity; all forms of praxis preserved; difficulty in denervating movements of the hand performed in sequence; ability to pronounce individual sounds and short words intact; great difficulty in pronouncing series of syllables, words, or sentences; clear signs of motor agrammatism.
5	Rž.	Wound inflicted by bullet entering the lower left frontal area and leaving through the left occipital area; right hemiparesis.	Severe motor aphasia; all forms of praxis preserved; profound disturbance of all attempts to carry out sequences of actions; apraxia of the speech apparatus absent; individual sounds pronounced easily, but series of syllables and words impossible; similar writing defects.
6	Abd.	Penetrating shrapnel wound in the left fronto-parietal and temporal areas with gross destruction of brain substance by a brain abscess; right hemiparesis.	Total motor aphasia; all forms of praxis preserved with obvious impairment of the ability to carry out serial movements; apraxia of the speech apparatus absent, but coordination of tongue and lip movements with respiratory movements impaired; preservation of the ability to repeat individual sounds and short words, but inability to remember or spontaneously use them; severe difficulty in repeating series of sounds or syllables; similar writing defects.

3. *The Syndrome of "Frontal Dynamic Aphasia"*

In all cases mentioned, the *external, phasic aspect of speech* suffered most, acoustic analysis was impaired, patterns of articulatory movements were disrupted, or the transition from one articulatory pattern to another was disturbed. There exist, however, forms of aphasia intimately related to those just described in which the external audio-articulatory organization of speech remains completely intact. The patient is able to distinguish speech sounds and talk (repeat words or name objects), but all the same he may show signs of aphasia which are even more profound than those we have described.

One such form of aphasia is the *frontal dynamic aphasia* which Goldstein has referred to as "central motor aphasia" in order to distinguish it from the "peripheral motor aphasia" described above. The essential symptom of frontal dynamic aphasia is that the patient is unable to use speech for generalizing or for the expression of thoughts and desires. It is as though such a patient's speech were deprived of its basic function, which Jackson characterized as the ability to formulate thoughts into sentences (propositionizing) and which Head referred to as "symbolic formulation and expression". This form of aphasia which dominated the attention of Jackson and which, in its pure form, also attracted the attention of A. Pick (1913, 1931), Head (1936), Kleist (1930, 1937), Ombredane (1951), and others, deserves special analysis.

The disturbances of speech which we are considering here are not frequently seen in a pure form. As a rule they arise as a result of *lesions involving the lower parts of the left frontal lobe just anterior to Broca's area.* In these cases there is destruction of a large part of the lower "speech" strip of the postero-frontal area without involving those parts of the premotor area, which, being closely connected with the posterior parts of the speech area, are directly involved in the execution of articulatory movements. The central feature of the disturbances in these cases is that, while the ability to utter words and even to repeat sentences remains intact, the patient is *completely deprived of spontaneous speech* and seldom uses it for purposes of communication.

It is extremely difficult to explain this syndrome in neurological terms, for we are still far from understanding its mechanisms. Thus what we have to say here must necessarily be limited to certain preliminary observations and impressions.

The area which is pathologically affected in this form of aphasia is one of the frontal cortical areas. It is well known clinically that lesions in this area produce "aspontaneity", "loss of initiative", "loss of purposeful activity", "impairment of active thought", etc. (Bekhterev, Bianchi, Kleist, Xoroško, Brickner, Penfield, Freeman and Watts and many others). Lesions of the anterior part of the left frontal lobe have often been found to produce a special type of "disturbance of verbal initiative" or "aspontaneity of speech" (Kleist). Despite the fact that these clinical observations are well established, however, the physiological interpretation of what Bechterev in the late 19th century referred to as the "psycho-regulatory function" of the frontal lobes remains a problem for future research.

Physiological investigations recently carried out on animals (Anoxin, 1949; Šumilina, 1949; Šustin, 1957; Pribram, 1957-58) suggests that with lesions of the frontal lobes an animal's behavior ceases to be subjected to the antecedent integrative system of associations which arise in the cerebral cortex and direct the behavior of the normal animal. As a result of this disturbance the animal with a frontal lobectomy is unable to perform delayed reaction tasks (Bianchi, 1926; Jacobson, 1935; Anoxin, 1949, Šustin, 1957, Pribram, 1957, and others). When placed in a situation demanding a choice between two stimuli, the animal lacking its frontal lobes immediately picks the most readily perceived stimulus, (Jacobson, Pribram, Šustin). Such an animal also has a tendency to make senseless mechanical movements between the two stimuli (Anoxin). This type of observation provided I. P. Pavlov the basis for suggesting that the dog whose frontal lobes have been resected is essentially an animal deprived of purposeful behavior (Pavlov, 1951).

In man the organization of the "antecedent syntheses" which determine active purposeful behavior is greatly complicated by the fact that for him a decisive role is played by associations which arise on the basis of *speech*. Thus the "active", "voluntary" "conscious", or "willed" behavior of man can by no means be considered as undetermined. It must be interpreted as behavior determined by a complex system of preliminary (antecedent) connections which arise on the basis of external and inner speech.

We have studied the development of the system of speech associations which plays so decisive a role in the development of further activity in a large series of special investigations.[10] These studies showed that such associations begin to form in the normal child as early as the third year but at this time are still very weak and require constant reinforcement by the child's *vocalization of his own self instructions*. Eventually such connections become quite stable, so that in simple cases inner speech may be relied upon at age 4 or $4\frac{1}{2}$ (Vygotskij, 1956; O. K. Tixomirov, 1958). It is these systems of connections developed on the basis of inner speech that disintegrate as a result of the weakening of excitatory-inhibitory processes in the cerebral cortex, e.g., in the cerebro-asthenic syndrome (E. D. Xomskaja, 1956, 1958). They are severely disturbed by frontal lobe lesions. Special investigations carried out in our laboratories (and published in a special book[11]) have shown that massive lesions in the convex parts of the frontal lobes (and primarily of the dominant hemisphere) produce no noticeable disturbance of the

[10] A. R. Luria, *Problems of Higher Nervous Activity of the Normal and Abnormal Child*, Vol. I (Moscow, 1956) and Vol. II (Moscow, 1958). Idem, *The Role of the Speech in the Regulation of Normal and Abnormal Behavior* (London, Pergamon Press, 1961).

[11] A. R. Luria and E. D. Homskaja (eds.), *Frontal Lobes and Regulation of Psychological Processes* (Moscow University Press, 1966).

phasic, lexical, or grammatical aspect of speech. They do, however, severely disturb the regulatory role of those connections which have been established on the basis of speech. By means of simple experimental techniques we were able to demonstrate a variety of features of the frontal syndrome. If a lesion involves both the convexity of the frontal lobe and its connections with the basal areas it may produce a syndrome of aspontaneity and defective behavioral control of such severity as to totally disrupt the patient's planned purposeful behavior. If it involves only a focus within the convexity of the left hemisphere, the disturbance of the regulatory role of antecedent input based on speech processes may be more subtle and appear only in situations where intellectual functions must be highly flexible and where the inhibition of immediate impulses is necessary for the correct solution of tasks. Finally, if the pathological focus is situated directly anterior to Broca's area and disrupts the normal regulatory function of inner speech without involving the audio-articulatory organization of external speech, one may observe the characteristic forms of speech disturbance which we are to consider next.

If the pathological focus, e.g. a tumor, arises within the premotor area and then gradually spreads to involve neighboring frontal cortex, one may clearly observe the successive development and close interaction of both syndromes. The first signs of disturbance in such cases are loss of motor habits and skilled movements. Later one observes involuntary movements and perseveration. Only a long time later does one observe a dissociation of activity from motives, difficulty in the voluntary performance of various acts and complete automatisms which are in no way determined by the patient's intentions.

Once we had the opportunity to observe a case which involved a slowly developing astrocytoma in the premotor area of the left frontal lobe. At first, the only sign was a virtually imperceptible weakness of the right hand accompanied by perseveration of movement in both hands, a definite decline in the smoothness of skilled movements, and a noticeable lack of smoothness in expressive speech. Subsequently, as the tumor expanded deeper into the premotor area these symptoms became more severe and were associated with simple automatism; when the patient tapped his finger, he was unable to stop even though it was clear that the movement was continuing against his wishes. Six months later when the tumor had clearly begun to expand into more anterior parts of the frontal lobe the syndrome changed considerably; individual movements were disturbed and a noticeable impairment of goal-directed activity became apparent. Sometimes this manifested itself as an instability of intention and "a forgetting of intention". The patient noted that he would go to the railroad station near his summer house only to find that he had "forgotten" why he was going to Moscow and would return home. Other times the disturbance would take the form of involuntary unmotivated actions. "I'm sitting here and I see the bell, and my hand is drawn to it. I ring and the nurse comes, I don't know why I called her." As time went on these uncontrolled actions became more common and inner purposeful intentions gradually disappeared so that eventually, as more and more of the frontal lobe became involved, we were dealing with a typical frontal lobe patient with a severe impairment of initiative and frequent automatisms inaccessible to voluntary control.

The results of trauma to this area run a similar course. If the pathological focus is located in the middle and upper central parts of the frontal premotor area it may not elicit severe speech disturbances. If, on the other hand, the lesion involves lower parts of the premotor area and spreads to neighboring areas of the frontal cortex, all of the changes described above may affect speech processes as well as simple motor activity. If the injury involves areas close to Broca's area, a severe motor aphasia may emerge as an initial symptom and the syndrome of "frontal", dynamic aphasia may only emerge later with the gradual disappearance of edema, resolution of the hematoma, and scar formation. When the lesion is located further anteriorly, one may observe only a mild motor aphasia; defects in the dynamic structure of speech processes associated with difficulties in carrying out verbally formulated intentions and frequent perseveration of simple speech patterns may predominate from the first.

We shall present two cases which clearly illustrate the two types of syndrome just described. Then we shall take up cases which show the "frontal" aphasic syndrome in a more pure form, i.e. cases in which the defects of "verbal initiative" and the disturbance of the dynamic structure of speech are the predominant symptoms.

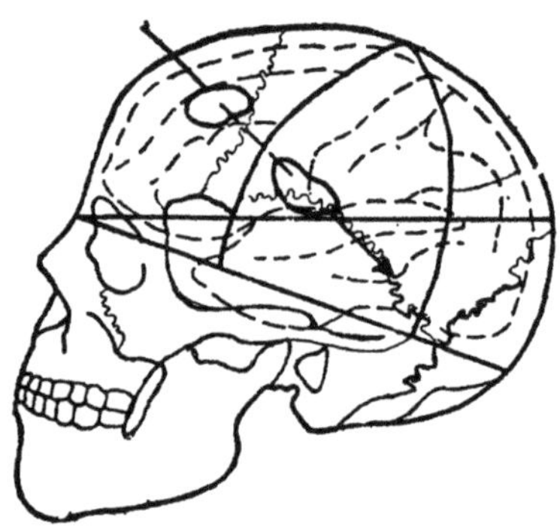

Patient Vav.: injury diagram (Case 7)

Case 7

On August 12, 1944, patient Vav. age 20 (case history no. 10112), an electrician with seven years schooling, was wounded by a bullet which entered the center of the left frontal area and emerged through the lower part of the left sensorimotor area. The following day an operation was performed to clear the area of bone fragments; 100 cc. of cortical tissue was removed. The recovery period was long and difficult and further brain substance was lost by extrusion from the skull defects.

Immediately following injury a right hemiplegia and motor aphasia were observed. The patient was placid. There was a loss of bladder control, but the patient's reaction was indifferent. The hemiplegia gradually disappeared giving way to a spastic hemiparesis which was most pronounced in the arm and accompanied by a sensory disturbance and altered reflexes. Three months later the patient's speech had also recovered to a considerable degree.

At the time of the first detailed examination four months after injury the patient was relatively active, somewhat apathetic, and somewhat euphoric. He answered questions easily, but was altogether incapable of narrative speech. Spontaneous expression and story telling were impossible. Articulation of words and sentences required great effort. Most of his answers consisted of single words or short sentences. Often he would utter the first two words of a sentence which he failed to complete.

The patient showed no signs of apraxia. He was easily able to place his hand in a given position and to fulfill tasks involving constructive activity. He showed no signs of apraxia of the speech apparatus. He showed noticeable difficulty, however, in carrying out sequential movements. Thus, when performing a single act he showed no signs of perseveration, but when required to execute a series of movements, he quickly forgot the correct order and often would repeat the same movement several times.

A similar phenomenon characterized his speech. He easily uttered individual sounds, but if required to repeat syllables in pairs or triplets he ran into difficulty. He would repeat one syllable several times and had a tendency to reproduce "pa-ba" as "pa-pa", or to reproduce "bi-ba-bo" as "bo-bo-bo". The repetition of meaningful syllables was easier, but still, in repeating the word "boroda" (beard), there was an obvious persistance of previously articulated speech patterns, so that after pronunciation of the word "brovi" (eyebrows) "boroda" was pronounced "borova". After correct pronunciation of the word "derevo" (tree) the word "perina" (featherbed) was pronounced "perevo"; and after "nogot'" (fingernail) he was altogether unable to repeat "derevo". In this case the two previously innervated articulatory patterns persisted to such a degree that the new word was impossible to pronounce. A series of two or three words was extremely difficult to reproduce, so that instead of "house-wood-cat" the patient had a tendency to repeat "house-wood ... house ...", as though he were unable to tear himself away from the persistent set. As a rule it was easier for him to repeat a series of words comprising a sentence than to repeat a nonsense series of words; thus after several attempts to reproduce the sentence, "Apple trees grew in the garden", he was able to do so with relative accuracy.

This loss of the ability to carry out sequences of acts and the tendency to perseveration emerged very clearly in the patient's *reading and writing*. He easily wrote individual letters in response to dictation, but it was much more difficult for him to write syllables or simple words. He was unable to write nonsense series of letters; his attempts were characterized by severe perseveration of the initial letters (Figure 36). The loss of the ability to maintain the sequence of elements and the accompanying tendency to perseveration were observed in his attempt to draw a series of figures of any type.

Similar defects appeared in his reading. He easily read individual letters and individual words, but when he came to connected text, e.g. a complete sentence, in which the first words were meant to create a certain mental set, he was unable to continue correctly. Instead, he might repeat the first words or substitute related "expected" words on the basis of his immediate associations. The following represents four attempts to read an address.

The patient also showed sign of instability in his attempts to carry out simple calculations. Thus, while he was easily able to write one and two digit numbers in response to dictation, he began to reverse digits and show signs of perseveration in writing three digit numbers. He might write 321 as 231 (reversal) and then write the next number 523 as 521 (perseveration). This perseverative tendency emerged most clearly when the patient attempted to make simple calculations. He might write "2 + 4" as "2 + 6" (anticipating the answer and substituting it for the second number to be added). Having correctly solved the problems "7 + 3 = 10", he was unable to shift from addition to

Text:	Moscow	EG505	Section 6	Ward 175
Trials:	Read as:			
1.	Moscow	5 . . .	Section 2 (perseveration of former address)	Vavilov (patient's surname)
2.	Moscow	2	Section	Va-vi-lo-vy (corresponding to digits 1-7-5)
3.	Moscow	Section 2	Ward 6	5,7,3 Ward
4.	Moscow	I don't know	Section 6	5,7,2 Ward

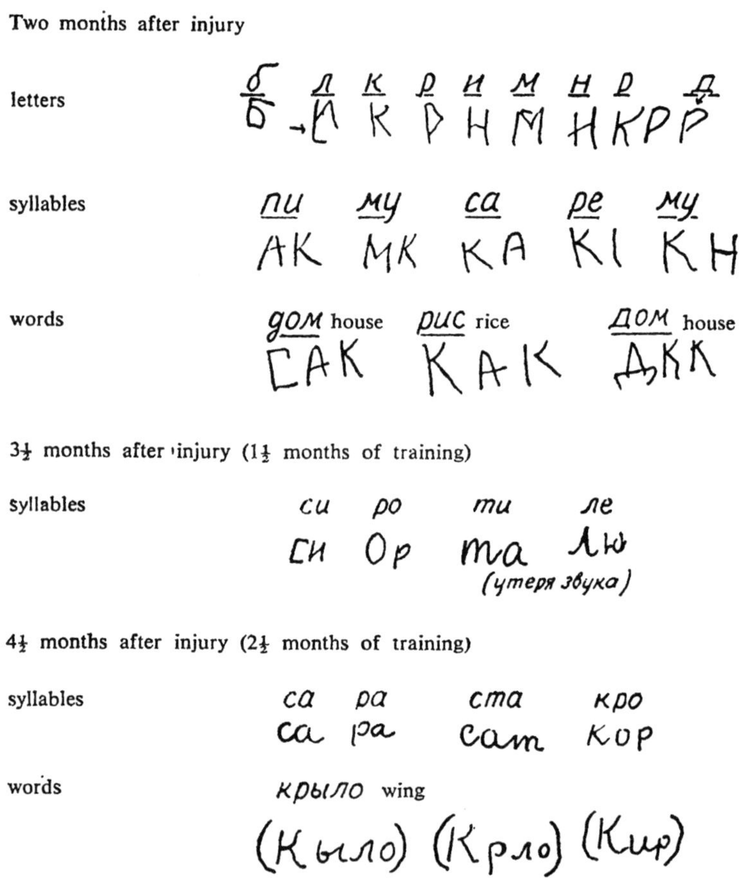

Patient Vav.: lesion of the left fronto-temporal area (translations see p. 205).

FIG. 36. Writing samples from Patient Vav.

substraction; thus, the next problem, "21 — 7", was written first: "21 + 7", and then "11 — 7". All of the symptoms observed during the initial period proved to be extremely persistent and remained for a long time after the initiation of therapy. Eight months after injury, however, the patient was able to repeat words, simple word lists, and sentences. With a certain degree of effort he was also able to convey the contents of a story and to talk spontaneously upon a given theme. His spontaneous speech was not

Two months after injury

letter	b	l	k	r	i	m	n	r	d
	B	B+L	k	r	n	m	n	kr	r

syllables	pi	mu	sa	re	mu
	AK	MK	KA	KL	KN

words	dom (house)	ris (rise)	dom (house)
	SAK	KAK	DKK

3½ months after injury (1½ months of training)

syllables	si	ro	mi	le
	si	or	ma	lyu

4½ months after injury (2½ months of training)

syllables	sa	ra	sta	kro
	sa	ra	sam	kor

words	krylo (wing)		
	(kylo)	(Krlo)	(Kir)

Patient Vav.: lesion of the left fronto-temporal area

Transliterations of FIG. 36. Writing samples from Patient Vav.

characterized by severe agrammatism. At this time he had noticeable difficulty in shifting from the recitation of one series of nonsense syllables ("bi-ba-bo") to another ("ba-bo-bi"); he also showed a tendency to perseveration and the repetition of sentences. Thus, having correctly repeated the sentence "the magpie loves anything that glitters", he reproduced the sentence, "No sooner does not he see something than he takes it away somewhere" as, "No sooner does he see something than he carries away anything that glitters." Only after several corrections was he able to overcome this perseveration. At this time he also showed a severe writing impairment characterized by an inability to maintain the sequence of letters in words and by a tendency to perseveration. Finally, he showed a severe reading disturbance growing out of a difficulty in analyzing the sequence of letters in words and tendency to impose his own meaning upon whatever he read.

The patient was released after seven months of therapy with mild residual symptoms of the syndrome described.

In this case the disturbances of speech dynamics, such as instability of intention and the tendency to perseveration, were accompanied by rather clear disturbances of speech itself. This appeared most clearly in writing and in the conscious analysis of the sound components of words. Lesions located somewhat more anteriorly and not affecting Broca's areas may give rise to a syndrome in which these symptoms are less prominent. In these cases a general akinesia of speech and thought and a persistence of more general kinetic patterns alter the flow of normal speech activity.

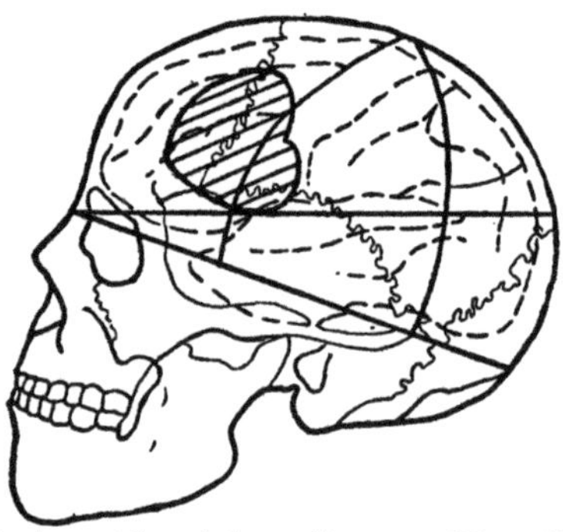

Patient Abr.: injury diagram (Case 8)

Case 8

On October 3, 1942, patient Abr., age 36 (case history no. 3069) received a penetrating injury in the inferior part of the premotor area; anteriorly a portion of the prefrontal lobe was involved; the lesion extended as far posteriorly as the Sylvian fissure and temporal pole. The patient was unconscious for several hours; there was no paralysis. A defect in the dura mater was observed at operation, and bone fragments were removed from the brain tissue. There were mild symptoms of a left hemispheric lesion in the form of a slight paresis in the right extremities with hyperreflexia. There were no sensory disturbances. Immediately following injury the patient suffered from a general akinesia, e.g. loss of bladder control. There was no motor aphasia. He seldom spoke and answered questions in a monotone, sometimes inappropriately.

At the time a detailed examination was carried out two months after injury the patient was somewhat improved. He was not very active, but his behavior was always appropriate. He complained that he had difficulty in following a train of thought and in carrying out intentions. He noted that this "speech did not always hold together", that "sometimes you say something that is not at all what you should say". He complained of great difficulty in writing. A careful examination elicited no signs of motor disturbance except that he showed a certain awkwardness in carrying out complex coordinated movements of the hands. The phasic aspect of the patient's speech was altogether intact. He had no articulatory difficulties and showed no signs of motor aphasia and no amnestic-aphasic symptoms in the naming of objects. His immediate memory for words was reasonable good, so that in memorizing a list of ten words he produced a satisfactory learning curve. Intellectual functions were intact; he was able to comprehend logical-grammatical constructions and to solve complex problems.

Against this relatively normal background, the patient showed a noticeable *disturbance of spontaneous speech.* He was unable to carry out any kind of involved narration. In telling a story his speech was limited to disconnected grammatically disordered word sequences. Severe disturbances were also seen in the repetition of groups of words or sentences. When he was asked to repeat the words "table-nose-house" he did so quite well, but when subsequently asked to repeat the words "cat-table-nose" he repeated (or wrote) "cat-nose-house", as though he were unable to overcome the inertia of the first word pattern. Even when instructed to copy the second group of words, he was unable to do so if the sample were erased before he had finished copying it. Always the second group was replaced by the group mastered first. A similar result was obtained when he was asked to reproduce sentences. He was able to repeat the first sentence relatively well, but instead of repeating the next sentence correctly, he inevitably produced a repetition of the first. The patient repeated the phrase, "In the garden there grew apple trees", correctly; but in attempting to repeat the second sentence, "On the wall there hung a coat", he was unable to shift to the new construction. His attempts were as follows: "in the wall there hung . . .", ". . . coat"; "In the wall there climbed . . . no"; "In the wall there hung . . .", etc. Perseveration was even more prominent in the patient's writing. The ability to write individual letters and words was not affected, but he was unable to make the transition from one sentence to another. Figure 37 shows that the patient was unable to write the simple sentence, "I was severely injured". Here he perseverated on the word "found" which had been part of a previous exercise and was unable to carry out the instruction.

1 sentence "Ja našel bol'šoj grib."
("I found a large mushroom")
(written correctly)

2 sentence "Ja byl tjaželo ranen."
("I was severely wounded.")

Transliteration:

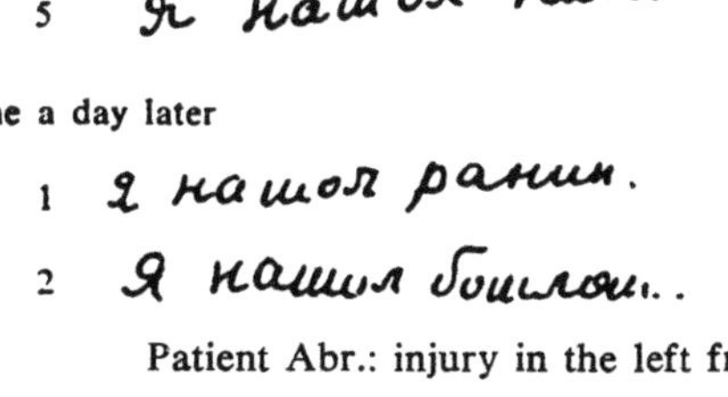

1 Ja byl . . .
2 Ja nabyl panin
3 Ja našel
4 Ja našol nanin
5 Ja našol nanin

the same a day later

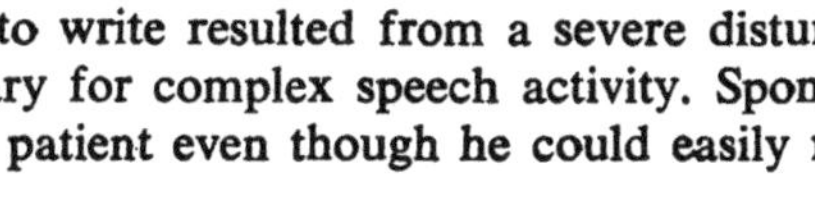

1 Ja nashol panin
2 Ja nasol bošlan . . .

Patient Abr.: injury in the left frontal area.

FIG. 37. A sample of writing by patient Abr.

The inability to write resulted from a severe disturbance of the denervation process which is necessary for complex speech activity. Spontaneous narrative speech was impossible for this patient even though he could easily repeat individual words and name single objects. Spontaneous speech was impossible for him because of the difficulty in formulating new sentences and because the schemata were disrupted by the perseveration of the schemata of preceding sentences. Thus, although the patient suffered no primary articulatory defects, he was, for all practical purpose, unable to talk.

In the cases just presented severe damage to the anterior parts of the premotor area and oral parts of the frontal lobe gave rise to the characteristic syndrome of "dynamic aphasia" in which impairment of spontaneous speech was associated with a sharp increase in the persistence or "inertia" of established speech sets. The loss of spontaneous speech is by no means always associated with the pathological persistence of speech patterns, however. There are also cases of frontal "dynamic aphasia" in which the perseverative tendency is absent or very slight, so that the major symptom is a disturbance of smooth spontaneous speech. Usually a loss of the unity of thought and speech underlies these disturbances and manifests itself as a great difficulty in the formulation of verbal intention. The causes of these two forms of "frontal aphasia" are not yet clear. Perhaps they result from the pathological involvement of cortico-subcortical connections disturbing the regulation of elementary motor processes which can be seen in the form just described.

As we saw earlier, lesions in the left premotor area destroy the ability to carry out action sequences. In particular there is a loss of the inner schemata of speech. Lesions located near the premotor area produce the same types of disturbance of sequential activity, but the motor aspect of speech itself offers no difficulties. The effect of disturbance of the dynamic schemata is shifted to an earlier stage in the formulation of speech, i.e. to a stage which *precedes* the speech act. Such a patient is deprived of those inner speech schemata which determine all the later stages in the formulation of statements. He can easily repeat a sentence or a word; he can read aloud; in conversation he is able to give simple answers to questions. This is especially true if the questions do not require more than a yes or no answer, or if it is possible to respond by repetition of a grammatical construction contained in the question itself. Whereas they show no signs of disturbance of the motor aspect of speech, these patients complain of a kind of "emptiness in the head"; they complain that their thoughts "stand still and don't move", and that they have great difficulty when they have to say something spontaneously. They indicate that they have no clear inner conception of what they are to say ("Before, I knew exactly that I wanted to say such and such; now I want to start, but nothing comes out . . . emptiness"). Since thoughts do not formulate themselves into inner speech schemata they do not get beyond the stage of general intentions and, while the patient is able to comprehend speech and retains the motor mechanisms necessary for speech activity, he shows a characteristic kind of "dynamic aphasia" which stands on the borderline between a speech disturbance and a disturbance of thought processes.

Even though a mild form of this type of disturbance creates severe inner conflicts for the patient, it may pass almost unnoticed to the casual observer. In its most severe form, however, it may intensify minor disturbances of expressive speech and create a picture identical with that of a severe motor aphasia or mutism. Relatively little investigation has been made of this phenomenon; the only descriptions of it are found in the work of Kleist and, to some extent, that of Goldstein (1948). Nevertheless it is not infrequently seen with lesions of anterior parts of the brain and is of considerable interest.

Here we shall present two typical illustrations of this form of disturbance. The first shows a mild disturbance of complex speech activity. The second demonstrates some specific defects of inner speech.

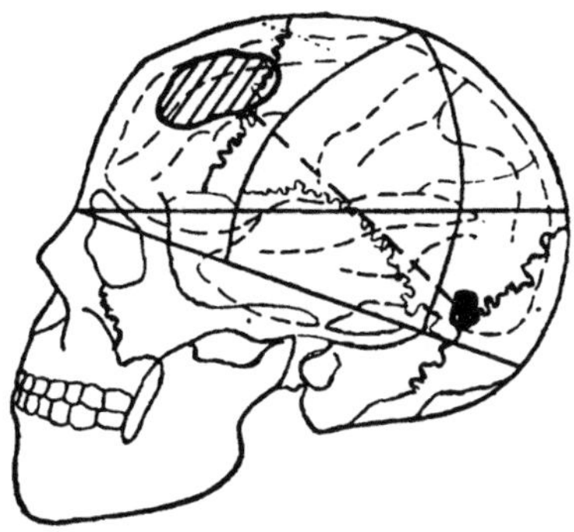

Patient Fr.: injury diagram (Case 9)

Case 9

On July 24, 1944, patient Fr., age 19 (seven years schooling) received a direct shrapnel injury in superior parts of the frontal area. By roentgenogram it was determined that a fragment had passed through the white matter of the entire hemisphere and come to rest in the occipital area at the border of the tentorium. At operation a day later extrusion of brain tissue was discovered and bone fragments were removed from the cortex; subsequently there was further extrusion of brain tissue.

The wound was not accompanied by paresis, but there was a long period of unconsciousness and a severe "motor aphasia". Two months elapsed before the patient spoke his first words. Subsequently, however, he was able to utter short sentences without great difficulty. He had no difficulty in articulation, in sentence construction, or in writing. Further recovery of speech was delayed by the patient's general lack of initiative. Four months after injury he began to suffer from occasional epileptic seizures of the adversive type accompanied by loss of consciousness.

Six months after injury the patient came under our observation and was examined in great detail. His behavior was appropriate but sluggish. He learned easily and carried out tasks with reasonable accuracy, but he remained silent and never took the initiative when participating in cooperative tasks. Sensation was impaired in the right leg (the right arm was amputated following the injury). There was no motor disturbance. Rhythms were reproduced with no difficulty and even very complex differential motor responses were easily established and stable. There was no severe defect in speech comprehension, writing, or calculation.

The clearest signs of disturbance were seen in the patient's speech. The only defect immediately apparent was a tendency to stutter. Certain words were pronounced unevenly and with effort: There was good retention of sequences; the patient was able to name the months in both correct and reverse order. He was able to repeat words, sentences, and even short passages with no grammatical errors. He named objects correctly. He showed no signs of having forgotten the meanings of words and correctly understood logico-grammatical constructions, though sometimes not immediately. In spite of all this, the patient's spontaneous speech was so disturbed that two way verbal communication with him was virtually impossible.

The patient quickly regained the ability to carry on a simple dialogue, i.e. he was able to answer questions quickly if they required only simple confirmation or negation or if the answer could be phrased in terms set forth in the question. He experienced severe difficulty, however, whenever the answer required the formulation of an entirely new statement. Thus, such a question as "Why?", or "For what reason?" was followed by an agonizing pause which sometimes lasted several minutes. Often he was unable to give any answer whatsoever.

The patient easily described the contents of a series of pictures providing the basis for familiar short stories. He was completely helpless, however, if a picture did not suggest a definite answer and if the narration required the preliminary formulation of an intention. He gave a coherent description of the contents of the picture "Ivan Susanin" saying, "This is easy, I know all about Ivan Susanin". He was totally unable, however, to make up a story about an unfamiliar picture in which a little girl lay beside an open window. In this case he limited himself to a simple enumeration of objects appearing in the picture: "A little girl . . . a bed . . . a window . . ." He said that nothing came into his head. Only after a very long pause was he able to continue a story which the examiner began: "One beautiful May morning, a little girl named Galja, . . ." He continued the story by saying, "One beautiful May morning a little girl named Galja woke up very early . . . opened the window, and looked out on the street . . ., but there was nothing in the street"; again, he terminated his story.

This defect arises from damage to the frontal areas and the disturbance of frontal diencephalic connections. It is essentially a disturbance of the inner "formulation" of a narration. It involves disturbances of both the inner schemata of thoughts and of the inner schemata of complex speech constructions. Any spontaneous use of speech is impossible. Though the patient may easily select a word which is opposite in meaning to one shown him, he is unable to select the pair of opposites from among several pairs of words. He is unable to produce a series of words by free association, cannot spontaneously formulate his thoughts, and is extremely limited in spontaneous intellectual activity.

This defect was extremely stable; in the course of many months of observations only minor changes were seen in the state of the patient.

This case permitted us to trace out the impairment of verbal thought which arises as a result of damage to the inner dynamic speech schemata necessary for any statement of an elaborative nature. Such extreme adynamia of thought is typical of damage to the frontal systems and is characteristic of many cases on the borderline between aphasia and the disturbances of thought which accompany frontal lesions. These disturbances appear limited to a loss of "thought initiative". The patients complain that nothing comes into their heads, that it takes them a number of hours or several days to write a simple letter, and that, having begun to write, they are unable to proceed beyond stereotyped greetings. In other cases the same picture is seen, inner speech is primarily affected. In these cases the severe disruption of verbal thought contrasts sharply with the perseveration of external speech. We shall present a short account of a case of "frontal aphasia" which was the object of special and long investigation.

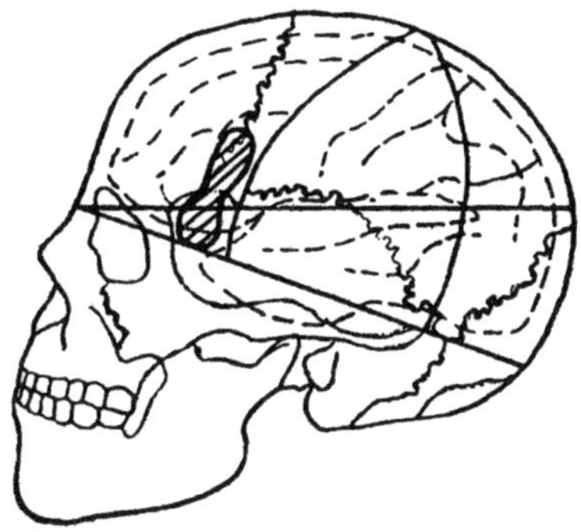

Patient Ger.: injury diagram (Case 10)

Case 10

Patient Ger., age 27, an instructor, finished university and was working for a graduate degree in history. In January, 1944, he received a direct penetrating shrapnel wound in the left frontal and antero-temporal area. The injury was followed by a loss of consciousness and a transient right hemiparesis with no sensory disturbance. It produced a noticeable but short-lived disturbance of connected spontaneous speech.

Examination of the patient was begun three months after injury. At this time he spoke rather freely. A slight slurring of individual sounds remained. He read easily and he was able to write, although in writing he made many orthographic errors which he attributed to "not paying attention" and which he corrected himself. Reading comprehension was good; he was well oriented and his behavior was appropriate. All forms of gnosis and praxis were intact. There was no sign even of those disturbances of the flow of speech which we noted in previous patients of this group. Mnestic-intellectual processes were also completely intact; he easily memorized a series of words (perfect recall of a ten word list on the fourth or fifth trial). He was able to master complex logical constructions and highly abstract material as shown by his ability to abstract, though somewhat slowly, the essential meaning of a passage. Given enough time, he could solve extremely complex relational problems of the Bertt type; he was able to analyze analogies and syllogisms; there was no noticeable disturbance in the structure of his intellectual processes.

The preservation of the structure of intellectual processes sharply contrasted with the severe disturbance of their *dynamics*. In his first visit to our clinic the patient complained that he had lost all spontaneity of thought. He felt that his "thoughts had come to a stop"; he felt such a "vacuum" in his head that any active intellectual process, e.g. writing a letter or carrying on a conversation, was impossible for him. It took him several hours to write a letter. Sometimes he spent days and still was unable to proceed beyond a few familiar and stereotyped expressions. The same difficulty arose in attempting to formulate his own conclusions regarding a passage which he read. He had difficulty in recognizing the basic meaning and in thinking of a name for it. "The bad thing is that I want to form my own conclusions, and I cannot", commented the patient, indicating the great difficulty he experienced in the spontaneous formulation of thought.

The impairment of this patient's mental processes manifested itself especially when he was instructed to carry out tasks requiring spontaneous thought and spontaneous narrative. He was able to describe a "situational picture" or series of pictures, but he was helpless when required to make up a story or to elaborate on a general theme. The intention did not coalesce into a definite schema and did not become embodied in definite constructions. The thought appeared torn into numerous fragments. Thus the patient declared that he was only able to enumerate individual elements and details of what he was thinking but was unable to combine these into a smoothly flowing narrative. "It's as though the material is all there at a distance ... as though it were all ready to go, but the minute you start to say it, it all scatters and it turns out there's nothing there ..." This defect emerged clearly when he was asked to write a composition on a given (familiar) theme. In so doing he was restricted to stereotyped expressions. There was a total absence of the usual smooth transitions which give unity to a written account. He experienced considerable difficulty in writing a short narrative. The individual words and thoughts which he wanted to express stood out clearly in his consciousness, but the schemata necessary for constructing sentences to express these thoughts were lacking. Thus he would pace for hours up and down the corridor uttering various combinations of words to himself; from these he was able to select the desired phrases.

This disturbance of inner dynamic schemata contrasted sharply with the preservation of comprehension of complex logical constructions. It affected both verbal and intellectual processes. Further investigation showed that the inner dynamics of sentence formulation were extremely disturbed. This was reflected not only in the difficulty which he had in formulating sentences, but also in his inability to catch immediately the relationships set forth in sentences. By reasoning the patient was able to understand any logical relationship, e.g. opposition, family-species, or cause-effect, but he was unable to grasp immediately to what category a given relationship belonged. First he had to pronounce the pair of words to himself. The same was true of his comprehension of complex grammatical constructions which have to be transformed in order to be understood. In these cases he analyzed the problem verbally and in a discursive style; having come to the correct solution, he would say, "All this is purely right logically, but all the same I don't have a real feeling for the meaning; the meaning isn't included; for me there is no unity of logic and meaning ..." It was extremely revealing to see in this patient such a well-preserved structure of intellectual function while the dynamic schemata of very simple grammatical relationships were severely impaired. He was unable to recognize immediately the relational significance of case, number, or gender. Only by means of long and conscious reasoning was he able to answer what would appear to be simple questions regarding grammar.

The patient had similar difficulties in practical intellectual activity. In the course of retraining he chose a new specialty and began to work in a construction bureau as a mechanical engineer. Here again, however, he noticed the same difficulty. He found that he had to spend much extra time in analyzing the defect in a piece of apparatus and how to correct it, because "the necessary hypotheses did not become immediately apparent". In every case he had to go through the entire discursive process, whereas earlier he had been able to rely on abbreviated propositions or hypotheses which arose as a result of "direct consideration of the facts". [11]

[12] For the full analysis of the case see in: A. R. Luria, *Human Brain and Psychological Processes* (New York, Harper and Row, 1966).

Figure 38 indicates the sites of lesions which most often give rise to such dynamic disturbances of verbal thought. Here one can see what kind of role is played in the organization of these processes by the "prefrontal area".

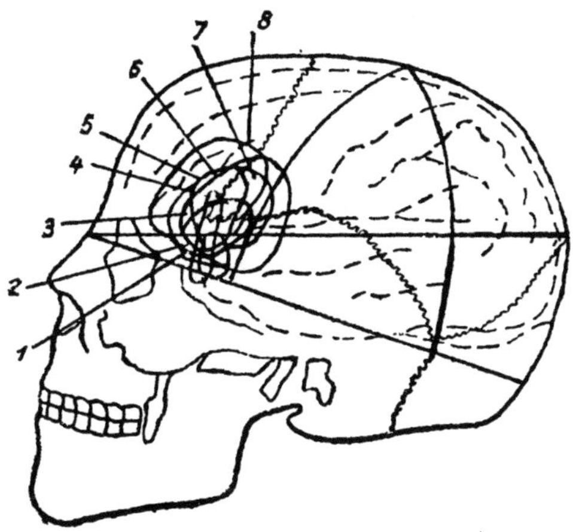

FIG. 38. Schematic diagram of lesions giving rise to frontal "dynamic aphasia".

In summarizing our findings regarding the disturbances which arise as a result of lesions in the *premotor and fronto-premotor systems* we might begin by pointing out that both of these areas tend to be considered typical "marginal" areas. Lesions of the premotor area produce a disturbance of complex kinetic schemata, i.e., disruption of the smooth integrated pattern of movements so that sequential movements are broken down into individual motor acts each of which must be produced by a special effort. This loss is accompanied by a disturbance of the process by which motor acts, once initiated, are denervated and consequently by an inability to shift from one link in the chain of actions to another.

In a large number of cases lesions of the premotor area of the left hemisphere affect speech activity. They give rise to a characteristic *dynamic aphasia*. When the lesion involves medial and superior parts of the premotor zone, this aphasia appears as a slight disturbance of smooth speech. Speech loses its automaticity and sometimes becomes agrammatical. In the most severe cases (usually resulting from lesions in the lower more specialized part of this area) one observes a severe disturbance of the inner structure of speech in which the same effort must be made to formulate thoughts as is necessary for the execution of smooth motor patterns. In some cases inner speech is so severely disturbed that one need only deny the patient the possibility of speaking aloud to deprive him completely of the ability to perform any kind of intellectual operation.

Lesions observed in cases of frontal ("dynamic") aphasia

Case No.	Name	Lesion	Speech disturbances
1	Syč.	Penetrating wound in the left frontal and temporal areas with no paresis or sensory disturbance.	Total retention of the phasic aspect of speech, reading, and writing; ability to name objects intact, but a notable amnesic disturbance of spontaneous speech; inability to follow a train of thought once initiated, a defect of verbal initiative. Phonemic hearing and speech comprehension intact.
2	Fed.	Direct penetrating shrapnel wound in the left frontal and temporal areas with no paresis or severe neurological symptoms.	Total retention of the phasic aspect of speech, reading, and writing; a noticeable lack of spontaneity of speech processes; inability to follow a train of thought; instability of verbal schemata; amnesic-aphasic difficulties manifest in spontaneous speech; phonemic hearing and speech comprehension altogether intact.
3	Mitzk.	Direct penetrating wound of the lower part in the left frontal area from a metal fragment which came to rest deep in the brain; no paresis or sensory defect.	Phasic aspect of speech preserved; difficulty in remembering words in spontaneous speech; akinesia of thought with a disturbance of the smoothness of speech processes.
4	Naz.	Nonpenetrating wound in the left frontal and temporal areas with pressure by the inner plate of the skull, damage to underlying brain tissue, and slight right hemiparesis.	Total retention of the phasic aspect of speech but a pronounced akinesia of verbal thought, interruption of thought processes, searching for words in spontaneous speech, and inability to maintain the sequential structure of verbal expressions; notable disturbance in the inner formulation of intentions.
5	Perm.	Penetrating shrapnel wound in lower parts of the left frontal area; very mild paresis of the right hand recovered gradually.	Motor aphasia which gradually disappeared; three months after injury the phasic aspect of speech was virtually intact, though there was slowing and difficulty in the verbal formulation of thought; spontaneous speech characterized by word searching and a certain degree of agrammatism; noticeable inertia of thought and difficulty in maintaining the schemata of sentences.
6	Porc.	Direct penetrating wound in the left frontal and anterior temporal areas with metal fragments embedded in the brain tissue; no paresis or sensory disturbance.	Inability to speak for ten days following injury, at which time phasic aspect of speech totally restored; reading and writing intact; severe disturbance of inner speech; spontaneous speech characterized by word searching; instability of sequential speech processes; total preservation of phonemic hearing and of the logico-grammatical structure of speech.

Case No.	Name	Lesion	Speech disturbance
7	Samor.	Direct nonpenetrating wound in the left frontal and anterior temporal areas with fracture of the skull and involvement of the dura mater; no paresis or sensory deficit.	Preservation of the phasic aspect of speech but a severe disturbance of inner speech and an inability to carry through sequential verbal processes; spontaneous speech frequently interrupted by search for words; defects of verbal initiative.
8	Belsk.	Oblique penetrating wound in lower parts of the left frontal area along its temporal border; no paresis; severe frontal syndrome.	Expressive speech, disturbed for a time following injury, recovered gradually; three months following injury phasic aspect of speech totally intact (easily recited tongue-twisters involving familiar phrases); profound disturbance of spontaneous speech with constant searching for words and loss of sentence structure during attempted narration.

If the injury is located in the lower parts of the premotor zone adjacent to the operculum, speech is the only function affected. The loss of skilled motor habits (exhibited in hand movements) may be very slight in these cases, whereas disturbances of speech activity emerge very clearly. The inner and external (phasic) organization of speech are affected, while the patient's phonemic hearing may be left intact. He may be able to break down the words he hears into sequences of articulatory elements. On the other hand, the word as a single serial structure in which audio-articulatory elements follow one another in a precise order may disintegrate. The patient is unable to analyze the sound sequences of words. He constantly omits or reverses the letters and consequently is totally unable to write. In the most severe cases patients even have difficulty in the articulation of individual sounds. These are the cases of "Broca's aphasia" in which the primary disturbance is a loss of the efferent schemata of words.

Once this primary defect has diminished, one can observe a more important consequence of the loss of the dynamic schemata of speech. The patient's inner speech is severely disturbed in that its predicative function is lost; it is reduced to the designation of individual objects without sentence structure. The formulation of thoughts into sentences becomes impossible and gives way to the enumeration of individual "content words" which is known clinically as "telegraph style".

If the injury is more extensive and, as some observations indicate, deep enough to involve the white matter and destroy cortical connections with the subcortical nuclei, the disturbance of smooth movement patterns is combined with severe difficulties of denervation. Any act once initiated tends to persist and the patient is unable to shift from one articulatory set to another. Thus expressive speech becomes virtually impossible. This type of "denervation difficulty" in motor aphasia may appear in various forms and with varying degrees of severity. Sometimes the inability to shift from one sound to another prevents the utterance of whole words. Sometimes, on the other hand, there is a persistence of whole sentence fragments which take on the character of "verbal emboli". These disturbances comprise one of the important components of severe "expressive motor aphasia" and probably constitute the greatest obstacle to normal articulate speech in the "motor aphasic".

Finally, if the lesion is located in the oral parts of the premotor and frontal area, the motor aspects of the disturbance emerge more clearly. The primary disturbance is more likely to involve general dynamic processes. The preliminary speech synthesis of inner speech is disrupted with little or no effect on the external phasic structure of speech. Thus a patient with such a lesion shows greatest difficulties in spontaneous narrative speech. He lacks the "initiating impulse" which sets verbal processes into motion as well as the dynamic schemata of inner speech necessary for the verbal elaboration of thought. This "akinesia of speech and thought" often merges gradually with the general picture of frontal akinesia and thus constitutes only one symptom of the broader frontal syndrome.

VIII

THE PATHOLOGY OF SYSTEMS INVOLVED IN SPATIAL ORGANIZATION OF PATTERN AND THE SEMANTIC APHASIA SYNDROME

So far we have been primarily concerned with disturbances of the *phasic aspect of speech*. Only in the last chapter did we go beyond this subject to discuss the more complex "frontal dynamic aphasia" referred to by Jackson and Goldstein as an aphasia "of a higher order". The speech disorders which one sees in traumatic aphasia may affect more than external speech, however. Clinicians have recognized for some time that in some cases of brain damage there is no impairment of the ability to recognize or pronounce individual sounds, no difficulty in word comprehension, and no reading or writing disorder. The external manifestations of inner verbal processes may remain altogether intact, and the patient may show no "general intellectual deficit". Despite this general preservation of external speech, however, his comprehension of complex grammatical constructions and his ability to employ logico-grammatical relations in his own speech may be extremely impaired. In such cases, the brain lesion disturbs the inner aspect of speech, i.e. the meaningful organization of speech. Linguists are well aware that words possess a very complex *cognitive* or meaningful aspect which may be lost, thus producing a characteristic form of speech disturbance. This disturbance is of considerable clinical interest. It has been referred to by a variety of terms but always with the recognition that it is one of the most complex and highest forms of speech disorder. The primary defect involves the semantic aspect of speech; thus, in order to understand the clinical picture which arises, it is necessary to review some basic linguistic principles.

A. THE MEANINGFUL ASPECT OF SPEECH AND THE PATTERNING OF SIMULTANEOUSLY ORGANIZED ELEMENTS

Basic to the meaningful structure of speech is the simplest of word functions, *viz.*, the *nominative* function, the function of "object representation". Every word represents some concrete or abstract object; pronunciation of the word calls forth some form of *image* of that object. The nominative function, however, is the simplest function of a word and does not constitute its entire meaning. Even a very common word does more than represent a single object. It also represents a certain *generalization*. For instance, the word "tree" designates not only a particular object, but also any of a variety of "trees".

Furthermore, the word "tree" can hardly be conceived of psychologically as a simple, vague, somewhat washed-out image which is stored in our memory. Behind every word there lie numerous potential connections and relationships into which the object may enter and in which our cognitive activity may place it. In other words, as has often been pointed out, the relationships connoted by a word play a role in the immense task of systematizing the phenomena of the outside world. By referring to an object as a "tree" we relate it to a particular category and activate potential associations, e.g., "living-nonliving", "a natural object", "swimming-nonswimming", "hot-cold", etc. By the process of naming we "classify the world" (Humboldt, Potebnija, Vygotskij, Bruner and others).

In some cases the structure of the word itself mediates the semantic function. Thus, the structure of the word "pepel'nica" (ashtray) indicates that we are dealing not only with ashes ("pepel-") but with an ash receptacle; for the suffix "nic" relates it to the category of receptacles. The same is true of such words as "saxarnica" (sugar bowl), "černil'nica" (inkwell), etc. While the generalizing function is sometimes mediated by the external structure of the word, it is often related to the subjective content or "internal structure of the word". There is no doubt that words both designate objects and play a role in the formulation of thoughts. We shall refer to this generalizing function of a word as its *meaning*. The more primitive the level of consciousness, the greater the degree to which words are tied to concrete practical situations. The more complex consciousness becomes, the richer and deeper are the various associations connected with individual words.

The complex relations and associations of words are the essence of speech as a second signalling system. They represent more, however, than the basic vocabulary of the language. Associations and relations may accrue to a word as a result of the way it is used in everyday speech; the establishment of such associations depends upon the logico-grammatical system of the language.

Thoughts are not expressed simply by stringing together words representing different objects, e.g., "door-wagon" or "father-brother". Prepositions, word order, and inflection set the objects in *specific relationships* to one another. Thus, "the door of the car" does not mean the same thing as "the door" or "the car" alone. It signifies a specific door associated with a specific car. "Father's brother" does not refer to each of the individual persons named; it refers to a certain relationship. Attention is shifted from the concrete words "father" and "brother" to a new concept which can be represented by a different word, "uncle". A change in the order of these words to give "brother's father" radically changes the meaning of the grammatical unit. In both cases the logico-grammatical system of the language determines the meaning of the words expressed, so that a genuine comprehension of their meaning can be achieved only by interpreting them in terms of the rules of the language. A simple grasp of the nominative meanings of the words is insufficient. For accurate comprehension it is essential to catch the *word-relationships*, the syntax, which is determined by the grammatical rules of the language.

The capacity of language to represent relationships among objects by means of grammatical word combinations is a result of a long developmental process and could hardly have been achieved in the early stages of linguistic evolution.

The work of several linguists, e.g., Humboldt and Sapir, ethnologists, e.g., Malinowsky, and psychologists, e.g., Bühler, have made it clear beyond a doubt that early in the development of language there was no grammatical structure and thus no way of representing relationships among objects or of expressing thoughts. Words were born of activities involving tools and gestures; they were originally used to designate specific objects. The meaning of a statement was conveyed by its "sympractical context", i.e., by an immediate action and associated gestures. Not until the combination of *two or more words* (syntax) first appeared was man in a position to do more than refer to objects by means of language. When syntax appeared he gained the ability to convey information about relationships among objects, events, or thoughts. Linguists and psychologists are of the universal opinion that this was a turning point in the development of language (Schuchart, Bühler). Language was transformed from a primitive form of "verbal pointing" to a means of expressing complex relationships.

The entire subsequent evolution of grammar has consisted of the development of means by which ever more complex interrelationships among objects can be expressed. This has been achieved by changing "the internal form of the word", i.e., by forming complex semantic systems based on roots and suffixes which permit the grouping of objects according to various characteristics and by developing rules whereby one word is subordinated to another, e.g., by inflection, or by manipulating conjunctions, prepositions, and word order. Thus have the various modern inflected languages become powerful means of thought formulation and expression.

The development of the semantic structure of language was by no means simple. Both the history of language development and the study of speech in everyday use both reflect the complexity of the process by which language has gradually achieved the capacity to go beyond the simple designation of objects to the expression of complex thoughts. Investigations of the primitive Paleoasiatic, American, and Melasian languages carried out in recent decades (see the works of Sapir, B. Malinowsky, Meščaninov, and others) have shown that these contemporary languages do not process all the means of expression characteristic of more highly developed languages. They have neither the numerous connecting particles nor the complex system of inflective relationships (tenses, conjugations, etc.) of more advanced languages. In many respects they have remained at the stage where individual substantives are strung together and the meaning of statements must be derived from the immediate (sympractical) situations in which they are uttered. The same was true of the modern inflected languages at earlier stages in their development. The history of language shows that the subordinate "hypotactic" forms required for expressing complex relationships developed considerably later than the coordinating "paratactic" forms whereby sentences simply designated things or events. We can find examples in Old German, Old English and Old Russian where the subordinate conjunctions were still not well established and were replaced by coordinating conjunctions: e.g., "Ergezet si der leide und ir (instead of 'die ihr') ir habet getan", (Nibelungen, 148, 6) or, "For yonders I hear Sir Guys horn blow and he (instead of 'who') hath slain Robin Hood", (from the Ballad of Robin Hood). These linguistic constructions reflect the psychological difficulty which attended the development of relative clauses. Languages long continued to designate individual objects without expressing their precise relationships. As a result one finds the paratactic designation of two objects together, "hendiadys", in place of the genitive case constructions used in present day writing, e.g., "mit Leidenschaft und Liebe" instead of "mit Leidenschaft der Liebe", or "προφυγονται μενος και χετρας Αχαιων" ("they evaded *the force and arms* of the Achaeans" instead of "the force of arms") or "Prince Oligerd refused to advance against the German hordes and force", instead of "the force of the German hordes" (16th century) etc. We have also gathered numerous examples of the use in popular everyday speech of such paratactic constructions in place of more complex relative constructions.[1]

Thus, it has been found that the history of language consists in the gradual development of grammatical rules whereby language can do more than merely designate objects. It has become possible to express complex meaningful relationships in the absence of "sympractical" context. Language has gradually become a complex system of codes which, like art, in the words of Leonardo da Vinci, "conceals within itself all means of expression".

What are the psychological conditions necessary for the mastery of a complex grammar? What sorts of brain mechanisms had to evolve in the course of historical development in order to make possible communication by means of language? It would be incorrect to look for the psychological prerequisites of language in the simple storage of "images" or "ideas" as was proposed by classical psychologists and philosophers. The "idea" concept would be sufficient to explain how a given word calls forth a given image but it is not sufficient to explain how one abstracts from individual images and perceives their interrelationships. In order to recognize these associations and relationships, man must be able to *simultaneously combine several related cues,* no one of which would directly evoke a clear image, but all of which taken together represent a certain *category or system.* Thus it is not the possession of a single idea, but the ability *to grasp the inner organization of a number of individual cues,* the possession of an "expanded field of attention", as it is described by Piaget, which permits the comprehension of structure and interrelationships.

B. BRAIN MECHANISMS UNDERLYING THE INTEGRATION OF SIMULTANEOUSLY ORGANIZED ELEMENTS (SIMULTANEOUS SYNTHESIS)

What might the physiological conditions be which permit one to combine numerous individual cues into a single perception? This is a question which deserves special attention. We have already discussed the concept originally set forth by I. M. Sečenov that there are two types of "synthetic", or integrative activity (Chapter 6). In the last chapter we considered how the brain mechanisms responsible for the

[1] A special analysis of the development of such constructions is given elsewhere, cf. A. R. Luria, *Studies in Aphasia*, part II. *Semantic Aphasia* (unpublished).

synthesis of sequential patterns give rise to dynamic stereotypes in the form of motor habits. Now we must consider what is known about the mechanisms underlying the unification of individual elementary impressions into simultaneous, for the most part, spatial *patterns*.

Neurophysiologists have long been concerned with the central organization of the processes where a unified image of the outside world is synthesized from individually perceived elements. These processes depend primarily upon vision, but they also involve the somesthetic and kinesthetic sensory modes. Further, they involve the coordination of eye and hand movements which are important for the perception of spatial relations.

The central cortical part of the visual system has often been likened to a screen on which a "point to point" representation of the retinal image is projected. In reporting his work on the structure of the visual cortex the famous Russian histologist Zavarzin (1955) pointed out the stratified architecture which is distinctive of the visual cortical area. He suggested that the visual cortex be thought of as a "screen like" structure. Investigations carried out more recently, however, have introduced certain changes into the conception of how this "screen" functions and have thus led to certain modifications of his theory.

It now seems more reasonable to think of vision, as a highly precise and active mode of perceiving, i.e., a complex activity with an efferent component. Retinal neural activity and eye movements are transformed at a central level into a dynamic structure of excitation which is capable of carrying information about simultaneously patterned events occurring in the outside world, thus giving rise to visual images. In other words, it appears that a whole series of processes is involved in the production of the visual image, and that as it has developed, it has become shortened and consolidated to form a simultaneous dynamic system capable of uniting numerous stimulation points into general patterns.

We still know very little about the electrophysiological nature of this process. On the basis of anatomical data Lorenté de Nó (1938) suggested the existence of closed reverberating circuits which unite groups of cells into different dynamic systems. With the advent of modern technology we are no longer restricted to theories whereby the visual system is thought of as analogous to a mirror. It can now be compared with a television camera in which a unitary image is derived by means of a moving, "scanning" electronic beam.[2] The formation of a visual image should by no means be considered a simple mirror-like or static event. Visual analysis and synthesis is a highly dynamic process which depends upon the problems faced by the organism at a given time and upon the field of cortical elements which are set at their optimal state of excitability. If a person looking at a painting of the Last Supper wishes to achieve a general impression of the entire picture his

[2] This case has been described in a previous publication. See A. R. Luria, "The Mechanisms of the Disturbance of Visual Perception with Lesions of the Occipito-Parietal Cortical Areas", *Brain*, 1959.

field of vision becomes very wide. If, however, he wishes to consider primarily the face of Christ, his eyes converge, the amount of information which he derives from the picture as a whole is greatly diminished; the peripheral parts of the visual field are inhibited, so that he perceives only that small area of the canvas toward which his visual attention is directed.

This type of dynamic change in the area of the visual field has been compared with the function of the diaphragm of an optical instrument. The ability of the visual field to expand and constrict is very important for simultaneous perception. The functions of the central parts of the visual analyzer consist in transformation of the stable visual field into a dynamic system. For instance, they play a role in altering the channel capacity of the system depending upon the task faced by the organism.

We have many reasons for believing that the unification of individual activated points into an overall pattern is not accomplished by having all parts of the visual cortex perform the same function. Investigations of the cellular architecture indicate that the primary projection area of the visual cortex (one of the "extrinsic areas" of Rose and Pribram) possesses a different structure from that of the secondary areas (the "intrinsic areas"). Whereas the first, Brodmann's area 17, has a dominant fourth layer, the secondary areas, Brodmann's areas 18 and 19, show a predominance of the second and third, projection-association layers.

There are electrophysiological differences between the two zones which correspond to these morphological differences. Dusser de Barennes and McCulloch (1944) showed that the excitation elicited by strychnine applied to a point in the occipital area is transmitted only a short distance, whereas the same type of stimulus applied to a point in area 18 or 19 gives rise to excitation over a much greater area (Figure 39). This indicates the great role played by the so-called "wide visual sphere" in the creation of dynamic systems involving widespread cortical areas.

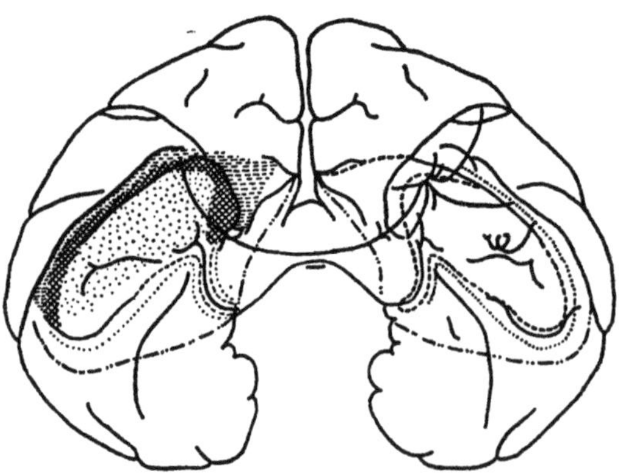

One hemisphere			Contralateral hemisphere		
17	18	19	19	18	17
ΔY	Y				
Y	YΔY	Y		Y	
—	—	YΔ	—	—	—

Δ Stimulus
Y Response

FIG. 39. Spread of excitation with strychnine stimulation of area 17, 18, and 19. (from McCulloch).

Similar data have been accumulated in experiments involving direct electrical stimulation of the visual cortex. In experiments by Pötzl and Hoff, Foerster, and Penfield, stimulation of the primary cortical area, or "narrow visual sphere" was found to produce only a general phosphene. On the other hand, stimulation of the secondary areas, "the broad visual sphere", produced formed images and, sometimes, dynamic hallucinations. Stimulation at the border of the temporal speech area sometimes gave rise to scene-like visual hallucinations. All of these observations testify to the complex synthetic functions of the secondary visual areas which constitute the zones of overlap between the cortical parts of the visual, kinesthetic, and auditory analyzers. Even more clearcut indications as to the integrative functions of the cortical areas lying between the occipital, parietal, and temporal areas can be drawn from the field of neuropathology. It has been repeatedly shown that damage to these areas, especially in the left hemisphere, may produce anything from a disturbance of eye movements to a very complex visuo-gnostic or visuo-spatial disturbance.

The patterning of eye movements is one of the prime prerequisites for tracing the outline of an object, orienting to it, and examining it. Impairment of such movements has been described by a number of authors as one of the major symptoms arising with lesions in the antero-occipital cortical areas, Brodmann's areas 18 and 19. Morel (1947), Buskaino (1946), Gordon Holmes (1918, 1938), Ettlinger, Warrington, Zangwill (1957), and more recently A. L. Jarbuss (1965), have pointed out the important role played by eye movements in the integration of spatial perception. These authors and numerous others have concluded that the disturbance of eye movements which accompanies lesions in the parieto-occipital areas may be one of major causes of the difficulty in spatial perception and patterned perception of objects in these cases (Bálint, 1909; Holmes, 1938; Kleist, 1934; Pötzl, 1938; and others). Similar findings based on animal experiments by Lashley and Tsang (1936) indicate that extirpation of the occipital area produces a nonspecific impairment of spatial integration processes even in cases where the visual system is not involved in the establishment of spatial habits.

The antero-occipital areas play an important role in the *transformation of sequential recognition processes into instantaneous recognition* (Goldstein) or in the *organization of individual visual traces into individual simultaneous systems* (Head). In fact, these may be considered the major functions of the "antero-occipital or occipito-parietal" systems. Perhaps we should describe in detail the disturbances of simultaneous visual integrative processes which may occur as a result of lesions in this area.

Patient Voit,[8] a 21 year old officer in the Polish army, was wounded in April, 1945. He received a direct bullet wound of the left parieto-occipital area. The bullet passed through the postero-medial portion of the left occipito-parietal area and came to rest in the inferior part of the right occipital area just above the posterior fossa (see injury diagram). Left hemiparesis and speech disturbance were noted immediately following the

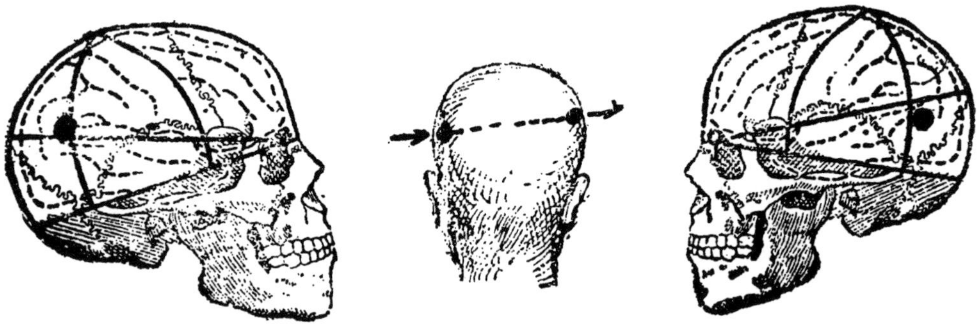

Patient Voit.: injury diagram

injury but the patient recovered rapidly. Six months later an operation was performed which involved trepanation in the right occipital area. It was impossible, however, to remove the bullet at that time. A year and a half later a second operation was performed at the Institute of Neurosurgery in Moscow and the bullet was removed. At the time of the second operation, the patient showed no signs of speech impairment. His speech comprehension was good; he was able to repeat a long series of words or digits without difficulty; he was able to carry out successive subtractions mentally and could solve problems involving logical operations. His only complaint had to do with a visual disturbance, *viz.*, an instability of the visual images of objects. It was difficult for him to grasp the contents of thematic pictures; sometimes he even had difficulty in telling how many elements, e.g., faces, were represented. He could read individual words, but, in attempting to read connected text, he would lose words or even lines and sometimes one word would suddenly "jump into the place of another". He had occasional epileptic seizures which were preceded by visual and kinesthetic auras and loss of consciousness. There was a distinct narrowing of the visual field and an impairment of binaural hearing. Further experimental investigation revealed that the basic disturbance consisted of *the fact that while the patient was able to perceive individual visual elements, he was unable to perceive two or more objects simultaneously.*

I. P. Pavlov described a similar patient reported by Pierre Janet as follows: "His visual attention was so concentrated that the visual cortex was under powerful inhibitory influence and was unable to accommodate two stimulus patterns simultaneously. When he was presented a stimulus pattern his concentration was directed to a single point, and the remaining points might just as well not have existed" Pavlovskie sredy ([Pavlovian Wednesdays], 1949 Vol. III. pp. 96-97).

This basic defect manifested itself in several different situations. If a card with two figures, e.g., a cross and a circle, was presented tachistoscopically he saw only one figure. After several exposures he might say, "I known that there are a cross and a circle there, but I only see one of them at a time." The origin of his disorder could not be said to lie in a simple constriction of the visual field; for, regardless of the size, he could never see more than one object.

He was unable to solve problems which required visuo-motor coordination. For instance, he was unable to place a dot in the center of a circle or at the juncture of two lines drawn in the form of a cross, for, while he could see either the figure or the tip of his pencil, he was unable to perceive both at once. He was unable to draw a floor diagram of his hospital ward from memory. In attempting to do so he had to look at his immediate surroundings repeatedly. Each time he recognized one or another element but he was unable to combine the various elements into a unified pattern. He had similar difficulty in grasping the significance of a thematic picture, for, here again, each element was recognized in isolation and a *single visual pattern* did not emerge.

The idea that we were dealing with a pathological "weakness" of the occipital cortex was tested experimentally. A 0.05-0.10 gram dose of a 10% solution of caffeine was injected subcutaneously. It is well known that caffeine raises the tonus of excitation in the cerebral cortex. Twenty-five or thirty minutes after the injection we noted a change in visual functions; the patient was able to perceive two or two and a half figures simultaneously; he had little difficulty in carrying out tasks involving visuo-spatial coordination, in estimating the number of elements in a group, in drawing a floor diagram of the ward, etc. On the basis of this we were able to attribute the impairment of visual integration to a drop in the tonus of visual cortical function resulting from trauma and subsequent inflammation.

In several cases lesions in the antero-occipital cortical area produced similar disturbances of *visual synthesis*. These disturbances consisted of loss of the ability to unite simultaneously occurring elements in a single act of recognition, which we consider to be the most important function of the occipito-parietal areas.

With left hemispheric lesions just anterior to the areas which we have been considering the impairment of simultaneous synthesis may assume an even more complex character. These are among the newest and most specifically human areas of the cortex. They constitute the zones of overlap between the cortical parts of the visual, somesthetic-kinesthetic, and auditory analyzers. Lesions in these areas give rise to deficits which involve different sensory modes and more complex memory patterns.

Everything that we have said up to this point regarding the more elementary cognitive processes has bearing upon the instantaneous organization of traces derived from our inner experience and the mastery of the semantic structure of speech. This is why the occipito-parietal and occipito-parieto-temporal areas must be intact if one is to go beyond the simple naming of images to master the *semantic system* of language. With this introduction we are prepared to analyze the syndrome of semantic aphasia.

C. THE SYNDROME OF SEMANTIC APHASIA

We have considered elementary disturbances of simultanous integration in the visual sphere. As we consider the pathology of more complex cortical structures we find the same types of disturbances, but at a higher level of organization. The infero-parietal or temporo-parieto-occipital area (the "tertiary zones" of Flechsig, the TPO zone of several authors, or Brodmann's areas 39, 40 and part of 37) has justifiably been considered one of the most complex areas in the posterior part of the brain. Phylogenetically, these were the last areas to develop. Their structure differs from that of other areas by the predominance of the superficial layers. Ontogenetically, they mature later than other zones. There are data indicating that they continue to develop through infancy and early childhood. The myelination of fibers occurs very late in these areas. We cannot accept Flechsig's suggestion that these zones constitute a "posterior cortical association center", for they have a great number of afferent and efferent connections with deeper structures. The fact that their vertical connections are directed toward secondary thalamic nuclei makes it possible to think of them as intrinsic areas of the afferent-efferent apparatus. This makes them part of a highly complex integrative, coordinative cerebral apparatus and is in accordance with the fact that they constitute the "zone of overlap" between the cortical parts of the three analyzers.

Electrical stimulation of this area gives rise to complex perceptual responses involving visual, kinesthetic, and auditory components. Such reactions are not, however, so clearcut and unambiguous as those elicited by stimulation of the occipital or temporal areas. The clinical symptoms arising as a result of lesions in these areas include important changes which bear on the phenomena of interest to us in this chapter. The symptoms of left parieto-temporo-occipital area lesions are always very complex. Damage to the more anterior parts produces the well known astereognosis in which patients lose the ability to synthesize a unified image of an object on the basis of tactile sensations. Damage to the occipito-parietal part gives rise to disturbances of spatial orientation. More widespread damage involving the temporo-parietal part gives rise to an extremely complex syndrome composed of semantic aphasia, spatial disorientation, acalculia, inability to name the fingers and a number of other signs and symptoms.

The one unifying factor in all of these disorders is the *disturbance of the capacity to unify individual stimulations into a single simultaneous pattern,* or, in the words of Head, *to combine separate details into a single whole.* We shall consider these various disturbances one by one.

Clinical investigation of cases involving damage of Brodmann's areas 18 and 19 have shown that there is little or no impairment of the ability to grasp the meaning of logico-grammatical constructions. The same is true of lesions in the anterior and superior parts of the parietal lobe (areas 7, 40, and perhaps the superior part of area 39). Damage to these areas produces disturbances of spatial orientation and tactile-kinesthetic recognition. The semantic and other disturbances emerge with great prominence, however, if the damage is more extensive or if it involves those specifically human parts of the left parietal area which border on the occipital and temporal areas. There is not sufficient clinical material to day to permit a precise description of the areas involved in the cases.

The impairment of complex perceptual and semantic processes was studied by Salomon (1914), Bonhoeffer (1923), Van Woerkom (1925), Head (1926), Conrad (1932), and others. Patients with such disturbances usually show no great impairment of direct visual perception. Usually they do not show the types of reading and writing which characterize the visual alexia and the temporal aphasic syndromes described above. In the most clear-cut cases, patients indicate that they have difficulty in combining letters to form words. They are only able to see two or three letters at a time, so that they consciously have to piece together the word from small groups of simultaneously perceived letters. Disturbances of tactile and kinesthetic perception are not very prominent. Usually it is difficult to note any signs of the ataxia and lack of coordination which accompany disturbances of deep pressure sense. Only with the more severe lesions does one observe signs of apraxia which, in these cases, consists of difficulty in placing the hands or fingers in given positions or difficulty in reproducing the spatial arrangement of objects. "Constructve apraxias" are not uncommon. A patient may be unable to reconstruct geometrical figures from memory; he may confuse directions and alter the spatial relationships of element patterns; for example, he may reproduce as or  and he may draw 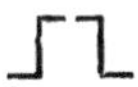 as 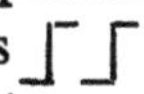 or 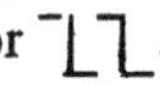. Such a patient has difficulty in performing the same types of operations mentally, and difficulties, for instance, to draw the mirror image of a simple geometrical figure or to reproduce the hand positions of a person facing him (as in Head's well known test).

If a picture or a pattern can be reproduced on the basis of a single image, it may be reproduced quite well. If, however, its reproduction requires a *grasp of relationships or a system of imaginary coordinates* the patient is helpless. Any task requiring a shift in spatial orientation with the preservation of relationships among the various parts is impossible. The same type of difficulty arises in tasks other than those involving constructive geometric principles. Bonhoeffer (1923) noted that such patients have difficulty differentiating between right and left. This may be responsible for the fact later described by Gerstmann (1924) that such patients make errors in naming their fingers, e.g., they confuse the index finger with the ring finger.

All of these symptoms reflect disturbances of inner schemata. Such disturbances are by no means, however, limited to spatial schemata. Perhaps even more well defined is the partial or even total loss of *conceptual and ideational schemata.*

Some of the most severe defects may be seen in the *computational processes.* One frequently hears such patients complain of difficulty in calculating. Although they are able to recognize individual digits, they become disoriented when confronted with numbers involving two or more digits. In reading multiple digit numbers they tend to confuse digit sequences and, in severe cases, read them as series of digits rather than as single numbers. If the examiner dictates a number which contains a zero, so that a certain part of the sequence is not expressed verbally, that part is omitted, e.g. "one thousand twenty three" is written 123 or 1000 23. Equally disturbed is the ability to differentiate between symmetrical numbers, e.g., 17 and 71, or the Roman numerals IV and VI. Such numbers are often perceived as the mirror images of themselves. It is clear that these patients are in no position to carry out any kind of mathematical operation, especially if it involves numbers greater than 10. Often they retain only the ability to perform operations which can be carried out by means of simple speech habits or on the basis of graphic images.[3]

The *speech disorders* have many features in common with the other disturbances. Patients who have been wounded in the occipito-parietal area have no difficulty in speaking smoothly or hearing and understanding individual words. Their phonemic hearing is usually intact. Unlike patients with temporal lesions, they show no signs of having forgotten word meanings. The only speech disturbance which the average observer may note is a tendency to forget the names of objects. The patients show a characteristic amnesic aphasia and confusion if the examiner confronts them with a somewhat complex or unusually constructed question. Neither of these symptoms is based on a true acoustico-gnostic or acoustico-mnestic disturbance. A patient unable to name an object has no difficulty if the examiner prompts him by uttering the first sound of the word. In this respect he differs from a patient with temporal amnesic aphasia who is unable to recall the word even if it is uttered almost in its entirity. This indicates that the causes underlying the "amnesic-aphasic" syndrome are not basically memory disorders. The patient who has difficulty in comprehending a complex sentence shows no great difficulty either in recognizing the individual words or in remembering what he has heard. He is able to remember simple concrete verbal constructions and is able to understand the general meaning of rather long sentence fragments.

The origin of this disturbance is not to be found in a hearing or memory defect or in a general dementia. Also, these disturbances differ considerably from superficially similar disorders observed as a result of lesions in the anterior cortical areas. In the latter cases there is a general cognitive inertia which makes it difficult for the patient to name objects or to comprehend complex logical constructions; he is essentially passive, so that he is unable to inhibit the flood of old associations which such problems evoke. In the cases we are considering here, however, the picture is quite different. The patient actively seeks the right answer. He is able to throw out inappropriate responses, but he is unable to find the correct one.

As one becomes more familiar with this syndrome one becomes more convinced that both the naming difficulty and the impairment of the comprehension of complex grammatical constructions arise from a *profound disruption of the semantic epistructure of words*. This defect may not be detected on cursory examination, but it becomes quite apparent on more careful investigation. The primary image represented by a word, i.e., its specific object relationship, remains intact. *But the system of relationships centered about the word is profoundly disrupted.*

In this group of patients the general meaning of speech may appear unaffected.

[3] A detailed study of the acalculia syndrome in cases of parietal lobe lesions had been presented in a dissertation by Z. Ja. Rudenko, *Disorders of Number and Calculation with Brain Damage* (Moscow, 1953).

The ability to grasp the general content of sentences is retained and in many situations the most important factors may be abstracted on the basis of context. In contrast to demented patients, these patiens are able to recognize such logical concepts as case, gender, and cause-and-effect. Their most prominent defect lies in the fact that the words which they perceive are excluded from the system of generalizations which ordinarily permits one to go from the words themselves to their semantic corollaries. Words can only evoke concrete images of objects or of overall situations. The movement from concept to concept, the movement according to a logico-verbal plan, or to use Bühler's expression, according to a "synsemantic" plan, becomes extremely difficult.[4] A word lacks its entire complex of associations and its meaning disintegrates. As a result it is easily forgotten. The patient, in searching for the word he wants, experiences the same difficulties as a normal person experiences inattempting to recall the name of a person; such a name is similarly lacking in logical associations. The patient often substitutes "random" paraphasias for the correct word. The amnesic-aphasic syndrome which the investigator observes is actually a result of this inner loss of the semantic structure of words.

The patient's intellectual processes are also clearly defective; operations involving relative structures are primarily involved. The motive force which directs his thought processes is intact. He never forgets the goal of his reasoning and, in contrast to the frontal patient, he has no difficulty in maintaining the direction of his thoughts for whatever time is necessary to solve a problem. He can easily pick out the essential elements in a given situation and never performs mental operations at random. The operations themselves, however, may be defective. This is especially true of operations which require the comparison of one thought with another or the elaboration of thoughts according to a conceptual plan. As long as the plan of thought involves only primary imagery and the mental retracing of concrete situations, he may show no signs of impairment. If, on the other hand, he is faced with having to follow a plan involving logico-grammatical schemata, he immediately shows signs of having lost the capacity for logico-verbal thought.

This loss in such a patient becomes most clear when, knowing only the primary meanings of the words involved, he is faced with a construction which is impossible to comprehend. He is unable to integrate the separate meanings into a logico-grammatical pattern, and thus becomes confused. He encounters difficulty whenever the sequence of images evoked by the words in a sentence diverges from its actual meaning, or, to paraphrase Spinoza, the moment "ordo et connexio idearum" ceases to correspond to "ordo et connexio verborum". Thus, while such a patient can easily grasp the meaning of a long, grammatically simple sentence such as, "Father and Mother went to the theatre, but the old nurse and children stayed

[4] A psychological analysis of this kind of cognitive activity was presented by L. S. Vygotskij in his book *Thought and Speech* published posthumously in 1934 (Chapter 7). See also Vygotskij, *Selected Psychological Investigations* (Moscow, 1956).

home", he can neither repeat nor comprehend such a long and grammatically complex construction as, "At the school where Dunja studied, there arrived a worker from the factory who was to give a talk". All attempts to rearrange the "expansive" construction of this sentence by altering its inner schema are unsuccessful. It is impossible for the patient to determine which of the persons mentioned in this sentence is the one who is to "give a talk". In order to understand this sentence he must transform it into a logical form according to the logico-grammatical code of the language. Since he has lost this code, the sentence remains to him a disorderly conglomerate of individual words. The primary difficulty lies in the integration of details into a single pattern, the recognition of relationships, the unification of individual elements into a single simultaneously-beheld system.

The same basic defect underlies all of the semantic disturbances which arise as a result of damage to the parieto-occipital systems. Not only is the comprehension of long grammatical constructions affected; a more simple form of the defect is seen whenever the patient encounters a two word construction which cannot be understood without recognizing their grammatical relationship. For instance, it is impossible to understand a construction which involves the genitive case. The expression "brother of father" should signify "uncle", but to a patient with a parieto-occipital lesion it is not different from the expression "father of brother". In trying to grasp the difference he may say over and over again, "Brother ... father ..." as though he is unable to see a meaningful relationship between the two words. Equally as difficult for such a patient are constructions involving other prepositions, e.g., "a circle under a cross", or constructions involving comparisons in which the actual meaning cannot be derived directly from the individual words, e.g., "less bright" or "less quiet". In all of these cases the patient is unable to grasp the semantic relationship, and he attempts to determine the significance of the construction by referring to the primary meaning of he words and their order in the expression. If asked to draw a "circle under a cross" he interprets the construction agrammatically and draws the figures as follows: (circle-under-cross). He is unable to mentally reverse the word order in a statement where it conflicts with the sequence of actions to be carried out. He similarly confuses the sequence of events expressed in such a statement as, "I ate after I read the newspaper". The disturbance of the ability to alter and manipulate the inner schemata of statements leaves the patient with speech which sounds relatively normal, but which is actually characterized by a severe *"receptive agrammatism"*. In other words, he is unable to process or decode incoming information according to the logico-grammatical code, or rules, of the language.

It is understandable that *verbal thought* should suffer as a result of this defect. The recognition of the grammatical relationships of words and the incorporation of words into general types of logical patterns are two processes involved in the logico-verbal operations of thought. Verbal thought is extremely difficult, because these processes are absent. A patient in this group is unable to understand such relationships as "Cate is darker than Mary, but lighter than Jenny", (from Burtt's series). The task of pointing out which of three circles of different sizes and colors is, "larger than the red one, but smaller than the blue one", is impossible for him. When he encounters such problems, he repeats the words over again to himself attempting to combine them in a meaningful way. After several attempts, however, he usually gives up and will say, for example, "I can't keep the whole thing in mind at once". He is often unable to construct analogies or syllogisms, so that in tasks where one might expect him to follow a sequence of operations based upon a logical plan, he does not do so. He lacks the normal operations of syllogistic thought. There is no doubt but that the patient's *entire previous system of knowledge has disintegrated.* As a rule, patients with temporal lobe aphasia eventually recover much of their previous knowledge; but patients with semantic disturbances show much less improvement of this type.

These are the symptoms of semantic aphasia which arise as a result of lesions of the cortical areas concerned with the patterning of simultaneous perceptual events. We shall present several examples of this syndrome. First we shall consider cases in which damage to the posterior parts of the parieto-occipital area give rise to a syndrome in which the visuo-spatial disturbances overshadow the accompanying speech defects. Secondly, cases of a more restricted form of semantic aphasia will be considered.

The data presented will illustrate the origin and characteristics of speech disturbances which arise as a result of lesions in the posterior systems of the left hemisphere associated with the recognition of simultaneous relationships. The syndromes produced by occipito-parietal lesions include a type of visual impairment which may be characterized as "visual asthenia". There is some degree of spatial disorientation; reading impairment occurs in 40-45% of cases; expressive speech disorders are by no means always present (Table 8). In the initial period following injury, speech disturbances are observed in 69% of cases. They persist into the residual period in only 23% of cases however, and they are always of a certain type. In no case where damage was limited to the parieto-occipital area did we observe a severe disturbance of auditory or motor speech. Patients complained of forgetting words and they often showed signs of alexia or visual agraphia. Only in isolated instances where cortical damage was more extensive was this picture complicated by impairment of the phasic aspect of speech. The same was true in the residual period. As a rule phasic disturbances played an even smaller role in the residual period than initially. The spatial disorientation and impairment of calculation, reading, and writing persisted, thus reflecting the disturbance of functions dependent primarily on the occipito-parietal systems.

TABLE 8

Frequency of Aphasic Disturbances with Wounds of the Parieto-Occipital Area

Site of injury	Total number of cases	Initial period			Residual period		
		severe forms (%)	mild forms (%)	total (%)	severe forms (%)	mild forms (%)	total (%)
Parieto-occipital area	55	46	23	69	23	16	39

Case 1

On March 23, 1943, patient Bas., a 29 year old surveyor with a higher technical school education received a superficial bullet wound in the left parieto-occipital area. The skull and dura mater were damaged. There was loss of consciousness for two hours following the injury. Right hemiparesis and sensory loss on the right were noted shortly following the injury, but these gradually disappeared. A rather severe speech disturbance was also noted shortly after the patient returned to consciousness: he was unable to remember words; he had difficulty in recalling his own surname; he could not remember the names and addresses of his relatives. The smoothness of speech was disturbed. He could name objects only after a long period of deliberation. He could neither read nor write; he could recognize individual letters but was unable to combine them into words. Mental calculations were impossible, for he was unable to remember the numbers he was working with. These difficulties lasted for about one and a half months and then they also gradually disappeared.

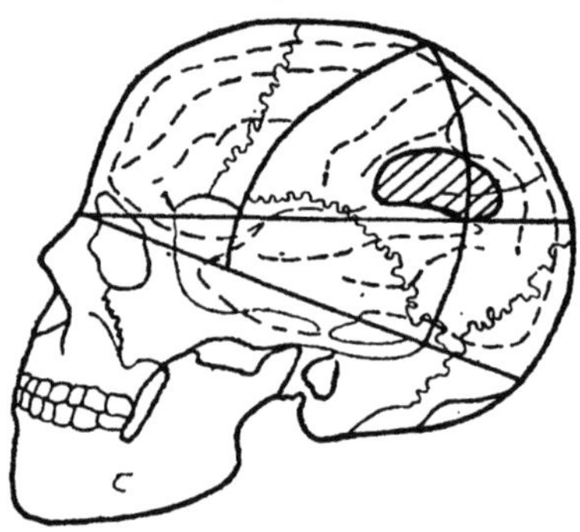

Patient Bas.: injury diagram (Case 1)

Three months after injury, when the patient underwent a thorough examination, his speech had largely recovered. He showed no signs of apraxia or of visual impairment. He read a great deal and did not complain of any impairment of speech comprehension. His only complaints were that he continued to experience considerable difficulty orienting himself. Despite his excellent knowledge of the principles of topography, he easily lost himself in the woods on the hospital grounds. A series of tests indicated that these complaints were well justified; he showed a severe disturbance of spatial orientation. When asked to draw a map showing the locations of important cities in the Soviet Union he made numerous mistakes reflecting the loss of spatial schemata (Figure 40).

This defect was rechecked many times and proved extremely stable. His impressions of the locations of and distances between cities were severely affected. Such a defect in a man whose specialty was topography was an impressive indication of the nature of the syndrome. This symptom persisted in the residual period even after difficulties in calculation became insignificant. In the residual period, the limited size of the lesion produced a correspondingly limited parieto-occipital syndrome which was uncomplicated by any detectable semantic difficulties.

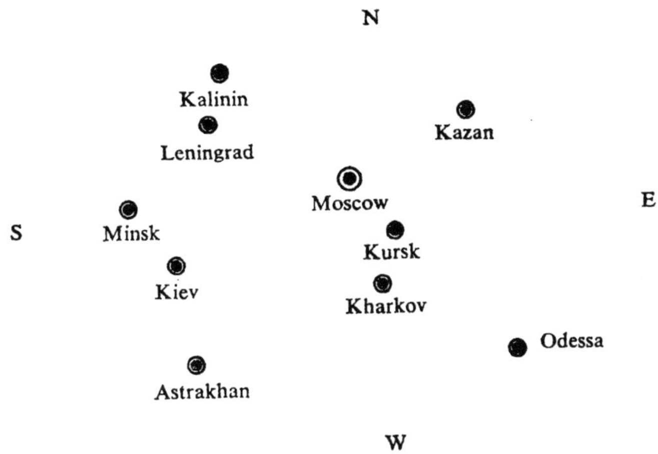

FIG. 40. Map produced by Patient Bas.

Case 2

On November 23, 1942, patient Ostr., a 20 year old nurse, received a penetrating shrapnel wound in the left parieto-occipital area. She was unconscious for several days following the injury. There was a right hemiparesis with a sensory disturbance. Vision was not seriously involved. The paresis soon disappeared from the hand, but the leg remained weak for a somewhat longer time. Initially the patient noted severe difficulty in recalling the names of objects and was unable to express her thoughts in words: "Nothing would come out; everything was blocked". She did not completely comprehend the speech of others; simple words and expressions were understood, but somewhat more complex constructions were impossible: "When the doctor said, 'grasp your left hand

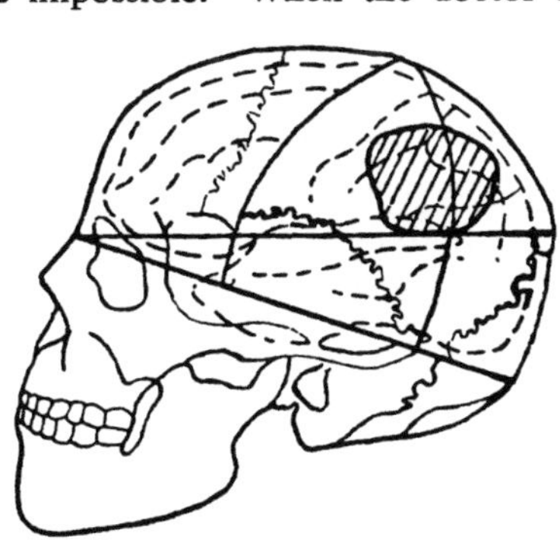

Patient Ostr.: injury diagram (Case 2)

with your right hand', I thought and I thought, but nothing happened". Accompanying these symptoms was a severe generalized amnesia. Gradually the amnesia disappeared and the ability to name objects and talk smoothly were regained. The disturbance of spatial orientation was considerably more resistant to improvement; difficulty in carrying out mental calculations also remained profound for a long time. When the patient came under our observation four months after injury she complained that after the injury she, "became extremely bad at mathematics", that she, "could not understand complex text", and that she was, "going to have to start studying all over again".

Careful examination revealed a very well defined syndrome. Neurologically the patient showed a mild right hemiparesis which was more pronounced in the leg, a disturbance of deep sensitivity, and astereognosis. There was no severe visual impairment and she had no difficulty in interpreting complex pictures. Only occasionally did she note a certain difficulty in spatial orientation, but this symptom was not very pronounced. Her speech was smooth and her vocabulary relatively rich. There were no signs of acoustico-articulatory or amnesic aphasia. Word comprehension and the ability to remember words and simple phrases were preserved, but the repetition of a complex sentence was made difficult by the fact that the different parts did not fit together into a general pattern. As a rule she was able to reproduce individual logico-grammatical constructions but if presented a sentence in which the sequence of verbal images did not correspond to the actual meaning of the sentence she had difficulties. Such problems as, "Jack is larger than John. Who is the smaller of the two?" or "Which of these two sheets of paper is less white?" were impossible for her. She had a great degree of difficulty in interpreting proverbs and metaphorical expressions. All of these symptoms disappeared in the course of three months of hospitalization.

The impairment of the ability to carry out mathematical operations was considerably more stable. The patient had no difficulty in carrying out subtractions such as 25-5, 28-4, etc. If the operations were made more complicated, however, so that certain steps had to be carried out "in her head", e.g., 31-14, 25-17, etc., she was unable to solve them. The failure of both oral and written attempts to solve these problems showed that the entire functional system necessary for computation had been lost. The presentation of mathematical problems did not evoke the inner schemata by which they might be solved. The operations of multiplication and division were totally absent; the understanding of fractions was also lost, as demonstrated by the fact that she was unable to estimate which of two fractions 7/8 or 8/7 was larger. Despite systematic retraining the patient still had great difficulty with mathematical calculations at the time she was released from the hospital three months later.

These cases are good examples. They show the effects of parieto-occipital lesions on spatial orientation in the one case and on calculational ability in the other. In both cases the basic functional disturbance was the loss or weakening of inner simultaneous schemata. In other cases this syndrome may take on more features and present as a full blown *semantic aphasia*. We shall consider three cases, one of which shows this syndrome in the earliest stages following trauma, and two of which illustrate the syndrome in the residual period of recovery.

Case 3

In August, 1941, patient Rožn. received a penetrating shrapnel wound in the left parieto-occipital area. He was unconscious for several hours. There was no sign of paresis, but a sensory deficit was noted on the right. There were disturbances of deep

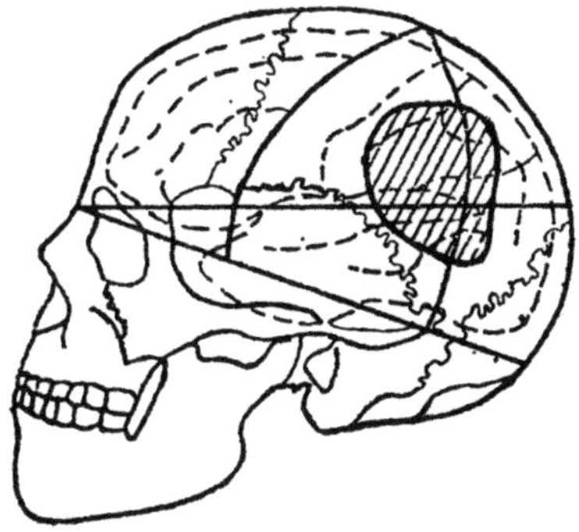

Patient Rožn.: injury diagram (Case 3)

sensitivity and astereognosis on the right with a pronounced right hemianopsia and apraxia on the right. Immediately, upon recovering consciousness the patient noted that his speech, "somehow couldn't get started; nothing would come out". It became difficult to read and write: "I couldn't even draw a simple circle"; the ability to calculate was also disturbed.

The patient was examined carefully two weeks following the injury. He was well aware of his condition and often asked if he would always be "so muddle-headed". Outwardly his speech appeared intact; there were no disturbances of phonemic hearing or of articulation; he easily repeated complex words and was able to repeat long sentences the first time he heard them. He had no difficulty in understanding individual words.

The first severe speech impairment was noted when we began to study the semantic structure of his speech. The patient easily responded to simple instructions, e.g., to point at a key or a pencil. He was unable, however, to understand combinations of inflected words. When asked to "point at the pencil with the key", he pointed first at one object then at the other: "Here is the key, and here is the pencil". In looking at a picture he could point out which of two persons was the mother and which the daughter, but he was unable to comprehend the expressions "mother's daughter" or "the daughter's mother"; he always pointed first at one person and then at the other. He was unable to "draw a triangle under a circle"; he interpreted the instruction agrammatically, drawing the triangle and then drawing a circle under it. He was totally incapable of explaining the difference between the questions, "What comes before, summer?" and "what comes after summer?". In both cases his answer was, "Fall". He retained the ability to name individual objects, but did not recognize the relationships among words in complex logico-grammatical constructions. The ability to calculate was similarly disturbed. While he easily recognized and interpreted individual digits, he was totally unable to carry out sequential mathematical operations. In addition to, or underlying, these disturbances there was a generalized and pronounced impairment of spatial orientation.

The patient showed signs of a severe ideational apraxia. He was unable to carry out actions according to an imaginary plan, i.e., he was unable to show how one lights a cigarette or stirs tea. He even had some difficulty in carrying out purposeful actions, since he was quite clumsy and often confused the directions of the movements he wished to make. Only after many attempts was he able to accomplish constructive tasks such as placing his two hands in certain relative positions. His ability to draw was greatly impaired. He could not even copy a triangle (much less draw one in response to verbal instructions).

This syndrome showed important differences from other mixed forms of aphasia, such as the syndrome of temporal lobe aphasia, even in the initial period after injury. Recovery took place gradually, but the basic combination of spatial disorientation and impaired comprehension of semantic relationships persisted for a long time.

This case illustrated the unitary syndrome comprised of spatial disorientation and semantic disturbances in the early stage following injury. In numerous other cases we had the opportunity to observe the same syndrome during the residual period of recovery.

Case 4

On January 3, 1942, patient Zas., a 23 year-old third year technical school student, received a shrapnel wound in the left parieto-occipito-temporal area with damage to the dura and cortex. After a long period of unconsciousness, the patient was found to have a right hemianopsia with a slight disturbance of epicritic sensitivity on the right. Also, immediately following recovery of consciousness he was found to have a speech disorder. Expressive speech was relatively intact, but he spoke little and noted that he "had few words left". Still, he was able to understand simple speech. His vision was considerably impaired in the initial period following injury: everything appeared dim and danced before his eyes, so that he was unable to read.

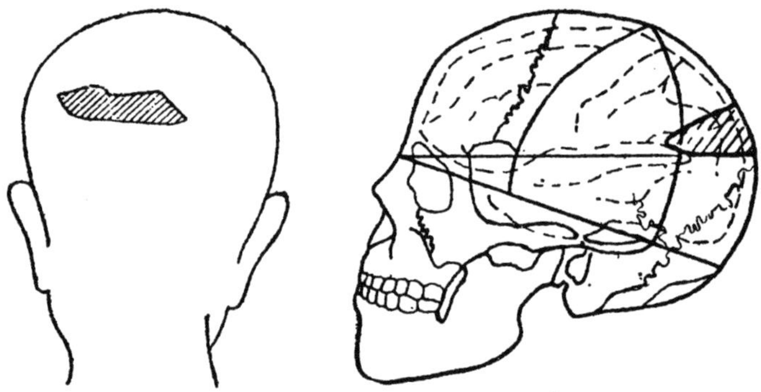

a b

Patient Zas.: injury diagram (Case 4)

The healing of the wound progressed favorably and we examined the patient two and a half months after injury. He was in good spirits but showed certain functional deficits. He complained that he was totally unable to read, that he had difficulty in writing, and that he was unable to count. He could not understand statements involving complex constructions and requiring logical analysis. He was able to copy complex figures rather well and showed no severe apraxia. His spatial orientation, however, was disturbed, so that he had to hesitate for some time before he could extend his hand to the position appropriate for shaking hands with the examiner.

When he was asked to draw a map he was unable to do so (Fig. 41). He confused the positions of the various cities and was even unable to point out different countries on a world map. It was clear that his inner spatial schemata were severely disrupted.

Perhaps the most severely disturbed function in this patient was the ability to calculate. He could neither recognize nor picture numbers to himself without reciting the whole series, 1, 2, 3, 4, etc., up to the number he wanted. When the number spoken corresponded to the one he was looking at he recognized it with no difficulty. He added and

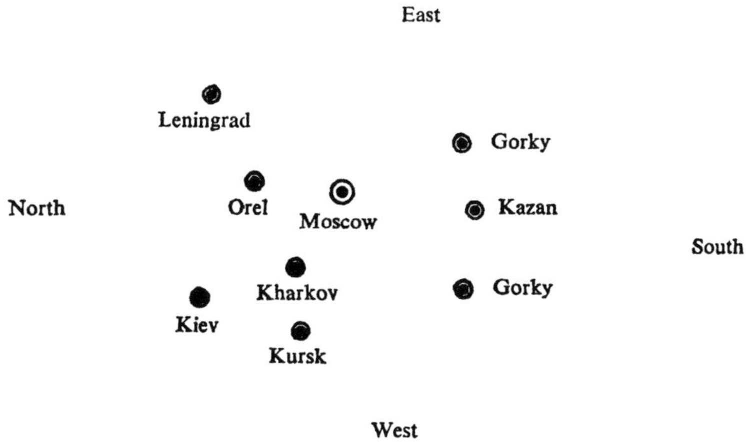

FIG. 41. Map produced by Patient Zas.

subtracted by counting up and down. He remembered his multiplication tables rather well, but he was totally unable to divide.

There was no disturbance of auditory analysis, but reading and writing were severely affected. He was only able to see two or three letters at a time and recognized each letter by reciting the whole alphabet until he found it. He recognized a letter only at the moment when he named it, so that reading was reduced to the sequential naming of letters which were never perceived simultaneously in a unified pattern. Similar disturbances characterized his writing. The semantic aspect of speech was also disturbed. Expressive speech was not greatly affected by this, however. Only occasionally was it interrupted by word searching. The patient showed good comprehension of the meaning of a literary selection so that, after a single reading he was able to summarize correctly the meaning of Tolstoj's fable "The Jackdaws and the Dove". In his words the moral was, "One should not strive to ornament oneself but to live honestly". The patient was able to grasp abstract relationships and, in some cases, succeeded in mastering such complex abstract operations as the naming of opposites, etc. At the same time, however, simple logico-grammatical constructions were impossible for him. It was surprising to find such well defined disturbances in the context of what appeared to be generally well-preserved intellectual status. The patient had no difficulty in pointing to objects named to him, e.g., a pencil or a key; but when asked to "point at the pencil with the key" he again pointed at each object in turn. He had difficulty in perceiving the relationships implied by inflective grammatical constructions. He could point out which of two persons in a picture was the mother and which the daughter, but he could not understand the meaning of the phrases "mother of the daughter" and "daughter of the mother". "I really know: there are two of them . . . I would imagine . . . mother . . . and daughter . . . but which of them!? I can't get it. It's so funny . . . daughter of the mother . . . it's related to mother or daughter . . . it's not clear; it just doesn't come to me." He was unable to compare the relative validity of two sentences containing identical words in different orders, e.g., "The elephant is larger than the mouse", and "the mouse is larger than the elephant", or "the sister of the wife" and "the wife of the sister". In each case he concluded that both were meaningful statements. Intellectual tasks of the type introduced by Bert, e.g., 'Which of the circles is larger than the red one and smaller than the blue one?" were completely impossible for this patient, for they required comparing two or more elements contained in the statement.

We were able to follow this patient for more than three years as the subject of a special investigation.[5] The impairment of reading and calculation as well as the amnesic speech disturbance became somewhat less severe. By means of special techniques to be described in a later chapter,[6] it was possible to retrain the patient to the point where he could comprehend certain types of complex logico-grammatical constructions. Even after extensive retraining, however, his comprehension of such constructions was derived by applying formal rules which he had memorized and learned to apply to specific forms of grammatical constructions. For instance, in interpreting the construction "the mother's daughter" he would reason as follows: "The word with the ending 'apostrophe s' is the possessive form of a noun modifiying the word 'daughter', the major element in the phrase." [7] In this way he was able to grasp the true meaning of the construction.

Case 5

On August 12, 1941, patient Gorjun., a 33 year-old teacher, philologist, and director of a large school in Leningrad was injured by a mine fragment which entered the parieto-occipital area close to the midline and came deeply into the left temporal area. The patient lost consciousness for a long period of time following the injury. There was a right hemiparesis with impairment of all modes of sensation. There was also an expressive speech disorder characterized by a lack of continuity. The latter gradually disappeared over a period of three months. Six months after injury all that remained was a slight hyperreflexia on the right, a reduction of epicritic sensitivity on the right, and right hemianopsia. Another form of speech disorder was noted which resembled an amnesic aphasia. Phonemic hearing was intact and there were no articulatory difficulties. The patient's speech no longer lacked continuity. Upon careful examination, however, it was found that he suffered from a severe form of semantic aphasia.

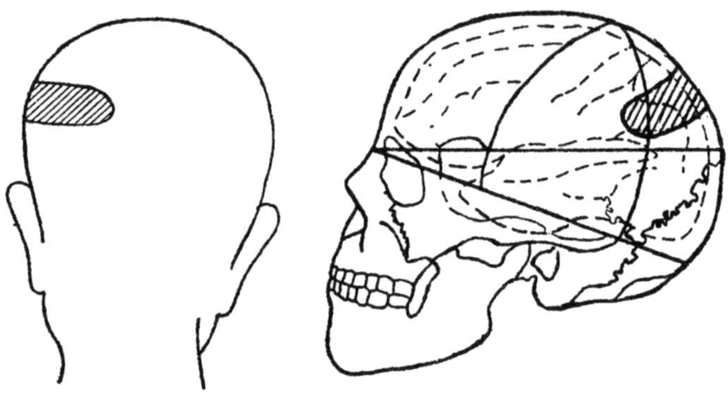

a b

Patien Goriun.: injury diagram (Case 5)

The patient came under our observation six months after injury. The wound had healed without complications. At this time he was uninhibited and unstable, he was sometimes euphoric and other times very depressed by the defect his injury had produced. He complained that when he was tired he was unable to remember words, and

[5] The author has a remarkable autobiography of that patient; he hopes to be able to publish it.

[6] See Chapter 16, Section 5.

[7] This quotation has been altered to fit the rules of English grammar rather than those of Russian grammar (trans.).

that he had difficulty in understanding long sentences. He attributed this to an inability to keep long statements in mind long enough to interpret them. He noted a difficulty in reading which consisted in an inability to identify the letter complexes which make up words. His ability to calculate was severely affected.

It was apparent from the first that the patient suffered no visual impairment. He easily recognized the significance of drawings whether they were realistic or diagrammatic, and he had little difficulty in identifying figures drawn against a background designed to mask them. Except for the hemnianopia, his visual field was not detectably constricted. He was able to perceive three or four figures at once when they were presented tachistoscopically. The first disturbances appeared when he was asked to interpret relationships and to carry out operations requiring spatial orientation. He experienced considerable difficulty when required to place one hand in a given position relative to the other. He was unable to draw or even to picture to himself a floor plan of his ward and other rooms along the corridor. He was unable to carry out any constructive operation involving the reorganization of elements in an inner schema derived from the direct perception of his surroundings. His attempted sketch of the profile of an object presented to him full face showed a dissociation of the component parts demonstrating the extent to which his inner geometrical schemata were disrupted.

Similar disturbances characterized the patient's attempts to calculate. He had no difficulty in recognizing individual digits, and he was able to count forwards. Counting backwards was extremely difficult for him, however. Beginning to count backwards he would reverse himself and start counting forwards, or he would simply name digits at random. It became clear that *he possessed no clear conception of the pattern of numbers arranged in increasing order of magnitude.* He also had difficulty in recognizing numbers composed of more than one digit. He could never recognize them immediately. Certain digit sequences which had been familar to him were preserved, but, in general, the relationship between patterns of digits and numbers was lost. He was able to write multiple digit numbers only if the digits were dictated to him one at a time. He also had difficulty in computation. He had little difficulty adding and subtracting numbers less than 10, but calculations involving numbers greater than 10 and requiring certain operations to be carried out "mentally" were impossible for him. Even subtractions such as 31-7 or 24-6 presented overwhelming difficulty when he attempted to solve them "in his head". Of course, multiplication, division, and all operations involving fractions were totally impossible.

The most severe disturbance seen in this patient had to do with verbal logico-grammatical operations. He retained a great deal from his previous intellectual experience, e.g., he was able to make use of the concept of categories and usually had little difficulty in solving problems involving the classification of objects. Similarly, he had little difficulty in identifying levels of generality such as the genus-species relationships in the series "birch-maple-tree-oak". Even here, however, he encountered a special kind of difficulty. He often could not remember the names of general categories. He gave 76% amnesic responses when asked to name general categories as opposed to 16% amnesic responses when asked to name concrete objects. In classifying objects he usually used concrete categories. This disturbance, however, was no more serious than what is often observed in mild cases of organic dementia. He showed extreme impairment of the ability to carry out intellectual operations requiring the *integration* of several details into a single meaningful pattern.

The patient had no difficulty in repeating and comprehending a grammatically simple sentence composed of 10, 12, or even 14 words. He was unable, however, to comprehend the relationship implied by a short phrase in which the order of the words was important.

Only with considerable help on the part of the examiner was he able to recognize that the logico-grammatical constructions "brother of father" and "father of brother" have different meanings. He had difficulty analyzing the significance of such a sentence as, "Jack was hit by John", this he interpreted as meaning the same as, "Jack hit John". He had similar difficulty with the sentence, "I ate after I brought in the firewood". Here he interpreted the sequence of events to be the same as the sequence of words in the sentence. He was unable to understand that "the less bright" of two figures is the darker of the two. In each instance the operation by which the initial structure of the statement could be modified to reveal the inner relationship between its elements proved to be impossible for the patient to perform.

Any intellectual operation requiring inner schematization served only to confuse the patient. He characterized his difficulty in relating his thoughts as follows: "There are probably numerous mistakes in the story which I wrote. I probably mutilated it to such an extent that it will be impossible to understand it. I write with no confidence in what I am saying. Before me there lies boundless ocean, speaking in less literary terms(!), in which I must swim, not knowing what I'll come up against . . ."

In view of what we have said one might expect to find that the patient's *system* of previous knowledge was greatly reduced. He retained certain fragments of previous experience and sometimes was able to show that he remembered things from his social science studies and philosophy, but to relate these to any logical, wellanalyzed system was impossible. Even such simple and familiar concepts as grammatical categories were severely affected. The categories of concrete experience such as number and gender remained intact, but the categories of relationships such as case, voice, etc. were severely disturbed. Thus, the patient was unable to conjugate verbs or analyze the grammar of sentences in order to determine the relationships which they were meant to convey. As might be expected this profound defect coexisted with relatively wellpreserved expressive speech. The only outward sign of the disorder was a difficulty in naming objects, one manifestation of the general disintegration of the system of word meanings.

These examples show that the disturbance of functional systems produced by damage to the posterior cortical zones associated with "gnostic" functions may produce severe aphasic disturbances. These disturbances differ sharply, however, from the disorders of expressive speech which arise with lesions in other areas. These lesions deprive the patient of the ability to relate several elements into a single pattern and to "unify separate details into a single whole". Loss of this ability leads to a disturbance of the inner schemata of geometrical relationships and, in extreme form, leads to a loss of logico-grammatical operations which are impossible without the capacity for inner schematization.

The syndrome just described is never seen with lesions in any other part of the brain. Lesions in other areas which do not affect the semantic aspect of speech give rise to symptoms of an entirely different character. Figure 42 shows the distribution of lesions in a series of cases of semantic aphasia. This figure confirms Head's finding that this syndrome is directly related to the occipito-parietal or visuo-gnostic portion of the cortex.

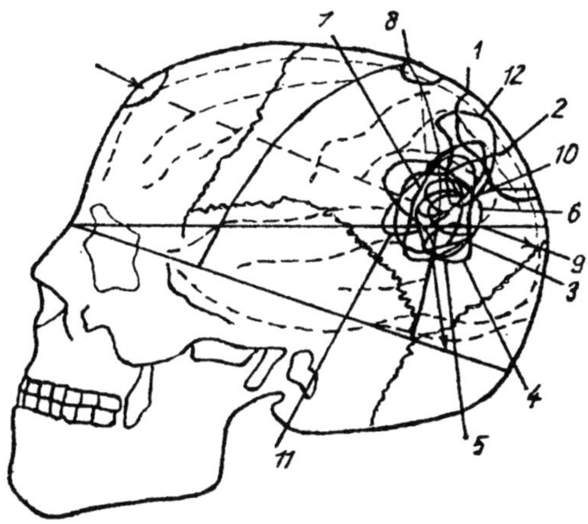

FIG. 42. Diagram of lesion sites in cases of semantic aphasia.

Sites of lesions in cases of semantic aphasia

Case No.	Name	Lesion	Speech disturbance
1	Bog.	Bullet wound, entering occipital area and emerging from the left parieto-occipital area.	Severe semantic aphasia with loss of logico-grammatical relations and amnesie-aphasic disturbances; clearcut disturbance of spatial orientation.
2	Pinč.	Grazing penetrating injury in left parieto-occipital area with extrusion of brain substance; no hemiparesis; minimal impairment of deep touch sensation.	Clearcut parietal syndrome with disturbance of spatial orientation; acalculia and severe semantic aphasia expressed in loss of logico-grammatical constructions; phonemic hearing and nominative function of speech intact.
3	Pryg.	Direct shrapnel wound in left infero-parietal area; no hemiparesis and only slight impairment of deep touch sensation.	Definite parietal syndrome with disturbance of spatial orientation but no serious impairment of computation; signs of severe semantic aphasia with loss of comprehension of logico-grammatical constructions and difficulty in naming objects.
4	Kov.	Direct penetrating shrapnel wound in left parieto-temporal area; no hemiparesis; astereognosis on the right.	Definite parietal syndrome with disturbance of spatial orientation; computation intact; severe impairment of comprehension of logico-grammatical relations which gradually diminished; phonemic hearing and writing intact.
5	Grexn.	Direct injury in left parieto-occipital area complicated by an abscess; sensory deficit on the right; slight loss of power in the right arm.	Definite semantic aphasia with difficulty in comprehending logico-grammatical relations and impairment of computation, both of which underwent gradual recovery; phonemic hearing and writing intact.

Case No.	Name	Lesion	Speech disturbance
6	Kar.	Missile entering superior part of left parietal area and emerging from left infero-parietal area; complicated by abscess; right hemiparesis.	Severe parietal syndrome with persistent disturbance of spatial orientation; agnosia for spatial relations; reading disturbance of verbal alexia type; persistent semantic aphasia; phonemic hearing and writing intact.
7	Sux.	Bullet wound, entering left frontal and emerging to leave area of major destruction in left infero-parietal area; right hemiparesis.	Clearcut parietal syndrome with loss of spatial orientation, disturbance of body image; impairment of computation and signs of severe semantic aphasia; phonemic hearing intact; reading and writing disturbed.
8	Don.	Penetrating injury in left parieto-occipital area; no hemiparesis.	Clearcut occipito-parietal syndrome with constructional apraxia, acalculia, difficulty in reading whole words, and mild disturbance of logico-grammatical relations.
9	Lar.	Penetrating wound in left tempero-parietal area with direct damage to brain tissues; right hemiparesis.	Severe semantic aphasia with disturbance of logico-grammatical aspects of speech and computation; signs of amnesic aphasia; relatively mild signs of impaired spatial orientation.
10	Zund.	Direct shrapnel wound in left occipito-parietal area; no hemiparesis; sensory deficit on right and right hemianopia.	Long-lasting amnesic aphasia with disturbance of logico-grammatical aspect of speech, acalculia, alexia, and constructional apraxia which underwent gradual recovery.

D. DISTURBANCES OF PARTICULAR BRAIN SYSTEMS AND GENERAL SPEECH DISORDERS: QUESTIONS UNANSWERED

We have considered the types of speech disorders which arise as a result of damage to specific brain systems and have determined what kinds of disturbance each imposes on the overall system of speech activity. We have observed the different ways in which speech suffers from the loss of various functions necessary for speech. This approach was chosen with full awareness of its difficulty and limitations.

In cases of brain damage inflicted by firearms one can often get only a rough idea as to the boundaries of the damaged area. Seldom does one have the opportunity to verify the anatomical site of a lesion as precisely as one might desire. In cases where it has been possible to section the brains of patients who have sustained war injuries, it has usually been found that the lesions were quite complex; often such lesions have given rise to complications leading to the death of the patient. In cases where anatomical verification was not possible it was obvious that many unrelated cerebral changes had occurred.

All of this tended to complicate the approach which we chose. On the other hand, carefully conducted clinico-psychological examinations of large numbers of wartime patients made this approach a desirable one: since large numbers of cases could be studied, it was possible to discover features common to all patients with a certain type of lesion. By analyzing the common symptoms in terms of modern-day knowledge of the structure and function of brain systems, is was possible to reach certain general conclusions. This method of analysis proved productive even in studying lesions of the "marginal" zones of the cerebral cortex. It permitted us to analyze disturbances which do not fit easily into the usual categories of aphasia.

The analysis which we have carried out has permitted us, first of all, to describe speech disorders not in terms of arbitrarily selected aspects of speech activity, but in terms of the primary components of brain activity revealed by experimental investigations in psychophysiology and brain pathology. This has a decided advantage over other approaches based on *a priori* assumptions about brain anatomy and the psychological principles of brain activity, for such assumptions can lead one to overlook or ignore large amounts of important clinical material.

On the basis of our approach we were able to distinguish the fundamental types of aphasia on the basis of their pathogenesis. Almost a century of intensive investigations has given rise to numerous classifications distinguishing an extremely large variety of speech disorders. One cannot deny the accuracy of the descriptions. On the other hand, one cannot help but see critical flaws in the majority of such classifications. Some authors, most of whom belonged to the period in which classical neurology was developing categorized aphasias on the basis of hypothetical anatomical schemes. This type of classification distinguished cortical and sub-cortical motor aphasias, cortical and sub-cortical sensory aphasias, and conduction versus transcortical aphasias. Soon after this scheme was proposed, however, it was found to be incompatible with the actual anatomy of the brain and recognized to be based largely on arbitrary theorization. Clinicians found that aphasic syndromes seldom fitted into these schemes; the real syndromes were generally much richer and much more varied than such classifications would admit. For this reason the majority of clinicians soon ceased to think of aphasia in terms of the early anatomical classifications. They turned to a purely descriptive psycholinguistic terminology which was more capable of reflecting the richness of clinical observation. Such terminology failed, however, to reflect the basic brain mechanisms underlying the syndromes which it described. Classifications of this type, reaching their logical extreme in the works of Head, made it possible to describe fine variations among different aphasic syndromes and thus to open such syndromes to psycholinguistic analysis.

The psycholinguistic division of aphasias into verbal, nominative, syntactic, and semantic types was not, however, widely accepted in clinical practice. There were two reasons for this lack of acceptance. First, basing a classification altogether on formal linguistic concepts could hardly be expected to prove successful. At the present time linguists are striving to overcome the limitations imposed by restricting their study to syntax and the nominative and semantic aspects of words. Thus, today more than ever before we have a reason to look with suspicion upon the idea that all speech disorders may be classified in terms of these arbitrarily defined aspects of language. Secondly, it seems unlikely that a classification of aphasia should be based upon phenomena which are totally divorced from actual brain processes and which ignore the primary pathogenetic basis of speech disturbances; this can only be discovered by a study of disturbances which arise when the functions of various cerebral areas are disrupted. These, then, are the reasons why classifications of aphasic syndromes which are based altogether on linguistic constructs are essentially formalistic and have proven inadequate in the face of actual clinical experience.

We have attempted to approach our study in a different way. By avoiding any *a priori* theory regarding the forms which aphasia might take we have attempted to discover the fundamental relationships among the functions of various cortical zones so that, on the basis of these functional characteristics, we might explain the speech disturbances which arise when particular physiological systems are destroyed. By adopting this approach we have taken a step toward a more rational classification of aphasic syndromes, i.e., toward a classification which is based upon actual *psychophysiological and pathological mechanisms of cerebral activity.* This approach should confirm the validity of some classifications and correct the shortcoming of others. Thus, in the study of motor and sensory aphasia it will provide more precision in the classification of symptoms which are basic to the two forms. On the other hand, it will introduce some essential changes in the study of the "amnesic" and "conductive" aphasias. "*Amnesic aphasia*" will cease to be classified as an independent clinical entity identified by some authors with lesions in the antero-parietal area and by others with lesions in the antero-temporal area. Instead it will become a symptom which can arise in any one of three types of speech disturbance, *viz.,* temporal-acoustic, parietal-semantic, or frontal-dynamic aphasia. Its particular functional structure is different in each case. In cases involving the temporal areas the symptom of amnesic aphasia proves to be one manifestation of an acoustico-gnostic defect which leads to a loss of word meanings. With lesions of the parietal area and the resultant semantic aphasia, the forgetting of the names of objects may be due to the loss of meaningful associations, making it difficult to find the verbal symbols for objects. Finally, in cases of frontal-dynamic aphasia, the inability to produce words in spontaneous speech arises as a symptom of the disruption of the dynamic schemata of sentences – a defect in the verbal organization of thought.[8] Thus, while in some respects this approach may give rise to a more complex classification, it provides a more accurate understanding of symptoms.

[8] See Chapter 11 for a fuller discussion of "amnesic aphasic" disorders.

The same situation holds with regard to the so called "conductive aphasias", the major feature of which is a difficulty in repeating sounds and words. Upon close analysis this symptom proves to be considerably more complex than one might expect. In some cases it appears as a mild form of acoustico-gnostic disturbance, in others as a defect of verbal articulation, and in still others as what Goldstein has described as a disturbance of the "abstract attitude" necessary for the voluntary repetition of words spoken by others.

The approach which we have taken does not, and need not, consist in an exhaustive classification of all the possible clinical forms which aphasia may take. In contrast to other attempts, it is designed to reveal the fundamental disorders which may combine in different ways to produce any number of complex clinical syndromes.

Here we come to the second advantage of this approach. By following it in the study of damage to the so-called "marginal" areas (adjacent to speech zones) we have succeeded in demonstrating disturbances of very subtle functions in a relatively pure form. This has usually been impossible in the study of syndromes arising as a result of lesions in these areas. The combinations of symptoms arising as a result of damage to the intermediate zones may be extremely diverse. Sometimes one, and sometimes another symptom plays a leading role. Different compensatory reactions come into play, so that superficially similar lesions may give rise to a variety of clinical syndromes. These can be better understood if one begins by analyzing individual symptoms with regard to their basic and common components.

Finally we come to a third advantage. The classical methods of analyzing aphasic syndromes were usually based upon an associationistic concept of speech activity. It was impossible for such analysis to reveal the general or systemic influence of particular defects. Yet it is perfectly obvious that local lesions have such effects and that they are extremely important. The loss of a specific function necessary for speech is never reflected in the loss of a single aspect of the speech process; it always has a more general affect on the functional system of speech as a whole. The loss of expressive speech arising from a disturbance of articulatory movements or a defect in the dynamic schemata of words is inevitably associated with a loss of unity of sound and meaning and impairment of speech comprehension. The disintegration of phonemic hearing which produces primarily a loss of word meanings leads secondarily to an expressive speech disorder; in milder cases one observes literal and verbal paraphasias, while in more severe cases there is a total block of expressive speech. Many of the disturbances which we have mentioned lead to the impairment of operations involved in reading and writing. Thus, each type of aphasia creates a certain *typical pattern of speech disturbances* many components of which have a complex indirect relationship to the primary disorder produced by the lesion. On the other hand, since the speech system always suffers as a whole, very diverse forms of aphasia may give rise to syndromes which are quite similar. In the final analysis, a complex pattern of speech disorders arises with the disturbance of any particular function (such as the loss of kinesthetic articulatory schemata), but one can never attribute a given syndrome *to the disturbance of a particular function* without analyzing it in great detail.

While this position is perfectly apparent to psychologists, physiologists, and clinicians alike, it deserves concrete analysis in terms of the approach which we have undertaken. While the loss of one or another function necessary for speech activity inevitably leads to the impairment of the speech system as a whole, the impairment need not be the same in all cases. Speech comprehension suffers in efferent (dynamic) motor aphasia, apraxic disorders, acoustico-gnostic disturbances, and semantic aphasias. In every case, however, it is affected differently. Expressive speech, reading, and writing also suffer in these types of aphasia; but, again, the disturbances differ from one another, since the basic cerebral defect varies from one another, since the basic cerebral defect varies from case to case. The approach which we have taken permits not only a description of the general systemic effects of particular disturbances but also an explanation of the specific forms which emerge in different cases. This problem will be taken up in the next chapter.

Several questions have remained unresolved in the course of our analysis. For the most part they have to do with phenomena not directly related to, or conflicting with the positions which we have set forth.

In some cases we observed disorders which clearly did not fit in any of the disturbance patterns we have described. Such observations included apraxias of the speech apparatus and the amnesia for speech movements which sometimes occurred with lesions in the anterior parts of the speech zone. These symptoms which Broca referred to as "aphemia", were observed to accompany lesions of the premotor and infero-frontal areas with the postcentral areas intact. In the majority of cases the difficulties in finding articulatory positions disappeared quite rapidly, especially if speech therapy was initiated; there was no doubt, however, that they were basically apraxic-amnesic in character. In the absence of precise morphological analysis it is possible that the lesion sites were not accurately determined. More likely the explanation lies in the fact that the afferent and efferent cortical areas associated with speech are so intimately connected with one another that damage to one can produce secondary effects on the other. Such a large number of observations running counter to the classification outlined above deserve further investigation.

A second group of unsolved problems has to do with observations which are not adequately explained by our theory and thus require the formulation of new hypotheses. For instance, there is a group of aphasic disorders in which the speech system is disturbed at a level higher than the articulatory one or the level of sound-meaning integration. We observed many cases of motor aphasia in which the major disorder was not an apraxic defect or a denervation difficulty, but rather a disorder which in classical neurological terminology would be referred to as "mnestic" in character. The patients easily repeated sounds and words; they showed no significant perseverative tendencies and, though they stuttered occasionally, they were able to pronounce the words they wished. Their difficulty lay in finding the words necessary for active speech. It was apparent that the primary defect responsible for this form of "mnestic" motor aphasia lay at the highest level of speech integration.

Similar observations occurred in the study of sensory aphasia. In some cases, (the majority involving the infero-temporal area) the patient showed no impairment of phonemic hearing, no literal paraphasia, and no writing disorder, yet they were unable to understand the meanings of words or to name objects. It was obvious that they had lost the meanings of words but the exact nature of their disturbance was not clear.

We should mention a third group of phenomena which demands special study. Goldstein suggests differentiating aphasias into two basic types. The "peripheral" type, involves a disturbance of such external aspects of the speech act, as articulation, etc., while the second, or "central", type involves higher levels of speech activity. The latter includes, for instance, disturbances of the nominative aspect of speech and impairment of categorical thought. In recent times Nielsen has reported observations indicating that aphasias may be thought of as disorders at "higher and lower levels" in the integration of speech processes.

Hughling Jackson was the first to put more emphasis on the level of speech activity disturbed than on the precise site of the underlying brain lesion. This approach came to be highly valued by such outstanding investigators as A. Pick (1913, 1931), K. Goldstein (1948), and Ombredane (1951). As a result, the analysis of speech disturbances in terms of the impairment of different levels of speech activity became very important. This same approach is implied in the Pavlovian conception of speech as a complex, specifically human, *second signalling system.*

How does all this relate to the approach which we have used in the analysis of aphasia? We are far from being of the opinion that the approach which we have taken is the only correct one, while the other is incorrect or inappropriate. Moreover, we have every reason to believe that the functional analysis of disturbances of the highly organized processes involved in the second signalling system is essential for a correct understanding both of normal speech activity and of speech disorders. At the same time, we have reason to think that any investigation of disturbances of higher levels of speech activity which does not go beyond considerations of the "voluntariness" or "categoric" aspect of the speech act and does not consider the relationship of the disorder to the site of brain lesion risks becoming a superficial exercise in description. By dissociating itself from its natural origins and by becoming wrapped up in a subjective terminology such a theory can become an obstacle to further scientific investigation.

The description of a disturbance of the highest, "voluntary", "conscious" form of speech activity is not the end but the beginning of a good investigation. Such a description is not an explanation of the clinical phenomena, it is only a statement as to what phenomena demand explanation. The real explanation should grow out of careful study of the pathological changes in neurodynamic processes which occur as the result of damage to local areas which are necessary for normal interaction and functioning of the second and first signalling systems. Such a study has not been presented in this book. An explanation based on the analysis of neurodynamic disturbances requires a careful preliminary analysis of the primary effects of localized lesions at different sites. Such a preliminary analysis was the goal of this investigation. The analysis of the changes produced by focal brain lesions is of clinical interest and, at the same time, serves as a starting point for more general pathophysiological analyses.

PART II

THE NEURO-PSYCHOLOGICAL EXAMINATION AND THE DIFFERENTIAL DIAGNOSIS OF TRAUMATIC APHASIA

IX

THE PROBLEMS OF NEURO-PSYCHOLOGICAL INVESTIGATION AND THE DIFFERENTIAL DIAGNOSIS OF TRAUMATIC APHASIA

A. GENERAL PRINCIPLES

Any investigation of traumatic aphasia must satisfy two criteria. First, it must help to differentiate between the patient's aphasic disturbances and speech disturbances of a nonaphasic type. It must distinguish true aphasia from reactive post-contusional deaf mutism, dysarthria, and such generalized cerebral disturbances as stupor and apathy. Secondly, it must allow the investigator to describe the type of aphasia with which he is dealing in the most precise manner possible. It must permit him to distinguish the basic defect from a host of secondary disturbances of speech and intellectual activity. This latter criterion is important not only for increasing the precision of diagnosis and locating the site of brain damage but also for the development of a rational approach to speech therapy.

The clinico-psychological investigation of traumatic aphasia should involve more than a simple description of the individual defects of perception, memory, speech, reading, writing, etc. which comprise a given syndrome. It should take into account just how each function is affected, the pattern of the disturbances, and what common factor unites the various symptoms. We have already indicated that the brain cannot be thought of as a system of "centers" which are responsible for specific "faculties". The destruction of a particular zone removes a precondition necessary for the proper functioning of the brain as a whole. The inevitable result is that in its absence a certain group of mental processes cannot be carried out. Any clinico-psychological investigation proposed to answer the questions of how mental processes are altered when different preconditions are removed and how one disturbance can give rise to different symptoms must take this fact into account. The first step is to arrive at a precise descripion and *psychological qualification of symptoms*; the second and equally important step is to explain the structure of the syndrome and to discover the "primary disturbance" underlying the diverse symptoms. As Goldstein has pointed out many times, clinico-psychological analysis is completed only when the primary defect has been determined and when the investigator is in a position to predict what changes will occur in the disturbed function in specific situations.

We shall consider one by one the speech disorders which arise as the result of brain lesions in different locations and will be concerned not so much with simply describing the functions lost as with analyzing the *type of disturbance* of neuro-mental functions and functional systems present. The first step will be to analyze the disturbances which may arise as a result of the impairment of non-speech processes (gnosis and praxis); the second step will be to analyze the disturbances of *speech activity* in an attempt to determine how the impairment of particular brain processes affects *expressive and receptive speech, the semantic structure of speech, and complex voluntary forms of speech activity.*

B. DIFFERENTIATION FROM NON-APHASIC SPEECH DISTURBANCES

Practically speaking, the differential diagnosis of traumatic aphasia requires only that it be distinguished from postcontusional mutism, dysarthria, and other conditions which may affect the patient's speech by producing cerebral asthenia, stupor, or, as is common in cases of frontal lobe injury, aspontaneity.

Reactive (postcontusional) speech disturbances are seldom encountered in peacetime. They differ sharply from traumatic aphasia in that they do not affect speech as a symbolic activiy; the primary defect lies in the functional "disconnection" of the entire phonational (auditory-articulatory) apparatus. Symbolic speech functions which do not involve *oral* speech may not be affected. A patient with postcontusional deaf mutism does not use his vocal and articulatory apparatus at all and he makes no attempt to use speech functions he retains as a means of communication. This picture contrasts sharply with that of the aphasic, who usually expends some effort in attempting to use whatever residual speech he may have. In reactive deaf mutism a generalized inhibition affects not only the articulatory system, but all systems involved in *phonation.* As a result the patient is not only deprived of the ability to form words; he can produce no vocal sound whatever. Attempts at vocalization may fail completely or result in generalized spasmodic contraction of the pharyngeal muscles. In either case no sound is produced. The phonational components of speech may reappear in later stages of recovery, but the major pathological feature of expressive speech continues to be *dysphonia* (stuttering, stumbling, inability to regulate the intensity of phonation) rather than impairment of the ability to articulate particular sounds which is characteristic of motor aphasia.

Thus, one difficulty of a patient with reactive postcontusional mutism is not so much a speech defect as a phonation defect, and this easily distinguishes him from the patient with traumatic aphasia. A second major difference is the *preservation of written speech.* An aphasia so severe as to totally disrupt the patient's speech is always accompanied by some degree of writing impairment. In cases of reactive postcontusional mutism, however, writing is usually intact, and the patient rapidly adopts it as a means of communication. He also seldom shows any difficulty in reading.

Sometimes reactive postcontusional *deaf-mutism* is treated as a sensory aphasia. In these cases, however, it is not difficult to distinguish the two types of disturbance. In sensory aphasia elementary auditory functions are partially or totally preserved and the patient makes as much use as possible of his residual auditory capacity; he listens attentively to what is said to him. The patient with reactive postcontusional deaf-mutism, on the other hand, *lacks any sign of conscious auditory activity*; it is as though he ignores the auditory environment completely.

Mixed cases in which primary aphasic disturbances are complicated by secondary reactive components were considered earlier (Chapter I, Section 5). The differentiation of traumatic aphasia from *dysarthria* sometimes presents great difficulty. While dysarthria usually signifies a bulbar or pseudobulbar lesion, it may arise with damage to the anterior part of the sensorimotor area bilaterally. This occasionally occurs when a bullet traverses the skull in a coronal plane. Dysarthria may also occur with deep injuries involving the subcortical ganglia of the left hemisphere. The signs of dysarthria differ from those of postcontusional speech disturbances in that they reflect a disturbance not of phonation but of articulation. It differs from the articulatory defects seen in motor aphasia in the same way that paresis, ataxia, and dysmetria of voluntary action differ from apraxia. In dysarthria, the general schemata of words are preserved, but the ability to pronounce many sounds is severely impaired. The articulatory disturbances result from a partial paresis of the vocal and articulatory apparatus or, if the extrapyramidal systems are damaged, from loss of the differentiation of articulatory movements. The speech of a patient with dysarthria is unclear and "mushy" due to the imprecise channeling of articulatory impulses. It is nasal in character. The pronounciation of lingual, pharyngeal, and labial sounds is severely affected as a result of impairment of the mechanisms responsible for closure of the vocal folds and the loss of tongue control.

Dysarthria affects all complex sounds equally; work on individual sounds usually proves of little help. The disturbance also affects both spontaneous and imitative speech. As a rule, injuries sustained in adulthood do not affect the patient's ability to write. This, again, indicates that the primary defect lies in the execution of speech movements.

It should be noted that a number of disturbances which are commonly classified as "dysarthria" vary considerably from one another. Perhaps future studies will reveal different components related to lesions of the subcortical, sensorimotor, and premotor systems, and a set of disturbances will be found intermediate between dysarthria and motor aphasia corresponding to the spectrum of disorders found in recent years to relate afferent paresis, dysmetria, ataxia, and apraxia.[1]

Special form of non-aphasic disturbances may arise as the result of damage to the

[1] In the latest years the differential features of dysartria and motor aphasia were carefully studied in our laboratory by E. N. Vinarskaya in her monograph of afferent motor aphasia (in print).

right, subdominant hemisphere. These disorders have not been studied to any large degree, but they appear to include disturbances of the smoothness of speech. Patients speak brokenly with a characteristic stutter and intonational defect (a "scanning" disorder or a disturbance of the melodious aspect of speech). The symbolic aspect of speech is apparently undisturbed. Perhaps the symptoms result from disruption of the dynamic "background" of motor processes which some authors, such as Goldstein and Penfield, have attributed to the right hemisphere. The lack of information regarding these disturbances precludes our describing them in detail at the present time.

The last major disorder to be ruled out in the diagnosis of traumatic aphasia is the *general brain damage syndrome* which involves asthenia, stupor, and aspontaneity. This syndrome frequently arises in cases of massive brain damage which involve subcortical structures or disrupt normal cerebro-spinal fluid dynamics. Changes in intracranial pressure may produce stupor and adynamia of such severity that the patient is unable to talk and thus create the impression of traumatic aphasia. Erroneous diagnoses of this type are most likely to be made in the period immediately following injury when general cerebral symptoms are most common.

The speech disturbances associated with generalized cerebral depression usually include the reduction and slowing of spontaneous speech, disorientation, and easy fatigability. The patient has difficulty in raising his hands and in speaking; his gaze is usually fixed; his eyes do not follow moving objects. Any actions he makes are apt to be slow and very restricted in range. Here the verbal adynamia represents just one aspect of a more general behavioral depression.

With damage to the *frontal systems*, the patient's speech exhibits all the signs of aspontaneity which are characteristic of the general brain damage syndrome. The patient has great difficulty in speaking if what he has to say is part of a general plan of action. On the other hand, he is readily able to repeat words or sentences spoken by others, and he utters familiar expressions with no difficulty. Sometimes his difficulty is discovered in the course of conversation when it becomes apparent that he has trouble formulating answers to simple questions. Sometimes it is seen as a total absence of narrative speech or an inability to solve simple problems. These disturbances arise most frequently with lesions in the left frontal area. In fact, they sometimes approach the form of frontal "dynamic" aphasia described earlier.

Anyone who undertakes the study of aphasia has to differentiate it from non-aphasic disorders and thus, faces fundamental clinical problems of this sort. He must be able to identify the precise *form of aphasia* with which he is dealing and the *site of the lesion* which gives rise to it. The latter is one of the most pressing problems which neurosurgical clinics face, whether during war or in time of peace. In order to do this in a rational way it is necessary to know how different aspects of non-verbal and verbal activity suffer in different forms of aphasia and exactly which symptoms can be considered reliable for differential diagnosis. The succeeding chapters are intended to clarify this question.

In accordance with the principles which we formulated earlier, we shall begin with a review of the methods for investigating the non-speech functions of gnosis and praxis. Then we shall consider techniques for investigating the basic forms of speech activity – receptive speech, expressive speech, reading, writing, and calculation.

X

THE INVESTIGATION OF NON-VERBAL FUNCTIONS: GNOSIS AND PRAXIS

Descriptions of non-verbal functions (gnosis and praxis) is generally not included as a part of the clinico-psychological examination for aphasia. It should, however, represent an important part of such investigation. Only by examining the gnostic and praxic functions can one discover the functional state of those cortical systems which, though not part of the "speech zones", may influence one or another component necessary for the organization of speech processes. An investigation of gnosis and praxis may indicate the type of speech disturbance to be expected in a given case.

Again, the primary goal of the investigation should not be simply to enumerate the various losses, but to *characterize the basic defects* which lead to the impairment of perceptual or motor activities. Sometimes gnosis and praxis can be investigated by a few special tests. Other times a disturbance of gnostic (afferent) synthesis produces an impairment of movements. In the latter case one can reach certain conclusions regarding the underlying disturbance of inner gnostic schemata by studying the disturbance of motor activity. Thus, the investigation of apraxic defects may involve description of the types of integrative disorders which have been referred to clinically as "apractagnosias".

A. THE INVESTIGATION OF GNOSTIC PROCESSES

For the present we shall omit consideration of special techniques for the investigation of auditory perception [1] and discuss general methods used in the study of the basic forms of afferent synthesis.

1. *The Investigation of Visual (Object) Recognition*

The study of object recognition is an important part of the investigation of speech activity in patients with brain lesions. First of all, the perception of objects in the

[1] The investigation of acoustico-gnostic processes associated with hearing and speech comprehension will be described below (Chapter 11).

environment is a prime prerequisite for the development of language and speech. Special investigations initiated by L. S. Vygotskij and R. E. Levina showed that the impairment of object perception at an early age prevents normal development of speech processes. A child lacking the ability to perceive objects in the world around him is deprived of the development of speech which would otherwise come to reflect these objects and their interrelationships.[2]

On the other hand, speech itself influences object perception. Speech is responsible for the constancy and generalizing character of perception and raises it to a higher level. This thesis has been set forth numerous times by both linguists and psychologists, (cf. Vygotskij, 1956, Rosengardt-Pupko, *et al.* 1947). Thus it is natural to expect that a speech disturbance should impair the generalizing and stabilizing character of object perception. This expectation has been borne out in investigations carried out by Goldstein and Gelb.

The study of primary and secondary disorders of object perception may be very important as a background against which to evaluate speech disorders. Such a study should establish (a) whether or not the patient retains the visual prerequisites for object perception, (b) whether or not he is able to carry out the integrative processes characteristic of normal object perception, and (c) whether or not his perception is capable of reflecting complex meaningful relationships of the type encompassed by image-based thought processes.

The investigation may involve a series of tests in which the patient is required to describe pictures of various objects and scenes. If he is unable to talk, he is allowed to point out pictures from another group which are identical to the ones presented. Usually the pictures are presented for a rather long period of time. If the investigator wishes to determine whether or not the patient is able to grasp the contents of a picture with normal rapidity he may present it tachistoscopically. If he wishes to determine the degree of retention of *images*, he may ask the patient to describe or draw the figure after it has been taken away.

The following is a series of tests usually employed in the investigation of object recognition:

a. *Recognition of Simple Geometrical Figures*

Such figures as squares, triangles, and circles are drawn with solid contours and dotted contours (Figure 43); then the same types of figures are *presented in groups*.

The patient's ability to perceive the figures is determined by having him name them, draw them, or select identical figures from a group on a separate card.

[2] This point has been dealt with in detail in the Russian psychological literature by S. L. Rubinštejn. See his work *The Fundamentals of General Psychology* (Moscow, 1946). In a special paper we already discussed the developmental results of early optic agnosia. Cf. A. R. Luria, "Vues psychologiques sur l'évolution des états oligophrènes", *1 Congr. Intern. de Psychiatrie Infantile.* (Paris, 1928).

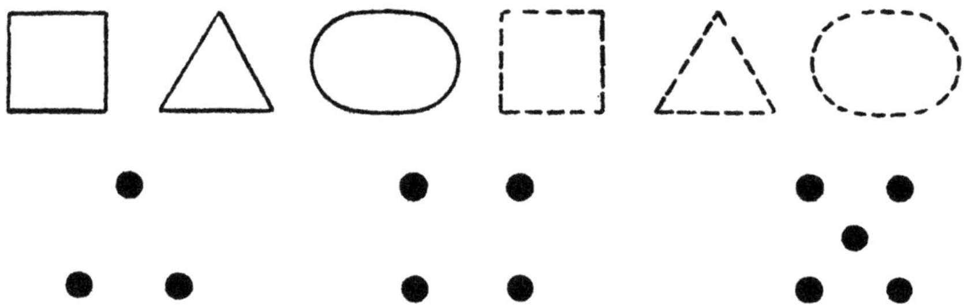

FIG. 43. Series of geometrical figures.

b. *Recognition of Pictures of Objects*

The patient is required to name or to identify objects by pointing them out in a group of pictured objects.

In order to determine the degree of stability of object perception and the extent to which the patient is able to abstract the imporant features of an object, he is asked to identify pictures in which the objects are represented with greater and lesser degrees of abstraction. The objects are represented by realistic sketches, line drawings, silhouettes, or by line drawings which are masked by random lines of varying complexity (Figures 44 and 45). A variation on this type of test suggested by Poppelreuter requires the patient to identify line drawings of various objects superimposed upon one another (Figure 46).

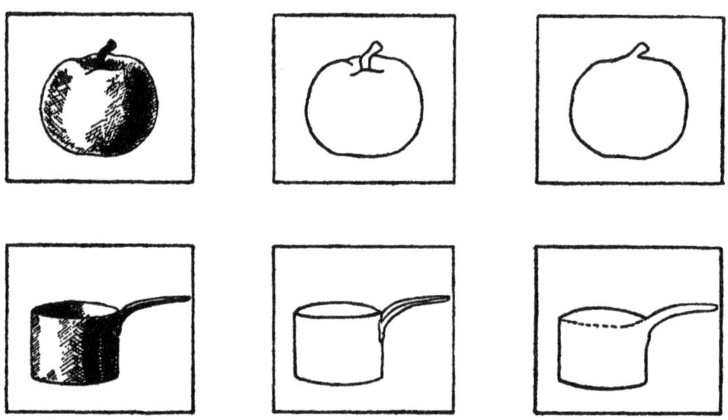

FIG. 44. Series of objects in pictures of varying complexity.

The Revault d'Allonnes test permits one to evaluate *active forms of perception.* The patient is required to trace out various patterns of squares, e.g., crosses and rectangles, on a checkerboard. The inability to do so indicates a defect of active perception or a disturbance of organized perception.

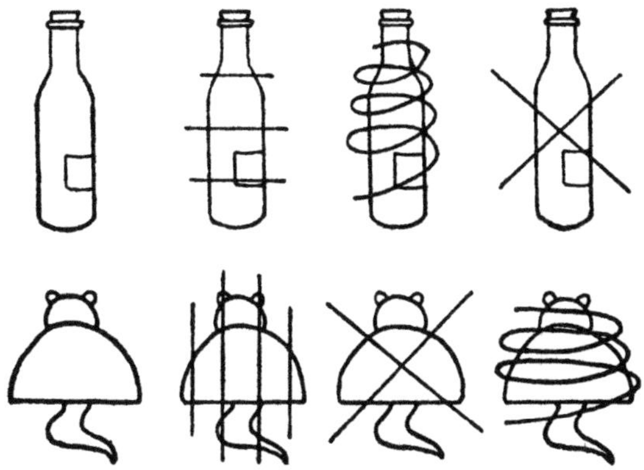

FIG. 45. Crossed-out figures.

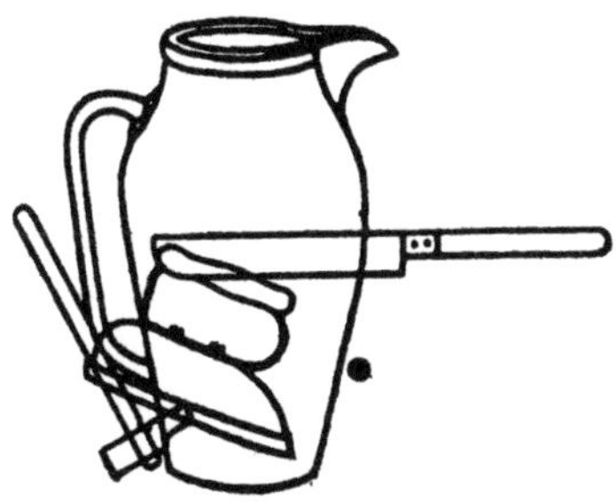

FIG. 46. Outlines of various objects superimposed on one another. (from Poppelreuter)

c. *Recognition of the Significance of Thematic Cards*

Pictures are presented containing numerous cues which together represent a meaningful situation. Usually, the first card shows a situation the meaning of which is easily apparent, e.g., a man cutting firewood or children ice skating; the last cards in the series show more complex situations, the meanings of which can only be ascertained by correlating several cues, and these can only be comprehended on the basis of complex psychological processes.

By using this series of tests one can learn a great deal about the adequacy of visual perception, both with regard to general disturbances of brain activity and specific deficits resulting from limited lesions of the cerebral cortex. *The perception of simple geometrical figures* is seldom affected by lesions localized near the cortical speech areas. A general depression of brain activity resulting from concussion, frontal lobe damage, long standing hypertension, intoxication, malignant hydrocephaly, or an abscess may greatly increase the time required to perceive geometrical figures and preclude the integration of lines or dots into a unified pattern. In extreme cases the patient may perceive the first figure quite well but then because of an abnormally persistent after-image, he may perceive all subsequent figures as similar to the first. He is apparently unable to separate himself from a perceptual set once it has been established. We have described this type of "sensory perseveration" elsewhere.[3] It can seriously affect perceptual activity and produce a secondary "dynamic agnosia" even in cases where there is no sign of a primary perceptual disturbance.

Another important defect is *constriction* of the perceptual field. With occipital lesions and often with adynamia of cerebral processes the perceptual field may be constricted, so that the patient can only see one or two figures simultaneously. The constriction does not involve any hemianopsic defect and is the same no matter what the size of the objects observed.

Total primary loss of the ability to perceive simple geometrical figures (not including the ability to appreciate complex spatial relations) is seldom seen; it occurs only with very severe lesions of the occipital area. Simple hemianopic defects usually do not noticeably impair the ability to perceive geometrical figures. Here, as Gelb and Goldstein have shown, good compensation for the perceptual deficit is often apparent.

One may observe diverse disturbances involving the *perception of visual representations of objects*. As a rule the lesions of the "primary speech zones" which produce disturbances of auditory speech do not give rise to any detectable impairment of simple object perception. The patient with motor or sensory aphasia usually has little difficulty in recognizing either realistic or schematic representations of objects; he can usually often line drawings masked by complex cross-hatching. Difficulty in the perception of such pictures occurs in cases where cortical damage abolishes processes necessary for visual analysis and synthesis, e.g., with localized lesions of the occipito-parietal systems. It can also occur in the presence of depression of cerebral activity resulting from the general types of disorders described above.

Normally direct or immediate recognition occurs only with very simple and familiar objects. The recognition of more complex, less familiar objects does not occur immediately. At first one receives only a vague general impression of the object or grasps certain individual features. From these alternatives one must select the most important, "leading" cues; only after considering these cues as a group does one develop an overall perception of the object. If a single step in this process is lost, one remains at the stage of "general impressions" and either says that he cannot recognize the object or identifies it incorrectly. Perception is a *complex meaningful process* in which it should be possible to distinguish various components.

The types of brain damage described above may also lead to the loss of complex

[3] A. R. Luria, *Higher Cortical Functions in Man*, part III (New York, Basic Books, 1966).

conceptual activity. The patient is either unable to select the important features of an object or he cannot evaluate a given cue correctly on the basis of the context provided by other cues. A drawing of an object which deviates slightly from a photographic representation may be identified incorrectly. The inaccurate perception of an object can usually be explained by the fact that one cue is considered without regard to other features of the object. A figure representing a pair of glasses may be seen simply as a pair of circles and consequently interpreted as a picture of a bicycle. A patient of this type also has difficulty in identifying objects concretely. A picture of a lion or a dog is simply identified as "an animal", for the patient is unable to identify the group of cues which are specific to a particular animal. All perception takes on a rather vague character. The patient is unable to identify figures which have been crossed out or to differentiate the line drawings of various objects superimposed on one another. In looking at such drawings, he groups various contours at random, so that recognition of the objects represented is impossible.

Defects of object recognition may occur in association with primary visual agnosias, damage to the frontal systems, or general cerebral disorders. The character of the disturbance depends to a certain degree upon which syndrome it accompanies. In cases of primary visual agnosia the patient actively attempts to identify the important features of the object. He may select inappropriate combinations of cues at random and thus interpret what he see inaccurately. On the other hand, with general depression of cerebral activity the active attempt to identify objects is absent. Incorrect identification occurs against a background of passivity and indifference. The most striking feature usually determines the erroneous conclusion which the patient reaches regarding the nature of the object he is looking at. Again, as might be expected, a figure which has been crossed out is especially difficult to identify. In these case the inability *to name* a given object is not a sign of a speech difficulty but a sign of a recognition disorder or of a dynamic defect lying beyond the realm of speech.

Disorders of cerebral activity which impair intelligent perception emerge with special clarity when the patient is asked to describe *thematic pictures*. This task differs from the simple recognition task described above in that the patient must consider a number of objects simultaneously, recognize meaningful relationships among essential cues, and ignore inessential features if he is to recognize the meaning of the picture as a whole. In order to do this he must first consider the various elements of the picture one at a time. In the normal person this systematic *review* of the picture is carried out very rapidly and is followed immediately by the *simultaneous integration of significant details into a single whole*. The picture is beheld in a single act of meaningful perception. It is obvious that this complex act of recognition is vulnerable to disruption by the disturbances of brain activity described above.

With a disturbance of visual recognition the patient is able to perceive individual details in a picture, but his perceptual field is incapable of accommodating them all at once. In the severest cases the impairment of the unifying function of perception may be so great that the patient is unable to perceive more than one object at a time. In other case the perceptual field is not so constricted, but there is a constriction of the inner "*mental field*", so that the patient is unable to accommodate several details into a single inner schema, i.e., he is unable to combine several cues into a simultaneous whole.[4]

Phenomena similar to these may be observed with depression of the general level of brain activity in association with frontal lesions or with the general cerebral disorders mentioned above. In such cases, however, the structure of the disturbances is considerably different. Here the process of active inspection is lost. The patient's gaze moves passively and randomly from one part of the picture to another. There is no attempt to correlate various details and the interpretation of the whole picture may be based upon a single striking or randomly perceived detail. The inertness of the mental processes underlying such a perceptual defect is emphasized by the fact that once a set has been established the patient will frequently insist that it is correct. He may refuse to turn his attention to other details or he may interprete all other details in terms of the one first perceived. With primary recognition defects there is disruption of the operation whereby details are integrated to form a single pattern. Here, however, a general dynamic disturbance precludes any form of intelligent activity or active perception.

The identification of these types of recognition disorders may greatly facilitate the interpretation of speech disorders arising as a result of focal brain damage. It permits one to evaluate the preservation of general perceptual processes and the degree of mental activity open to the patient. In this way it helps in the evaluation of the patient's speech which may reflect an inabiliy to perform simultaneous synthesis or a disruption of the general dynamics of mental processes.

2. THE INVESTIGATION OF SPATIAL INTEGRATION

Evaluation of the patient's ability to recognize spatial relationships is as important as the evaluation of other forms of recognition. Orientation in space involves more than visual functions. The ability to recognize the positions of objects in space and their spatial relationships to one another as well as the ability to tell up from down and right from left involves more than visual perception. These functions require the integration, or synthesis, of visual information with information from the vestibular, somesthetic, and kinesthetic systems.

The vestibular system is the primary sensory apparatus concerned with spatial

[4] Cf. A. R. Luria, "The two forms of Synthetic activity of the Human Cortex". In: A. R. Luria, *Human Brain and Psychological Processes* (N.Y., Harper and Row, 1966).

orientation; the somesthetic and kinesthetic sensory modes are essential for the precise manipulation of objects. Spatial orientation is organized in terms of a set of symbolic coordinates, *viz.*, right-left, up-down, before-behind, which develop on the basis of practical experience and language. The integration of inputs whereby spatial orientation is established requires that the parieto-occipital area and in particular, the tertiary zones of the inferior parietal gyrus be intact. The investigation of spatial integrative functions is often of crucial significance in diagnosing generalized disorders of reading, writing, computation, and the semantic aspect of speech.

The investigation of processes involved in spatial integration includes the following tests:

a. *Orientation of the Patient in Space*

The patient is observed as he proceeds to and from his bed, makes his bed, puts on his robe, etc. It is important also to determine whether or not he had difficulty orienting himself in familiar places or in distinguishing right from left before injury.

b. *Reproduction of Geometrical Figures*

The elements of these figures have a specific spatial orientation (Figure 47). The patient may draw the figures, reproduce them with match sticks, or position figures drawn by the experimenter. These tests involve both gnosis and praxis and will be considered in greater detail below.

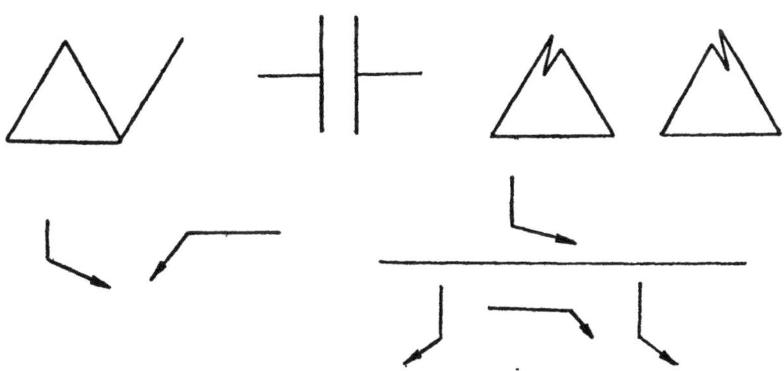

FIG. 47. Figures used in the investigation of spatial orientation.

c. *Mental Reorientation of Geometrical Figures in Space*

The patient is asked to reverse the position of a geometrical figure about a given axis (Figure 48). Also included in this group are Head's well-known tests in which the patient must reproduce the hand positions of a person facing him; he must mentally reverse the positions so as to produce a mirror image of the positions as he perceives them (Figure 49).

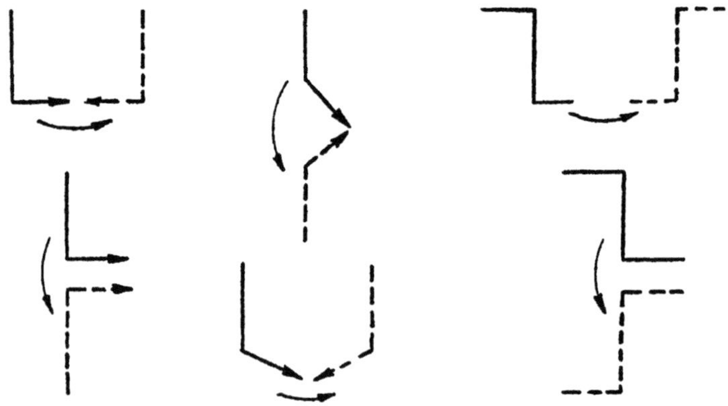

FIG. 48. Task requiring mental reversal of spatial relations.

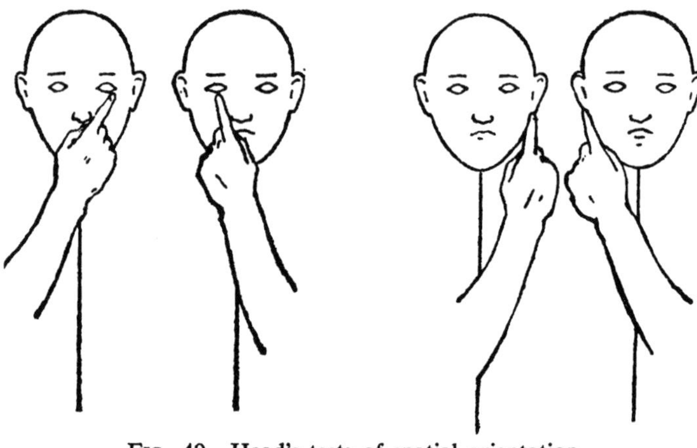

FIG. 49. Head's tests of spatial orientation.

d. *Diagramming Spatial Relationships*

The patient is asked to draw a rough map of the world or of a region which he knows well, a floor diagram of the hospital ward, a floor plan showing how to go from one ward to another, etc.

e. *Differentiation of Symbolically Represented Spatial Relationships*

This includes testing the patient's ability to identify his right and left hand and the right and left hand of a person facing him. It also involves testing his ability to point to fingers of his own hand as they are named by the experimenter, to name his own fingers (so-called "finger recognition"), and to identify Roman numerals which differ only in the spatial orientation of their elements (IX and XI, IV and VI).

The tests just enumerated permit one to describe some typical disturbances which are of value in localizing the site of brain damage. Neither general cerebral depression nor focal lesions lying outside the occipito-parietal area usually give rise to disturbances of these functions. Lesions in the inferior parts of the parietal area and marginal occipital zones may produce a clear-cut disorder of spatial orientation and impair the recognition of spatial relationships with no detectable impairment of primary visual recognition. In severe cases the signs of this disturbance are obvious. The patient confuses directions, steps to the right when he should stept to the left, and is unable to tell his right hand from his left. In less severe cases the disturbance can be demonstrated only by special tests. Although the patient may copy simple figures with no difficulty, he makes gross errors in reproducing figures with a specific spatial orientation; his reproduction may reverse the orientation of the object presented. In another type of test he may select the wrong figure as being identical to the one presented.

Even more difficult for such a patient is the task of mentally reversing the positions of spatial maps. Since he is unable to orient a figure of the type shown in Figure 48 to an *inner schema* he either produces an exact copy or gives up completely. He is unable to draw a rough map or to comprehend a diagram involving spatial relationships. In attempting to draw a map he may reverse the positions of east and west: E$\overset{N}{\underset{S}{+}}$W. He is unable to locate landmarks familiar to him and easily gives up trying to draw a floor plan of his ward. Sometimes the verbal schemata of spatial coordinates are retained and dissociated from the disturbed visuo-spatial schemata. For instance, when one patient, who had been a surveyor, was asked to draw a map of European Russia he began, saying, "Yes, I know that East is to the right and West to the left". On this basis he drew the points of the compass correctly. But then he reversed the positions of the Black Sea and the Caspian Sea. Saying, "The Volga flows into the Caspian Sea", he drew the Volga as running to the Caspian Sea, but in direction opposite to the correct one.

Usually such a patient is unable to name his fingers or to identify them as the examiner names them ("finger agnosia"). He is unable to differentiate between Roman or Arabic numerals composed of identical elements in different order (IV and VI, 67 and 76, etc.). He also makes characteristic errors in reading and writing.

All of these signs taken together are known clinically as the "parietal syndrome" and have recently been studied in detail by A. Ja. Kolodnaja. They are very important for the understanding of aphasic syndromes. By removing essential prerequisites for the appreciation of spatial organization, such disturbances inevitably produce a loss of complex mnestic and intellectual processes, for these processes are impossible in the absence of the ability to differentiate and remember *directions*.

Figure 50 shows an example of the loss of spatial orientation which resulted from a lesion of the parietal area.

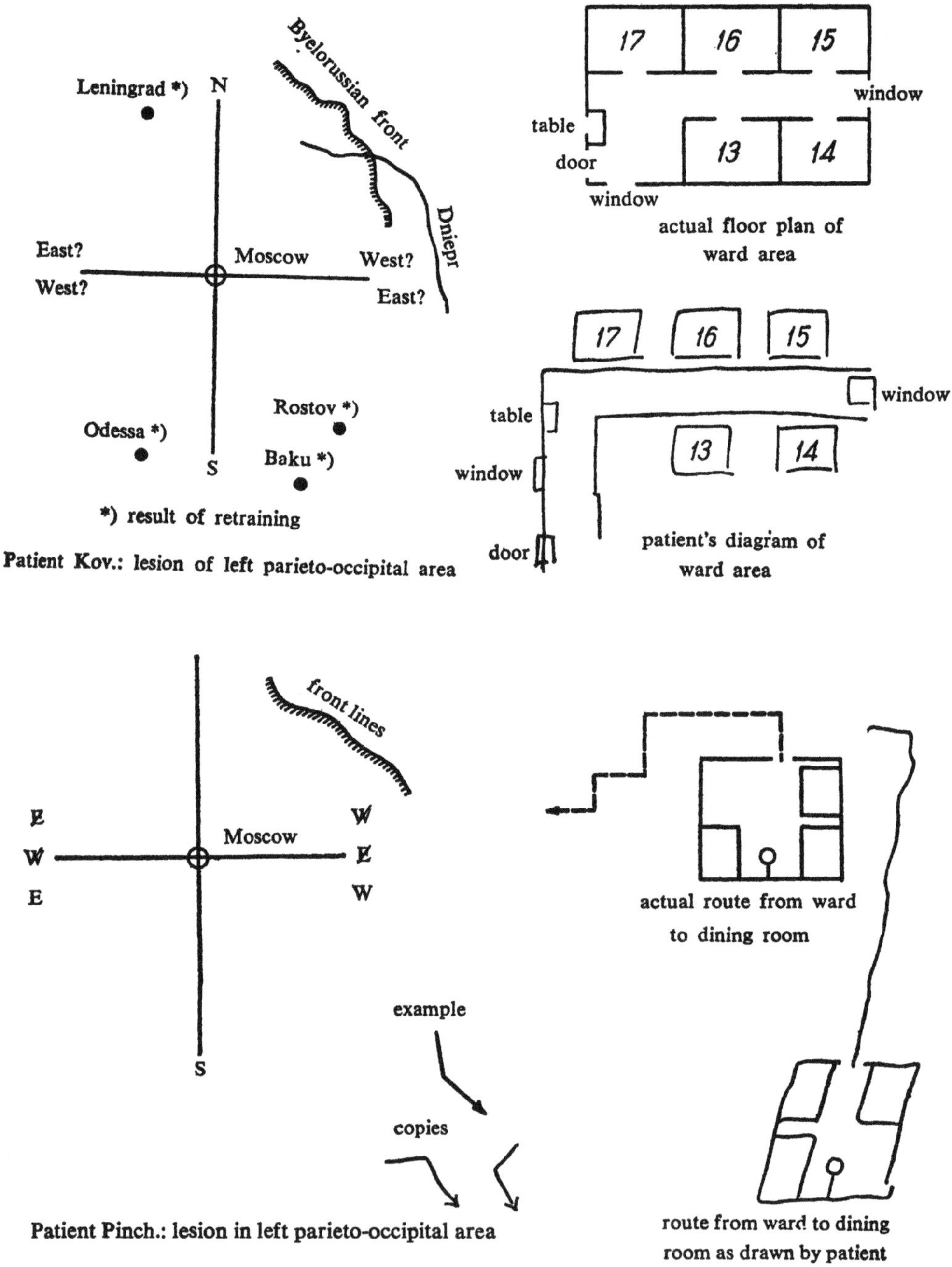

Patient Kov.: lesion of left parieto-occipital area

Patient Pinch.: lesion in left parieto-occipital area

FIG. 50. Illustrations of loss of spatial orientation in a patient with damage to the parietal systems.

3. *The Investigation of Sequential Integration*

Whereas the investigation of object recognition and spatial orientation has long been a part of the clinical examination, the investigation of sequential integration was, until recently, a completely untouched area. The investigation of this aspect of cerebral function, however, is extremely important.

The cerebral cortex performs not only simultaneous (spatial) synthesis, but also sequential (temporal) synthesis. A series of excitations is integrated into a single sequential system; the pattern of such a temporal sequence serves as a starting point for the subsequent development of "kinetic melodies." The investigation of a patient's ability to recognize and recall sequential patterns is thus a no less important part of the functional investigation of cerebral activity then the investigation of spatial orientation. The significance of this investigation for the localization of brain lesions has been increased by the observation that sequential integration is accomplished by a completely different system of cerebral zones than that responsible for spatial integration. This was demonstrated by Lashley (1937) and later in our own laboratory.[5] The cortical areas primarily involved in this form of integration are not located in the parietal and occipital lobes, but in the temporal and fronto-temporal areas.

The most convenient clinical method for investigating sequential integration is a series of tests involving the *perception, retention, and reproduction of rhythms.*

A. The examiner taps out a rhythm with his finger or a pencil. The patient listens to such a rhythm consisting of groups of two or three beats separated by a pause (// // // or /// ///) and is asked to tell of how many beats the pattern is composed. For more precise investigation the rate is varied; trials with patterns of two and three beats are presented several times in random order.

B. After the first test has been carried out the patient is asked to tell the number and force of beats in a complex rhythmical pattern where some taps are accented more than others (for example: //' or /''' or '/'). After several repetitions of a given pattern the patient is asked to describe it. For example, he should say, "Two loud taps and one soft," or, "two taps and then one more."

C. No matter whether the first two tasks are performed accurately or not the patient is asked to reproduce the rhythms presented. He should attempt to imitate two beat or three beat rhythms or more complex patterns such as //''', '''/, or '/'. If these rhythms are reproduced incorrectly the examiner should note to what extent the patient is aware of his error.

Control studies have shown that normal subjects even of a relatively low cultural level are able to perform these simple tests. Only in exceptional cases do they show difficulty in evaluating or reproducing the more complex rhythms. On the other hand, patients with brain lesions may show great difficulty, the degree of which depends largely upon the site of the lesion. Lesions of the occipital (visual) areas

[5] F. M. Semernickaja, *Rhythm and its Disturbance with Various Brain Lesions* (1945, dissertation).

generally do not impair the perception or reproduction of such rhythmical patterns. Sequential integration is likewise preserved in patients with lesions in the sensorimotor area. Lesions in the parietal areas, however, may give rise to distinct and very specific disturbances. The patient usually has no difficulty in imitating a given rhythm, but he may be unable to estimate the number of beats involved, especially if the rhythm is rapid. The explanation probably lies in the fact that damage to these systems makes it difficult to carry out simultaneous integration, i.e., to consider the sequential elements simultaneously. As a result it is impossible to count the elements of which the pattern is composed (F. M. Semernickaja).

Impaired perception of sequential rhythmical patterns may, on the other hand, result from certain neurodynamic disturbances which give rise to perseveration. These disturbances emerge most clearly with frontal lesions. The patient appears unable to suppress the sequential pattern which results from hearing a given rhythm. In other words, he shows "sensory perseveration". He may estimate groups of two to be composed of three beats and groups of three to be composed of four. This over-estimation is seen most clearly if one of the taps is made stronger, or if the tapping is done more rapidly. The inertia of neurodynamic processes is often generalized to affect the motor sphere also. The patient may tap out the rhythm // // // as /// /// /// without recognizing his error.

The most important disturbances of sequential integration are the *primary* disturbances which arise as a result of lesions in the temporal areas. In these cases the patient can neither perceive nor imitate rhythmical patterns. His interpretation of sequential patterns is chaotic, and he is unable to remember them. Having repeated a given rhythm once, he immediately loses it and begins to tap at random. The presentation of a complex rhythmic pattern involving accentuation of certain elements complicates the problem even more so that the patient perceives no rhythm at all. Here, as in certain other cases, the acoustical structure may be recognized if speech mechanisms are invoked so as to raise the task to a higher functional level.[6] Figure 51 illustrates a disturbance of sequential integration which resulted from a lesion in the temporal area.[7]

Investigation of the impairment of sequential integration does more than indicate possible sites of brain damage. It also provides information regarding the ability to recognize, store, and reproduce the types of sequential patterns characteristic of human speech, the highest and most complex form of sequentially organized function of the brain. By considering the speech defects which involve or result from

[6] The role of speech in organizing elementary sensorimotor processes is not dealt with in this volume, but it has been considered in detail elsewhere. See *Problems of Higher Nervous Activity of the Normal and Abnormal Child*, Vol. II (Moscow, 1958); chapters by O. K. Tixomirov and E. D. Homskaja.

[7] It appears that the most clear-cut impairment of sequential integration occurs with lesions in the *anterior parts of the temporal area*. This impression is supported by the observation of amusia in such cases.

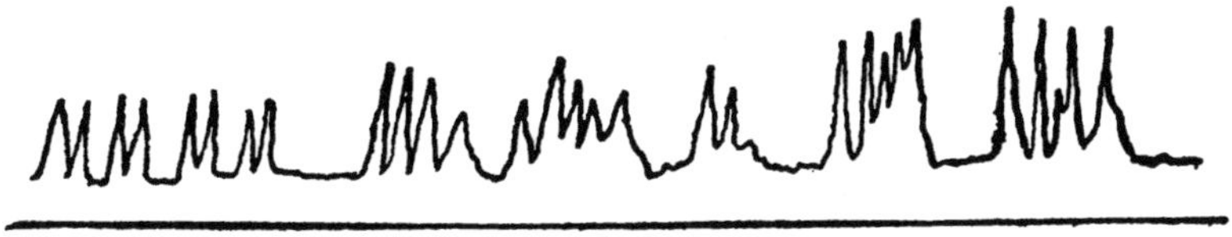

Rhythm // // // Rhythm /// /// /// "I can't follow it . . ."

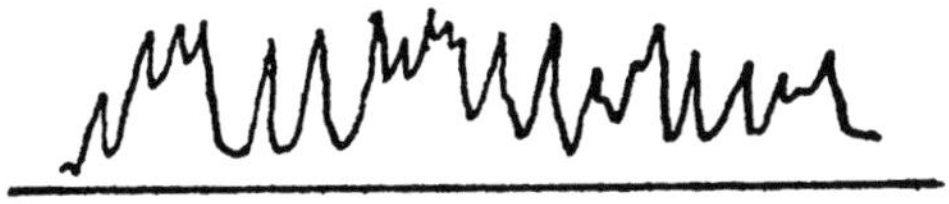

Rhythm // /// "I can't, I don't know how . . ."

Patient Osip.: lesion in left tempero-parietal area.

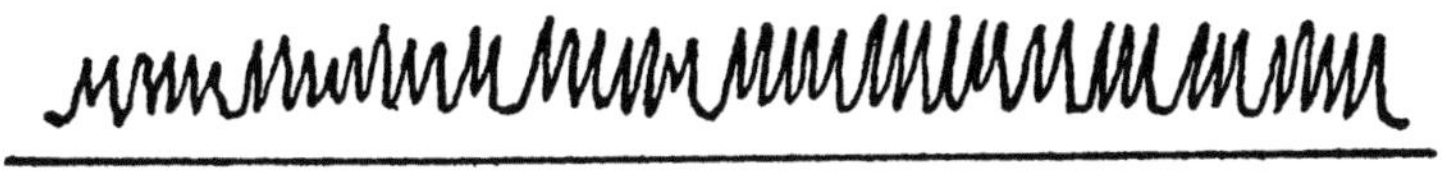

Rhythm /// /// /// "I can't break out of it . . ."

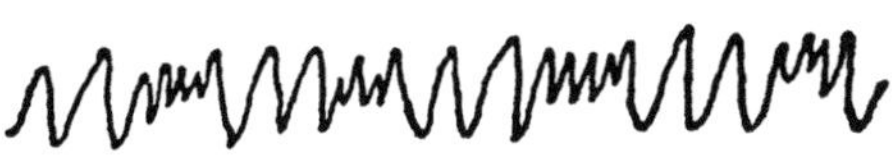

Rhythm // /// "It won't stop . . ."

Patient Burs.: lesion in the left temporal area.

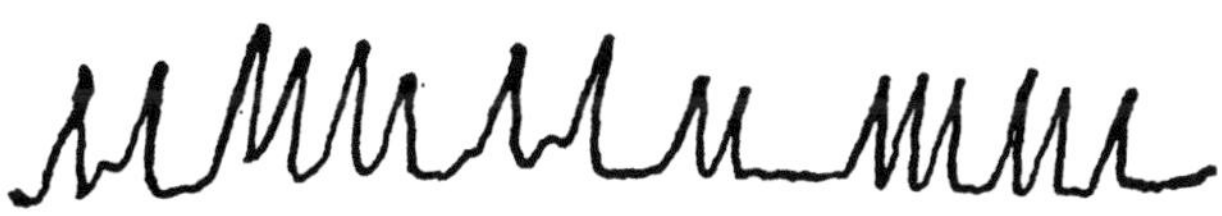

Rhythm // // // (gives up)

Patient Samorod.: lesion in left fronto-temporal area.

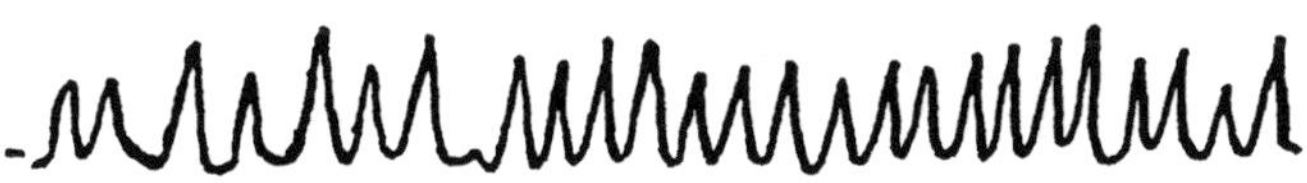

Rhythm // // // (gives up)

Patient Porc.: lesion in left fronto-temporal area.

FIG. 51. Production of rhythms with loss of sequential syntheses.

the impairment of sequential organization, we shall be able to further evaluate the significance which the investigation of this aspect of brain activity has for understanding the cortical mechanisms of different aphasic syndromes.

B. THE INVESTIGATION OF MOTOR ACTIONS

The foregoing description of afferent integrative processes brings us directly to the investigation of the organization of *motor processes* which are evoked and conditioned by afferent influences. We shall omit from this discussion the partial forms of apraxia which occasionally masquerade as primary speech disorders. We shall discuss how one assesses the *spatial organization of movements* at different levels and the *dynamic organization of movements* which is associated with the efferent parts of the brain.

1. *Investigation of the Afferent Organization of Movements*

As was shown by Liepmann, and later by N. A. Bernstein, disturbance of the integration of afferent impulses always affects motor processes, i.e., invariably produces corresponding apraxic symptoms. Since afferent integration may be disturbed at different levels, it is possible to distinguish three basic types of afferent motor disorder: *spatial apraxia proper, apraxia of pose,* and *object-symbolic apraxia.* The first two types correspond to disturbance of the schemata of the environmental space and of the body image respectively; the third results from impairment of a higher level of afferent integration which prevents the formulation of intentions for appropriate movements.

All three forms of apraxia usually arise as a result of lesions in posterior parts of the cortex. Disturbances of the spatial organization of movements arise most commonly with lesions of the occipito-parietal systems and correspond to the role played by the visual system in the development of schemata representing the outside world. Apraxia of pose is more often seen with lesions involving the post-central areas and is sometimes associated with a disturbance of kinesthetic schemata. It is difficult to localize precisely the lesions which give rise to symbolic apraxias. It should be noted, however, that symbolic apraxias are seen most frequently with complex lesions accompanied by speech disturbances and general impairment of the organization of behavior.

Investigation of the *spatial organization of movement* begins with the tests described above which are designed to evaluate the ability to integrate spatial cues. To these are added tests which assess the ability to imitate movements within a given system of spatial coordinates. These include several tests of the ability to reproduce hand positions. If paresis prevents the patient from using his right hand he may use his left. Imitating the examiner he places his hand first in a horizontal plane, then in a frontal plane, and finally in a sagittal plane (Figure 52). With damage to the spatial (parieto-occipital) systems these tasks become difficult and the patient tends to confuse frontal and sagittal, or horizontal and frontal hand positions. Apraxic disorders of this type arise most often as a result of lesions in the left (dominant) hemisphere and affect both the contralateral and ipsilateral hands. If the right hand is not weak, the best method of investigation is the bimanual test. The two hands are placed in different positions relative to one another, i.e., in different spatial planes (Figure 53). The disturbance of spatial orientation is revealed when the patient is unable to find the appropriate positions immediately.

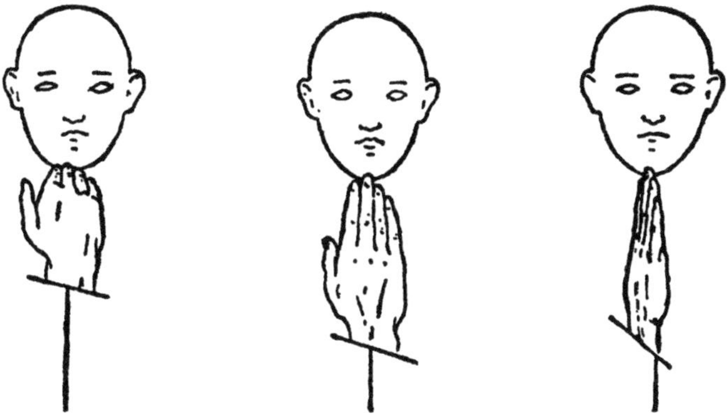

FIG. 52. Single-handed tests for disturbance of the spatial organization of movements.

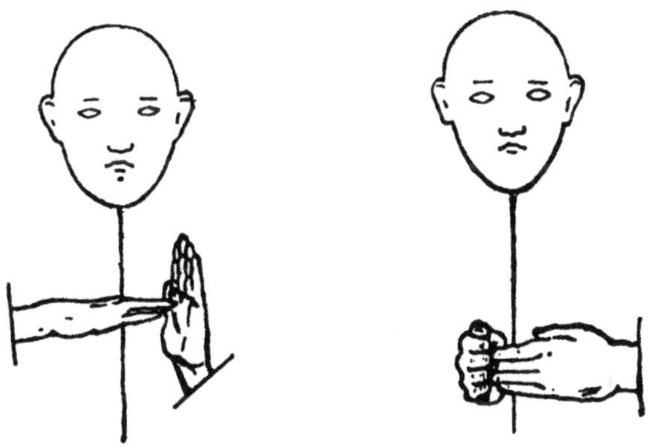

FIG. 53. Bimanual tests for disturbance of the spatial organization of movements.

The great difficulty in performing the bimanual tasks lies in recognizing the *simultaneous relationship* of the two hands. This may be associated with constriction of the perceptual field which frequently occurs with damage to the areas involved in visual recognition. Disturbances of the spatial organization of movements are not associated with impairment of the phasic aspect of speech, but they may be related to semantic aphasic defects. They may enter into a syndrome involving semantic aphasia, acalculia, reading disorders, and, sometimes, writing defects.

Other techniques of investigation are required for evaluating an *apraxia of pose*. One has the patient reproduce different hand positions which can only be done if he can integrate proprioceptive impulses in terms of an inner schema of the body or "body-image". Only in terms of this schema is it possible to carry out the precise channelling of impulses necessary to produce the required positions. These tests involve extension of the fingers in various patterns, e.g., extension of the second and third or second and fifth fingers (Figure 54), or apposition of two fingers to form a ring. In a severe case the patient with an apraxia of pose is totally unable to place his fingers in such positions. With a milder, more subtle disturbance the patient may be able to find the correct position, but he requires several attempts to do so. In testing for postural apraxia, one should consider primarily the ease with which the patient is able to find the appropriate innervational schemata, and not whether or not the hand as a whole is oriented correctly in space, e.g., in a supine position instead of a prone position. The latter is a symptom of spatial apraxia. As a rule unilateral lesions produce bilateral postural apraxias, though, to be sure, the disturbance is more apparent in the contralateral hand. As with spatial apraxia, the symptoms are most striking when the lesion involves the left, or dominant, hemisphere. The significance of postural apraxia for the origin of speech disturbances consists in the fact that it is sometimes associated with an apraxia of the speech apparatus and thus can give some indication as to the factors underlying some cases of afferent motor aphasia.

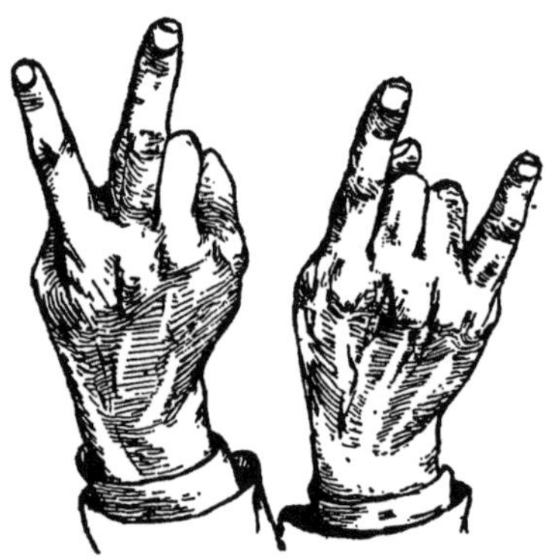

FIG. 54. Tests for positional apraxia.

The foregoing tests have dealt with the patient's ability to organize a series of motor acts by imitating the examiner. In the investigation of *object-symbolic apraxia* one studies the patient's ability to formulate a pattern of actions necessary for the intelligent use of objects or for the performance of symbolic activities. The patient does not receive an example of the movements he is to carry out. He must adapt himself to an actual situation, e.g., button a jacket, strike a match, or, more importantly, carry out an action appropriate to an imaginary situation. In order to test the latter function he is asked to show by means of a *descriptive gesture* or pantomine, how one does such things as rolling a cigarette or hammering a nail. Similarly he may be asked to demonstrate *meaningful gestures* such as waving his finger threateningly or crooking a finger as though he were beckoning to someone.

The difficulty in these cases lies in formulating an imaginary plan and submitting one's actions to the conditions it imposes. The task is impossible if one is unable to find the appropriate schemate for using objects or executing symbolic acts. Object-symbolic apraxias resulting from brain lesions have not been studied sufficiently. It appears, however, that they may assume various forms depending upon what component is lost. It has been observed that disturbances of symbolic gesture may result from the impairment of at least three different factors. In some cases the ability to handle objects is not affected, but the patient is unable to reach the level of "abstract" behavior and to carry through the actions appropriate to an imagined situation. Classical examples of this type of disturbance are found in cases of generalized brain damage or lesions of the frontal systems. In other cases, patients have no difficulty in detaching themselves from the immediate situation, but they lack the processes necessary for working with or imitating the use of external objects; they lack the precise motor schemata which are necessary for conscious and voluntary actions. Patients of this type can show how to carry out a certain acton only by outlining in a general way the different movements involved. They cannot find the positions necessary for demonstrating movements. In the third type of case, gestures demonstrating how one uses objects are retained, but the patient loses the ability to produce the symbolic gestures which express subjective relationships and emotional states. For instance, he is unable to beckon, to wave his finger threateningly, or to shake his head to express negation.[8] The loss of such symbolic gestures usually occurs in association with aphasic disturbances, and it may be that with more careful analysis it will be found that in some cases the nominative aspect of gestures is lost, while in others, only the predicative aspect is disturbed. A comparative semantic analysis of apraxic and aphasic disturbances must be carried out if we are fully to understand the brain mechanisms of these disorders.

It is true that spatial apraxia or apraxia of pose may prevent the successful fulfillment of these latter tasks. If spatial apraxia is involved, the patient may place his fingers in the correct position for a threatening or beckoning gesture, but the movement of his arm in space may be inappropriate. On the other hand, if apraxia of pose is present, he may be unable to place his fingers in the position appropriate to either gesture.

[8] Investigations by A. V. Zaporožec, 1959, concerning the origin and pathology of "inner patterns" have contributed much toward an understanding of these disturbances.

Having considered the motor disorders which result from the disturbance of afferent integrative processes we come to the last group of disorders, *viz.*, disturbances of *movements of the speech apparatus.* These disorders have special significance for the study of aphasia. The impairment of movement of the speech apparatus is frequently referred to as impairment of "oral praxis." In some cases it occurs in association with an apraxia of pose and a general symbolic apraxia; in others it occurs independently. Apparently, oral apraxias are explained by the fact that one can produce the correct combination of lip, tongue, and oropharyngeal positions only if the appropriate kinesthetic schemata are intact. If such schemata are absent, there is a kind of "postural apraxia" of the speech apparatus which can interfere with oral speech. Movements of the speech apparatus differ from movements of the extremities in that they are based upon a different system of afferent integrative processes. Oral praxis involves acoustico-gnostic schemata, and since it is part of the speech system, it is carried out at the level of complex symbolic activity. Thus a positional apraxia of the speech apparatus removes only one of the prerequisites for control of oral movements and, in some cases, does not produce a severe defect. Further, the segmental organization of the secondary motor areas suggests that in certain cases apraxia may involve the hand without affecting the schemata of oral movements.

Before testing for apraxia of the speech apparatus, the examiner should test the patient's ability to recognize the position of his tongue when it is passively moved from one position to another. The investigation of apraxia should include the following series of tests. The patient is instructed:

(1) to imitate several "postural" movements as they are demonstrated by the examiner, e.g., touch the upper lip with the tip of the tongue, place the tongue between the upper lip and the teeth, etc.;

(2) to carry out the same movements in response to verbal instructions;

(3) to reproduce meaningful symbolic acts, e.g., to produce the oral movements appropriate to spitting, kissing, whistling, clicking the tongue, etc.

A patient with no apraxia of the speech apparatus is able to carry out these instructions without difficulty. A patient with oral apraxia, on the other hand, is unable to do so. Usually this results from damage to the postcentral areas and inferior parts of the sensorimotor area. It is important to note that an apraxia of the speech apparatus does not affect the execution of "postural" movements of the lips and tongue as much as it does the execution of simple acts which are symbolic in nature but dissociated from the system of speech, e.g., spitting, kissing, etc. The patient may be able to produce such movements involuntarily in situations which are appropriate to elicit them, but he is unable to produce them voluntarily in a context where they have no practical significance. The inability to mobilize the necessary coordinative processes at this level of functional organization is very clear. This symbolic apraxia of the speech apparatus is probably very similar to afferent motor aphasia in its psycho-physiological mechanisms.

2. *Investigation of the Dynamic Organization of Movements*

Precise afferent integration is not the only prerequiste for the execution of complex movements. Another necessary process is what Professor N. A. Bernštejn refers to as "re-coding" of the spatial, simultaneous schemata of movements into the *dynamic schemata* by which the are carried out. This involves the creation of flexibe patterns of coordination and the organization of sequential kinetic schemata so that one phase easily gives way to the next to produce a smooth pattern of action through time.

An assessment of these flexible dynamic schemata is obtained by studying the ease with which elementary motor patterns are established, i.e., the ease with which individual motions may be combined to produce a smooth pattern of movement. As was pointed out above (Chapter VII, Section 2) the loss of these kinetic patterns may severely affect the execution of speech processes. Thus, it is important that they be investigated before one begins to study the retention of speech activity itself.

A disturbance of dynamic praxis may appear in the extremities either contralateral or ipsilateral to the site of the lesion. Therefore, the investigation of "dynamic apraxias" may involve both bimanual tests and tests using only one hand. It usually consists of the following series of tests: [9]

a. *Motor Test of the Ability to Reproduce Rhythms*

This test has already been described in connection with the investigation of sequential integration. It consists in the imitation of a rapid rhythm tapped out by the examiner, e.g., *// // //, /// /// ///, // // //*, followed by reproduction of a complex rhythm such as *//‴, //‴*, or *‴// ‴//*. The patient taps with his finger or a pencil, or taps a key so that the rhythm he produces may be recorded. The examiner notes how easily the rhythm is mastered and retained, whether or not it degenerates with several repetitions, and whether or not extraneous taps are introduced. He also notes whether or not there is perseveration of one rhythm as the patient attempts to produce a second, and whether or not the patient is able to detect his errors.

b. *Test of the Ability to Shift from one Motor Pattern to Another*

This test consists of a series of changes in hand position. The most commonly used sequences are as follows:

(1) In the "fist-palm-side test" (Figure 55) the patient strikes the table top three times, first with his fist, then with his open palm, and then with the side of his hand. (For some patients, the sequence "fist-side-palm" may be more difficult to produce then the sequence "fist-palm-side").

[9] A detailed description of these tests is given by E. G. Škol'nik-Jarros, in: A. R. Luria and E. D. Homskaja (eds.), *Frontal Lobes and the Regulation of Psychological Processes* (Moscow, University Press, 1966 [Russian]).

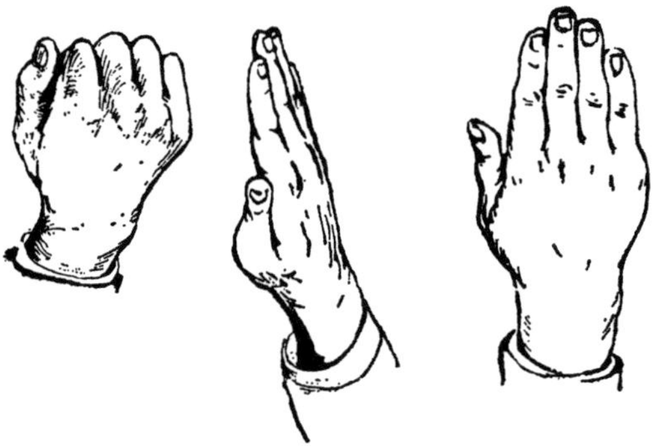

FIG. 55. Test of successive shifts in hand position.

(2) In the *"fist-ring test"* the patient is instructed to extend his arm several times, first with his hand in a fist then with thumb and forefinger apposed to form a ring. With successive extensions of the arm he alternates between these two positions (Figure 56).

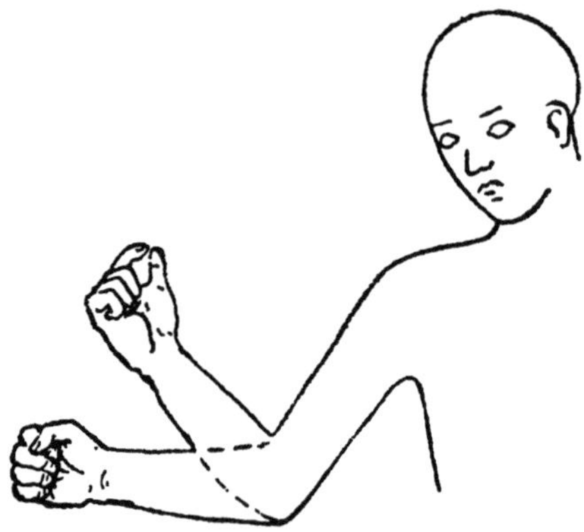

FIG. 56. Test of coordinated reversal of movements ("fist . . . ring").

(3) *Graphical tests of alternation,* the patient draws a figure composed of two alternating components (Figure 57). So far as possible he should not remove his pencil from the paper. This test may be carried out with the eyes either open or closed.

(4) *Test of reciprocal coordination.* This is a bimanual test first described by N. I. Ozereckij. The patient places both hands on the table, one in a fist, the other palm down. Then he is instructed to rapidly alternate the positions of the two hands (Figure 58).

(5) *Test of the ability to shift patterns of finger movements.* The patient is instructed to place his hand on the table as though he were playing a piano. He taps the table with two fingers at a time as though he were playing two chords in alternation, do-mi and do-so, i.e., alternating between fingers 1-and-2 and 1-and-5. For a more sensitive test, the examiner may instruct him to do this first silently and then with verbal self-instruction: "first and second, first and fifth, first and second . . ."

In all of these tests the examiner observes the ease with which a given movement is established and notes any lack of smoothness, disturbance of coordination of the individual motor components and any difficulty in the denervation of movements once they are established. Denervation difficulties may make it impossible to shift smoothly from one movement to another and manifest themselves in the perseveration of established motor patterns.

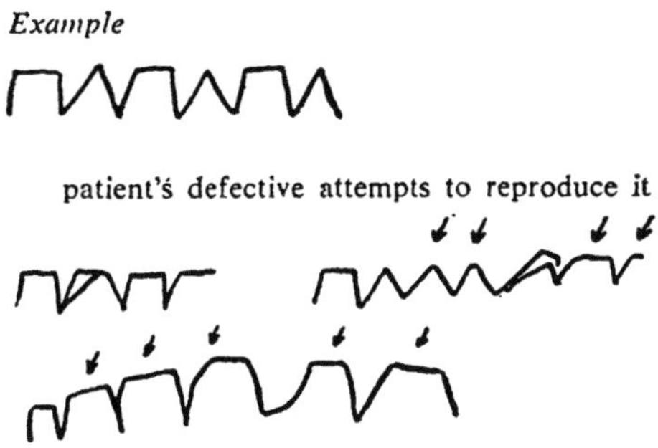

FIG. 57. Pencil test of alternation.

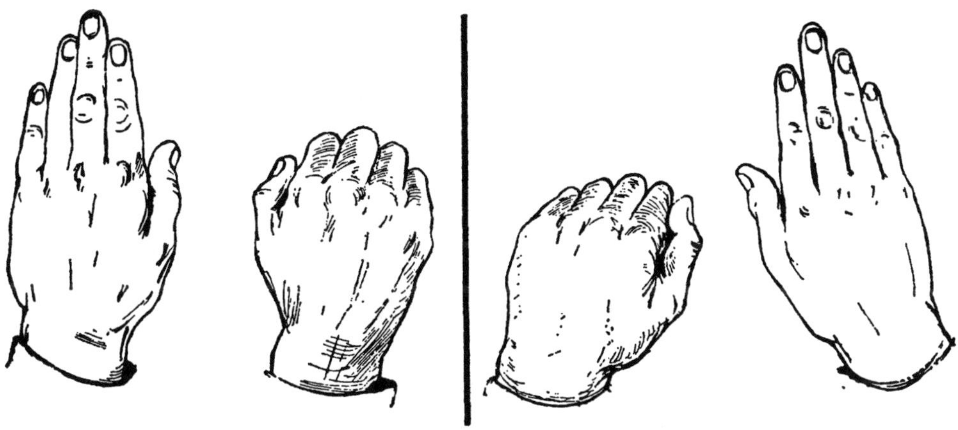

FIG. 58. Test of reciprocal coordination.

Normal subjects show no difficulty in mastering these types of movements; after one or two attempts they are able to carry out any of the tasks described easily and smoothly. The tests are equally easy for patients with lesions in the posterior afferent parts of the cerebral cortex. Because of the impairment of afferent integrative processes such patients may have difficulty in placing their hands in given positions; their coordination, however, is usually not affected.[10]

[10] G. I. Poljakov has described this type of disturbance in a special unpublished study of the reciprocal coordination test. He has pointed out that with kinesthetic disorders one may observe a tendency for reciprocal movements to be replaced by identical movements of the two hands, whereas with lesions of the premotor systems there is simply a loss of synchrony in the execution so that the hands move to reciprocal positions but not simultaneously.

An entirely different picture is seen with lesions in the anterior parts of the cerebral cortex, particularly with lesions involving the premotor areas. As was pointed out above (Chapter 7, Section 3) a patient with a premotor area lesion has no particular difficulty in placing his hand in a desired position, but he is unable to master new motor habits. He understands perfectly well the movement to be carried out, but he cannot excute it smoothly. Here there is a loss of generalized dynamic schemata, so that a special impulse is required for the execution of each link in a chain of movements. The overall motor pattern loses its normal smoothness. Motor perseveration emerges with great clarity signifying impairment of the ability to denervate movements once they have been established.

In the rhythm tests there is a deautomatization of the kinetic pattern; sometimes superfluous beats are introduced which the patient recognizes as erroneous, but which he is unable to inhibit. In the reciprocal coordination tests one hand may not function at all. Each component of a complex act, for instance, the formation of the fist or ring, is executed independently. One of the components may drop out altogether. Sometimes a movement established in a previous task may perseverate so that the whole pattern is disrupted.

These difficulties signify dynamic disturbances the effects of which are seldom limited to the motor sphere. In cases involving the dominant hemisphere, speech activity is often affected also. Thus, the discovery of a disorder in the dynamic organization of cortical processes is of immense significance in the investigation of aphasia.[11]

The series of tests described above permits one to obtain a rather clear impression of the types of functional disturbances present even before one investigates the speech processes themselves. It provides a background against which one may assess disturbances of speech *per se*. As a rule, the analysis of speech activity involves the evaluation of *expressive speech, hearing and speech comprehension*, and *written speech* (reading and writing). Also important in the diagnosis of aphasic disturbances is the investigation of *computation processes*. We shall consider the symptomatology and analysis of the disorders in this order.

[11] We analysed these data in details elsewhere. Cf. A. R. Luria, *Higher Cortical Functions in Man* (New York, Basic Books, 1966) and *Human Brain and Psychological Processes* (New York, Harper and Row, 1966).

XI

THE INVESTIGATION OF SPEECH PROCESSES: EXPRESSIVE SPEECH

A. PRELIMINARY EVALUATION OF SPONTANEOUS SPEECH

The investigation of speech processes usually begins with an evaluation of the patient's *spontaneous speech*. This in itself contributes greatly to the understanding of his underlying speech difficulties. The patient is asked to relate the events surrounding some episode which is familiar to him, for instance, the circumstances under which he was injured, or the types of things he does when he is at home. The examiner carefully records his responses. Patients with occipital and parieto-occipital lesions rarely show any marked disturbance of this form of speech activity. If they have an amnesic aphasia, they may have some minor difficulty in finding words. Thus their narrative speech may not be altogether smooth. In general, however, their spontaneous speech is well preserved. On the other hand, patients with *motor and premotor aphasic* disturbances usually show significant signs of difficulty with connected speech. In severe cases speech is altogether absent; in less severe cases or in the residual stages of recovery such patients may speak brokenly. They appear to have to expend a special effort with the utterance of every word. In severe cases of motor aphasia the impairment of spontaneous speech is obvious. Characteristically, the loss of the dynamic schemata of sentences renders the speech agrammatical. The predicative functions of speech suffers greatly, so that patients are often left with only individual substantives, or "designative" words. All of the dynamic elements of sentences, e.g., predicates, connectives, etc., are omitted. Patients show the type of speech disturbance which is frequently referred to in the literature by the term "telegraph style". The nominative character of such speech persists into the late residual phases. The patients have a tendency to begin sentences with nouns and to omit verbs, adjectives, and connective elements such as prepositions and conjunctions. Characteristically their speech loses its intonational features and becomes fragmentary, monotonous, and inexpressive.

In the residual stages of motor aphasia and, also, in the "dynamic" forms of frontal aphasia, the phasic and grammatical aspects of speech may show no detectable disturbance; but still the speech becomes passive and inert. In these cases connected speech may be limited to the use of familiar expressions and, in dialogue, the imitation of the grammatical structure of concrete questions. One never hears the spontaneous utterance of statements formulated in complex grammatical terms. Characteristically, the relation between intention and speech is defective. The patients show great difficulty in expressing thoughts and in choosing the words to use in spontaneous speech. They have no difficulty, however, in naming objects. The processes involved in pronunciation and in the utterance of structured phrases are not as severely affected as is the active formulation of thoughts in verbal form. This is the impairment of verbal thought which was described in such great detail by Hughlings Jackson.

Patients with signs of "afferent motor aphasia" have difficulty in pronouncing speech sound and, thus, are unable to produce any form of complex spontaneous speech. In the residual stages of recovery, however, they often regain their mastery of spontaneous speech. A typical sign of this disturbance is the expenditure of great effort in spontaneous speech as the patient turns all of his attention to the pronunciation of individual phonemes within words.

Great changes in spontaneous expressive speech are also observed in patients with lesions of the *temporal* systems. The "sensory" aphasia which arises in these cases results from a disturbance of phonemic hearing and loss of the precise auditory images of words. For such patients words have no stable structure; they lose their nominative function and, thus, their basic meaning. As a result, nouns virtually disappear from the vocabulary and spontaneous speech becomes primarily predicative in function. It consists of opening words and phrases and substitute words bound together by normal intonational patterns which give a certain psychological unity to the "sentences". The patients are able to pronounce words without detectable articulatory difficulties, but the appropriate nouns may be replaced by verbal and literal paraphasias, the meanings of which can often be guessed on the basis of intonation. Comparison of the nominative speech of the motor aphasic with the predicative speech of the sensory aphasic gives a clear picture of the differences between these two disorders. According to Jakobson's interpretation (1956) the first involves disturbance of *context,* whereas the latter involves loss of the lexical *code* of the language.

Patient Cap.
(lesion in the anterior part of the speech area; motor aphasia)

Patient's account of his injury

"Oh ... the front ... a German ... go ... mouth ... attack ... then ... head ... well ... wounded ... hand, leg ... well ... ugh ... o-pe-ra-tion ... talking ... nothing! ..."

Patient Af.
(lesion in the left temporal area; sensory aphasia)

Patient's account of his injury

"I just don't know anything ... well at the beginning there were a lot of them ... and well ... wham! – and then nothing ... and then all of a sudden I can see, and I see! and so (pointing at his head) – and that's what! and then again nothing ... and then little by little, just a little bit ... and now, already it's ok! ..."

B. THE INVESTIGATION OF SEQUENTIAL SPEECH

The analytic investigation of expressive speech begins with a study of common speech processes which occur automatically in the adult patient. Many years ago Hughlings Jackson pointed out that impairment of the active symbolic aspect of speech is not always associated with disturbance of the ability to pronounce words and that, in some cases, the lower levels of speech may be preserved. In such a case the patient is unable to formulate propositions, but he is sometimes able to name objects or repeat words; he may retain a few familiar speech expressions. He is able to utter spontaneous exclamations and to tell what his name is; he may even be able to run through certain speech sequences which have become automatic for him. Any speech pattern which might be used for the expression of a thought is impossible, but speech processes which are not a part of this system, i.e., those which involve simple verbo-motor habits or which express affective states, may be retained. Of course these forms of verbal activity do not constitute speech in the true sense of the word.

The extent to which elementary verbal habits are preserved may be demonstrated by an investigation of habitual expressions which do not involve verbal thought mechanisms. Such an investigation usually consists of a few very simple tests.

A. The patient is asked to recite a familiar *number sequence,* e.g., 1, 2, 3, 4, etc., or *some other automatic sequence* such as months of the year or days of the week. During the course of these tests, the examiner notes not so much the clarity of pronunciation as the degree of preservation of the sequence itself.

B. The patient is asked to *recite the same sequences, but in reverse order.* If he is unable to do so, he is asked "control" questions in order to determine to what extent the difficulty lies in a disturbance of the logical schemata of sequential structure and to what extent it is due to primary inability to remember the original sequence. If, for instance, the patient has difficulty in naming the months backwards the following questions will reveal any impairment of directional orientation: "What comes after summer? Spring, Fall, or Winter?" "What comes before summer?", etc. Difficulty in answering these questions indicates that the difficulty is cognitive in nature. Whereas the first test permits one to evaluate the patient's ability to carry out elementary speech processes, the second test permits evaluation of the ability to go beyond such elementary processes. In order to fulfill this test the patient must be able to handle the sequence at a more voluntary level and to manipulate it consciously in a form which is of practical significance. This is the form which he was able to use such information before he was injured.

It is customarily assumed that brain lesions which disturb higher levels of speech activity do not affect familiar automatic sequences. This is only partially true, however. It is true that when a lesion disturbs the higher level processes of perceptual integration, complex intelligent speech becomes impossible for patients in whom familiar and habitual expressions may still be preserved. Everything that a patient with such a lesion does is based upon well ingrained speech patterns. Thus, if there is severe derangement of the acoustico-gnostic systems and inability to maintain the constancy of word meanings, or if there is a disruption of inner simultaneous speech schemata, the simple verbo-motor ability to recite sequences of numbers or months usually remains intact. But even this more elementary process is disturbed if the patient is required to deal with the sequence in a more conscious way, i.e., if he must analyze the sequence rather than simply rely on the verbo-motor pattern which he mastered previous to his injury. If, for instance, he is asked to begin counting at some place other than the beginning he often loses the correct order of numbers, omits numbers, or returns to the beginning. He is unable to work with the sequence at a higher level. In some cases, especially those involving lesions in the posterior cortical areas, the dissociation of automatic verbal habits and consciously directed speech functions may be so great that the patient is unable to name a given number, month, or day of the week except by reciting the entire sequence in which it is embedded. In these cases the execution of automatic verbal habits offers the only means of compensating for the defective active speech processes.

An entirely different picture is seen in cases involving lesions of the anterior parts of the cortex, i.e., the areas associated with the integration of dynamic processes. Damage to the anterior portions of the speech zones renders the utterance of familiar sequences extremely difficult.

It is understandable that any form of motor aphasia (including the afferent form) should create great difficulty in the utterance of familiar sequences simply because of the defective articulation. With lesions in the premotor systems, in particular with those giving rise to efferent motor aphasia, there is also a loss of "kinetic melodies", i.e., of motor patterns. The persistence of set arises, blocks the shift from one articulatory pattern to another, and thus prevents the smooth recitation of familiar sequences. Frontal lesions which produce a loss of higher level dynamic integration also disturb the reproduction of familiar sequences in another way. The intentions which guide the utterance of long sequences are disturbed. The patient repeats the instruction given him in an echolalic fashion; he reproduces the example given, e.g., "1, 2, 3, 4", or "1, 2, 3", and can proceed further only with further prompting and by reproducing the rhythm of the examiner's speech, e.g., "1, 2, 3 . . . 4, 5, 6 . . . 7, 8, 9 . . . 10, 11, 12 . . .", etc.

One observes more severe disturbances as one shifts from the automatic recitation of familiar sequences to conscious, voluntary utterances. This shift to a higher psychological level occurs when the patient is asked to recite a familiar sequence in reverse order. In this test he must not only recognize the logic of the sequential structure, but he must also overcome the tendency to stereotypy which is created by the automatic repetition of sequences.

When only articulatory processes are defective, as in the apraxic type of motor aphasia, reversal of the order of recitation produces no significant change in the overall picture of speech impairment. When, however, the aphasia involves a higher level of organization of speech processes, this task presents considerably greater difficulty. This is true both of perceptual and of *dynamic* disturbances. Thus almost any form of aphasia affects the ability to recite sequences in reverse order, but, as we shall see below, the effect is different depending on the type of aphasia.

In cases of efferent motor aphasia associated with defects of inner speech the primary obstacle to the recitation of sequences in reverse order lies in the loss of inner dynamic schemata. This difficulty reveals itself as a general loss of sentence structure preventing the patient from considering the sequence as a whole. For such a patient the utterance of one element in this sequence does not give rise to a series of subsequent elements but is viewed as though it were totally removed from the sequence. "For you Thursday is always followed by Friday and Wednesday always comes before Thursday", said one patient in the residual phase of recovery from a disturbance of dynamic speech, "but for me the slots before and after Thursday are completely empty, and I don't know where to go from there . . ." Because of this difficulty such a patient frequently refuses to carry out the tasks required of him. At best he makes halting attempts to recall the sequence as he knows them and then by this roundabout method, discovers the appropriate elements. In cases involving *frontal* lesions this strategy is impossible. Here patients may be able to reproduce series as they have learned them, but they are unable to get away from the original order and repeatedly recite sequences as originally learned rather then in reverse order as instructed. Occasionally, they recognize the fact that they are not responding correctly, but they are unable to correct their errors. Over and over again they fall under the influence of the original sequence.

One observes an entirely different type of difficulty in patients whose aphasia results from a primary disturbance of the auditory speech system. The disturbances of auditory integrative processes occurring with temporal lesions usually prevent the patient from being able to retain verbal sequences. Various elements drop out, their meanings become unstable, or they become totally incomprehensible. Thus, while a patient may recite a familiar verbo-motor sequence with perfect accuracy, he can neither retain nor reproduce the reverse sequence; he cannot picture to himself the sequential pattern of elements. Here one sees a patient who can only produce the reverse sequence by repeating the original sequence many times in order to recall successive elements. "Saturday . . . I can't go any further . . . Monday, Tuesday, Wednesday, Thursday, Friday, . . . ! Friday. Monday, Tuesday, Wednesday . . . Thursday ! . . . Monday, Tuesday . . . Wednesday !", etc.

In cases involving the loss of inner logico-grammatical schemata, i.e., in semantic aphasias, other causes are responsible for the inability to recite sequences in reverse order. Conscious manipulation of sequences is impossible because the patient is unable to grasp the relationships of individual elements as components of a single, simultaneous structure. Some patients are incapable of differentiating the simple categories of "before" and "after". As a result they lose their orientation in time. For them, the sequence of elements is lost altogether so that they tend to recite the elements in random order. Here, as in the previous cases, the patients may be able to use the original, automatic verbo-motor series as a means of compensating for their defect.

It is apparent that lesions of several different cerebral systems may produce an inability to consciously manipulate the elements of a familiar sequence, but this common defect has *different causes* and involves *different psychological mechanisms* in the different cases.

C. THE INVESTIGATION OF IMITATIVE (REPETITIVE) SPEECH

The foregoing series of tests dealt with the investigation of familiar verbal habits not involving the auditory aspect of speech. With the investigation of imitative (repetitive) speech the object of analysis is the auditory organization of speech.

By asking the patient to repeat a series of syllables or words we place him in a very special position. He must ignore the usual communicative aspect of speech as a means of thought expression, i.e., he must concentrate his attention not so much on the meaning of words as on their acoustical structure; he must analyze the auditory constituents of the words which he hears. Secondly he must be able to retain the sequential sound patterns, and finally, he must be able to reproduce the original pattern by his own articulatory processes. If any one of these subprocesses is disturbed he is unable to repeat the sound complexes which he hears.[1]

Although the following techniques are quite simple, they are capable of evaluating several different factors which contribute to the successful execution of complex speech processes. In order to isolate and investigate the various factors separately the investigation may be so organized that different series of tests reveal disturbances of the three components mentioned above.

The simplest investigation includes the following tests:

1. *Repetition of Individual Sounds and Syllables (Including Vowels and Consonants)*

The patient is asked to repeat after the examiner the sounds and syllables, "a, o, u, i"; "b, k, s, d, r"; "ta, na, ra, sa". The examiner notes the degree of clarity with which the patient differentiates the various sounds and the ease with which he articulates them.

In order to differentiate articulatory defects from defects of auditory discrimination patients who are unable to repeat sounds orally are asked to write them down or to identify them in a list of written sounds. It may be that such a patient can pronounce the sound if he carefully observes the tongue and lip movements of the examiner.

The ability to write or recognize the letter accurately and the inability to pronounce it except by following the examiner's articulatory movements is usually indicative of an articulatory rather than an auditory defect.

[1] Careful studies on imitation and conscious repetition of speech sounds were recently made in our laboratory by E. N. Vinarskaja ("Studies in afferent motor aphasia", in print).

2. *Repetition of Similar, (Correlative) Phonemes*

The patient repeats such pairs of syllables as "ba-pa" or "pa-ba", "da-ta" or "ta-da", "za-sa" or "sa-za". This is a more sensitive test for the preservation of auditory acuity. Again, in order to determine more precisely whether inability to fulfill this test results from a disturbance of auditory discrimination or from an articulatory defect one may ask the patient to *write down* the sounds dictated or to locate the syllable in a list of syllables. Finally, one can ask the patient whether he considers the sound sequences "b-p" and "p-b" to be the same or different. If the patient performs this control test accurately one may presume that the difficulty in repeating similar (correlative), phonemes indicates an articulatory rather than an auditory defect. Conversely, difficulty in carrying out these tests indicates a disturbance of phonemic hearing.

3. *Repetition of Series of Syllables*

By having the patient repeat series of syllables, such as "bi-ba-bo", "bo-ba-bi", or "bi-bo-ba", one can establish the extent to which he is able to retain elementary series of speech sounds which differ from one another by a single vowel. One can also assess the degree of ease with which he is able to reproduce such series and the ease with which he is able to go from one series to another, e.g., from "bi-ba-bo" to "bo-ba-bi". This test largely eliminates difficulties in the discrimination of similar phonemes and thus tests as specifically as possible the ability to retain sound sequences. In order to determine whether or not difficulty in carrying out these tests results from an inability to perceive and retain sound sequences or from an impairment of expressive speech, such as a persistence of articulatory patterns or a transition difficulty, the examiner notes the nature of the patient's errors. An inability to maintain the order of vowels, e.g., repetition of "bi-ba-bo" as "bo-bo-bo", usually indicates a defect in the denervation of established articulatory patterns. This interpretation is confirmed if, after having correctly repeated one series of syllables, e.g., "bi-ba-bo", the patient is unable to shift to another pattern, e.g., "bo-ba-bi". He may continue to repeat the first series. This type of pathological persistence of established articulatory patterns is never seen in primary disturbances of the ability to grasp or retain sound sequences.

4. *Repetition of Simple and Complex Words*

By instructing the patient to repeat such words as "cupboard", "image", "lemonade", or "general", it is possible to determine the degree to which he can pronounce complex articulatory complexes and to observe the role that meaning plays in his ability to differentiate, retain, and reproduce syllable sequences.

In order to determine whether a patient's success in this test results from the meaning of sound patterns or is independent of meaning, he is asked to repeat syllable patterns which are of equal complexity but which are less frequent, e.g., "parenthesis", "chronoskopy", or "Haurizankar". If, after several presentations, there is a great difference between his ability to pronounce real words and to pronounce such complex words, one has evidence for a defect in the organization of complex auditory processes. In this case it becomes apparent that the factor of "parenthesis" plays a considerable role in helping the patient to compensate for his auditory defect.

Of special note are patients who respond with distorted versions (literal paraphasias) of the words presented or who replace the correct words with other words, e.g., substitute the word "chicken" for the word "canary." These responses may vary in origin, but they usually indicate impairment of the precision of speech hearing and sometimes reflect a compensatory mechanism whereby imitation is based upon the meaning of the word rather than its acoustical characteristics.

5. *Repetition of Short Series of Words*

By having a patient repeat series of words such as "house-wood", "house-wood-cat", or "cat-house-wood", it is possible to determine the degree to which the ability to retain and to reproduce short series of meaningful sound patterns is preserved. Major attention is given to the question of whether or not the patient is able to retain short word sequences and to what extent he is able to reproduce words in their correct sequence. The evaluation of symptoms arising in this case is similar to that in the tests described above (Test 3).

6. *Repetition of Full Sentences*

By having the patient repeat such sentences as, "In the garden beyond the high fence there grew apple trees," or "At the edge of the wood the hunters killed a wolf," it is possible (1) to evaluate his ability to retain meaningful statements and (2) to assess the extent to which groups of words held together by meaning are more easily understood than groups of unrelated words.

In order to determine whether or not difficulties observed in this test result from a difficulty in retaining long series of words or from an inability to master and retain their grammatical structure, the patient is asked to repeat sentences which vary in degree of grammatical complexity. A long, but simple sentence would be, "Father and Mother went to the theater, but the children remained at home"; and an example of a complex sentence would be an extended construction such as, "The mountain on which the house stood was high", or a descriptive sentence such as, "One clear spring morning the singing of the birds filled the air".

Equal difficulty in repeating the two types of sentences indicates a primary defect in the ability to retain long verbal sequences; ease of pronunciation of simple grammatical sentences in a patient who has difficulty in repeating grammatically complex sentences indicates that the primary defect lies beyond the auditory sphere and is rooted in a disturbance of the grammatical organization of speech.

One seldom sees impairment of imitative speech as the sole symptom of traumatic aphasia. Usually it is associated with difficulties in spontaneous expressive speech, as though it were combined with or derived from inability to recall sound patterns. When this symptom is clearly present, one is dealing with what has classically been referred to as "conductive aphasia". It is seldom explained by a disturbance of voluntary "categorical" behavior preventing the patient from grasping the meaning of the instructions to repeat a given word. Much more often the imitative speech is associated with one of the factors which we have mentioned above. In some cases the difficulty in repeating long sequences originates in the impairment of acoustico-gnostic processes, so that the sounds lose their clarity and stability with multiple repetitions. In other cases it results from the fact that the sounds lose their sequential organization. Finally the disturbance of imitative speech may arise from an efferent defect arising from an inability to find the necessary articulatory position or to preserve the appropriate schema of words and to denervate articulatory sets once they have been established. Thus, one finds that imitative speech may be disturbed by almost any form of aphasia, though the origin and mechanisms of the disturbances observed in different cases are not always the same.

The loss of *efferent speech schemata* and difficulty in denervating established articulatory patterns are characteristic of "efferent motor aphasia". Patients with this syndrome have no difficulty in repeating individual sounds if they are allowed to do so slowly. Significant difficulties arise only when they are asked to pronounce syllables or complex sound patterns. There is a perseveration of established articulatory innervational patterns which acts as an obstacle to the articulation of subsequent sounds. Sometimes this disorder manifests itself as a type of stuttering. In mild cases one observes difficulty only in the second of the tests above, where the patient is required to read pairs of oppositional phonemes. The first syllable is pronounced with no difficulty, but it is impossible to shift smoothly to the next one. Thus "ba-pa" is pronounced as "ba-ba" or "da-ta" as "da-da". A feature of this disorder which immediately distinguishes it from a disturbance of phonemic hearing is that the patient is fully aware of his error by slowly and carefully pronouncing the syllables he may be able to correct himself. He has no difficulty in writing pairs of oppositional phonemes. The fact that patients show extreme difficulty in repeating series of syllables which differ only in their vowels tends to confirm the contention that the basic defect lies in an inability to shift from one articulatory position to another. In test 3 such patients are unable to grasp the intonational unity of the syllable series "bi-ba-bo". Thus they either fail to go beyond the first or second syllable, or show profound perseveration of the first syllable so that the second and third syllables are pronounced the same as the first. In mild forms of this disorder patients who succeed in mastering the pattern "bi-ba-bo" are unable to shift to a different triplet and continue to repeat "bi-ba-bo" throughout succeeding trials. There are two simple confirmatory tests which may be used when this occurs. If a greater interval of time is allowed between responses it becomes much easier for the patient to shift from one triplet to another. Secondly, he may be instructed to write down the sounds which he hears instead of repeating them orally. This may reveal that the difficulty is not primarily auditory in nature.

Patients with efferent motor aphasia have clear-cut difficulty in repeating meaningful words. Since they are unable to shift from one articulatory pattern to another they show various types of pronunciation defects; elision, reversal, antiposition, and assimilation. Thus instead of "muka" (flour) they may say "mu-ma", instead of "galstuk" (necktie), they often say "gal-gus". In less severe cases these defects may not appear. Still, one may detect the difficulty in shifting from one element to another by the fact that the patient pronounces the first word of a phrase correctly but distorts the pronunciation of the next word by repeating part of the first word with it, i.e., by perseveration of all or part of the first word. As a rule the tendency to perseverate is less marked with the pronunciation of meaningful words. It emerges quite clearly when the task requires shifting from one speech unit to another.

A different type of difficulty arises when a patient in this group attempts to repeat a sentence. If, as occurs with lesions in the premotor areas, the loss of inner dynamic schemata involves only external motor processes the defect observed in the repetition of sentences is a lack of smoothness. The utterance of each word requires a special effort. On the other hand, in cases where the loss of inner dynamic schemata is the basis for the efferent motor aphasia the patient is totally unable to repeat sentences. There is a disturbance of the predicative aspect of speech; the over-all structure of the sentence disintegrates, and the patient, retaining only the nominative function of speech can only repeat its substantive components. He is unable to repeat the sentence as a grammatical and "melodious" whole. In attempting to repeat a sentence such a patient frequently repeats only the nouns; verbs and combining elements are lost. The repetition of a sentence is reduced to the reproducton of a single word which may convey the general sense of the statement but lacks all grammatical structure. For instance, on presentation of the sentence, "Yesterday the weather was bad", such a patient may respond with the single word, "Weather", or he may make more concrete the meaning of the whole sentence by saying, "Rain". Of course, the repetition of complex predicative and descriptive constructions as well as the repetition of sentences involving extended or inverted constructions is impossible for him. The origin of the difficulty is not a memory defect but a disturbance of the predicative function of speech and loss of the inner structure of sentences.

Different disturbances of imitative (repetitive) speech are also observed in cases where the primary defect is loss of the inner schemata of articulatory movements. In cases of *afferent motor aphasia* patients even have difficulty in repeating individual speech sounds. The ability to hear speech sounds is generally not affected. The patient encounters great difficulty, however, whenever he must recall a certain sound, differentiate it from similar sounds, and produce the articulatory position necessary for its utterance. In the most severe cases patients are completely unable to find the articulemes necessary for pronouncing the speech sounds. In less severe cases, or in the late phases of recovery from severe disorders, the patient may only confuse sounds which have similar articulatory patterns. Thus he may pronounce "d" as "l" or "n" (the palato-lingual group) or he may pronounce "b" as "p" or "m" (the labial group).

Patients in this group often try to make use of visual aids in articulating speech sounds. They can pronounce sounds considerably better if they watch the face of the experimenter or observe their own articulatory movements in a mirror than if these aids are not available. It is as though they were unable to pronounce sounds on the basis of inner articulatory schemata. Sounds produced by oral movements which are clearly visible, e.g., the vowels "a", "o", and "u" and the consonants "b", "m", and "p", are rapidly remastered, whereas those which are not associated with easily visualized oral movements, e.g., the vowel "i" or the consonants "k", "x", "š", etc., are much more difficult to recover. Also characteristic of these patients is the fact that, having mastered one articulatory position appropriate for a given sound, they are not necessarily able to pronounce different variants of the same sound. Thus a patient who has remastered the sound "t" may be able to pronounce it relatively easily in hard syllables, e.g., "to" or "tu", but still have difficulty in pronouncing it as part of soft syllables, e.g., "te" or "ti". As a result, he may have great difficulty in going from the pronunciation of individual sounds to the pronunciation of syllables. His difficulty lies not in the denervation of words or in the running of words together but in finding the appropriate articulatory position for the pronunciation of a known sound in different syllables. In severe cases this defect may preclude expressive speech altogether; in milder cases or in late stages of recovery the forced character of articulation always remains. It is distinctive of the speech of patients who have had some form of "kinetic aphasia". The most important difficulties in these cases arise in finding appropriate articulatory positons for individual sounds. Thus, no really new difficulties are revealed by subsequent tests involving syllables and words. It makes no difference whether the material to be repeated consists of phonemes, syllables, words, or sentences; the ability to repeat them depends upon the degree to which the patient is able to produce the appropriate articulatory patterns.

The disturbance of articulatory schemata results not only in an inability to find the positions of the speech apparatus which are appropriate to the different speech sounds; it also produces difficulty in recognizing spoken phonemes and assigning them to precise articulatory groups. The patient may not only be incapable of articulating a sound which he hears but he may have considerable difficulty in picking it out from a list of several sounds. This indicates that the articulatory schemata play an important role in the recognition of speech sounds. We shall consider this defect further when we describe disturbances of word comprehension, reading, and writing.

The primary disturbance of *acoustico-gnostic processes* associated with lesions in the left temporal area is the loss of phonemic hearing. It produces an extreme impairment of imitative speech. The auditory reception of speech in these cases is so imprecise that the patient, who may have no articulatory difficulties whatever, is unable to differentiate the various speech sounds which he hears and hence cannot repeat them correctly. Often he perceives them as random noises, so that his attempts to pronounce them reflect little more than a process of trial and error. He confuses similar sounds and is never certain that the sound which he utters is correct even though it may be so. Not infrequently a patient unable to analyze a sound or syllable attempts to identify it as part of a meaningful word and thus to compensate for his primary auditory defect. Even these attempts, however, do not lead him to any degree of confidence that he has repeated the sound correctly. For instance, he may grope for the sound "k" as follows: "k? . . . š? . . . č . . . k? . . . s? . . . x? . . . x? . . . k . . . x . . . koška (cat) koška . . . x? . . . k?". This type of response is typical of a patient with sensory aphasia.

The most important test for identifying patients in this group is that involving the repetition of oppositional phonemes. As was pointed out above, even patients with mild forms of temporal lobe aphasia are unable to differentiate such phonemes. They usually pronounce them both the same, e.g., "ba-pa" becomes "ba-ba" or "pa-pa", or they repeat the sounds in reverse order, e.g., "pa-ba". In either case they remain uncertain as to whether or not their responses are correct. Characteristically these patients give erroneous responses no matter what the medium of expression. It makes little difference whether they respond orally, choose the sounds which they think they have heard from a list, or write down what they hear; they are usually wrong. This indicates that the underlying disturbance is a *sensory* defect and distinguishes it from the types of aphasia in which the errors are perseverative in nature. In some cases, the unambiguous identification of this symptom alone is sufficient to warrant a diagnosis of temporal (acoustic) aphasia.

Tests in which the patient is required to repeat a series of syllables all beginning with the same consonant, e.g., "bi-ba-bo", reveal another form of disturbance in cases of temporal aphasia. The difficulty which the patient has in carrying out this test is determined not only by the extent of damage to the phonemic structure of speech, but also by the degree of instability and loss of sequential auditory patterns in general. He tends to forget certain components of a sound sequence or confuses their order. Unlike a patient with motor aphasia, he does not produce a perseverative response. Instead, there is a pronounced lability and instability in the sound patterns which he attempts to reproduce. The disturbance of phonemic hearing affects the reproduction of meaningful words as well as of nonsense syllables. The repetition of simple familiar words, such as "house", "hand", etc., is affected only in severe temporal lobe aphasias with profound disruption of speech comprehension. In these cases, the patient does not recognize words, and sound patterns rapidly disintegrate for him. In attempting to keep words from getting away from him he may repeat them or similar sounding words several times; e.g., if the word "golos" (voice) is presented, he may repeat, "Kolos (ear of grain) . . . golos (voice) . . . glos (meaningless) . . . xols (meaningless) . . . xolst (canvas) . . . glos (meaningless) . . . gols (meaningless)" as though he were unable either to recognize the original word or retain its sound structure. He may complain that the word vanishes the moment it is spoken.

The patient, unable to pronounce the word, immedately begins to analyze its sound structure, but in trying to analyze it he becomes more confused. As a result of the shift of attention to the sound structure of the word, he produces numerous literal paraphasias. He may pronounce such a word as "muxomor" (death-cap) as "muxoron ... muxorop ... muxor ... muxoren ... muxorek", etc. (all meaningless). He is unable to settle one sound pattern as being acceptable to him. Such instability emerges very clearly with the repetition of an unfamiliar word or a combination of nonsense syllables. The lack of meaning removes the one factor upon which the patient might base his ability to repeat it. The necessity to shift his attention to the analysis of the sound structure of the word places him in a very awkward situation, for it leaves him totally unable to repeat complex combinations of phenemes. A patient with impairment of the acoustico-gnostic systems is unable to repeat words unless the act of recognition can be mediated by the word meanings. The moment attention is shifted to their sound structure, the chances of accurate repetiton disappear because auditory analysis is impossible.

Disturbance of the acoustico-gnostic systems produces more than a loss of phonemic hearing. It also renders auditory traces extremely labile and creates an obstacle to the retention of sequental sound patterns. Thus, even the repetition of a series of syllables, as "bi-ba-bo", or a word becomes difficult. The typical result is that when the patient attempts to repeat sound sequences on the basis of his unstable impressions, he may utter the phonemic components in random order, and the order may change with each new attempt.

The difficulty which we have been describing emerges most clearly when one tests the ability to repeat sentences. In severe cases of temporal aphasia this test is impossible and the patient usually comments that, "There are too many words", that they create a chaotic conglomeraton from which he is unable to remember anything. In the late phases of recovery from temporal aphasia the patient may make unsuccessful attempts to repeat sentences. He may able to retain the intonational pattern of a sentence, but he is unable to fill in the correct words. He may remember the general meaning of a sentence but forget the exact words and thus respond with a meaningful paraphasia, e.g., instead of "in the garden" he may say "in the woods", instead of "apple trees were growing" he may say "pears ... well these ... were hanging", etc.[2] In attempting to reproduce a sentence by concentrating on the phonemic structure of the words he again loses the constancy of the sound pattern and produces typical literal paraphasias. For instance, "bazarom" ("bazaar", instrumental case) or "bazorom" (meaningless) instead of "zaborom" (fence, instrumental case); "rešili" (solved)) or "lešni" (meaningless) instead of "rosli" (grew); etc. Multiple presentations of the same sentence do not help such a patient; he is still unable to repeat it correctly. The inability to retain whole sentences is most profound in cases where the lesion involves the tertiary acoustico-mnestic systems of the temporal area. In these cases the ability to repeat individual words usually remains intact, but the patient shows signs of severe disturbance

[2] A detailed psychological analysis of cases of this type was published by M. S. Lebedinskij (1941), and later by Ė. S. Bejn and S. M. Blinkov.

when asked to repeat long word sequences. Even after several presentations of a given sequence he can only repeat the first two or three words, indicating that the rest of the words have disappeared from his span of consciousness.

The difficulties in imitative speech which we have described make up one of the most important group of symptoms of temporal lobe aphasia. In terms of this discussion it is possible to consider some cases of so called "conductive" aphasia as simply mild forms of temporal lobe aphasia. Spontaneous speech is relatively unaffected, but whenever the patient shifts his attention to the phonemic composition of words he shows great difficulty in producing the appropriate articulatory positions and this gives rise to a striking disturbance of imitative speech.

Patients with semantic aphasia, who have lost the simultaneous schemata of speech, show no characteristic disturbance of imitative speech. Usually they are able to repeat individual sounds and syllables without difficulty. They show no impairment of the ability to differentiate similar, "oppositional", phonemes. Only occasionally does the constriction of their inner perceptual field lead them to have difficulty in retaining the order of syllables or words in long sequences. These patients can repeat long sentences provided they do not involve complex logico-grammatical constructions. Because of the loss of logico-grammatical schemata, however, it is impossible to repeat equally long sentences, or even considerably shorter ones, if they involve complex grammatical constructions. In contrast to motor aphasia, in which loss of the predicative aspect of speech underlies the majority of errors, one does not observe in semantic aphasia the reduction of sentences to strings of unrelated nouns. Instead, there is a confusion of similar grammatical constructions and, in general, simplification of the grammatical constructions used in spontaneous speech. The difficulties in imitative speech observed in these cases do not result from a disturbance of the phasic aspect of speech. We shall further analyze the agrammatism of semantic aphasia in a later section.

D. INVESTIGATION OF THE NOMINATIVE FUNCTION OF SPEECH

The ability to name objects is one of the most important functions involved in spontaneous speech processes. This, together with the predicative functions, constitutes the basis of the meaningful aspect of speech. A disturbance of the ability to name objects can produce a profound impairment of the entire speech system. Recalling the name of an object, action, or situation is by no means a simple act. Naming is always a process of classification, generalization, or, as is commonly said, "a categorical act". It would be incorrect to assume that whenever a person gazes at an object the word representing it pops directly into his consciousness. It is a well established psychological fact that the first thing to appear in consciousness is a general sphere of meaning in which a great complex of names or characteristics are bound together. From this the appropriate name is selected out. If the process of differentiation is impaired, the patient may easily substitute another name for the appropriate one, and the name he chooses will indicate the general sphere with which it is associated, e.g., instead of "elbow" he may say "shoulder" or "knee".

The complexity of the naming process becomes apparent to a normal person whenever he attempts to name an unfamiliar object, define a general concept, or remember a word in an unfamiliar language. It is understandable that any disturbance of "categorical" thought, i.e., the abstraction of primary features and their association with the appropriate category, should impair what would otherwise appear to be the simple function of naming objects.

Another psychological characteristic of naming objects is that it requires not only the ability to find the appropriate concept but also the ability to pronounce the corresponding word. The auditory image of the appropriate word does not occur to the subject in its finished form; in order to pronounce it he must be able to call forth the corresponding inner phonemic schema. It is obvious that if the auditory image of the word is unstable or diffuse the pronunciation of the name will be impossible. In this case the patient will be forced to grope randomly for the appropriate phonemic pattern or will have to substitute a word of similar sound structure for the correct one. This is how various forms of "paraphasia" arise (M. S. Lebedinskij, 1941; È. S. Bejn, 1947, 1957, 1959).

Assessment of the ability to name objects thus gives one the opportunity to determine both the degree of preservation of the nominative, generalizing function of speech and also the preservation of the phonemic images of words. The techniques used in investigating this function should be so structured that the investigator can distinguish which of these two components of the naming process is disturbed.

The technique used to investigate the nominative function of speech is very simple. It usually consists of the following tests:

1. *Naming Objects Presented Visually*

The patient is presented a series of common objects or pictures of objects and asked to name them. The examiner notes the readiness with which he is able to respond and if errors arise, he notes whether they are phonemic or semantic in character. Special attention should be given to whether or not the patient has to grope for the appropriate phonemic structure of words. For instance, in naming a comb (rasčeska) he may respond. "Ras ... četka ... raščovka ... rasčestaka ... rasčeska?" He may show a tendency to replace the appropriate noun by a non-nominative word or phrase, e.g., instead of "comb" he may say, "For combing one's hair." Instead of "elbow" he may say "knee" or "shoulder", instead of "nurse" he may say "teacher", etc. In order to determine whether the difficulty results from a disturbance of the stable phonemic images of words the examiner may prompt the patient. If hearing the first syllable of the correct word pronounced by the examiner does not help him, one has evidence that the underlying disorder is acoustico-gnostic in nature.

2. *Naming Objects Described Orally*

The examiner describes an object to the patient and asks him to name it. For example, he may ask, "What do you call a bird which pecks trees?" or "what kind of metal are light dishes, pots, and frying pans made from?"

This test is, of course, only used in cases where speech comprehension is relatively intact. If the examiner's question elicits a whole complex of associations, one can gain some idea of the degree of differentiation in the semantic sphere and of the patient's ability to use language as a means of sharpening his discriminatory capacities.

3. *Naming Categories*

The simplest and most widely studied test is that which evaluates the ability to name various shades of a given color. A similar type of test involves the naming of general groups of objects in a given class, e.g., "chair", "table", "divan", and "chest" are all members of the class "furniture".

A great discrepancy between the ability to name concrete objects and to name categories indicates that the underlying disturbance involves the semantic aspect of speech.

The nominative aspect of speech is disturbed in several forms of aphasia. In the early stages of traumatic aphasia almost any speech defect is accompanied by difficulty in the spontaneous naming of objects. This phenomenon is apparently due to a profound dissociation of the auditory and semantic aspects of words and to a disturbance of the system of meaningful associations attached to words (V. M. Kogan). This phase passes rapidly, however, and the various aphasic syndromes soon begin to differentiate out. Characteristically, lesions in the anterior (dynamic) systems are accompanied by disturbances of the predicative aspect of speech, while lesions in the posterior (perceptual) systems disturb primarily the nominative aspect of speech.

In a patient with motor aphasia the nominative function of speech is not particularly affected. Such a patient experiences the same difficulty in naming objects as he does when attempting to repeat the words presented orally. Only in cases involving massive lesions or in the early phases of cases involving efferent motor aphasia is the spontaneous recall of names apt to be more difficult than simply repeating the same words presented orally. Here the patient is able to derive benefit from hearing the sound pattern or observing the articulatory movements of the examiner. In these disturbances the meanings of words become very narrow, so that a word used in one concrete situation ceases to have any meaning if the situation is altered. The ability to recall the meanings of words is impaired. The constriction of the word meanings has been shown by O. P. Kaufman to occur quite frequently in cases of motor aphasia. Other forms of aphasia show defects of the meaningful structure of words which are similar in nature. In motor aphasia, however, these disorders are usually related to difficulty in recalling the articulatory images of words. The patient may distort words by omitting syllables, altering their order, or substituting one sound for another. Rarely does he produce verbal paraphasias involving the substitution of one whole word for another.

In efferent motor aphasia patients characteristically have little difficulty in naming objects presented visually. They have great difficulty however, in formulating any kind of spontaneous thought. This is not so much due to loss of the nominative function of speech as to loss of the generality of verbal meanings (see above) and disturbance of the predicative aspect of speech and the verbal formulation of thought which we shall consider below. Finally, the ability to name objects may be made quite difficult as a result of the perseveration of preceding words. For instance, having pronounced the word "kryška" (lid) a patient may have great difficulty in finding the word "pila" (saw) because of his tendency to repeat "kryška": "Ko . . . no . . . koš . . . no . . . ko . . . no !" He may combine the two words to form a single one: "Pška . . . net (no)! . . . piš . . . net (no) . . . piš . . . la ! . . . net (no)!" The patient recognizes his errors, but he is unable to overcome the persistent recurrence of the first word.

A disturbance of the acoustico-gnostic, visuo-gnostic, and simultaneous perceptual systems can produce equally severe disturbances of the nominative aspect of speech. Close investigation shows, however, that the defects arising in these cases involve different mechanisms.

A patient with impairment of phonemic hearing resulting from a temporal lobe lesion can neither repeat nor remember words. The instability and diffuseness of the auditory images of words and the associated "loss of word meanings" (Chapter 12) may be so great that he is completely unable to remember the appropriate words. In some cases the disturbance is so severe that the patient is unable to retrieve any part of the appropriate word, e.g., "Well . . . this . . . well I know . . . uh . . . well . . ." In other cases, he utters several phonemic word fragments, but they are often inappropriate and convey only the general intonational pattern of the word. The sounds which he remembers are not stable. Hence, in attempting to piece out the rest of the pattern, he produces more and more erroneous variations which sometimes retain one or another component of the original sound pattern. In his attempts to find or retain the correct sound pattern the patient often drifts into the utterance of meaningful words which sound similar to the one he seeks. Thus, what was a literal paraphasia (distortion of the phonemic structure of the word) becomes a verbal paraphasia (substitution of another word for the correct one). The patient's auditory image of the word he seeks is very imprecise; so that he can be prompted with virtually the whole word and still not recognize or recall it. An illustration of a literal paraphasic response to a picture of a small case (futjar) might go as follows: "Fljurt . . . fljar . . . fultjar . . . fulter . . . fljar . . . flir . . . fljur . . .", etc. A verbal paraphasic response to the word "pila" (saw) might be, "Želeso (iron) . . . lopata (shovel) . . . net ne lopata (no not shovel) . . . lita . . . plita (flagstone) . . . net ne plita (no not stove) . . . pila (saw) . . . pilo . . . pila (saw) . . . železnaja pila (iron saw)!" The first is an auditory type of paraphasia; the second is a semantic type of paraphasia. It is important, however, that the semantic paraphasia continues to bear traces of a severe disturbance of the inner structure of the word. Since the root parts of words are much more seriously disturbed than the grammatical parts (prefixes, suffixes, etc.) the verbal paraphasias are characterized by a particular type of "contamination." The grammatical appendages of the word are combined with the root part of some other word to produce for instance, "konfetnik" (meaningless) instead of "kofejnik" (coffee-pot), "stixtuški" (meaningless) instead of "častuški" (couplet), or "plokhoda" (a combination of the words "plokhaja" and "pogoda" ("bad" and "weather") instead of "doždlivaja pogoda" (rainy weather).

The psychological mechanisms underlying such contaminations has been studied recently by È. S. Bejn (1947), S. M. Blinkov, and others. Disturbance of the constancy of word images leads in many cases for a radical reorganization of the naming process itself. The patient may unconsciously replace the appropriate word by one which reflects some important feature of the given situation. For instance, he may say, "The sister did not approach the child for a long time", instead of ". . . did not approach the patient for a long time". M. S. Lebedinski (1941) has pointed out that such paraphasias can be understood only by taking into account the entire situation in which they are uttered.

It is important to note that in the cases which we have been describing, literal and verbal paraphasias may appear together. Which of the two will occur in a given situation depends upon the attitude of the patient. If he works with the fragmentary auditory images which he retains, his attempts to find the correct sound patterns result in literal paraphasias. If he abandons this approach and attempts to express the same meanings by other words, he produces verbal paraphasias. Sometimes both strategies occur simultaneously, and the paraphasia which results is quite complex.

Patients in this group tend to compensate for their difficulty in the direct naming of objects by producing the appropriate names in common verbo-motor contexts. For instance, in attempting to find the word "lopata" (shovel) such a patient may say "ložka" (spoon) . . . net, ne ložka (no not spoon) . . . koška (cat) . . . net (no) . . . taška (meaningless) . . . net, net (no, no) . . . že . . . železnyj (iron) . . . železnaja iopata (iron shovel) . . . vot (there)!" Or in attempting to produce the word "lampa" he may say, "Èto (this) . . . kak eto (how does it), nu (well) . . . ke . . . kerosin (kerosine) . . . net ne kerosin (no not kerosine) . . . a ètot (but this) električestvo (electricity) . . . električeskaja lampa (electric lamp)!"

The basic disturbance underlying loss of the nominative function of speech is not always a loss of the auditory schemata of words. It has been found that lesions of lower parts of the left temporal area (usually resulting from abcesses of wounds in the third temporal gyrus) impair the ability to find words not so much by reducing the precision of auditory schemata as by producing a general inconstancy of such schemata. Thus, a patient with an acoustico-mnestic disturbance does not produce the literal paraphasias which would indicate loss of the auditory schemata of words. All the same he is unable to find the words and may produce a number of verbal paraphasias. The mechanism of this disturbance is rooted in the acoustic-gnostic sphere, so that prompting with part of the correct word is usually of no help. Even if the patient finds the correct word, it is very unstable; if he is presented the same object several minutes later he must go through the same difficult recall process as before.

In this case the disturbance of the nominative function of speech arises from a disturbance of the precision and stability of auditory speech schemata. In other cases, however, the disturbance may be related to loss, *not of the auditory, but of the semantic aspect of speech.* This occurs primarily with impairment of the cortical functions responsible for the creation of simultaneous schemata. It becomes impossible to consider any object as a meaningful whole and to associate it with the complex connections and relationships which are appropriate to it. The disturbance of this function is seen most clearly in semantic aphasias, where selectivity of the "net of alternatives" in which words are imbedded is disturbed. The meanings of individual words appear to be constricted and they do not fall into clear-cut logical categories. The boundaries between different semantic groups are blurred. This is why patients with semantic aphasia have difficulty in defining the categorical meanings of words. Their disorder is reminiscent of the type of difficulty which any normal person experiences in attempting to recall the forgotten name of a friend. Such names are not usually part of any clearly defined logical categories. A patient with a primary disturbance of the nominative function of speech rarely distorts the phonemic structure of words. He is more likely to replace the categorical name of an object by predicative description of an action appropriate to it. For instance, instead of "pen" he may say, "This . . . well, you write with it." He may produce a verbal paraphasia by replacing the word representing an object such as a knife with other words which have some meaningful associative link with it: "This . . . well, a hammer; no, not a hammer . . . well . . . no, not a spoon, a knife . . ." A good indication of the semantic nature of this disturbance is the fact that prompting is immediately recognized by the patient and usually elicits the correct word. The difficulty in finding names to represent categories, e.g., the generic names of colors, is much greater than the difficulty in naming objects.

This discussion of disturbances of the nominative function of speech would not be complete were we not to mention one other origin of such disorders. With lesions in the visuo-gnostic systems of the occipital area there may be no severe signs of visual impairment; yet the perceptual constancy of objects and pictures of objects is lost so that the patient has difficulty in naming them. If such a patient is presented a slightly blurred, but still recognizable, picture of an object he is totally unable to name it, or he refers to it by a term which is too general, e.g., instead of "dog" he may say "animal". It is as though he were unable to grasp the specific features of the picture and has to base his judgment only upon its most general features. Cases of this sort usually involve lesions along the border between the temporal and occipital cortical areas and have been described in the literature as "visual aphasias." They are characterized by an impairment of visual perception which prevents the categorical naming of objects. This feature makes such disorders similar to the agnostic disturbances and forces one to consider them to be disturbances occupying an intermediate position somewhere between the agnosias and the aphasias. L. S. Vygotskij and R. E. Levina have shown that deprivation of the perceptual prerequisites for speech at an early age adversely affects further speech development and may lead to alalia. O. P. Kaufman has shown in our laboratory that certain lesions in adults can produce difficulties in the naming of objects but leave more abstract and categorical terms intact.

Regardless of their origin, all of the disturbances of the nominative function which we have described above are extremely difficult to overcome. Direct attempts to rememorize the names of various objects are generally unsuccessful. Thus, it is important to be aware that patients who have lost the nominative function of speech are able to compensate for this disorder by reproducing familiar expressions or contexts in which the desired words are imbedded. A patient unable to remember the word "star" may have no difficulty in repeating the sentence, "Red stars shine above the Kremlin". By using a narrow meaning of the word it is possible to circumvent the difficulty of direct naming and thus to compensate for the primary defect (see Chapter 16).

On the basis of the above discussion one can reach certain conclusions which are extremely important for the clinical study of aphasia. A special form of "amnesic aphasia" involving difficulty in finding words has been described by a number of authors (Henschen, Nissl von Meyendorf, Kleist, Economo, and others). Some associate it with infero-temporal lesions, while others (Pötzl and Kroll) identify it with lesions in the parietal area. On the basis of the material which we have presented it is possible to conclude that amnesic aphasia is not so much a special form of aphasia as a symptom which arises as a result of lesions in various locations and thus can result from diverse pathological mechanisms. It is seen most clearly in cases involving temporal and infero-temporal lesions which give rise to the syndromes of temporal or acoustico-mnestic aphasia. It also occurs, however, with parietal lesions which give rise to semantic disturbances. Analysis of the mechanisms underlying the various disturbances permits one to understand how a single type of symptom may arise following lesions in several different cortical areas.

E. THE INVESTIGATION OF PREDICATIVE (NARRATIVE) SPEECH

Whereas the foregoing tests were designed to investigate the nominative, designitive function of speech, the following series of tests should determine the degree of preservation of predicative, narrative speech processes. The expression, or more precisely, the formulation of thought is certainly the most important function of speech. It appeared much later than the nominative function and is associated with that stage in the history of language development when grammatical sentence structure first appeared. This function makes it possible not only to represent particular objects but also to convey thoughts by means of words.

The formulation of a statement may occur at any one of several levels and in different psychological systems. The most simple function involving statements is *dialogue*. Here the semantic frame of reference is created by the interlocuter. The subject's response which may involve naming an object or conveying a thought, is largely reactive in character. Much more complex is the act of *recitative (reproductive) narrative* in which the speaker verbally reproduces some perceived or recalled scheme. In this case speech is more fully developed and more spontaneous. It continues to meet conditions placed on it by a semantic frame of reference determined by a specific perceptual experience or group of memory images. Finally, the most complex level of speech is *productive narration* or *discursive speech* in which the speaker himself develops a narrative theme or verbally elaborates a certain line of reasoning. Whereas the second form of speech consists essentially in the description of a remembered or imagined situation, the third form expresses verbal thought processes in the true sense.

The grammatical forms used in the various types of spontaneous speech may not be identical. In some cases they may consist of very short propositions which do little more than designate objects or situations; in other cases they consist of complex grammatical constructions in which the nominative component ceases to play a leading role or is incorporated into a pattern of interrelated words so as to permit the expression of thoughts. For this the nominative function of speech is not sufficient. Here the *predicative* function is of major importance. Hughlings Jackson, A. Pick, L. S. Vygotskij, and others, showed that the relationship of the predicative speech function is closer to inner speech than that of any other function. In order to be expressed it must be clothed in a propositional pattern formulated in terms of a particular linguistic system, i.e., in grammatical speech. A loss of inner speech or a disturbance of antecedent propositional schemata precludes the elaboration of predicative linguistic patterns and reduces speech to a purely nominative function. Individual words are left intact, but the patient is deprived of genuine speech, i.e., of the speech processes whereby thoughts are formulated.

The investigation of predicative speech should establish whether or not the patient retains predicative speech functions and at what level he is able to uitilize them. It includes several tests of different degrees of complexity.

1. *Dialogue*

The patient is asked a series of questions. Some are so structured that his answer can be phrased in the same way as the question; thus it is unnecessary for him to formulate a new sentence structure in order to respond, e.g., "Have you eaten today?" or, "Do you know how to read?" Other questions do not provide a pattern which can be used in the answer. The patient must employ certain of his own speech processes in the formulation of new statements, e.g., "How were you wounded?" or, "How did you get along after the injury?"

2. *Recitative Narrative Speech*

The patient is shown a rather simple picture or series of pictures the contents of which he is to describe in narrative form. The same purpose may be served by having him repeat the contents of a story which he has heard or describe a situation which is very familiar to him.

3. *Spontaneous (Productive) Narrative Speech*

The patient is asked to make up a short story on a given theme or to suggest the meaning of a picture which does not contain sufficient detail to evoke an obvious interpretation. In supplementary tests he may be given two or three words, e.g., "river", "boat", and "money", from which he is to construct a grammatical sentence. A more complex form of test is to have the patient dictate a business letter; this leaves the choice of the sentences themselves up to the patient.

These tests usually provide a sufficient basis for the assessment of narrative speech. The investigator, of course, pays greater attention to the degree of spontaneity, complexity, and grammatical accuracy of the patient's speech than to the precision of articulatory patterns.

It is to be expected that any form of aphasia will produce some disturbance of narrative speech. Damage to the different cerebral systems, however, produces very diverse forms of impairment. Whereas lesions in the posterior perceptual systems produce disturbances primarily of nominative speech function, impairment of inner speech usually results from lesions in the anterior, dynamic cerebral systems. The disruption of inner speech is responsible for severe disturbances of the predicative aspect of speech. Patients with such disorders have great difficulty in going from naming objects to formulating thoughts. In severe cases they may be unable to formulate any form of predicative statement. In dialogue, their answers are usually limited to simple confirmations and negations. In responding to questions which require more complex answers, they are largely limited to the nominative, designative representation of objects and actions. Even in expressing desires they do no more than name objects; there is no predicative aspect to their statements. As might be expected, the reproduction of narrative speech is difficult, but spontaneous narrative speech is even more impaired. If such a patient attempts to interpret a picture he is able to do little more than enumerate the objects or actions represented. This is the form of aphasia to which Jackson referred when he indicated that a patient could be deprived of speech even though he were not deprived of words.

The severe disturbance of the predicative function of speech which is characteristic of efferent motor aphasia often remains even in the late stages of recovery. After long and intensve retraining, a patient whose speech has been reduced to the naming of individual objects and actions – so called "telegraph style" – may retain signs of a "nominative agrammatism". In formulating a sentence he utters only a series of isolated words each of which designates some action or thing; strictly speaking, he does not formulate a sentence at all. As was indicated above, such a patient may be unable to repeat whole sentences. He is able to repeat several of the meaningful phrases involved, but they lack grammatical context. He is unable to generate the "intention" for a whole sentence; his grammatical "feeling for the language" is defective, so that sometimes he may sense the inadequacy of his sentence structure, yet he is unable to identify what it is about the sentence that is incorrect. He is aware of individual meaningful elements but these elements never coalesce into the intonational pattern of a sentence. Even though the patient's statements may outwardly appear to be cast in the form of sentences, they actually remain disconnected references to objects and actions. Grammatical analysis of such statements reveals no content other than the logical subject and predicate. An example of this type of agrammatism is seen in the following statement about the war: "Yes ... soldiers ... and troups ... and ... we are there ... and cannons ... and Germans ... oh ... that's all ... I really cannot ... yes ... that's that ..." In the late stages of recovery, after long periods of retraining, patients may succeed in mastering the external schemata of sentences, but for a long time they still show a tendency to utter the substantive parts of speech at the beginning of the sentence and to leave the nonsubstantive, predicative, or explanatory parts to the end. Sometimes the latter parts may be omitted altogether. Generally this type of sentence structure never disappears altogether in a patient who has a severe efferent motor aphasia.

Loss of the grammatical structure of sentences is not the only disorder which may disturb predicative narrative speech. In cases involving the more advanced parts of the anterior speech areas, bordering on the prefrontal area, the grammatical structure of sentences may remain intact while the nominative function is altered. In the cases which we have described above as forms of frontal dynamic aphasia the patient retains only his reproductive narrative speech. The grammatical structure of his speech is correct and appropriate, though somewhat less rich than before injury. He can only use it however, to describe the individual details in thematic pictures or to repeat stories he has heard. Occasionally he is able to give a fuller description of a thematic picture or of the circumstances presented in a certain short story, but he is never able to go beyond the discussion of a concrete subject to productive, spontaneous speech. The active formulation of a narration is impossible for him. He may note that, for him, the overall plan of the narrative never crystallizes. Any attempt to undertake a spontaneous narrative results in the mechanical utterance of sentence fragments or stereotyped expressions which he has memorized. A typical example which might be added to those already presented (Chapter 7, Section C) is that of a patient who, when asked to write a composition about the North, wrote, "There are bears in the North . . .", and after a long pause concluded his composition by writing the common stereotyped phrase, "This I bring to your attention!"

The disturbance of inner speech is seen here not in a loss of the predicative structure of sentences, but in loss of the overall schemata of active narration. Whereas lesions in the dynamic cortical systems destroy the predicative organization of speech, lesions in the *posterior perceptual areas of the brain* produce just the opposite picture. Here it is common for the predicative function of speech to remain relatively intact, so that a patient in whom the nominative aspect of speech is impaired preserves the intonational patterns whereby speech is used for the expression of thoughts. The predicative structure of speech may be affected by impairment of the nominative function, since the latter leads to frequent interruptions as the patient searches for words. Careful analysis shows, however, that these interruptions do not reflect difficulty in the expression of thoughts but in recalling their nominative contents. The speech of such a patient flows most smoothly when the surroundings are appropriate to the thoughts expressed, and when the patient is able to use familiar phraseological constructions. On the other hand, when he consciously wishes to transmit new information or to give a literal recitation of something he has memorized, a new complicating factor is added to the task. In this case he is unable to use familiar phrases and shows a noticeable impairment of speech. The contrast between the relatively good preservation of familiar speech patterns and the severe disturbance of abstract or recitative speech was noted long ago by Jackson and later by Gelb and Goldstein.

Two factors are capable of disturbing narrative speech with lesions in the posterior perceptual brain areas. With temporal lobe lesions which produce primary damage of the acoustico-gnostic systems narrative speech may be impaired by the loss of the nominative function and the inability to retain long sequential verbal constructions. The patient is unable to compose sentences of words which are phonemically and semantically vague to him. His basic problem becomes one of finding words to replace the ones he has lost. The words he wants often have to be replaced by others, the precise meaning of which he may also have forgotten. Thus, his verbal activity is characterized by a general sense of uncertainity. The word sequences which he wishes to utter are very unstable and quickly disappear from his consciousness, so that the intonational structure of his sentences is left devoid of substantive content. A special investigation carried out by È. S. Bejn has shown that this explains the discontinuity of the patient's speech. His speech is constantly interrupted by the search for substantives and is distorted by substitutive expressions, e.g., "Well this . . . well . . . as he . . . well then when this was . . ." There is a sharp contrast between the high degree of preservation of the intonational schemata and accompanying gestures and the severe disturbance of the nominative content of sentences. Only when the patient is able to speak in stereotyped phrases does this contrast disappear. Then the intonational pattern may embody more or less appropriate content. Characteristically these difficulties affect reproductive and spontaneous narrative speech equally. This is unlike the frontal aphasias in that there is no increase in difficulty as the patient goes from recitative narration to spontaneous narration.

In cases where disturbance of the nominative aspect of speech results not from a loss of the phonemic constancy of verbal images but from a disturbance of meaningful associations narrative speech may be disturbed to an equal degree, but the mechanism underlying the disturbance is altogether different. Special investigations which we have carried out with V. K. Bubnova have shown that one almost never observes a true expressive agrammatism in semantic aphasia. The patient shows no loss of "feeling for the language", no signs of "telegraph style", no difficulty in the proper use of grammatical rules, and no disturbance of the substantive content of sentences. Here again, however, the intact intonational patterns appear in conjunction with great difficulty in finding the words which make up the substantive content of sentences. The distinctive feature is that the difficulty is not limited to the search for words of a substantive nature but also involves the formulation of grammatical relationships. The patient complains that his thoughts are "disjointed" and that he is unable to formulate the grammatical constructions which are essential for normal speech.

These defects reflect disorders of the semantic aspect of speech and emerge most clearly when patients attempt to go beyond concrete events to deal with complex logico-grammatical relationships. Here, as in the cases of temporal lobe aphasia described above, the patient attempts to compensate for his defect by the use of stereotyped expressions and familiar speech patterns. By this means he can often conceal his speech defect in everyday conversation and thus create the impression that his spontaneous speech processes are intact.

XII

THE INVESTIGATION OF SPEECH PROCESSES: RECEPTIVE SPEECH

The investigation of hearing and speech comprehension despite its importance has not been given its due as part of the routine neurological examination. Usually the examiner determines only how well the patient understands single words and instructions. Such a superficial evaluation of his ability to understand speech is altogether inadequate. Modern linguistic and psychological investigations have shown that speech comprehension is a complex process and that it may be disturbed in a number of ways.

In order to understand the speech of others, the preservation of *phonemic hearing* is essential, otherwise, one cannot recognize the speech sounds and grasp the primary meanings of individual words. Lesions which disturb this prerequisite lead to imprecise word perception, loss of word meaning, and disturbance of processes basic to the comprehension of speech.

The preservation of phonemic hearing alone, however, is not sufficient for understanding words. Equally important is the breadth and stability of the *meanings* which words represent. If the words lose their general meanings, retaining only their narrow, concrete meanings they can be understood only in specific familiar situations. When they are used in other situations they are incomprehensible. L. S. Vygotskij and his students showed that the lack of speech comprehension in children often results from the fact that words have much less generalized meanings for them than for adults. Defective speech comprehension in deaf mute children has been studied by Morozova, Goldberg, Boskis and others. Again, the defects were found to result from the unusually narrow and concrete meanings which words have for such children.

In addition to this group of disorders which has to do with the nominative aspect of speech, there is a second group which is related to the predicative aspect, i.e., to preservation of the ability to comprehend the background and intentions which underlie verbal statements.

Investigations of the psychology of language (Bühler, Malinowsky, Vygotskij, and others) have shown that at least two factors are involved in the comprehension of verbal statements. These factors appear differently in different types of statements. In order to understand the speech of others one must be aware of the concrete conditions to which the statement is related, i.e., in what kind of setting the statement occurred. If this condition is met a person may catch the meaning of a statement even though it is expressed in very fragmentary form. Knowing the context, one can easily understand fragmentary comments which, taken out of context, would have no meaning. Conversely, if this condition is not met, separate words and separate sentences which a person hears may reach his consciousness, but the general *meaning* of the statement is completely lost; the statement is empty, deprived of its inner meaning. Thus knowledge of the context and grasp of the sets underlying statements are important for speech comprehension in everyday communication.

This is not the only condition which must be met for the comprehension of complex grammatical oral or written speech. It is also essential that a person be able to recognize the connections and interrelationships among the individual words in *grammatical constructions*. Without understanding of these logico-grammatical relationships, complex statements degenerate into mere sequences of words. A person who lacks such understanding can only guess at their overall meanings. The more complex the statement, the more divorced it is from immediate practical circumstances; the closer it comes to discursive speech, the greater the importance of the comprehension of logico-grammatical relationships.[1]

These are the primary prerequisites for normal speech comprehension. Every act of comprehension involves all of the conditions which we have enumerated. It is necessary to study separately each aspect of the comprehension process.

A. HEARING AND THE DISCRIMINATION OF SPEECH SOUNDS

The perception of speech sounds depends not only upon auditory acuity. In order to differentiate the sounds of which speech is composed and to distinguish a given sound from others which have similar physical characteristics a person must be able to identify those distinctive features which are important for distinguishing different words. He must be able to relate all of the sound patterns which bear given sets of distinctive features into precise and stable groups. Investigation of phonemic hearing must reveal the degree of preservation of auditory processes involving systematizations appropriate to the phonetic system of a given language. It must show to what extent the patient is able to pick out the stable speech cues in the flow of sound which he perceives. Investigation of phonemic hearing may be carried out once a preliminary audition test has established the absence of true deafness, the presence of which would complicate the study of phonemic hearing.

The methods to be used in the investigation of phonemic hearing have been partially

[1] In the latest years important statistical studies of word frequencies as factors of understanding were performed. We are unable to mention here these important studies (cf. H. Shuell, 1965 and others). We are unable to mention here important studies of information theory and its significence for the perception and understanding of speech (cf. G. Miller, 1951, D. E. Broadbent, 1958 and others).

described above; they may be supplemented by other special methods. Techniques used in the investigation of speech hearing include several groups of methods.

1. *Discrimination of Disjunctive and Opposite (Correlative) Phonemes*

Discrimination of disjunctive and opposite (correlative) phonemes, i.e., discrimination of sounds which differ from one another by several or by a single distinctive feature respectively. Examples of disjunctive phonemes are "d" and "s" or "k" and "t", examples of opposite (correlative) phonemes are "b" and "t" or "t" and "d". The sounds are presented in pairs of disjunctive, opposite, or identical phonemes. Examples of disjunctive phonemes are "ka-ta" and "na-la", of oppositional phonemes are "pa-ba" and "ba-pa"; and examples of identical sounds might be "pa-pa", "na-na", and "za-za". The patient is required to repeat, write, or point out from a list the syllables which he hears. (For a more detailed description of this test see Chapter II, Section C).

Important for the study of phonemic hearing have been experiments involving the conditioning of differential motor responses to pairs of phonemes – in particular to pairs of oppositional phonemes. The patient is presented a particular phoneme, e.g., "b" and is instructed to lift his hand (or his hand is lifted passively) until he has learned to raise it whenever he hears the sound "b". Once this response has been conditioned, the conditioning of an inhibitory response is begun. An altogether different phoneme, e.g., "r", is presented and he is instructed or shown that he should not lift his hand in response to this sound. Once the response system has been well established the primary experiment can begin. Instead of being presented disjunctive phonemes of the type "b" and "r" he is presented oppositional phonemes, such as "b" and "p". If he has difficulty in responding differentially to these phonemes one has evidence of a phonemic hearing disorder.

For a more precise analysis of the hearing disorder one can introduce greater complexity. The rate at which sounds are presented may be varied, or the pitch at which the two phonemes are spoken may be different. The latter technique may help in determining whether the subject responds primarily to phonemic or to non-phonemic features of the speech sounds.

2. *Production of Words Beginning with Given Letters and Evaluation of Incorrect Pronunciation* *

The patient is presented a given letter and asked to name several words beginning with that letter. The examiner notes whether or not he erroneously names words beginning with an oppositional phoneme. Next the examiner pronounces a series of words, some correctly and some incorrectly; for instance he may say, "guino" instead of "kino" (movie) or "tym" instead of "dym" (smoke). He notes whether or not the patient catches the errors. If the patient does not differentiate between the correct and incorrect pronunciation of the words, there may be a disturbance of phonemic hearing. Further techniques for determining the degree of preservation of phonemic hearing will be presented in connection with the investigation of reading and writing.

Disturbances of speech perception may occur with lesions of several different systems, especially with damage to the areas involved in the integration of acoustico-gnostic processes. In addition, they may appear secondarily with articulatory dis-

* This method was first proposed and used by R. E. Levina and R. M. Boskis.

orders. This is explained by the fact that in order to recognize, identify, and remember speech sounds one needs not only primary auditory analysis but also an active component of auditory perception, *viz.*, silent reproduction of the articulatory schemata corresponding to the sounds heard.

The most severe loss of phonemic hearing is seen with lesions in the left temporal area. As we described above (Chapter 5) a patient with such a lesion may indicate that he is unable to recognize speech sounds. If the lesion is massive, he is unable to identify the phonemes imbedded in the flow of speech. His attempts to reproduce speech sounds show that he tends to confuse phonemes which have one or more features in common but which are otherwise quite different. The common feature which he relies upon may be quite irrelevant in terms of the phonemic system of the language. For instance, patients frequently confuse the two unvoiced stop plosives "k" and "t". That the defective reproduction of disjunctive phonemes is not due to an articulatory defect but to a defect of auditory differentiation is shown by the fact that the erroneous response is produced with no articulatory difficulty whatsoever.

In less severe cases this particular defect may be absent. As a rule, however, any disturbance of the acoustico-gnostic systems is accompanied by a certain amount of difficulty in the differentiation of oppositional phonemes. The patient perceives the phonemes as variants of one and the same sound. In contrast to this, pairs of sounds in which the constants are identical, e.g., the hard and soft "t' " 's in the sounds "to" and 'te" are almost never perceived by these patients as variants of the same sound. The soft "t" is more often confused with "c" or "s" than with the hard "t".

If one adds the instability of inner auditory images to the inability to recognize individual sounds it becomes clear that the disturbance of auditory perception removes an essential prerequisite for the reliable perception and comprehension of oral statements. Impairment of the phonemic organization of hearing is not the only factor which may disturb the precise perception of speech sounds. It has been found that a less severe but easily detectable defect of auditory discrimination may arise as a result of the loss of inner articulatory schemata which occurs in afferent motor aphasia. The patient with afferent motor aphasia shows clear-cut signs of difficulty in differentiating similar speech sounds; he makes the same mistakes whether he repeats them orally or writes them down. He has difficulty in distinguishing the phonemes themselves and thus, in distinguishing the words in which they appear. The most characteristic feature of speech perception in such a case is that the patient tends to confuse not only phonemes which sound alike but also phonemes which are articulated similarly, the so called "homorgans", e.g., "t", "n", and "l", or "m", "b", and "p". These errors are observed most clearly in the patient's writing. Words which include sounds that are articulated similarly cease to be accurately differentiated. As a result, the patient shows secondary impairment of the ability to identify speech sounds and to recognize the sound patterns of meaningful words. These defects show that the active articulatory processes play a role in speech perception just as singing to oneself or tapping out the rhythm plays a role in the appreciation of music.[2]

B. COMPREHENSION OF VERBAL MEANINGS

The ability to recognize the meanings of words develops relatively early in childhood and represents one of the most stable speech functions. If certain conditions necessary for the accurate recognition of word meanings are removed, however, this function may be severely disturbed. The disturbance may take one of two forms. The phonemic pattern of the word may lose its constancy; it may become vague, so that "primary identification" of the word is impaired; the sound pattern of the word may become diffuse, or it may be forgotten altogether. On the other hand, the auditory aspect of the word may be preserved while its meaning becomes very narrowed; the system of generalizations surrounding the word may be so reduced that it retains its meaning only in certain very concrete situations. The investigation of word comprehension gives information not only about the disturbance of verbal meanings but also permits one to describe the nature of the disturbance and its underlying mechanism. Evaluation of the inability to recognize word meanings must take into account the conditions under which the disturbance of word comprehension occurs, the stability of verbal meanings and what factors help to compensate for the defect.

The investigation of word comprehension involves the following series of tests:

1. *Preservation of the Nominative Function of Words*

The patient is presented the names of a number of objects. He must recognize the names and point out the corresponding objects or explain in words or by means of gestures what the words mean. In order to determine how well the meanings of words are preserved, the degree of constancy of word meanings, and the factors which help to compensate for any defect present three further tests may be carried out:

(a) One should determine whether the meanings of words are preserved only when the objects they represent are present or *whether the meanings of words are always present.* First the examiner names a series of objects which are lying before the patient. He is asked to point out the objects as they are named. In a control test the examiner names objects which are not present in the patient's visual field and which he must either find somewhere in the room or describe by means of words and gestures. One may present relatively rare words or words which have several syllables in common, e.g., "zausenica" (hangnail) or "lossosina" (salmon). If the meaning of the word is

[2] Careful studies of factors of sound perception in aphasia were made recently in our laboratory by E. N. Vinarskaja.

unstable the patient has no difficulty in carrying out the first task, but if he cannot combine the word with simultaneous perception of the object he may have considerable difficulty in recognizing the word.

(b) One should determine whether the word retains its meaning *in inner speech* or whether the patient can only recognize it when he speaks it aloud. First the patient is asked to point out objects named by the examiner without repeating the names aloud. In the control test he repeats the name aloud and then points to the object. Inability to carry out the first test with a patient who has no difficulty with the second test indicates that the defect of comprehension is associated with a disturbance of inner speech.

(c) One should determine whether or not the patient recognizes the meanings of words *in isolation* or whether they must occur in a meaningful context. If the patient is unable to recognize words presented individually he may be asked to define their meanings on the basis of their use in meaningful sentences. If words are only recognized when imbedded in sentences there is a severe disturbance of the nominative function of speech with preservation of the comprehension of semantic constructions.

2. *The Stability of Nominative Word Function*

This group of tests should determine the stability of word recognition under conditions of varying complexity; it consists of three basic tests:

a. *Tests of the Stability of Word Meanings with Repeated Use*

This test reveals the degree to which inhibition may affect the stability of word meanings. The examiner names several objects, e.g., eye, ear, and nose, many times in random order and the patient is instructed to point at the objects as they are named. If the word meanings are sufficiently stable the patient can continue to follow such instructions for a long time. If the stability of word meanings is not adequate however, the patient will cease to recognize them after the first three or four trials and will begin to point at random or to perseverate the meaning of past words.

b. *Test of the Stability of Word Meanings as a Function of the Amount of Information to be Retained*

The patient is asked to point out one, two, or three objects which are all named at once. If his perceptual field is reduced he will be able to recognize only one of the words. The second and third will either lose their meanings or be quickly forgotten.

c. *Test of the Stability of Word Meanings in Time*

This test approaches the investigation of *memory function*. In this case the patient is given one or two words. At the end of a given time interval he is to point at the corresponding objects. Disturbance of the stability of the memory traces of words is revealed when the words lose their meanings under delayed response conditions, i.e., if they or their meanings are forgotten after a short time.

3. *The Structure of Word Meanings*

In contrast to the foregoing tests, this series concerns not the stability of the primary meanings of words but the breadth of the generalization which lie behind them. The patient is asked to define words when they are used in a broad or metaphorical sense. Here it is useful to assess the depth of such concepts as "liquid", "surrogate", "transport", etc. Similarly, one investigates the comprehension of methaphors, e.g., "an iron fist", "a golden head", "the forest sings", etc. Comprehension of the direct meanings with an inability to understand words used in less concrete situations or in a metaphorical sense indicates not a disturbance of the stability of the nominative functions of words but a loss of their inner semantic structure.

In studying the preservation of word meanings the examiner may derive great benefit from tests in which the patient is asked to point out objects fitting the meanings of given words, e.g., "building", "tree", or "vehicle". If the patient is able to choose objects which fit into a given category the structure of meanings associated with the corresponding word is intact. Restriction of the selection, so that, e.g., only military vehicles are categorized under the term "vehicle" indicates a constriction of word meanings. The inclusion of objects which might be associated with the given word in certain concrete situations, e.g., the inclusion of such objects as "stove", "pipe" and "furniture", in the category "building", indicates a loss of the categorical meaning of the word. The generalizations behind the word have taken on a "complex" concrete character.

Similar methods for investigating word meanings by having patients classify various objects have been developed by Gelb and Goldstein (categorization of nuances belonging to a certain color), Vygotskij (classification of art figures corresponding to a given word), Weigl, and others. Thus this type of technique is quite valuable for the clinico-psychological investigation of aphasia.

The preservation of stable word meanings presupposes a high level of integration of cortical processes. Without such integration neither the unity of the sound pattern of a word nor the meaningful category which it represents can exist. Thus it is understandable that both in the initial period of traumatic aphasia, when important systems of the speech areas are not functioning, and in cases of massive damage to these systems word comprehension is unreliable. V. M. Kogan has observed that patients with such disturbances are unable to recognize word meanings; they hear the words but find them empty of meaning. They recognize the meanings of words only when they are simultaneously able to observe the objects which the words represent. If the objects are removed, the words immediately lose their meaning. Such patients usually have an expressive speech defect. Only in very serious cases does the absence of the inner constancy of word meanings persist for a long time. Usually a period of total loss gives way to a period in which words regain their meanings, but the meanings are very unstable and the inner semantic structure of words remains constricted. At this stage patients recognize the meanings of words only in a very narrow concrete sense. Any generalization, abstraction, or use of words in other than a concrete sentence is incomprehensible to such patients. Thus the range of events about which they can communicate is severely restricted. Simple recognition of these disturbances does not help one to evaluate the roles played by the various individual functions in the loss of comprehension of verbal meanings. In order to do this one must look for the specific features of disturbances arising as a result of lesions in different areas.

The *impairment of auditory perception* which results from lesions in the left temporal area removes an important factor needed for the comprehension of verbal meanings. A word which loses its precise phonemic structure also loses its precise meaning. A patient who has "lost the meanings of words" is able to repeat words as they are presented, but he is unable to identify their meanings. Simultaneous presentation of the objects which words represent may also be ineffective. The patient continues to repeat the word without recognizing its meaning.

Loss of word meanings as a result of loss of the acoustico-gnostic structure of words may not be absolute. The word meanings may merely become vague and unstable. Observations made in our clinic by È. S. Bejn have shown that in these cases word meanings become diffuse; words may be confused with other words which have similar sound patterns. Thus the word "metka" (sign) may, on various presentations, be perceived as with "med" (honey), "metla" (broom) or "metall'" (metal). Usually the meaning of the root part of the word suffers more than suffixes or inflective aspects. Thus a patient who has forgotten the direct meanings of words is still able to relate them to the proper semantic categories.

In many cases, loss of the phonemic structure of words may be relatively mild compared to the loss of word meanings. The patient is able to repeat words with little alteration of phonemic patterns, but he is still unable to understand them. He retains a certain feeling of familiarity with a word and knows the "sphere" to which it is related, but if he is to use it he must either guess at its precise meaning or analyze it etymologically. The following are typical responses of patients with impairment of the acoustico-gnostic systems when asked to define particular words. For the word "elbow" the patient may point at the shoulder, elbow, head or fingernail and say, "Something having to do with the arm". In the most severe cases of temporal aphasia, disturbances of this type may be revealed by tests involving very simple words. In more subtle cases, however, more sensitive tests are required, e.g., tests involving the repetition of one group of words several times. One indication of the degree of impairment is the rapidity with which the words lose their meaning. Figure 59 depicts the increase in the stability of word meanings which occurred as postoperative edema disappeared over a two week period in a case involving the left temporal area. As was indicated above, the *words which a patient is unable to comprehend singly may regain their meaning if they are incorporated into meaningful verbal context*. Thus a patient who does not comprehend the word "death" when it is spoken by itself may be able to understand it in the context "death at the hand of the German occupants". This phenomenon is explained by the preservation of comprehension of phraselogical structure which is typical with damage to these areas.

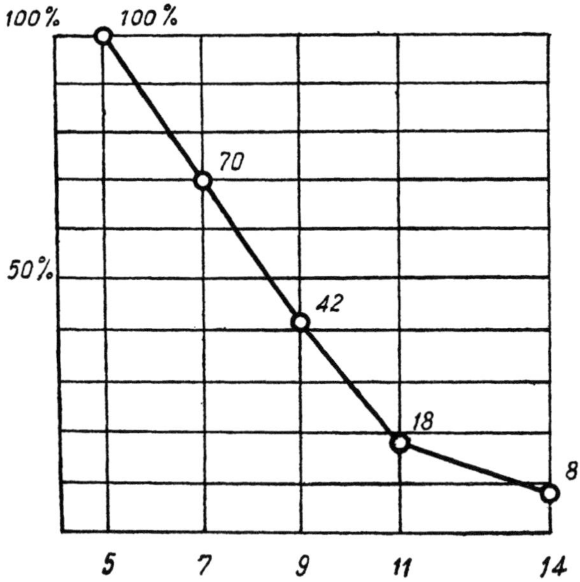

FIG. 59. Percent of word meanings lost after an operation of the temporal area.

In temporal lobe aphasia the disturbance of speech comprehension resulting from primary loss of the acoustico-gnostic structure of words affects all words equally; the constriction of word meanings, or loss of their categorical structure, is not typical of temporal aphasia. Recognition of the meanings represented by the words may suffer not only as a result of damage to the acoustico-gnostic systems. In some cases severe impairment of *expressive speech* may produce a secondary disturbance of word comprehension. Clinical observations of our own and separate experiments by O. P. Kaufman and L. K. Nazarova have shown that these disturbances may have either of two origins. In some cases they are associated with loss of the inner articulatory schemata which are normally involved in speech perception, i.e., which take a part in what Wernicke referred to as the "primary identification of words". Thus patients with severe afferent motor aphasia may have difficulty in the immediate recognition of words. This is most apt to occur with words which are not very familiar or which are so complex that their recognition requires precise analysis of phonemic structure. Patients who lack the normal "innervational sensations" and thus are unable to differentiate sounds which are similar in articulation are unable to carry out an adequate auditory analysis of words. The component phonemes of words are not adequately differentiated. Consequently the patient receives vague impressions of the words rather than precise perceptions. Such vague impressions are devoid of precise meaning. The source of the disturbance becomes especially clear if one compares word comprehension when the corresponding object is present with comprehension when the object is absent. Similarly one may compare comprehension when visual analysis of the examiner's articulatory movements is present and when the opportunity for such analysis is absent. A typical motor aphasic with a clear-cut disturbance of articulatory schemata may perform as follows: when all external articulatory movements are suppressed (by pressure applied to the tongue) he recognizes only 30% of the words presented; when he is allowed to pronounce the words and observe the oral movements of the experimenter he recognizes 80%; when the objects named are present in his visual field he is able to recognize 100% of the words.

This experiment brings us to the effects of *impairment of inner speech* on the comprehension of verbal meanings. By observing patients with efferent motor aphasia and severe impairment of inner speech it was found that the process of primary word identification may be severely affected if external speech is suppressed. Patients in this group may be able to recognize words only if they repeat the words aloud. The examiner can sometimes block the primary recognition of words by depressing a patient's tongue. Instead of genuinely understanding words such a patient often guesses at their meanings on the basis of a few features; sometimes his attempts are characterized by perseveration. Thus a disturbance of motor speech and its inner schemata may, under certain conditions, lead to a "pseudosensory" disturbance of the ability to understand verbal meanings.

In all of the cases described so far the source of the disturbance was an impairment of the primary identification of words. Disruption of the acoustico-gnostic systems led to a vagueness and instability of word meanings; motor aphasia produced a temporary loss and sometimes a constriction of word meanings. Cases have been observed, however, in which lesions of the tertiary perceptual areas of the cortex left the phonemic structure of words intact but at the same time produced distinct changes in word meanings. This situation arises in *semantic aphasia.* Outwardly the comprehension of words may be preserved. The patient easily hears and recognizes words; he has no difficulty in pointing out the objects which they represent. He shows no signs of having forgotten the meanings of most words. Only when asked the meanings of words which represent specific relationships, e.g., the prepositions "over" and "under", or "right" and "left", does he show any difficulty. Here, however, he tends to confuse one term with another. Close observation reveals that behind this disorder there lies a disturbance of the generalizations or connotations which comprise part of the actual meanings of words. Simple tasks requiring the definition of such concepts or the comprehension of metaphorical expressions immediately reveal the loss of word meanings in these patients.

They define concepts in very narrow and concrete terms; usually they recognize only the simplest functional characteristics of objects. Not infrequently they have difficulty in recognizing words used in a figurative sense; they tend to recognize only the literal meanings of words. They often show the disturbance of "categorical thought" which has been studied in detail by Goldstein. Words are used only to refer to concrete situations; they lose their abstract or categorical significance. This is shown by the fact that the patients tends to relate all the objects associated with a concrete situation to a given word. On the other hand, they are unable to relate a word to its categorical equivalents. The meaning of a word loses its generalizing character, thus giving rise to the way of handling meaningful material characteristic of patients with semantic aphasia.

C. COMPREHENSION OF GRAMMATICAL STRUCTURE

The investigation of receptive speech involves more than a test of the ability to comprehend verbal meanings. Even more important is investigation of the ability to *comprehend grammatical structure and the predicative aspect of speech.* As pointed out above, the ability to comprehend statements as a whole is not necessarily a sign that the patient is able to master all the grammatical constructions which may be used in the communication of thoughts. In a situation where the practical significance of a statement is obvious the patient may be able to understand it, even though its formulation is very fragmentary. If the examiner points to the open door through which the patient has entered and says, "The door?" this fragmentary statement is capable of conveying the same meaning as the sentence, "The door should be closed; you have forgotten to close it". Here only one component of the statement has been expressed verbally; the predicate of the message lies outside the verbal statement, i.e., it lies in the concrete surroundings supplemented by the gesture of the examiner.

The fact that the meanings of statements may be comprehended without genuine grasp of their grammatical structure has not been given adequate attention in many clinical investigations. Such common instructions as, "Open your mouth", "Extend your tongue", and "Raise your hand", may be understood even though the ability to grasp the grammatical structure of sentences is severely diminished. The clinical examination itself is well enough structured so that hearing the single word "mouth !" is sufficient to induce the patient to open his mouth; hearing the word "tongue" is sufficient to have him extend it; hearing the word "hand" may lead the patient to raise it automatically. An examiner who concludes that speech comprehension is intact on the basis of such tests may acquire a quite false impression of the patient's receptive speech.

In order to investigate the true limitations of speech comprehension, tests must be so constructed that the patient is unable to derive the meanings of the statements from his surroundings. The meaning of his verbal instructions should be comprehensible to him only if he is capable of grasping the grammatical relationships of words in the statement. The comprehension of individual words is, of course, not sufficient to guarantee genuine understanding of expansive statements. Two other conditions must be met. The patient must grasp and retain the *sequence of words,* for word omission or alteration of word sequence may change the meaning of the statement. Secondly he must grasp the *significance of grammatical relationships* which bind together the individual words of complex statements. These two prerequisites of speech comprehension may be disrupted by various brain lesions to produce a loss of complex receptive speech. A special series of tests has been developed for the investigation of these functions.

Methods for the evaluation of a patient's ability to comprehend complex speech include the following tests:[3]

1. *Comprehension of Simple Inflectional Forms*

The patient is presented three objects, e.g., a key, a pencil, and a comb, and is asked to point out the objects as they are named. He is then asked to name the objects himself in any order. Next, a grammatical element is introduced into the instruction regarding the order in which he is to name them. Finally, the grammatical structure of the instruction is made more complicated. The three phases of this experiment are carried out as follows:

(a) The patient is asked to point out pairs of objects as they are named, e.g., "pencil-key", "key-comb", "comb-pencil", etc. The results of this test show the degree to which he is able to perceive the words and to preserve their order.

(b) With no pause or change in intonation the patient is presented the same pairs of words, but this time, with inflective endings, e.g., "With the pencil, point at the key", "with the key, point at the comb", etc.[4] In this test the patient must not only remember the words in their correct order, but he must also grasp the grammatical relationships imposed by the instrumental case suffix. If he ignores the suffix one has evidence for a disturbance of the ability to grasp the logico-grammatical significance of inflective relationships.

(c) Again, without pause or change in intonation, the order of the words is changed. Whereas in the previous test the order of words always corresponded to the order of actions, e.g., the patient was to use the first named object pointing at the second, the order of actions in this test is different from the order of words; the relationship is in-

[3] The tests included in this outline include techniques introduced both by H. Head and by ourselves through many years of clinico-psychological investigation. A psycholinguistic analysis of these tests was presented elsewhere (A. R. Luria, *Studies in Aphasia*, part II. *Semantic Aphasia*, unpublished).

[4] In Russian a noun is placed in the instrumental case simply by adding a suffix. Thus the only difference between the instructions "Point at the key, ... at the pencil", and "Point with the key at the pencil" is an instrumental case ending on the word for "key". The sentence, "Point at the key, ... at the pencil" is "Pokažite ključ, ... karandaš"; the phrase "Point with the key at the pencil" is "Pokažite ključom karandaš". (trans.)

verted. Such instructions as "Point at the pencil with the comb", or "point at the key with the pencil" belong in this category. In order to carry out such instructions correctly the patient must inhibit his immediate tendency to point at objects in the order in which they are named. He must grasp the second object and point at the first. In order to carry out the inverted instruction he must not only understand the grammatical relationships of the words, but he must overcome a tendency to carry out the instruction according to the direct sequence of words. He must resist the impulse to grasp the first object and point at the second.

2. *Comprehension of Attributive Constructions*

Comprehension of attributive constructions: the patient is asked to explain simple constructions consisting of two words so related that one represents an object while the other represents a qualitative characteristic of the object. Such constructions include the following types: (1) constructions involving possessive adjectives, e.g., "mother's daughter", "daughter's mother", etc.; (2) constructions involving the genitive-attributive case, e.g., "the daughter of the mother", "the brother of the father", "the father of the brother", "the brother of the boss", "the boss of the brother", etc.

In each case the patient must recognize the grammatical construction and ignore the direct meaning of one of the words if he is to comprehend the meaning of the construction as a whole. The task usually takes either of two forms. In some cases the patient looking at a picture representing for instance, a woman and child, is asked to tell, "Which is the mother?", "which is the daughter?" and then, "which is the mother's daughter?" and "which is the daughter's mother?" The second type of task is similar to the first except that no picture is involved. The patient must either explain the construction or define the difference between two constructions which are similar to one another; e.g., "The brother of the boss" versus "the boss of the brother". Finally, one may present nonsense constructions, such as, "The wife of the sister" to be compared with the meaningful construction, "The sister of the wife". The task in this case is to tell which of the two is the nonsense construction.

It has been shown experimentally that patients with a third grade education, and sometimes even less, have no difficulty in understanding such constructions. Inability to comprehend the grammatically determined relationships becomes apparent when a patient asked to point out "The mother's daughter" points instead at the two figures in turn and says, "Here is the mother, and here is the daughter", or when he considers the two constructions "brother of the boss" and "boss of the brother" to have the same meaning. Such responses indicate a disturbance of the comprehension of inflective relationships.

3. *Comprehension of Relationships Expressed by Prepositions*

The patient is asked to draw "a circle under a triangle" or "a triangle under a circle". An inability to grasp the meaning of this instruction or failure to carry it out correctly indicates a difficulty in the mastery of grammatical relationships. Another form of the same test is to present the two instructions and ask the patient to define the difference between them.

A more complicated form of the same problem involves the "triple construction". The patient may be asked, for instance, to "draw a circle under a triangle and above a cross" or to "place the fountain pen to the right of the key and to the left of the comb". Inability to carry out such an instruction is again, symptomatic of the loss of comprehension of logico-grammatical relationship.

4. *Comprehension of Comparative Constructions*

The patient is presented two sentences expressing comparisons of the following type: "An elephant is larger than a fly"; "a fly is larger than an elephant". The patient is asked to explain the difference between the two statements and to tell which of them is correct. In a similar, but more complex test he is presented two slips of paper of differing colors and asked to indicate which of the two is lighter, which is darker, which is less light, and which is less dark. The same may be done using weights. In this case he is to tell which is heavier, which is lighter, which is less heavy, etc. If the patient has a receptive agrammatism he will show a tendency to perceive the individual words in a given statement separately. Thus instead of understanding the construction "less light" correctly, he may understand it as less in size and lighter in shade.

A more complicated task involves triple construction of the type used by Burtt: "Mary is fairer than Ann and darker than Jenny; who is the fairest?" Similarly he may be presented three circles of different sizes and colors: red, green, and blue. He is asked, "Which of the circles is larger than the red one and smaller than the blue one?"

5. *Comprehension of Inverted Constructions*

Comprehension of the logico-grammatical statements presented in this test requires that the patient mentally reverses the order in which words occur in the instruction. An example of such a grammatical construction is the passive statement, "The earth is illuminated by the sun". This construction may sound less correct to the patient than, "The sun is illuminated by the earth", simply because the order of words does not correspond to the usual subject-predicate-object pattern. A more complex type of problem which requires the same mental inversion is, "I ate after I chopped some wood. Which did I do first?", in which the connective "after" reverses the chronological order of the events named. An inability to grasp the real meaning of these constructions is a sign of receptive agrammatism.

6. *Comprehension of Complex Grammatical Constructions*

Whereas the preceding tests are designed to assess the comprehension of different grammatical elements, this series of tests is designed to evaluate the ability to comprehend complex grammatical speech as a whole. The patient is presented two long sentences, one of which is grammatically simple while the other involves complex grammatical and logical relationships.

An example of a simple sentence is the following: "Father and mother went to the theatre, but the old nurse and the children stayed home". The patient reads this sentence twice and then is asked, "Who left? who remained home?" The examiner notes whether or not the patient is able to comprehend and remember the meaning of the statement. A complex sentence is one which cannot be comprehended without considering it as a whole and recognizing the grammatical interrelations of the parts. The best sentences for this purpose involve expanded constructions in which related phrases are separated by qualifying and subordinate clauses. Other such sentences may involve complex types of cause-effect relationships. An example of an expanded construction is the following: "To the school where Dunja studied a worker came from a factory to give a talk". The relationships between the individual meaningful elements in this sentence cannot be arrived at by guessing; they can be comprehended only if the ability to understand grammatical relationships is intact. The patient is presented a sentence of this sort several times and then asked such questions as, "Who gave the talk? Where was the talk given? Who studied at the school?" In order to determine whether failure to understand such a sentence results from an inability to remember or an inability to recognize grammatical relationships one may allow the patient to answer the questions with the sentence written on a sheet of paper before him.

Retention and comprehension of simple sentences with noncomprehension of the relationships implied by complex grammatical constructions indicates that the patient lacks the ability to recognize grammatical relationships.

7. *Comprehension of Fables*

This last group of tests is designed to evaluate the patient's ability to grasp the *general meaning* of a written passage without regard to the mastry of individual grammatical constructions. A simple story with an underlying moral is read to the patient several times. A very useful passage for this purpose is Tolstoy's story of "The Hen Who Laid the Golden Eggs". "A farmer had a hen who laid golden eggs. One day he wanted more gold; so he killed the hen. He expected to find a treasure of gold inside her, but he found nothing; for inside she was no different from any other hen". The patient is asked not only to repeat the contents of this story but also to tell its underlying meaning. He must attempt to generalize from it and to comprehend the motives underlying the action of the farmer. Finally, he should be able to tell the moral which the story illustrates. The ability to recognize the general meaning of such a story indicates preservation of the ability to go beyond the concrete content of a passage and to relate it to underlying motivation.

As with other disorders, disturbance of the comprehension of grammatical constructions may result from lesions in different brain areas and thus may appear as one aspect of several different types of aphasia. In each type, however, the basis for the comprehension defect is different; the mechanisms underlying the disburbances vary from case to case.

In patients with temporal lobe aphasia disturbance of acoustico-gnostic processes with the loss and instability of word meanings may produce considerable difficulty in understanding connected speech. The origin of the difficulty is by no means an impairment of the ability to grasp logico-grammatical constructions but simply the loss of the nominative aspect of words. The vagueness of word meanings and the rapidity with which words are lost from consciousness makes it extremely difficult for the temporal aphasic to understand connected sentences. His difficulties become apparent in the first test, which, in a sense, serves as a model for all tests of the ability to comprehend logico-grammatical constructions. When asked to "point at the pencil and the key" such a patient often fails to recognize the meanings of the words and points randomly at various objects; "Here is the pencil", (pointing at the key); "here is the key", (pointing at the comb). Sometimes the patient is unable to retain the word order but remembers the objects named in the instruction and points them out in some other sequence. Sometimes he simply forgets one of the words and has to ask over and over again, "Key . . . but what else? ! . . ." This last type of response is most often seen in cases of acoustico-mnestic disturbances in which there may be no loss of word meanings, but the ability to retain verbal sequences is severely impaired.

The comprehension of grammatical relationships may be undisturbed in cases of acoustico-gnostic disturbances or it may suffer secondarily as a result of loss of word meanings, imprecise recognition of inflective features, or inability to remember verbal sequences. Thus, in the test just described, the patient may grasp the inflective relations with little difficulty. For him the first signs of difficulty may arise when he is asked to interpret long or complex sentences. If he is able to recognize and remember the meanings of words, the grammatical construction can be mastered without difficulty. If he is unable to overcome the vagueness and instability of word meanings, the comprehension of complex grammatical constructions in subsequent tests is of course, impossible.

An altogether different type of comprehension difficulty arises in cases of motor aphasia, especially in those accompanied by disturbances of *inner speech.* A. Pick, L. S. Vygotskij (1934), and, more recently, A. N. Sokolov and others have noted that inner speech is an essential link not only between the emergence of intention and its transformation into external speech, but also in the processing of auditory speech antecedent to the comprehension of verbal statements. Grammatical speech which is complicated by expanded constructions, inversions, or length must be condensed by processes of inner speech. Inner speech is responsible in some cases for bringing the meaningfully related elements of sentences closer together, for assigning emphasis to the important parts, for establishing the predicative sense of statements and for transforming sentences into thoughts. It is easy to understand that a disturbance of this inner functional link may severely impair the ability to comprehend statements. Thus motor aphasics in whom inner speech is severely impaired have difficulty with the tests we have just described.

O. P. Kaufman has shown in investigations carried out in our laboratory that comprehension difficulties associated with disturbance of inner speech manifest themselves as an inability to grasp the meanings of statements immediately upon presentation. Often a patient must hear or read a sentence several times and repeat it to himself or better, aloud, before its meaning becomes clear to him. That which a normal person grasps immediately, the patient achieves only through a process involving a great deal of effort.

Further analysis shows the underlying cause of this difficulty. On first reading a sentence a patient, who has lost the predicative aspect of speech but who retains the designative, nominative aspect, is able to grasp only the objects and actions involved. He still does not know exactly what the sentence means. If, at this point, one prevents him from using external speech by having him open his mouth or hold his tongue between his teeth, the disturbance of inner speech prevents him from proceeding beyond the recognition of individual words; he is prevented from grasping the general meaning of the grammatical constructions involved. He can fulfil this task only if he is permitted to use external speech. If the sentence is so constructed that the use of external speech can be of no assistance, he will still be unable to comprehend it. Thus, in the first of the tests described above he may easily point out two objects as they are named and succeed in using one to point at the other. It is very unlikely, however, that he will be able to grasp the meaning of inverted constructions, i.e., to "point at one object with a second". In order to do this he must be able to abstract the proper relationship from the inverted word sequence and, by means of inner speech, formulate a sequence of actions which is the reverse of the sequence of words in the instruction. With special training he can learn to recognize such constructons, and by memorizing logical formulae he can learn to derive the proper relationships. Typically the first impression of such a patient as to the meaning of inverted logico-grammatical constructions is incorrect, but he can learn to make secondary corrections of his first impression. The primary defect lies not in the structure of meaning but in impairment of the *process* by which the meanings of grammatical constructions are derived.

The types of speech comprehension disturbance described so far have all been "pseudo-semantic" in character. The primary disorders of speech comprehension arise as a result of lesions in the tertiary perceptual systems and manifest themselves as the syndrome of *semantic aphasia.* In semantic aphasia the nominative and predicative aspects of speech are preserved. The patient has no difficulty in recognizing the names of individual objects and understands simple statements. He shows signs of difficulty only when the words in a statement are related grammatically to one another in such a way that the overall meaning cannot be derived on the basis of their concrete meanings. He has lost the ability to integrate all the aspects of a sentence into a single meaningful whole. Consequently, he is unable to grasp the meaning of relations. He is perfectly aware of the fact that certain words in the sentence must be combined to yield the meaning which he seeks, but he is unable to grasp their inter-relationships. External speech is of little help to him. The more he attempts to reason out the significance of what he has heard the more confused he becomes. Even after multiple attempts he cannot reach the proper conclusion.

In a patient with severe semantic aphasia the comprehension of logico-grammatical relations may be so disturbed that his disorder is exposed by very simple tests. He may fulfill the instruction, "Point at the key and the pencil", but be unable to tell the difference between this instruction and the inflected instruction, "point with the key at the pencil". If he does not perceive the relationship expressed by the inflected construction he points again at the two objects in turn: "Here is the key, and here is the pencil".

Difficulties emerge also with attempts to comprehend the other types of grammatical constructions described above. When confronted with attributive relationships the patient shows a similar inability to go beyond the concrete meanings of words. In attempting to understand the expression, "Mother's daughter", he is left with the impression that two different subjects are referred to, a mother and a daughter. He recognizes no difference between the expression, "brother of the boss" and "boss of the brother". The only difference which he sees is that the order of the words is different in the two expressions.

The comprehension of constructions involving prepositions presents extreme difficulty. When the patient is asked to draw a circle under a square he usually begins by drawing a circle and then, under it, he draws a square. As he does so he may say to himself, "Circle ... under ... square ...", thus revealing the "receptive agrammatism" which thwarts his attempts to comprehend grammatically complex instructions.

The same types of difficulties arise when a patient with semantic aphasia attempts to understand comparative constructions. Here again, the major difficulty lies in getting away from the nominative aspect of words. The individual terms "light," "dark," "lesser" and "taller" present no difficulty, but he is unable to carry out the process of abstraction necessary for comprehending such an expression as "less dark." It is impossible for him to understand that "less dark" refers to the lighter of two shades of a color rather than to an object which is less in height and dark in color.

It is to be expected that the comprehension of inverted and expanded constructions should be severely disturbed in these cases. Characteristically patients with semantic aphasia make multiple helpless attempts to recreate or recognize the proper logico-grammatical relationships by rearranging the words of a sentence.[5]

These disturbances constitute a great obstacle to the comprehension of grammatical speech in patients with semantic aphasia. Such "technical" obstacles by no means deprive them of the ability to understand the general meaning of some statements. They are assisted in this respect by preservation of the ability to grasp the significance of the general settings in which meaningful statements are uttered and by preservation of certain familiar phrases and logical operations of thought. Since they are perfectly well oriented to the practical significance of their sur-

[5] A detailed psychological analysis of speech comprehension in patients with semantic aphasia has been reported by V. K. Bubnova in her work, *Disturbance of the Comprehension of Logico-Grammatical Constructions with Brain Damage* (1946, dissertation).

roundings, such patients have difficulty in grasping the intentions underlying statements. Thus, they can often reconstruct the meanings of fragmentary statements, fables, or anecdotes, despite the fact that they are unable to analyze grammatically the verbal constructions involved. With this type of compensatory mechanism intact, the semantic aphasic finds himself in the same position as a person attempting to grasp the general meaning of sentence fragments in a language, the grammar of which he knows very poorly. The fact that such compensation is possible indicates that there is a great difference between the processes by which the grammatical meanings and the practical contextual meanings of statements are recognized.

On the basis of the above it is possible to understand a clinical observation which might otherwise appear paradoxical. Patients with disturbances of the acoustico-gnostic process, as well as patients with semantic aphasia who are unable to comprehend simple logico-grammatical constructions, are generally capable of grasping the general meaning of statements and fables. This observation is explained by the fact that comprehension of the motives underlying statements or the general meaning of statements is essentially a different process from that of comprehending individual words and sentences. Grasping the intent behind a statement can often occur on the basis of very fragmentary perception of the words or sentences involved. It involves psychological and cerebral mechanisms which are apparently preserved with the receptive forms of aphasia, but which are severely disturbed in, for instance, certain cases of frontal lobe damage.

XIII

THE INVESTIGATION OF SPEECH PROCESSES: READING AND WRITING

Disturbances of reading and writing are probably the most common symptoms of traumatic aphasia. The investigation and clinico-psychological classification of these symptoms is far from simple and must be based upon psychological examination techniques. Reading and writing can by no means be broken down into two entirely separate processes as was often attempted by the classical neurologists. What one attempts to evaluate is the *conscious utilization of speech processes* and the *conscious manipulation of phonemes* which are basic to both. Reading and writing is a *special level of speech activity,* the psychological structure and functional characteristic of which are considerably different from those of oral speech.

Spontaneous oral speech serves as a direct means of transmitting concepts or thoughts. In writing, however, one must deal not only with sounds, but with letters, the symbols which represent sounds. Even when writing has become a highly skilled process, the analysis of a dictated or internally generated word into individual sounds, the selection of the appropriate letters to represent these sounds, and the arrangement of letters into proper sequence continues to occupy the consciousness of the writer. The same is sometimes true of reading. Thus, writing differs from oral speech in its functional characteristics. Normally a person is not conscious of the process by which he pronounces sounds in oral speech. On the other hand, writing is a conscious process. The conscious direction of attention to letters (or, in reading, to syllables) is most pronounced during the early stages of learning to write. With the development of writing habits the consciousness of individual elements may give way to awareness of whole words. All the same, this conscious feature continues to distinguish reading and writing from oral speech.

Finally, the origins of these processes are considerably different. Whereas oral speech develops as a direct result of imitating and communicating with others, written speech develops as a result of conscious study, and continues to bear traces of its origin even in its most advanced stages of development.

Psychologically the writing process involves several steps. The flow of speech is broken down into individual sounds. The phonemic significance of these sounds is identified and the phonomes represented by letters. Finally, the individual letters are integrated to produce the written word. The only difference between this process and reading lies in the order of the steps. Thus, it is clear that the investigation of reading and writing should begin not with concern for the ability to read or write letters or words but with an assessment of the patient's ability to carry out the conscious *auditory analysis and synthesis* which are essential to both reading and writing. Once these prerequisites have been evaluated, it is possible to study the processes of reading and writing *per se*.

A. THE INVESTIGATION OF ACOUSTIC ANALYSIS AND SYNTHESIS

Acoustic analysis and synthesis are among the most important prerequisites for reading and writing. Several tests may be used to evaluate them. The patient must be able to extract phonemes from the smooth flow of speech sounds. The various sounds merge with one another and assume different auditory characteristics depending upon the sounds appearing before and after them. Thus each speech sound may have several "variants". The patient must be able to recognize the different variants of a given phoneme as being equivalent to one another and as being represented by a particular letter. Once the phonemes have been identified they must be retained so that, in writing down a given word, each letter may be appropriately combined with other letters to form a syllable. Finally, combinations of letters must be combined to form words. This is the process of acoustic analysis and it is an extremely important psychological prerequisite for writing.

It would be wrong to consider acoustic *analysis* a psychologically simple process. It requires that person be able to ignore the meaning of a word and turn his full attention to its auditory characteristics. He must be able to break down the complex of sounds and perceive the word as something other than a random flow of sound. He must be able to accommodate the word as a whole in his sphere of consciousness; otherwise he is unable to maintain the correct sound sequence.

The act of acoustic *synthesis,* the first step in the *reading* process, is no less complex than that of acoustic analysis. Here the individual sounds corresponding to the different letters must be brought into relation with other sounds to form more complex units. The pure sounds represented by the different letters must be modified to fit their context. Thus, the soft "t' " sound in the word "tina" (mud) is acoustically different from the hard "t" in the word "Tanja" (a girls name). In reading the words a person is able to make this distinction by means of acoustic synthesis. In order for such synthesis to be carried out, the various sounds must be clearly perceived. A given sound must be perceived the same each time it is heard; it should change only as is appropriate in relation to the preceding and succeeding letters. Only if these conditions are met is it possible to recognize set sequences of sounds and, in turn, to understand the meanings of whole words.

These two aspects of acoustic analysis and synthesis can be studied separately. Their investigation usually involves the following tests:

1. *Analysis for the Number of Sounds in Individual Words*

The patient is presented a word consisting of three, four, or, occasionally, five letters, e.g., "kot" (cat), "dom" (house), or "most" (bridge), and is asked to tell how many letters there are in the word. In order to show whether or not the patient is able to carry out this task by means of inner analysis the examiner asks him to analyze the word to himself. External speech can be blocked, for instance, by having him hold his tongue between his teeth. Inability to carry out this task without repeating the words aloud indicates a disturbance of inner analysis of the phonemic composition of words.

2. *Naming of the Sounds Represented in Words*

The patient is asked to tell what sounds are present in given words. He may be required to name the letters in a particular order which does not correspond to their order in the word, e.g., he may be asked to tell what the first, second, third, and fourth letters are in that sequence.

Ability to carry out the first task with inability to carry out the second indicates that the general intonational images of words are preserved but that their precise phonetic-articulatory content is disturbed.

3. *The Synthesis of Syllables and Words from Individually Pronounced Sounds*

The patient is presented several sounds in a series which taken together, form a syllable. In order to avoid direct sensory merging of the sounds each is separated from the next by a word, e.g., the examiner says, ' 't' then 'o' ", or " 'k', then 'r', then 'o' ". The patient is asked to tell what syllable is formed by these combinations of sounds. Testing the ability to synthesize short words is carried out in a similar fashion. Here such words as "k-o-t" (cat) or "n-o-s" (nose) are appropriate.

In order to determine what factors facilitate auditory synthesis these tests may be carried out first with and then without external speech. In another variation the patient may be allowed to observe the lip movements of the examiner as he pronounces the words.

A consideration of acoustic analysis and synthesis in various types of disorders helps in identifying the basic types of disturbance which affect the perception of auditory stimuli and thus give rise to writing difficulties.

The disturbance of *acoustic perception* associated with lesions in the temporal area seriously affects the process of acoustic analysis. The sounds of which the normal flow of speech is composed seem so chaotic and unstable to a patient with this type of disorder that he gathers only a vague impression of the individual phonemes. He hears words as conglomerations of sounds. Thus it is impossible for him to represent the sounds by letters. Although he may recognize the meaning of a word in context, he is usually unable to recognize its sound structure and is completely unable to break it down into its phonemic components. In severe cases patients may refuse even to attempt to tell how many letters there are in a word or they may give answers which are clearly conjectural. In either case it is obvious that they are unable to picture words to themselves. It is equally impossible for them to tell what sounds words are composed of. They have difficulty in breaking down complex sound patterns; they may substitute one sound for another or feel they hear distortion where a normal person perceives only the common softening or hardening of a consonant. Sometimes such patients have difficulty in preserving the order of sounds; all that they remember of a given word may be a disordered set of phonemes. These defects are observed even in late stages of recovery in temporal aphasia; so that accurate acoustic analysis remains a difficult problem.

Patients in this group also have great difficulty with acoustic synthesis. Their acoustic images of sounds are very vague and unstable. Often they confuse sounds which are similar to one another. Sounds, once heard, rapidly disappear from consciousness, and they do not fit together into any type of overall auditory pattern. Thus the patient whose acoustico-gnostic processes are impaired has difficulty with auditory synthesis and often attempts to compensate for his defect by guessing what the word might be on the basis of the sound fragments which he is able to catch.

Acoustic analysis and synthesis are affected in a different way when the basic disorder is a loss of articulatory schemata. As a rule, patients in this group are able to tell the number of sounds comprising different words much more easily than patients with auditory perceptual disturbances. Only in very severe cases is auditory analysis completely impossible. Significant difficulty arises in the recognition of words in which several consonants occur together, e.g., "Pskov" (a city) or "portnoj" (tailor). It can also occur in cases where the disturbance of articulatory schemata makes it difficult to break down sound complexes, thus preventing the patient from being able to tell how many individual sounds there are in different words. The major defect emerges however, when the patient attempts to identify the sounds of which words are composed. Here he has great difficulty due to the disturbance of articulatory schemata. If, for instance, the articulatory schema for the sound "n" is not sufficiently differentiated from the schemata of the sounds "l" and "t", it is natural to expect that he should sometimes pronounce the second letter in the word "snop" (bundle) as "l" or "t". Similar errors may occur when he attempts to identify other consonants and vowels, e.g., to differentiate "m", "b", and "p", or "o", and "u". In this situation he may perceive the word "sup" (soup) as consisting of the sounds "s-o-m" (a type of fish); or he may identify the word "slon" (elephant) as consisting of the sounds "s-t-o-l" (table). In severe cases the loss of articulatory schemata may make it difficult for patients to differentiate between sounds which are articulated quite differently from one another. He may correctly state the number of sounds in a word but be unable to name any of the sounds involved.

It is extremely interesting that in this type of case one of the best methods of compensating for the articulatory defect is observing the oral movements used to pronounce the words. A patient who is unable to recognize a single sound with his eyes closed may be able to do so if he observes the examiner's pronunciation or follows his own articulatory movements in a mirror.

Acoustic synthesis offers no additional difficulties to the patient who has lost the articulatory schema of sounds. The typical errors described above can be explained in terms of the role which the articulatory schemata normally play in sharpening and fixing the speech sounds. The disturbance of articulatory schemata and the partial loss of phonemic hearing affect primarily the ability to recognize speech sounds, to differentiate them from other sounds, and to fix them in memory. There exist, however, cases in which the basic defect is not in the identification of individual sounds but in loss of the sequential schemata of whole words. Though they may occur together with other syndromes, these disturbances are seen most clearly in efferent motor aphasia. They affect both acoustic analysis and acoustic synthesis. A patient who is able to recognize the number of sounds in the word may be unable to tell the order in which they occur. When asked the order of letters in a word, such a patient gives an answer which is based more on the intensity of the various sounds then on their actual positions in the word. He may not even be able to tell which letter comes first. For instance, he may say that the first letter of the word "okno" (window) is "k". Such a patient is totally unable to tell the order of letters in a word in which several consonants appear together. In some cases he may succeed in figuring out the sequence of sounds if the words are spoken loudly and with very distinct articulation; but this is difficult because of the loss of the inner schemata of words.

The patient's difficulty becomes more extreme when he is asked to synthesize or to combine individual sounds into syllables or whole words. As a rule he is unable to do so. He either combines the sounds in a random fashion, e.g., "k-t-o (who), 'kot' (cat)? . . . 'tok' (current)? . . . 'kto' (who) . . . 'otk' (meaningless)? . . .", or he attempts to guess its meaning.

Characteristically, this inability to recognize the order of sounds in a word persists even after the patient regains oral speech. The ability to recognize the order of sounds appears very late in comparison to re-acquisition of the practical use of speech. It is a long time before the patient is able to raise the acoustic synthesis of words to a conscious level. Until he is able to do so he must compensate for this defect by mechanically repeating words to himself and listening to the sequence of sounds.

Finaly we should consider the changes in acoustic analysis and synthesis which arise with damage to the parieto-occipital systems, i.e., the systems concerned with simultaneous perceptual integration. Perhaps on the basis of what we have said earlier these systems may be expected to play little or no role in the integration of auditory stimuli. This is not true, however, for loss of the patterning of simultaneous excitation affects the simultaneous organization of verbal processes. We have frequently observed that patients with damage to the occipito-parietal systems and severe simultaneous agnosia may be able to name the sounds of which a word is composed in correct sequence but unable to answer such questions as, "What is the third sound in the word? . . . what is the second sound?" etc. This task requires the ability to picture to oneself the structure of the word as a whole and is impossible for such a patient to perform. He may be able to compensate for his defect by naming all of the sounds in order until he arrives at the correct answer, but it is clear that the process of auditory synthesis is totally lacking. Although he is able to repeat the entire sequence of sounds he is unable to combine them into a single, simultaneous pattern from which he can extract the desired element.

B. THE INVESTIGATION OF THE WRITING PROCESS

Writing disorders accompany almost every form of aphasia. Only in a very few of the several hundred cases which we studied did the writing process remain intact. These involved primarily lesions of the infero-temporal and infero-parietal areas. Only in two or three cases did we find writing unimpaired in patients whose lesions involved the primary speech areas and who showed severe disturbance of the phasic aspect of speech.

The writing disturbances which we observed were quite variable in character. In some cases the cause of the writing disorder was a loss of the visual schemata of letters (graphemes) with no detectable disturbance of the acoustic analysis of sounds. In others the basic disturbance was a loss of preliminary auditory analysis resulting from inability to extract phonemes from the flow of connected speech, to categorize the sounds and to identify their place in the overall structure of words. In a third group of cases these two functions were not disturbed, but a writing disorder developed due to loss of patterned movements and inability to denervate motor patterns once they were established. These different writing disturbances resulted from damage to different primary functions. Thus, the primary functions should be considered individually.

The investigation of writing must take into account one factor which was not pertinent to the investigation of expressive and receptive speech. Whereas the automaticity of oral speech does not vary greatly from one person to another, the skill with which different subjects write varies greatly. The psychological organization depends upon the degree to which it is automatized. In a person who has just learned to write the auditory analysis of words and the determination of what constant phonemes are involved constitute a large part of the writing process. Major attention is directed to the correct formation of individual letters. Preservation of the proper order of letters requires secondary corrections which are frequently made by spelling the words aloud. By way of contrast, a person for whom writing has become almost an automatic process directs his attention not so much to individual letters as to whole words or sound-letter complexes. What to the inexperienced person is the major object of conscious effort becomes a less conscious, automatically executed operation. Analysis of the positions of phonemes in a word is carried out automatically. In the words of N. A. Bernštejn, the placing of letters becomes the "object of primary correction". With further development certain words, e.g., one's signature, come to be written automatically, on the basis of unitary motor engrams.

The investigator describing writing disorders must never forget that knowledge of the psychological structure of the writing process previous to trauma is significant for the evaluation of writing defects. In different cases the same "symptom" may have different causes.

For purposes of investigation writing is broken down into *copying* and *writing per se*. Evaluation of the ability to copy written material tests for preservation of the visuomotor prerequisites of writing. The investigation of *writing per se* includes tests of the ability to write very familiar words, to write to dictation, to write down the names of objects, and finally, to write narratively.

1. *Copying Letters and Words*

The patient is asked to copy letters or words presented in various types of print and written in various styles of longhand. The examiner notes whether or not the patient copies letters as though he were reproducing a drawing, i.e., with rigid adherance to all features of the letters without regard to their significance. This type of copying is to be contrasted with copying based upon genuine recognition of graphemes. Easy reproduction of printed and handwritten words indicates preservation of the phonemic symbols. A similar purpose is served by having the patient read the stylized letters and point them out from a printed alphabet.

In order to determine the degree of stability of visual images the patient may be shown a word and then asked to write it from memory.

2. *Automatic Writing*

The patient is asked to write his signature. He may be asked to write his address also. Preservation of the ability to write such familiar words in a patient who is unable to write to dictation indicates retention of highly automatized motor components of the writing process.

3. *Writing Individual Letters to Dictation*

The examiner dictates individual letters and the patient writes them down or points them out from a printed alphabet. In order to evaluate various factors which may help him to compensate for his writing defect this test is carried out first with the exclusion of external speech, secondly with the patient repeating the letter aloud, and, finally, with the patient observing the movements of the examiner's lips as he pronounces the sound.

This test will reveal any difficulty which he has in recognizing sounds.

4. *Writing Simple and Complex Words to Dictation*

The examiner dictates simple open syllables, such as "ba", "ta", "po", and "ti"; closed syllables such as "at", "ot", "ir", and "uk", and complex syllables including two or more consonants, such as "kru", "tro", and "stra". In each case the patient writes down the syllable or points to the corresponding letters in the alphabet. If he has difficulty with this test the examiner may clarify which factors are responsible for the difficulty by having him carry out the task first silenlty, then repeating the syllables aloud, and, finally, observing the lip movements associated with production of the sound.

If a patient has no difficulty writing down individual letters to dictation but has difficulty with this task it can be said that he shows a disturbance of the schemata of sound sequences.

5. *Writing Words to Dictation*

The patient is asked to write several words which vary in the complexity of phonemic structure, e.g., "noga" (leg), "okno" (window), "stročka" (stitch) or "prostranstvo" (space). This test differs from the previous one in that the phonemic patterns constitute meaningful words. Thus, they are easier to remember and preservation of the visual images of the words may assist the patient in writing them down.

6. *Naming Objects and Expressing Thoughts in Written Form*

The patient is asked to write down the names of objects presented to him. In a more complex task, he may be asked to write a letter or to write down the contents of a passage he has read. The goal of this task is to determine the degree to which he retains the inner, auditory schemata of words and the extent to which he can use them in writing words and sentences. (Testing of the ability to write spontaneous narrative is not part of the initial investigation of writing.)

In spite of the fact that different writing disorders accompany almost all forms of aphasia, their origins are not usually difficult to establish. Primary disturbance of the *visual schemata of letters* is reflected in a very distinct type of writing impairment. Investigations reported by a number of authors, including O. P. Kaufman of our laboratory and B. G. Anan'ev of the Leningrad University, have shown these disturbances to take one of three forms. In some cases the patient retains individual elements of various letters but is unable to combine them to form whole letters. The letters which result are fragmentary and distorted. Often there is simply a loss of the visual pattern and of the spatial orientation of letters. Examples of this type of disturbance are presented in Figure 60. In the second group of cases there is no loss of the visual images of individual letters, but spatial orientation is so impaired that the patient may write letters backwards. Often he does not recognize his error. We have noted this together with impairment of spatial orientation in several cases in which a formerly right handed patient was required to write with his left hand. The same phenomenon was described at the turn of this century by Pick and has been described more recently by S. M. Blinkov and his coworkers. A. Ja. Kolodnaja analyzed such cases as part of our investigation. In Figure 61 we present an example of this type of writing disorder from a patient with a well defined parietal lobe syndrome.

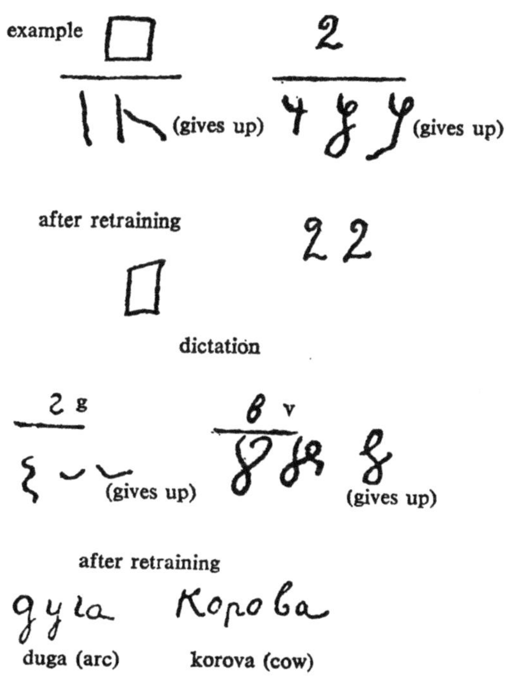

Patient M.: lesion of left parieto-occipital area; visual agraphia

FIG. 60. Writing disturbance in visual agraphia. Case involving loss of the visual structure of the letters.

copying writing to dictation

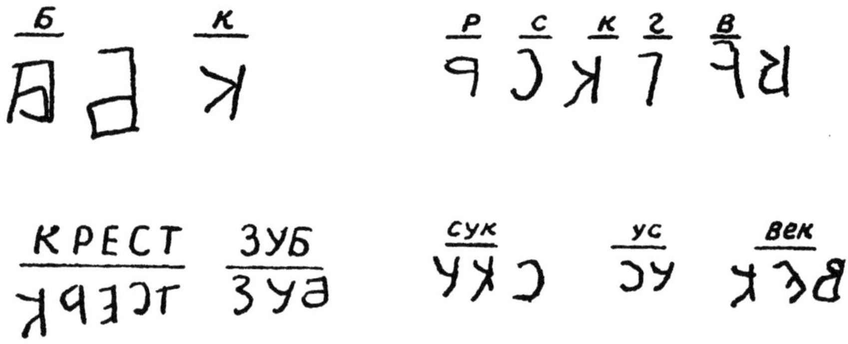

Patient Sm-Sok.: lesion of left postcentral area; parietal syndrome

transliteration:

B K R S K G V

KREST ZUB SUK US VEK

FIG. 61. Writing disturbance in visual agraphia; "mirror writing".

In a third group of cases described in detail by O. P. Kaufman we found a defect which involved not so much loss of the visual patterns of letters as loss of their symbolic significance. These cases usually involved lesions of the occipital area and were accompanied by severe defects. The visual images of letters were preserved, but the meanings were forgotten, so that the patients would match letters with the wrong phonemes, even though they perceived the letters perfectly well. In Figure 62 we present several examples of this disorder. In all three groups the auditory analysis of words remains intact. The only disturbances have to do with the visual representation of letters and recognition of the sounds which they represent. They occur most frequently as a result of lesions in the occipito-parietal (visuo-gnostic) systems of the left hemisphere. In the most severe cases there is a loss of graphemes or of their meanings; in less severe cases, and in late stages of recovery, patients seldom have any difficulty in remembering which letters represent which sounds. It is not uncommon however, for such patients to continue to have difficulty in writing familiar letter sequences, words and ideograms.

writing to dictation

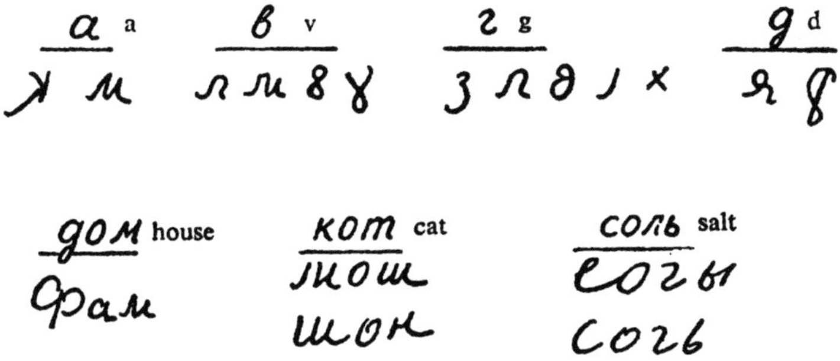

Patient Sam.: lesion of left parietò-occipital area; visual agraphia.

transliteration:

writing to dictation

a	v	g	d
(?) m	l m 8 (?)	z l d (?) x	ja 8

dom	kat	sol
fam	moš	sogy
	šon	sog

FIG. 62. Writing disturbance with visual agraphia; loss of letter meanings.

It is known (and we shall come back to this below) that loss of the ability to analyze the auditory content of words as a result of damage to the temporal or opercular parts of the speech zone abolishes those forms of writing which require precise auditory analysis. Patients with such lesions, however, retain the ability to write familiar ideograms, such as signatures, the names of famous cities, or friends' names. Lesions in the occipito-parietal systems, on the other hand, do not affect the auditory analysis of words; here the ability to reproduce familiar visual ideograms is more apt to be impaired. The writing disorder in this case may be especially severe if the patient writes in a relatively nonphonetic language such as French or English, i.e., in a language in which the spelling of words often does not correspond to the pronunciation.

The following is a case which clearly illustrates the type of writing disorder which may arise with a lesion of the occipito-parietal area.

Patient Falt., a 42 year old naturalized French citizen of Polish origin, received a direct shrapnel injury at the occipital border of the left inferoparietal area. He was a journalist and had served for some time on the staff of the French newspaper "L'Humanité". He took part in the Spanish War as a member of the international brigade and, in 1937, was wounded at Saragossa. The injury gave rise to an aphasia which lasted for a long time but which gradually disappeared leaving severe reading and writing disorders. The patient indicated that for six months he read nothing. Though he was able to recognize individual letters, he was unable to recognize words. His writing remained disturbed for a considerably longer time. For nine years he remained in a special school for the handicapped. He was a polyglot who spoke French and Russian with equal facility and during this time he regained the ability to write in Russian, but he remained totally unable to write in French. In other words, he recovered the ability to write phonetically, but he was unable to write in a nonphonetic language. This occurred despite the fact that before the injury he had written in French much better than in Russian.

Careful investigation showed that the auditory analysis of words gave him no difficulty whatsoever. Thus, he was easily able to write such Russian words as "okno" (window), "koster" (bonfire), "strax" (fear), and "step'" (steppe). His ability to write in French, however, was limited to words in which the sequence of letters could be determined on the basis of phonetic analysis. Words which had to be spelled on the basis of visual ideograms were impossible for him. From his attempts to write in French it became apparent that he did not retain even such a familiar ideogram as his own signature. Signing his name in French he would often insert Russian letters or say that he had forgotten how to write certain letters. The confusion of Russian and French letters resulting from severe visual agraphia was noted in his attempts to write a number of other words. The impairment of writing emerged most clearly when he was required to write words according to their conventional transcription. He was unable to spell correctly the name of the newspaper (L'Humanité) even though he had worked as a journalist on its staff for several years. In stead he wrote the name "Himanite". He made mistakes in writing the name Couturier and wrote instead "Coutiriez". Finally, he completely lost the ability to recognized the "orthograms" which distinguish the meanings of French homophones. Thus on the basis of phonetic analysis he would write "le metre" (meter) and "le maître" (teacher) identically. Similarly, he spelled "l'été" and "il était" as identical. Similar loss of visual ideograms were revealed by his attempts to write other words. Figure 63 gives several samples of his writing.

The disturbances outlined above result from disruption of the visuo-gnostic process and usually accompany lesions in the occipito-parietal areas. A large number of other aphasic writing disturbances observed in our clinic arose from *loss of the acoustic analysis* which precedes the act of writing and which is consequently an important mechanism underlying the writing process. Disorders in this group usually occur with disturbance of the *acoustico-gnostic systems* resulting from lesions in the temporal areas. The ability to copy is seldom disturbed in these patients; they are commonly able to copy complex material. It is noteworthy that their spelling errors sometimes reveal the preservation of certain familiar rules of syntax and spelling. They usually have no difficulty in writing their own names, and sometimes they can write their addresses. The major difficulty arises when they are required to write to dictation. Under these conditions it becomes clear that copying

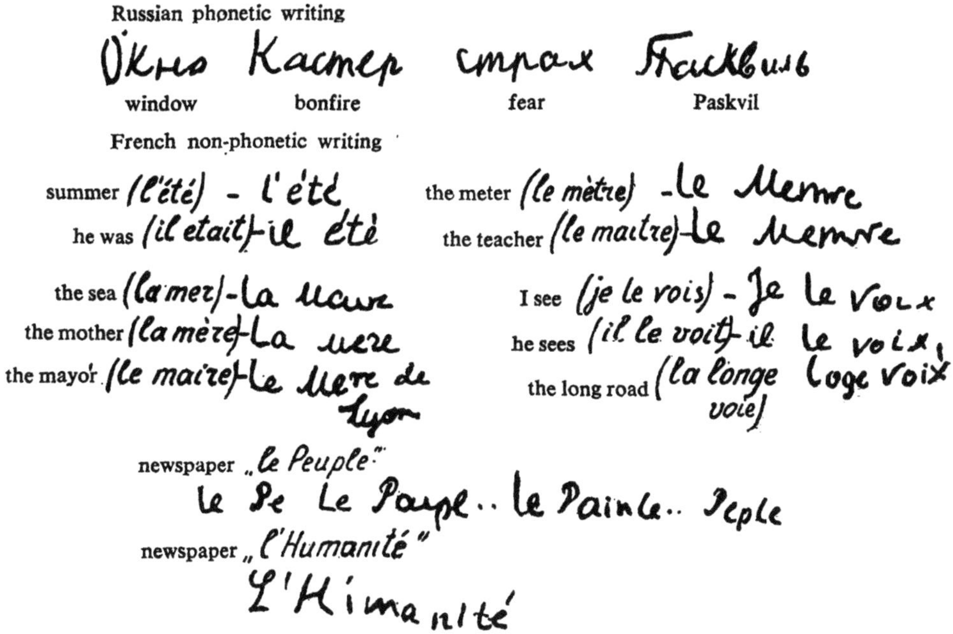

Patient Falt.: lesion in the left postero-parietal area

FIG. 63. Writing disorders in Russian and French as written by patient Falt.

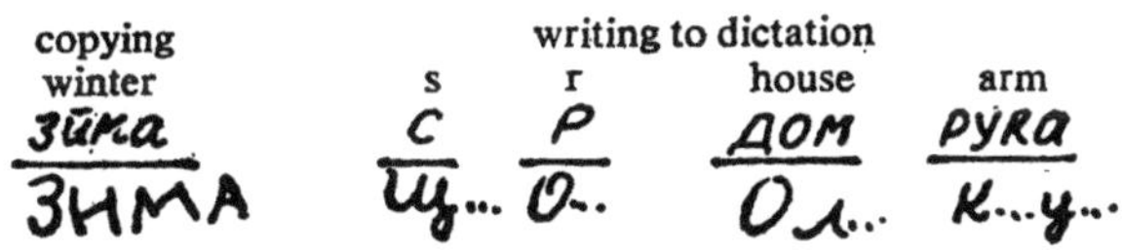

Patient Afon.: lesion in left temporal area

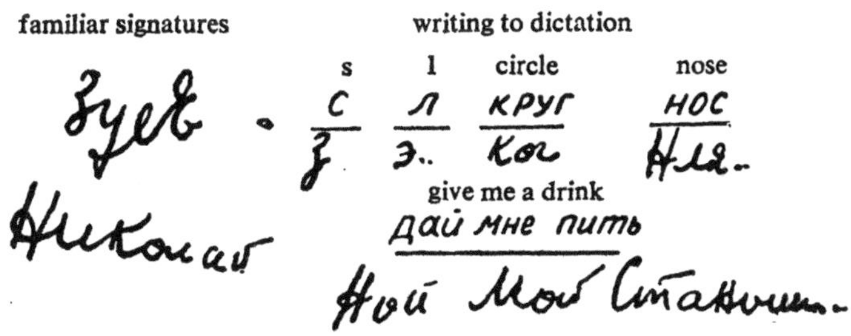

Patient Zuev.: lesion in left temporal area

FIG. 64. Copying, "automatic" writing, and writing to dictation by patients with loss of auditory analysis as a result of lesions in the left temporal area.

transliteration of Fig. 64

copying	writing to dictation			
ZIMA	S	R	DOM	RUKA
ZIMA	ŠČ	O...	OL...	K... U...

Patient Afon.: lesion in left temporal area

familiar signatures	writing to dictation			
Zuev	S	L	KRUG	Nos
Nikolaj	z	è	Kog	Nlja

give me a drink
Noj Moj Stanym

and signing one's name have nothing in common with genuine writing, for the latter can be severely disturbed with little or no impairment of the former. Figure 64 presents two protocols in each of which the two types of writing are compared. It is apparent that the patient's difficulty arises the moment he is deprived of visual or motor cues and has to write words on the basis of auditory analysis of the flow of speech sounds. Often, if one allows him to copy the first part of a word and then removes it from his field of vision he will fail to write the remainder correctly.

The impairment of auditory analysis is so severe and the inner auditory images are so disrupted that the patient may be unable to write individual letters to dictation. In such a case syllables and words offer even greater difficulty. If the impairment of auditory perception is less severe the patient may be able to write some words to dictation. In this case he is most likely to have difficulty in recognizing the phonemes in syllables consisting of several consonants in a row. He characteristically confuses phonemes which sound similar to one another, i.e., oppositional phonemes. He may write "kot" (cat) as "got" (meaningless) or as "god" (year). Similarly, he may write "bulka" (roll) as "pulka" (meaningless) or "burka" (coat); he does not recognize his own errors. In Figure 65 we present several examples of such temporal lobe dysgraphias.

A patient with temporal aphasia is not helped by repeating the words aloud to himself or by observing the lip movements of the examiner. Frequent exercises over a long period of time are required before he is able to compensate for his

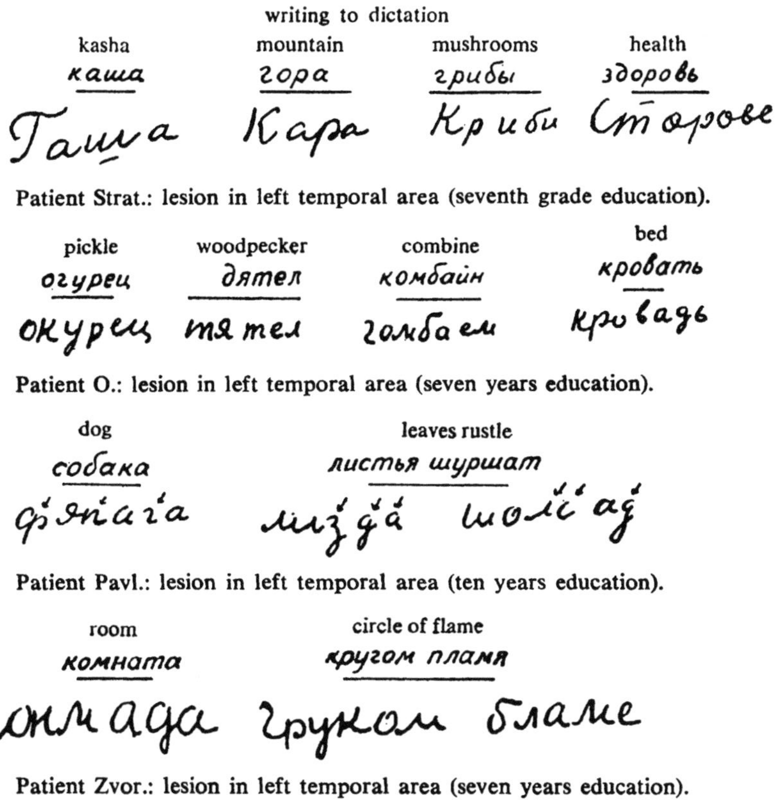

FIG. 65. Phonemic substitutions in the writing of patients with temporal aphasia.

transliteration of Fig. 65.

writing to dictation

kaša	gora	griby	zdorov'
Gaša	Kara	Kribi	Storove

Patient Strat.: lesion in left temporal area (seventh grade education).

ogurec	djatel	kombajn	krovat'
okurec	tjatel	gombaem	krovad'

Patient O.: lesion in left temporal area (seven years education).

sobaka	listja šuršat
fopaga	lizda šolsad

Patient Pavl.: lesion in left temporal area (ten years education).

komnata	krugom plamja
gonmada	grukom blame

Patient Zvor.: lesion of left temporal area (seven years education).

FIG. 65. Phonemic substitutions in the writing of patients with temporal aphasia.

inability to analyze words and to recognize their phonemic structure. During retraining he is continually uncertain as to the accuracy with which he identifies the phonemic constituents of words. The underlying lability of phonemic hearing is revealed by constant self correction which never terminates with an altogether confident assertion as to the nature of the word. Figure 66 (taken from the work of Ė. S. Bejn) gives an example of this type of uncertainty as manifested in the writing of a patient with temporal lobe aphasia.

writing to dictation

„летит птица" "the bird flies"

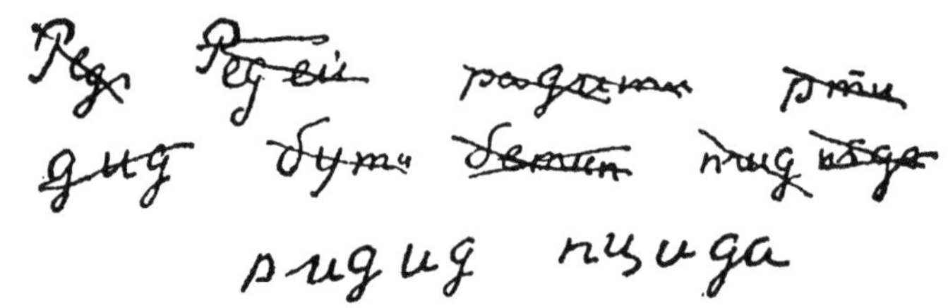

Patient Pavl.: lesion in left temporal area (seventh grade education).

FIG. 66. Uncertainty as to the sound analysis of words as revealed by the writing of a patient with temporal asphasia.

transliteration:

"letit ptica"

Red	Redrej	raditi	rti
did	buti	betip	tidtda
	ridid	pcida	

Impairment of the ability to recognize phonemic structure and to write down the corresponding letters occurs not only in cases involving primary loss of phonemic hearing. It is seen in an equally clear-cut form with the loss of inner *articulatory schemata*. If the loss of articulatory schemata is so extensive that the patient is deprived of oral speech, writing becomes impossible also. He is unable to distinguish nouns which are similar in articulation, and thus tends to make mechanical spelling errors. He substitutes homorganic phonemes for one another. Even after such a patient has largely recovered from the impairment of oral speech imposed by the afferent motor aphasia, he may continue to have great difficulty writing. Though he can tell the number of phonemes in a word, he is unable to identify the individual sounds and consequently cannot represent them by the appropriate letters. He even has difficulty in writing individual letters to dictation. If he attempts to repeat a sound so as to recognize what phoneme it represents, he tends to shift to another sound which is similar in articulation. He may pronounce "l" as "n" or as "d"; he may write "t" as "l" or "n". Exactly the same types of errors emerge when he writes syllables or whole words. Here the basic difficulty is not so much an inability to retain the correct order of sounds as a difficulty in representing them by the correct letters. Mistakes which might otherwise appear to be the result of random

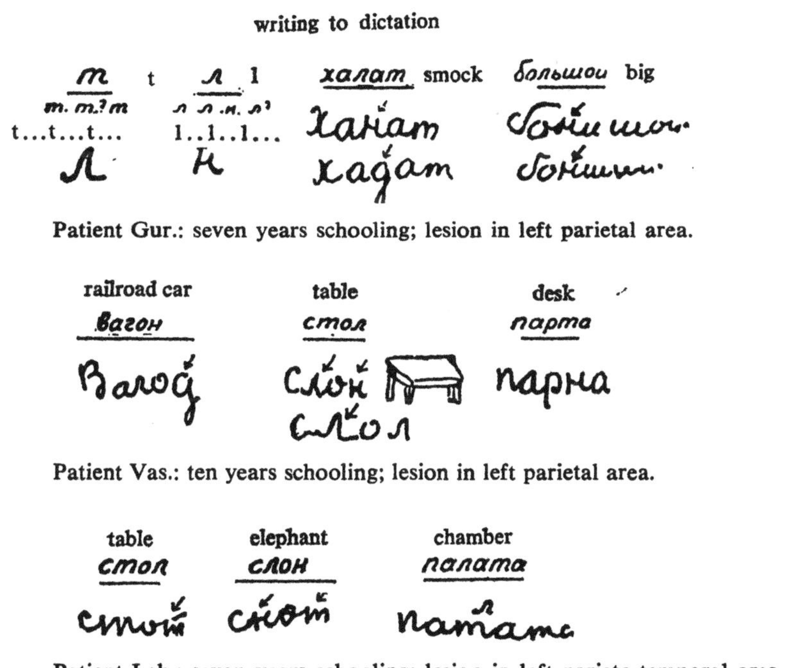

FIG. 67. Letter substitutions in the writing of a patient with a loss of articulatory schemata.

transliteration of Fig. 67.

t ... t̄ ... t ... l ... l̄ ... l ...	xalat / xanat / xadat	bol'šoj / bonišoi / bonšii

Patient Gur.: seven years schooling; lesion in left parietal area.

vagon / vagod	stol / slon (elephant) / slol	parta / parna

Patient Vas.: ten years schooling; lesion in left parietal area.

stol / stot	slon / snot	palata / patata

Patient Leb.: seven years schooling; lesion in left parieto-temporal area.

FIG. 67. Letter substitutions in the writing of a patient with a loss of articulatory schemata.

substitution, e.g. the writing of "slon" (elephant) as "stol" (table) or "sup" (soup), become understandable once one analyzes the articulatory relationships between the letters substituted and those they replace. The sounds "l-n-t", "p-m-b", and "o-u", are poorly differentiated by patients in this group. Figure 67 is taken from the work of L. K. Nazarova and shows several examples of the types of substitution made by a patient suffering from an articulation defect. In some cases the difficulty recognizing individual sounds is so great that the patient only catches a few of the letters making up the words he hears. He is able to represent the remaining letters, however, by dashes, thus indicating that he is aware of the total number of letters and that his difficulty lies only in their precise identification. Figure 68 presents several examples of this phenomenon.

The mechanisms underlying all of these disorders become clear when we investigate the various factors which can help the patient to compensate for his defect. Observations by S. M. Blinkov have shown that the exclusion of external speech accomplished by holding the tongue between the teeth produces a total disruption of the ability to write. He refers to this phenomenon as "kinesthetic agraphia". The sites of lesions which have been shown to produce kinesthetic agraphia are presented in Figure 69. Our observations have shown that if such a patient is allowed to observe the lips of the examiner as he pronounces various

Beginning of retraining

Dictation without visual aids

that	pipe	there is smoke
та	*труба*	*там дым*
-а	-р---	-а- Д--

with use of articulatory diagram

та тр--- -а- ды-
тру-а -ам дым
труба Там дым

after seven months retraining

Здравствуйте дорогие родные
мама, Нина и брат Геля. По-
лучёл от Нины письмо и
большой спасибо. Шлю я вам
сердечный привет

Hello dear family, mama, Nina, and brother Gelya. I received the letter from Nina and thank you very much. I send you sincere greetings.

Patient Xol.: lesion in left parietal area.
Afferent motor aphasia.

FIG. 68. Omission of certain sounds in the writing of a patient who lacks articulatory schemata.

transliteration of Fig. 68.

Beginning of retraining

Dictation without visual aids

ta	truba	tam dym
-a	-r---	-a-d--

with use of articulatory diagram

ta	tr---	-a-dy-
	tru-a	-am dym
	truba	tam dym

after seven months retraining

Zdravstvujte dorogie rodnye
mama, Nina i brat Gelja, Po-
lušel ot Niny pis'mo i
bol'šoj spasibo. Šluj ja vam
serdesnyj privet.

Errors here:
"Polušel" should be "Polučil" "bol'šoj" should be "bol'šoe"
"serdesnyj" should be "serdečnyi" (trans),

Patient Xol.: lesion in left parietal area.

Afferent motor aphasia

FIG. 68. Omission of indefinite sounds in the writing of a patient who lacks articulatory schemata.

words or if he is allowed to observe his own articulatory movements in a mirror, his difficulty in recognizing the acoustical components of words is greatly reduced. These measures can help him to write letters and words correctly. The data presented in Figure 70 give a convincing demonstration that the writing defect in such a case lies in imprecise recognition of sounds as a result of the loss of inner articulatory schemata.

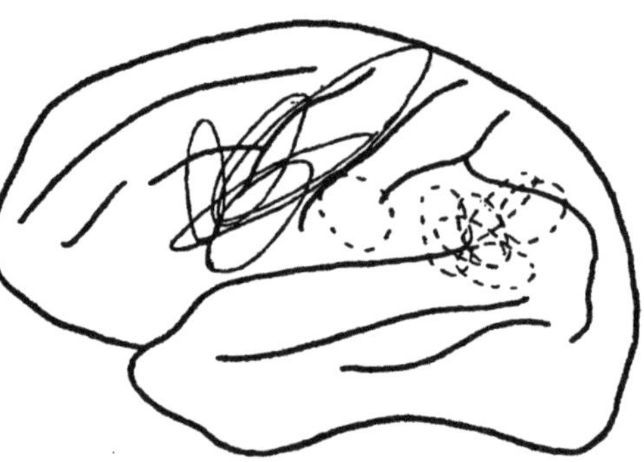

—— sites of lesions in cases where the exclusion of oral speech does not produce a writing deficit

- - - - sites of lesions in cases where the exclusion of oral speech produces a writing deficit

FIG. 69. The influence of excluding external speech on the writing of patients with afferent motor aphasia. The localization of lesions in these cases (from S. M. Blinkov).

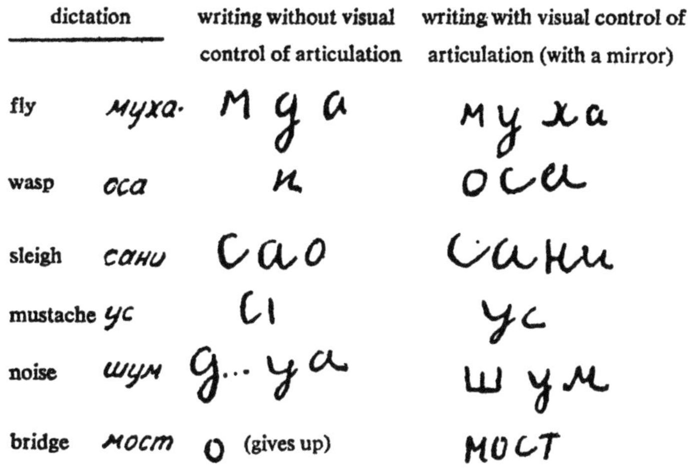

transliteration

dictation	writing without visual control of articulation	writing with visual control of articulation (with a mirror)
muxa	mda	muxa
osa	i	osa
sani	sao	sani
us	s(?)	us
šum	d . . . ua	šum
most	o (gives up)	most

Patient Nas.: lesion in left postcentral area; afferent motor aphasia.

FIG. 70. The influence of visual control of oral movements on the writing of a patient with afferent aphasia.

Patients in both groups characteristically attempt to compensate for the difficulty in identifying sounds by fixing and retaining them in indirect ways. The *contextual relationships of letters* play a large role in compensating for such writing disorders. Patients often turn their attention to the semantic context of a letter in attempting to identify it. For example, a patient recognizing the letter "z" at the beginning of a word may say, "Z . . z . . . ah, z ! . . . zajac (rabbit)"; or recognizing the letter "n" in a word he may say, "Na . . . n . . . ah, n ! . . . it's Nina !"

The basic difficulty in these two groups is a disturbance of the primary identification of phonemes. In addition to these two there is a large group of writing disorders which do not involve any difficulty in writing individual letters. Here the difficulty results from a disturbance of the *sequential patterns of sounds* making up syllables or words. Our observations have shown that though these disturbances may result from a loss of simultaneous perceptual schemata, they are seen most frequently in efferent motor aphasia. As a rule, patients in this group have no difficulty in writing individual letters to dictation. If, however, they are required to write syllables, i.e., to write series of letters in which the sequence is important, they make many errors. It becomes apparent that the ability to recognize and retain the sequential pattern of sounds is severely disturbed.

In the early phase of this type of traumatic aphasia a patient may be able to retain only one of the letters of a two or three letter syllable. The remainders are forgotten or replaced by repetition of the first letter. Perseveration occurs as the patient goes from writing individual letters to writing syllables and words to dictation. Several examples of such perseverative writing in the early stages of efferent motor aphasia are presented in Figure 71. At later stages (or with less severe injuries), when the stagnation of neurodynamic processes becomes less profound, the loss of sequential sound schemata emerges quite clearly. It becomes apparent that the patient is unable to find the schemata of simple syllables or words. In trying to write letter sequences he gropes helplessly for the correct sequence by repeatedly altering the order of the letters. Even though he may produce the correct sequence he is unable to recognize it. Figure 72 presents several examples of writing by patients who have lost the sequential schemata of syllables and words; all are from cases of efferent motor aphasia. The first example was taken from the examination of an engineer whose motor aphasia and agraphia resulted from a neck wound involving the left carotid artery. He had suffered for four years from a writing disorder secondary to loss of the sequential schemata of words. This defect had prevented him from performing his previous functions as a construction engineer; with three months of retraining the writing disorder was removed. In his writing, initial vowels (the articulation of which involves no clear-cut kinesthetic component) were frequently omitted. Thus the following consonants appeared at the beginning of the word. The word "okno" (window) was written as "kono", or "nako". Similarly, the word "most" (bridge) was written "mst" or "stom". In neither case did repeated effort produce the correct letter sequence. In attempting to write the name of the city "Pskov" he wrote „Psok" or "Psvok"; only after several attempts did he arrive at the correct spelling.

Multiple repetition of a dictated word or observation of the examiner's lips as he pronounces it are of little assistance to a patient of this type. Eventually he resorts to the one means he has of compensating for his defect; he pronounces the word aloud to himself and writes the letters corresponding to the sounds as he utters them. By pronouncing words aloud he avoids the necessity of relying upon inner

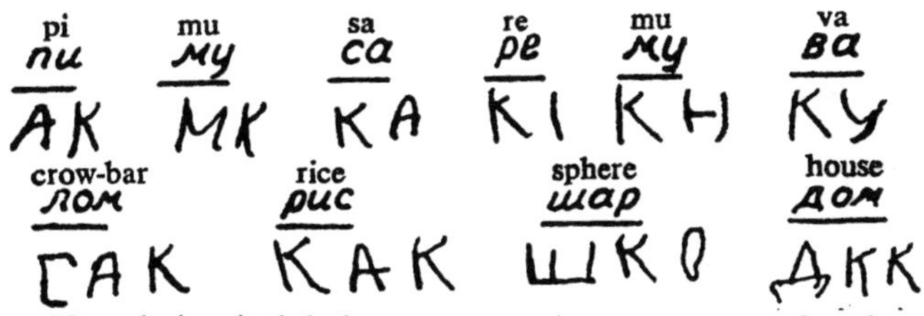

Patient Vav.: lesion in left fronto-temporal area; two months after injury.

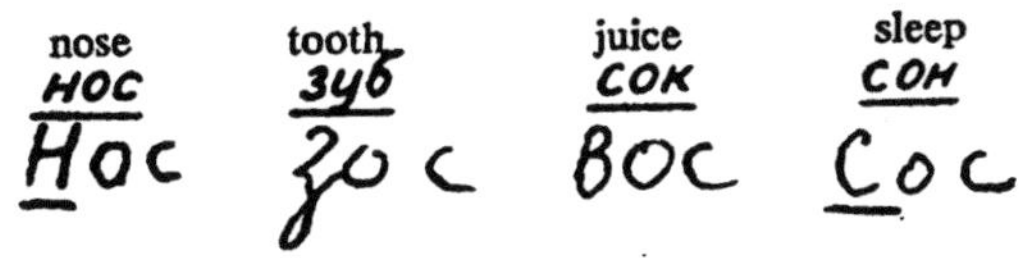

Patient Dim.: lesion in anterior speech area; two months after injury.

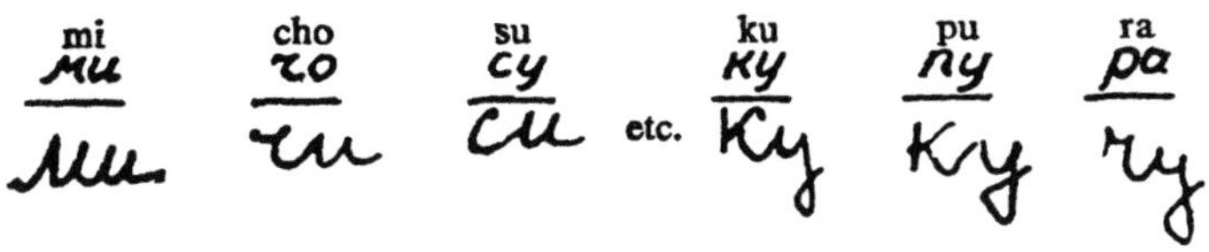

transliteration

pi	mu	sa	re	mu	va
AK	MK	KA	K(?)	KN	KU

lom	ris	shar	dom
SAK	KAK	ŠKO	DKK

Patient Vav.: lesion in left fronto-temporal area; two months after injury.

nos	zub	sok	son
Nos	zos	vos	Sos

Patient Dim.: lesion in anterior speech area; two months after injury.

mi	čo	su	ku	pu	ra
mi	či	si etc.	ku	ku	ču

Patient Plotn.: lesion in left fronto-temporal area; two months after injury.

FIG. 71. Perseveration of syllables and words in the early phases of motor aphasia.

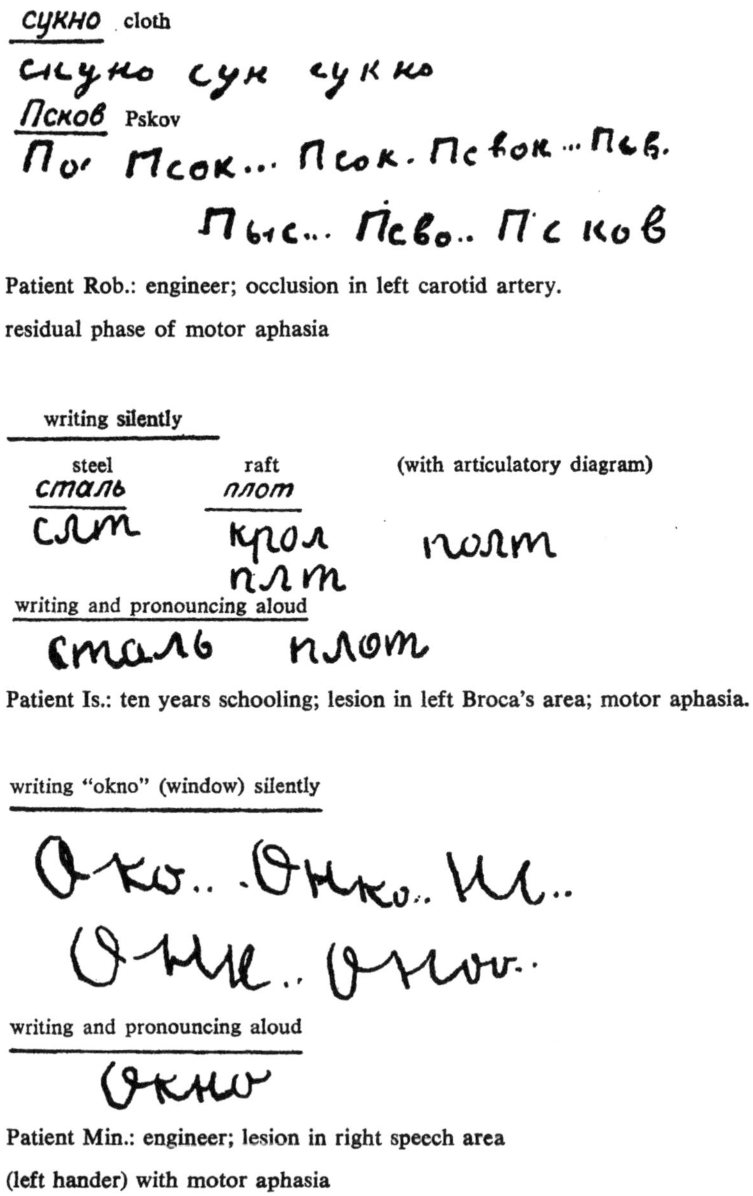

FIG. 72. Loss of syllable and word schemata in the writing of patients with motor aphasia.

sequential schemata and thus circumvents the only obstacle to his writing accurately. For this reason, the exclusion of external speech is capable of greatly intensifying his writing difficulty. In contrast to the cases mentioned previously, however, this effect results from interference not with the primary identification of sounds but with production of the correct sound sequence.

transliteration of Fig. 72.

sukno
skuno suk sukno

Pskov

Po Psok ... Psok. Psvok ... Psv.

Pys ... Psvo .. Pskov

Patient Rob.: engineer; occlusion of left carotid artery.
residual phase of motor aphasia

writing silently

stal	plot	(with articulatory diagram)
slt	krol	polt
	plt	

writing and pronouncing aloud

stal' plot

Patient Is.: ten years schooling; lesion in left Broca's area; motor aphasia.

writing "okno" (window) silently

Oko .. Onko .. n (?) ...

Onk .. On (?)

writing and pronouncing aloud

Okno

Patient Min.: engineer; lesion of right speech area
(left hander) with motor aphasia

No matter what area of the brain is damaged, patients for whom writing is not an automatic process suffer greater impairment than others. A person who, previous to injury, has acquired many automatic written words and phrases may preserve the corresponding motor patterns and thus be able to write even though his phonemic hearing, articulatory schemata, or sequential integrative processes are profoundly disturbed.

C. INVESTIGATION OF READING

With traumatic aphasia the incidence of reading disturbances is somewhat less than that of writing disturbances. This is partly because the reading process is inherently less difficult than writing and partly because in the cultured adult reading becomes more automatic than writing; thus it comes to depend on much simpler psychological mechanisms.

While reading has much in common with writing it also has some important differences. Its distinguishing characteristic is that the letters representing sounds are supplied directly to the reader; he must supply the corresponding phonemes. Whereas in writing one extracts phonemes from the flow of speech and transforms them into letters, in reading one transforms the phonemes representing individual sounds into the appropriate articulatory variants depending upon the context of letters. This makes the process of sound-letter synthesis extremely important for reading. The reader must constantly be running ahead as he perceives the individual letters so as to be able to pronounce them correctly in context. Investigations by D. B. Ėlkonin have shown that without this synthetic function the process whereby sequential phonemes melt into one another is impossible.

Analysis and synthesis constitute only the first stage in the reading process, however. As the initial reading habits become automatized they quickly give way to another type of reading function which is simpler in organization. The experienced reader ceases to extract individual letters or syllables. He quickly learns to recognize words "as individuals"; words are transformed into visual ideograms. Recognition of the meanings of words may occur with no reference to their sound structure. The experienced reader grabs only the general countour of a word and the characteristic configuration of its major letters which usually constitute its root part. On the basis of this he guesses the meaning of the word as a whole. He is helped considerably in this process by the context of the word. In some cases the context may be such that the number of distinctive features required in the word itself for accurate recognition may be reduced to almost zero. The reader is able to recognize it on the basis of some very minor feature. Of course, this characteristic of the automatized reading process implies a greatly simplified psychological structure and helps to explain why a patient may be able to recognize written words even though the analytico-synthetic operations are severely disturbed.

Investigation of the reading process should begin with an evaluation of the patient's ability to recognize letters (graphemes). It should show whether or not he can remember the sounds corresponding to given letters and whether or not by taking context into account he can pronounce the sounds correctly. Finally, it should show to what degree he can integrate groups of letters into whole words. An important part of the investigation is the study of how well the patient understands the words which he reads when he does not pronounce them aloud to himself (so-called "silent reading"). During the entire series of tests the investigator should keep in mind that unfamiliar words are read by analysis and synthesis of their sound components, while more familiar words may be read on the basis of direct recognition.

The investigation of reading includes the following tests:

1. *Recognition of Individual Letters*

The patient is presented individual letters written in various types of print and long hand. He must either read them aloud or point out the same letters from a list written in a different kind of print. For instance, having read "D" he should be able to recognize "*D*" or "*d*" as being identical. Similarly, having read "B" he should be able to pick out "*B*" or "*b*" from a list of letters. Inability to carry out these tasks indicates a disturbance of the primary identification of the meanings of letters. Inability to carry out the second task, i.e., to choose identical letters from a list indicates a loss of visual graphemes.

2. *Reading Simple and Complex Syllables*

The patient is required to read syllables which vary in phonemic complexity, e.g., "to, ta, te, pa, pe", or "kro, kri, stro", etc. The purpose of this test is to determine whether or not he is capable of integrating the individual letters into complex syllables and of pronouncing letters appropriately depending upon the context. The investigator notes whether or not he pronounces syllables as a whole or spells them out as series of letters.

3. *Reading Simple and Complex Words*

The patient is required to read familiar words and abbreviations which are likely to have become visual ideograms for him and which he might he expected to recognize directly, e.g., his own surname, "Moscow", "USSR", "Lenin", etc. Then he is presented less familiar words which are likely to be read on the basis of auditory analysis and synthesis, e.g., "bonfire", "cupboard", "defense", etc. First he is asked to read the words silently and point at the corresponding objects. If this is impossible he is allowed to read aloud. Finally, if reading the words aloud does not help him to understand their meanings he is allowed to observe the lip movements of the examiner or to follow his own lip movements in a mirror as the words are pronounced. By carrying out these three variations of the basic test it is possible to determine which factors help the patient to compensate for his reading disorder.

4. *Reading Sentences*

The patient is asked to read sentences some of which establish a set helpful in the reading of the component words, e.g., "I clean my boots with a brush", while others create a set making it more difficult to read the individual words, e.g., "At the front I was injured by a bullet in the knee". On the basis of this task it is possible to evaluate the effectiveness of the reading process as a whole, for when the set established by context conflicts with specific words within sentences, the reader is forced to correct the set by conscious analysis of the individual words.

Primary damage to the visuo-gnostic systems arising as the result of a lesion of the occipital area produces the clear-cut syndrome of *visual alexia.* This syndrome may take either of two basic forms (if one ignores peripheral visual disturbances which are not legitimately classified with the alexic disturbances).

The most clear-cut form of visual alexia is the so-called "literal alexia" which has been described many times and which has recently been subjected to careful psychological analysis by B. G. Anan'ev and Ž. I. Šiff. These authors conclude that in literal alexia the letters are either not perceived with sufficient clarity or are confused with one another, e.g., "p", "d" with "b", "’" with "q", etc. Sometimes the letters are perceived accurately but their meanings are lost. This "literal amnesia" is the most absolute form of loss of graphemes. The patient is not only incapable of reading letters presented to him, but he is unable to identify the same letter when it is written in different hands or different types of print. He confuses letters on the basis of secondary features. We have observed several such patients; in every case this symptom was part of a larger syndrome involving fine visuo-gnostic disturbances. Every patient was able to compensate for his defect by manually or visually tracing the borders of the letters and thus incorporating a kinesthetic component into the perceptual process.

The second group of visual alexias are classified as verbal, or simultaneous, alexias. The patient whose processes of auditory analysis and synthesis are relatively intact is unable to integrate the letters which he perceives into a single, simultaneous pattern, e.g., he is unable to recognize them as making up whole words. Even familiar words which are usually perceived as visual ideograms are not recognized by such a patient. In reading words he tends to name the individual letters rather than combine them into a meaningful whole. If he combines them, he does so only by an indirect process. First he translates the letters into sounds, and then, by running these sounds together he arrives at the appropriate sound pattern of the word.

This group includes disturbances in which the major defect is in the visual processes underlying reading. In many years of observation we have noted that with lesions in the occipital area the "reading field", i.e., the number of simultaneously perceivable letters, may diminish to a degree which is out of all proportion to the degree of constriction of the visual field as ordinarily measured. Frequently the patient notes that he is unable to perceive more than one or two letters at a time. Beyond these one or two, all letters appear in a dim undifferentiated visual sphere. Further, data compiled by N. S. Preobraženskaja have shown that the origin of this defect is not a simple constriction of the visual field. The patient perceives only one or two letters regardless of their size or location; in other words, regardless of what part of the visual field they occupy. This disturbance is apparently a defect in the simultaneous organization of visual material. When such a defect is present, the patient is forced to carry out the process of word synthesis not in the visual mode but in the auditory mode; he reads the syllables aloud and thus, compensates for his primary defect. In Figure 73 we present a summary diagram showing the sites of lesions in several cases involving constriction of the "reading field".

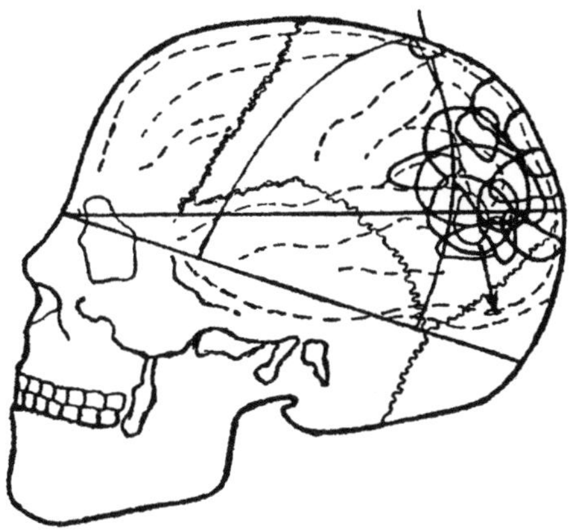

FIG. 73. Localization of lesions in cases involving constriction of the "reading field".

In none of the cases presented so far have the reading disorders involved defects of nonvisual processes.[1] In all the following cases the reading disorders are associated with disturbances of speech processes and particularly with diturbances of the auditory analysis and synthesis of words.

Lesions of the temporal area which disrupt the *acoustico-gnostic systems* provide a valuable source of material for understanding the mechanisms of reading disorders. Temporal lobe lesions less frequently produce reading disorders in adults than in children (R. E. Levina). This is explained by the fact that the automatization of reading habits transforms reading from a sound-letter, analytico-synthetic process into a process of direct visual recognition in which the sound structure of words is largely ignored. A patient with temporal aphasia may recognize familiar words even though he is unable to read individual letters or syllables. When con-

[1] We shall omit cases involving changes in the relationships between the central and peripheral visual fields, inability to follow lines on the page, and disturbances of the inhibition of peripheral excitation described by Pötzl. These symptoms are seen often but are not pertinent to our investigation.

fronted with individual letters his attempts to identify the corresponding sounds are usually unsuccessful. He repeatedly gropes for the appropriate sounds and with each attempt remains uncertain as to whether or not he has reproduced the letter correctly. His difficulty is most acute when he is confronted with nonsense syllables or unfamiliar words in which there are no meaningful ideograms to assist him. Sometimes the difference between a patient's ability to read on the basis of auditory analysis and on the basis of ideographic cues is so great that the examiner has no

reading sounds

A	S	M	N	BREAD	HAND
a	gives up	s?	gives up	forest? no, I didn't recognize it	no, I don't know reading ideograms

reading ideograms

AFONIN	SAŠA	USSR	LENIN
(immediately) +	+	I know, here!	I know ... I know ... he was - - - but he's not here now

Patient Af.: lesion in left temporal area; sensory aphasia.

reading sounds

O	S	CRASH
I don't know	now ... no sound - - - there's no sound	no ... I don't know ... there's no sound ...

reading ideograms

LONDON	VOLGA	BENEŠ
I know ... I know ... a city ... a large city ... eight ! .. the biggest city ...	a large body of water ... a river ... our ... Volga ... Volda ... our ! .. the biggest ! ..	an old man .. he was not ... but now he has gone there ... not ... a military man ... before the war he left ... erriot? no ... doesn't seem ... Masarik ! no ... Beneš ? no ... Beneš ... Beneš ... there, that's better ! ..

Patient Levsk.: hematoma in the left temporal area after a local contusion; sensory aphasia.

FIG. 74. Examples of patients with temporal aphasia attempting to read sounds and ideograms.

difficulty in telling which words he reads by which method. M. S. Lebedinskij noted the interesting fact that in ideographic reading the patient often recognizes the meaning of a word even though he is apparently unable to pronounce it. We also have studied this phenomenon. The patient makes errors which can only be classified as semantic in character. For example, he may read "aircraft" as "airplane", or he may read "Kiev" as "Kharkov" or "Odessa". In Figure 74 we present examples of the reading errors which occur with temporal lobe aphasia.

It is to be expected that the impairment of reading should be more pronounced in patients with poorly automatized reading habits than in patients who read well, i.e., patients whose reading is based primarily on the recognition of visual ideograms.

Although auditory analysis plays a large role in the primary identification of letters, an equally important part is played by the *inner articulatory schemata.* The articulatory schemata permit the reader to find the precise meaning of a given letter and to differentiate it from other sounds which are phonetically similar or which are articulated similarly. Thus, a patient with afferent motor aphasia, who has lost the inner articulatory schemata of words, has difficulty not only in writing, but also in reading. A patient with a mild afferent motor aphasia tends both to read and to write "n" as "l" or "d". Consequently, he may read such a word as "sup" (soup) as "som" (fish), "sito" (sieve), or "silo" (meaningless).

It is very interesting that these errors affect the patients ability to read even when he reads to himself. A patient who is unable to identify the phonemic significance of letters when he reads aloud is equally unable to do so when reading to himself. Consequently, a patient with afferent motor aphasia has as much difficulty reading silently as reading aloud. If he comes upon a somewhat unfamiliar word which has not attained the status of an ideogram he is unable to grasp its meaning. He may recognize some individual letters correctly; others he may replace by letters which are similar in articulation. After several unsuccessful attempts to analyze an unfamiliar word he may simple guess at its meaning on the basis of whatever syllables he is able to recognize.

In general, a patient's ability to read is greatly enhanced if he reads aloud. This is especially true if he pays careful attention to his own articulatory movements or follows the articulatory movements of the person with whom he is talking. By this method he is able to establish dependable cues by which he can differentiate the different articulatory patterns and thus he attains the ability to identify the various speech sounds. It is instructive to observe how the patient comes to recognize a given word and how he loses it the moment he is deprived of external speech. External speech is the only substitute he has for the articulatory schemata which he lacks. These difficulties are seen, of course, only in cases where reading is based upon the auditory analytic and integrative processes. They do not arise when the patient reads words which, for him, are visual ideograms. Figure 75 presents several examples of reading difficulties associated with loss of the inner articulatory

Visual recognition of graphemes:

(patient underlines identical letters)

Reading letters aloud:	Š	R	L
	oh . . s . . no . . .	s . . no . . r . . .	m . . m . . s . . l . . n . . l !

Letter recognition:	D	P
	Is it "m" ? no . . . "k" ? no . . . "r" ? no . . . "d" ? uh . . . uh . . . (uncertain)	Is it "s" ? no . . . is it "b" ? no . . . I don't know (uncertain) . . is it "m" ? yes . . no . . (uncertain) . . is it "n" ? no . . yes . . n . . (uncertain)

Reading words:	FLY	SKIS	DUCK	CAT (kot)
	gives up	gives up	gives up	skates ? . . . (konki ?)
	NINA	FIELD (pole)	CART (telega)	
	Di-na . . Ni-na . . Ti-na ? . . .	Mu . . mu . . li ? . . .	Te . . li . . xa . . Te . . nika . . (did not understand) Te . . ni . . xa . . (uncertain)	

Patient Nasedk: lesion in left postcentral area; afferent motor aphasia.

Reading letters:	B	L	T
	I don't know . . is it "m" ? I don't know . . is it "s" ? I don't know . . is it "b" ? I don't know . . .	n . . n . . s . . l ! . .	s . . m . . t . .

Reading words:	LIP (guba)	SITO (sieve)	GRANDMOTHER (Babuška)
	gu . . ma . . guma ? . .	S . . si . . lo . . silo ? . . . si . . si . . l . . l . . silo ? ! . .	Ma . . muška ? . . . Ma . . buška . . . . Babuška ? . . .

Patient Gur.: lesion in left postero-parietal area; afferent motor aphasia.

FIG. 75. Reading difficulties with the disturbance of inner articulatory schemata.

schemata of words. It also shows what factors can facilitate or complicate word recognition.

In the above cases the origin of reading difficulty lay in impairment of the ability to remember the phonemes represented by different letters. An entirely different type of reading disorder is observed in cases of efferent motor aphasia which involves a disturbance of dynamic schemata. Here the patient has no difficulty whatsoever in reading individual letters. His difficulty arises when he is required to read groups of letters forming sequential patterns, for he has lost the schemata whereby letters appearing in sequences unite to form syllables. He is unable to look ahead and by noting the context of a given letter, pronounce it correctly. The process responsible for smooth transition from one sound to another is disrupted. Thus, while he is able to read the letters "t" and "e" separately, he is unable to read the syllable "te" correctly, because the presence of the "t" gives the vowel "e" an entirely different sound. The patient has even greater difficulty when faced with reading complex syllables composed of several letters. He may comment that he knows each letter separately but that he is unable to combine them into a single whole; he frequently treats letter sequences as though they were randomly. In the early phase of traumatic aphasia this difficulty is complicated by the fact that he is unable to keep more than a very few letters in mind at once. The traces of letters which have just been perceived merge with traces of preceding letters so that the preceding sounds enter into the process by which subsequent sounds are integrated and give rise to perseveration. In later stages of traumatic aphasia this perseverative tendency may disappear, but the difficulty in integrating individual letters into stable sequential patterns remains. As a result, the patient is unable to deal with words of any great complexity.

With the loss of word schemata the patient shows a compensatory tendency to rely on the context provided by other words to help him recognize the meanings of words which he is unable to recognize directly. This is why such a patient often appears to substitute guessing for genuine reading. Absence of the sound-letter schemata of words also prevents him from performing the normal "secondary check" on what he guesses to be the words he is reading. Consequently, his reading sometimes diverges widely from the actual text. This discrepancy can be exaggerated by having him read a text which establishes a set of expectations that do not correspond to specific words imbedded in the next. He reads the words according to the pre-established set and experiences no doubt as to the accuracy of his performance.

Finally, we come to the reading disorders seen in patients with damage to the *frontal systems*. In these cases reading consists almost entirely of guessing. The secondary correction mechanism is lost completely and the patient recognizes no discrepancy whatever between his reading and what is printed in the text.

Several examples of the types of reading defects observed with efferent motor aphasia are represented in Figure 76. The analysis of reading disorders which accompany various aphasia syndromes has shown that this complex form of speech activity may be severely impaired with various types of brain lesions. But here again, the type of disturbance and its underlying mechanism depends altogether on which cerebral system is damaged.

Reading letters:	no difficulty!			
Reading syllables:	RO	KO	SO	PRO
	r, o.. together? revo?..	k..ko-- no,.k..o..	s..to?.. s..t..s..?	p, r, o.. poroda (race)?
Reading words:	LUK (onion)	SNEG (snow)	OKNO (window)	KARAS (carp)
	l, u, k together? I don't know	(gives up)	..kino (movie)? ..okino (meaningless)	together? together? krasnyi (red)?
Reading word-ideograms:	ROKOSSOVSKIJ (name)		U MITI ŠČENOK (Mitya has a puppy)	
	Komissariat?!		U Mamy ščuka.. (mama has a fish)? (uncertain)	
	LENIN	USSR	PRAVDA	
	+	+	+	

Patient Xoruž.: lesion in left premotor area; residual phase of motor aphasia.

FIG. 76. Reading disturbance with afferent motor aphasia.

During the last years a careful study of defects in reading with different forms of brain lesions was made in our laboratory by L. S. Cvetkova. These studies, which add new and significant data will be published elsewhere.

XIV

INVESTIGATION OF CALCULATION

The investigation of processes involved in calculation is an integral part of the clinico-psychological study of aphasia. It is important in two ways. The number system is a symbolic system just as is speech. It is perhaps narrower than the speech system and does not depend upon phonemic hearing to the same degree, but otherwise it has much in common with speech. Written symbols represent given quantities. The decimal system of notation permits communication regarding a quantity of any size by means of a small number of symbols. Mathematical operations serve as a model for other intellectual functions. They involve a goal which must be preserved throughout the rational process of calculation. The goal is set forth in terms of specific conditions which must be taken into consideration at all times. Solution of a numerical problem requires that a series of operations be carried through and sometimes this involves a long chain of reasoning. Thus, in studying the changes in psychological processes which accompany aphasia it is useful to test for preservation of the concept of number and for the ability to carry out computational operations.

The investigation of numerical operations can be broken down into two parts: *evaluation of the concept of number or rank order, and evaluation of computational processes* (mathematical operations in the true sense of the word). The first group of tests is designed to determine to what degree the patient retains numerical concepts and the ability to use the decimal system of notation. It is well known that the concept of number as expressed in the decimal system is a relatively late psychological development. A child of pre-school or elementary school age is able to name any number; but to him each number represents a distinct entity. To an educated adult on the other hand, the number "49" represents possible relationships (4 tens plus 9 units, 5 tens minus 1 unit, 7 sevens, etc.) For a child it simply represents a large, vague quantity.

The first object of the investigation is to find out whether or not numbers retain their complex meanings for the patient. The second problem is to analyze psychologically the types of computational mechanisms which he retains. The numerical concepts retained are revealed by the computational processes which remain available to him. Thus, it is important to determine whether he is able to carry out computations on the basis of inner plans, i.e., appropriate sequences of operations;

further, one must determine what mathematical operations he retains and whether or not he is able to organize these operations into sequential plans capable of solving meaningful problems. It is important at every step to note whether he can perform mathematical operations orally or in written form. The investigation of disturbances of computational operations usually includes the following tests:

A. READING AND WRITING ONE-DIGIT NUMBERS

If the patient is able to talk and comprehend oral speech, problems may be presented in verbal form; if not, he may be shown different numbers of objects and instructed to write down how many he sees; or he may be shown a written number and asked to point out a group containing the corresponding number of objects. First the numbers are presented in the order "1, 2, 3, etc."; then they are presented in random order. In either case the patient is required to write down the number of objects he sees or to hold up the number of fingers corresponding to the digit he sees.

B. READING AND WRITING NUMBERS INVOLVING MULTIPLE DIGITS

This is designed to investigate whether or not the patient still comprehends the decimal numerical system. He is presented complex numbers in which one or two of the digits are zero and thus are not pronounced when the number is read, e.g., one thousand twenty three or eight thousand three. If he omits zeros in reading numbers, this constitutes evidence for a disturbance of the comprehension of decimal notation. A second test to clarify the patient's concept of number requires that he tells which of two numbers is larger. He is presented a pair of numbers. In one number the hundreds digit is large, while the tens and unit digits are small. In the other, the hundreds digit is small, while the tens unit digits are large, e.g., 601 and 589 or 201 and 196. An incorrect comparison of the number pairs indicates that the patient estimates the size of numbers by weighing the various digits equally rather than on the basis of the decimal system of notation.

C. DIFFERENTIATING SYMMETRICAL NUMBERS

The patient is presented two numbers, e.g., 17 and 71, and asked to tell whether they are equal or not. A special form of this test is to present *Roman numerals,* particularly symmetrical pairs, e.g., VI and IV or XI and IX. If his comprehension of the number system is intact, he perceives the difference between two such numbers. If he has lost the concept of numbers, he sees them as identical. This often results from an impairment of spatial orientation, in which case he may sometimes read numbers backwards, e.g., he may read 36 as 63.

The investigation of *computational processes* involves the following series of tests:

D. AUTOMATIC CALCULATIONS

The goal of this test is to determine whether or not the patient remembers the elementary operations of addition and subtraction and the multiplication tables up to ten. These operations should be sufficiently simple and familiar so that they can be carried out on the basis of established habits. In studying these processes the examiner notes the degree to which they are automatized and what psychological systems are primarily involved in their execution, e.g., visual, verbo-motor, etc.

E. COMPLEX CALCULATIONS

These are operations which require that several components be present in the field of consciousness at once. The most convenient task used in studying complex oral calculations is subtractions by a digit less than ten, such that the tens digit is reduced by one, e.g., 31 minus 7. A more complex problem is the subtraction of a two digit number from a two digit number, e.g., 41 minus 17. The problem "31–7" requires two or three steps: 31 — 1 =30; 30 — 7 = 23; 23 + 1 = 24. If the problem is solved in this manner the smaller number is subtracted from the remainder of a preceding subtraction and the "1" is subsequently added back (23 + 1 = 24). Another way of solving the same problem is to break down the subtrahend into two parts and to subtract them separately: 31 — 1 = 30; 30 — 6 = 24. In either case the solution is reached by following an inner plan or sequence of operations. If the patient has difficulty he should be allowed to attempt solving the same problem on paper. Much of his difficulty may disappear when he is allowed to treat the problem in written form. A second group of problems in this group involve the division and addition of fractions. These operations are more complex however, and they are usually less useful in the study of computational processes.

One other special method is to present simple written addition and subtraction problems with the numbers represented in unconventional ways. For instance, one may present problems in which two digit numbers to be subtracted from one another are written vertically, e.g., $\begin{array}{r}1\\8\\-1\\\hline 4\end{array}$ or in which the subtrahend is written above the minuend, e.g., $\begin{array}{r}17\\-24.\\\hline\end{array}$

The patient must overcome the impulse to carry out the operations as first suggested by the layout of the problem. If he is to conform to instructions he must show that he is genuinely aware of the relationships of the digits in terms of the decimal system of notation; otherwise he will be unable to perform the numerical operations required of him.

F. SEQUENTIAL CALCULATIONS

This series of tests is designed to show the extent to which the patient is able to carry out successive mathematical operations. In order to perform sequential calculations he must be able to retain the numbers derived from preceding operations long enough to use them in subsequent operations. The most useful tests in this series are the following:

1. Multiple subtractions of 3 or 7 from 100.
2. Addition or subtraction of three numbers, e.g., 12 + 6 — 3.

If a patient is able to do all types of problems except sequential calculations one can infer that the difficulty lies not so much in the loss of numerical concepts as in disruption of the inner dynamics of numerical operations.

G. RECOGNITION OF THE RELATIONSHIPS REPRESENTED BY MATHEMATICAL SYMBOLS

This study involves comparison of the patient's ability to solve two different types of problems. In one type of problem, e.g., 8 + 2 = . . . or 8 — 2 = . . ., the calculations are carried out at a practical level. In the other type, e.g., 8 (?) 2 = 10, or 8 (?) 2 = 6. The result is given and the patient's problem is to indicate what operation must have been used to produce it. Inability to recognize the arithmetical operations by which given answers are generated in a patient who is able to solve problems at a practical level indicates that relatively well automatized habits are retained but that the ability to recognize numerical operations has been lost.

Investigation of the patient's ability to solve arithmetical problems of practical significance is quite interesting, but it involves computational defects which are not common accompaniments of traumatic aphasia and are thus not included as part of the usual clinico-psychological examination.

The disturbances of numbers and calculations which accompany brain lesions may result from a number of different factors.[1] In some cases the disturbance of numerical concepts and computational operations are nonspecific in character. As pointed out above, they may result from loss of the meanings of visual or auditory symbols, memory disorders, or disruption of the dynamics of mental activity. In other cases, the perceptual processes on which computation is based remain unaltered, but the intrinsic structure of numerical concepts and computational operations are severely disturbed. We shall consider these two types of disturbances separately.

Calculation difficulties may result from loss of the *concept of number*. This syndrome is not often seen; when it occurs, however, it usually accompanies a lesion in the occipito-parietal area of the dominant hemisphere. This disturbance may take either of two forms. One is purely visuo-gnostic in character. A lesion in the occipital area produces a loss of the visual images of numbers, so that they appear distorted just as letters appear distorted in visual alexia. The patient has difficulty in recognizing numbers, and tends to confuse digits which look similar to one another, such as 6 and 9 or 3 and 8. Some patients completely forget the meanings of the various numbers, so that when asked to write one number they write another. They make similar errors when reading numbers. This disturbance may be similar to the constructive and spatial agnosias; or it may be seen as one aspect of a more general memory disturbance. In either case, oral calculation may be relatively intact. There is a certain vagueness and imprecision in the use of numbers which will be considered below in connection with the calculational disorder accompanying semantic aphasias.

[1] We have presented a detailed investigation of this problem elsewhere. See A. R. Luria, "The Disturbance of Number and Calculation with Lesions of the Brain", *Proceedings of the Academy of Pedagogical Sciences*, Vol. III (1946). See also Z. Ja. Rudenko (dissertation, Moscow, 1951).

The second group consists of cases in which the disturbance of numerical concepts is much more general in character. Here the defect involves more than the visual images of numbers. They are poorly recognized no matter how they are represented. Such words as "seven", "three", or "nine" sound to the patient like vague sound patterns devoid of any definite meaning. This may occur without loss of the meanings of words representing objects and without any impairment of phonemic hearing. It frequently results from lesions along the temporal border of the occipital cortex and sometimes arises with lesions in the parietal area. Sometimes a patient is able to recognize the meaning of a number only if he reaches it by counting from zero. He may be forced to name all of the preceding numbers if he wishes to recall the meaning of a given number or if he wishes to name a number presented to him in digit form. Figure 77 shows the sites of lesions which have been found to give rise to this syndrome. As might be expected, such a disturbance severely limits the patient's ability to calculate and may lead to other disturbances; the character of such secondary disturbances will be considered in greater detail below.

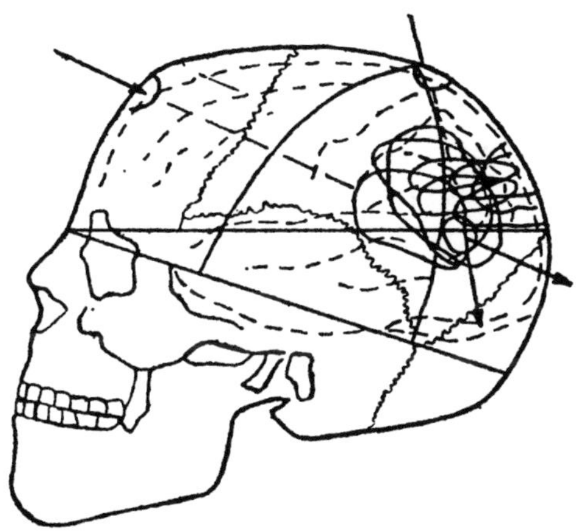

FIG. 77. Localization of lesions giving rise to a primary loss of numbers and computational operations.

The meanings of numbers may be disturbed in a different manner, *viz.*, the *acoustico-gnostic aspect* may be disrupted. This usually is a result of a left temporal lobe lesion. The meanings of numbers pronounced aloud are lost and the patient cannot identify them, much less subject them to any kind of mathematical manipulation. Sometimes there is no obvious loss of the meanings of spoken numbers, but the acoustico-gnostic disturbance manifests itself in a general instability of numerical operations. In such a case the patient is unable to remember long numbers. When he attempts to repeat a number with several digits he forgets both the digits themselves and their order. He is unable to remember two numbers or to understand the meaning of such mathematical terms as "minus", "plus", or "multiply". The partial loss of word meanings is not sufficient to account for the severe loss of mathematical operations in such a case, for if the patient is allowed to solve problems in written form the results are entirely different. As a rule he has little difficulty in recognizing simple and complex numbers. He accurately evaluates the meanings of digits representing units, tens, and hundreds; and he is able to carry out relatively complex operations on paper. He shows signs of difficulty only when his written calculations must be supplemented by certain operations mediated by internal speech. This occurs, for instance, when a three digit number is divided by a two digit number. Such a problem is impossible for the patient not because there is a loss of comprehension of the decimal system of notation, but because of the instability and diffuseness of his speech processes.

Secondary disturbances of computational processes may occur as a result of *motor aphasia,* especially if the aphasia involves a disturbance of *inner speech.*

The disturbance of computational operations in these cases is almost always the same. The recognition of individual digits is usually well preserved, although the severe disturbances of inner speech may affect even this function. If the patient hears a number pronounced he does not have an immediate concept of the quantity it represents. Often he hears a number simply as some kind of amorphous sound complex. The pattern becomes meaningful only if he pronounces to himself. In so doing he analyzes its meaning; he sorts out the individual digits and thus determines its meaning. He may also recognize the meaning of a number if he is allowed to see it in written form. It appears that external speech or a visual image is necessary for objectivization and sharpening of any number which he hears. When one of these factors is incorporated into the perceptual process the precise concept of the number becomes clear. Thus, one cannot say that the primary defect lies in loss of the concept of the number.

One also finds dynamic disturbances in the computational processes of such a patient. Almost every patient with a clear-cut motor aphasia complains of some difficulty in carrying out calculations "in his head". If he is prevented from using external speech, addition and subtraction become difficult, and more complex operations become altogether impossible. The psychological basis of these disturbances does not involve loss of the numerical operations themselves, but rather an inability to conceptualize numbers and loss of the automaticity of simple computational operations. The first difficulty makes it impossible to perceive or remember the numbers on which mathematical operations are to be performed. When the patient attempts to carry out an operation the numbers disappear, disintegrate, or are displaced by the perseveration of numbers previously operated upon. Thus the problem $29 + 17$ may be transformed into $29 + 27$ or $29 + 19$. The patient is uncertain as to whether he remerbers the numbers correctly or not. As might be expected, calculations involving three digit numbers are impossible for such a patient. The numbers become conglomerations of digits which he is unable to organize and retain in proper sequence. Such a patient is characteristically aided by pronouncing the numbers aloud. By uttering them aloud, he is able to analyze them, his concept of the numbers he is working with is sharpened, and he is better able to apply the proper operations.

The second source of difficulty is loss of the automaticity of computational processes. This is typical of lesions of the premotor systems in general and of the anterior parts of the speech areas in particular. As a rule, even highly automatized computational habits are disturbed in these cases. The patient completely forgets the multiplication tables and attempts to compensate for his loss by means of addition. Less automatic operations also suffer. In the most severe cases patients are unable to carry out the most familiar and simple arithmetical operations. The problem "7 + 3" does not immediately elicit the response, "10"; "11–2" does not evoke the immediate response "9". Loss of the automatic character of computational operations often forces the patient to count on his fingers in order to solve simple problems. It is obvious that problems involving change in the tens digit, e.g., 31–7, thus a two step solution, is extremely difficult. Often the patient will carry out only one step and assume that he has reached the answer. It is as though he forgets the second step altogether. Problems in which the solution can be reached by several steps, e.g., 12 + 6–3, have shown that patients in this group are unable to retain the inner plan of operations required to solve such problems. All elements which they are required to retain in consciousness tend to run together, to be displaced by perseveration of preceding elements, or to disappear altogether.

These defects are not structural but dynamic in nature.The patient still comprehends the decimal system of notation and is able to carry out individual numerical operations. He is able to derive great benefit from external speech for by naming the numbers and operations aloud he reduces the instability of the number images and numerical operations whereby the numerical information is processed. If allowed to solve problems on paper he has virtually no difficulty. A patient who cannot solve a single numerical problem "in his head" may be able to carry out quite complex computational operations under conditions which permit him to avoid the use of inner speech and mathematical habits which he has lost.

Disturbance of the conceptualization of problems as a whole occurs most commonly in cases involving lesions in the *frontal area* just anterior to the speech zone of the left hemisphere. Massive lesions in this area do not affect the concept of number or such elementary computational operations as addition and subtraction of numbers less than ten. Difficulty arises, however, when the patient is required to solve problems which can only be solved by adherence to planned sequences of calculations, i.e., which require him to solve certain sequences of "sub-problems". When he has to solve a problem in his head he frequently omits steps. He is unable to organize his mathematical operations according to a plan by breaking down the overall problem into a series of sub-problems. This defect becomes obvious whenever he attempts to substract one two-digit number from another, e.g., 41–27. Ordinarily the solution to such a problem would involve a series of sub-problems, e.g., 41–20 followed by subtraction of 7 from the remainder. He has difficulty in dividing because he is unable to make the preliminary approximation which it requires. Finally, he is unable to carry out multiple subtractions of 7 from 100. Here again, the minuend at each step is the remainder from the previous operation. Completion of the step 100–7 = 93 must immediately set the stage for the next step 93–7 = 86. Many patients with frontal lobe lesions are unable to transform the answer from one operation into a given for the next operation. Often they end up by substituting a simple stereotype sequence of responses for the correct subtractive process, e.g., "100–7 = 93 . . . 83 . . . 73 . . . 63 . . . etc."

Impairment of the ability to conceptualize the sequence of operations necessary to solve simple problems obviously prevents the solution of more complex problems. Often patients with massive frontal lobe lesions are unable to devise a proper sequence of operations; thus they substitute a random combination of mathematical operations for the appropriate rational sequence. As might be expected this usually leads to nonsensical results.[2]

In all of the above cases the disturbance of calculation has been secondary to some other disturbance. The primary structure of numbers and numerical operations remained intact, but the execution of computational operations was hindered by such factors as instability of acoustico-gnostic process or disruption of the dynamics of mental processes peripherally involved in calculation. Cases have been observed, however, in which there was a *primary loss* of the structure of numbers and consequent disruption of all computational operations. This "primary acalculia" is almost always present with *semantic aphasias* and frequently arises as a result of lesions in the left occipito-parietal area.

Patients with semantic aphasia retain the meanings of simple numerical symbols. They have no difficulty in writing numbers to dictation and are able to read numbers composed of one or two digits. On close examination, however, it becomes apparent that only such elementary numerical processes are intact. Comprehension of the decimal system of notation is profoundly disturbed. Thus, while the digits retain their direct meanings, they lose the meaning which they would gain on the basis of their context if the patient retained his understanding of the decimal system. Loss of comprehension of the decimal system of notation gives rise to severe impairment of numerical concepts.

Patients in this group have no difficulty in *counting*, but if they attempt to count backwards, they make numerous mistakes, e.g., they omit numbers. Patients with

[2] A complete psychological analysis of this type of disturbance is beyond the scope of the present investigation. We have presented more observations pertinent to this syndrome elsewhere. See A. R. Luria and L. S. Cvetkova, *Neuropsychological Analysis of Problem Solving* (Moscow, Prosveščenie, 1966 [Russian]) (the French edition: *Troubles de solutions des problèmes neurospychologiques*, Paris, Gautier-Villars, 1968).

severe injuries may have difficulty in counting forwards, not uncommonly their counting goes, "11, 12, 14, 17, 18, etc.", indicating that they have lost the sequential pattern of the numbers. This defect emerges most clearly when there is a change in the tens digit. Here again, the patient may skip a digit to produce such a sequence as, "78, 79, 90, 91, etc." Such patients never detect their own errors.

The patient's greatest difficulty arises when he attempts to *read or evaluate numbers of more than three digits*. Usually he is unable to read numbers involving more than one digit. For instance, he may read 17 as "1 and 7", or he may read 264 as "2, 6, and 4", as though he is unable to integrate the individual digits into a single number. The only multiple digits which he can perceive are such round numbers as 100, 500, etc. These are apparently perceived as numerical ideograms and can be recognized without the processes necessary for numerical synthesis. With much practice the patient can learn to read multiple digit numbers, but his comprehension of the relationships between digits defined by the decimal system of notation remains defective. As a result, his attempts to evaluate numbers continues to produce gross errors. He estimates the size of a multiple digit number on the basis of the individual digits rather than on the basis of their significance in terms of the decimal system. To him 398 appears larger than 401; he estimates 189 to be larger than 203. If the examiner asks him which digit represents tens, which represents hundreds, and which represents units it soon becomes apparent that he has completely lost the concept of decimal notation. He makes frequent mistakes in writing numbers to dictation; he tends to write the digits in the order in which they are pronounced rather than in accordance with the decimal system, e.g., he writes "seventeen" as "71". Sometimes he writes the digits in the wrong sequence for no apparent reason, e.g., he may write "three hundred forty two" as "324". He makes frequent errors in writing numbers which contains zeros. For instance, he may write "one thousand twenty three" as "123" or "100023". He makes the same types of mistakes when he reads numbers, so that even after a long period of retraining he may read 1003 as one hundred three. He perceives complex numbers not in terms of he decimal system but simply as groups of numerical ideograms.

Characteristically, the most persistent defect in patients in this group lies in differentiating between symmetrical numbers. Thus the numbers 69 and 96 are estimated to be identical in value. The Roman numerals IV and VI or IX and XI may be confused or evaluated incorrectly. These difficulties arise because of loss of the sequential structure of multiple digit numbers. A loss of directional orientation prevents the patient from distinguishing visual stimuli which differ only in the order of symbolic elements. This cannot help but influence his ability to calculate. As a rule the only operations which remain are those which have become highly automatic. In contrast to patients with efferent motor aphasia who are unable to recall the multiplication tables, patients in this group show no detectable impairment of motor-speech. Calculations which have not become automatic, however require that mathematical operations be carried out at a conscious level, and these operations are lost.

These patients also lose the system of alternatives which allow one to recognize immediately the relationships of a given number to other numbers. Thus it is not immediately apparent to them that 16 may be looked upon as 20–4, 15 + 1, or 4 x 4. Having lost the sets of equivalents, they are unable to carry out simple numerical operations with normal facility and are sometimes forced to resort to doing addition and subtraction on their fingers, whereas a normal person would be able to give an immediate answer.

The ability to add and subtract two digit numbers may remain severely impaired long after other defects have disappeared or been compensated for. Any calculation involving a change in the tens digit is capable of exposing the fact that the patient no longer recognizes the meaning of the decimal system of notation. He combines units and tens as though he were unable to keep the digits in their appropriate sequence. The difficulty does not result from a memory defect but from an inability to recognize the significance of sequence. This becomes especially clear if the patient is required to calculate the answers to problems presented in an unconventional manner. For instance, if the problem 12 plus 14 is written so that the digits appear in a vertical column the patient simply adds all of the individual digits together without paying any attention to the order. He may identify the numbers incorrectly in which case he is apt to make one of the following types of mistake:

$$\begin{array}{r} 1 \\ 2 \\ +1 \\ 4 \\ \hline 8 \end{array} \quad \text{or} \quad \begin{array}{r} 1 \\ 2 \\ +1 \\ 4 \\ \hline 53 \end{array} \quad \text{or} \quad \begin{array}{r} 1 \\ 2 \\ +1 \\ 4 \\ \hline 35 \end{array}$$

As might be expected, such a patient is totally incapable of working with fractions. In attempting to subtract one fraction from another he confuses the minuend and subtrahend. Characteristic errors resulting from this type of disturbance are:

$$\frac{1}{4} + \frac{1}{4} = \frac{2}{8}\ ;\ \frac{1}{2} + \frac{1}{3} = \frac{2}{5}\ ;\ \text{etc.}$$

The origin of the computational difficulties in these cases lies in a loss of spatial orientation. In solving such a problem as 31–7, the patient must first subtract 7 from the round number 30 and then add 1 to the result. In solving this problem, however, he will frequently answer, "30 minus 7 equals 23; 23 minus 1 equals 22". His concepts of mathematical operations are lost, so that he is often unable to supply the missing mathematical symbols in such problems as 8 (?) 2 = 10. He confuses subtraction with addition and division with multiplication. He is unable to differentiate between such statements as " x is so-*much* larger than y" "x is so-*many-times*-larger than y". In either case he is apt to write (x + y = . . .).

These are the computational disturbances which are seen to accompany lesions in the parieto-occipital system. They are usually not accompanied by general dementia. They are simply one aspect of the semantic aphasia syndrome which results from the loss of inner simultaneous schemata. In this sense they are analogous to the speech disorders seen in semantic aphaia.

CONCLUSIONS

On the basis of this outline of aphasic syndromes we can draw certain general conclusions regarding the principles which one should follow in assessing the psychological symptoms of focal brain damage. Careful study has convinced us that damage to any area of the cerebral cortex which plays a role in the integration of one or another form of cerebral activity inevitably affects the overall system of psychophysiological processes. Thus we have pointed out that almost any cortical lesion leads to some motor or perceptual deficit, some impairment of expressive speech or speech comprehension, or some reading, writing, or computational disorder. This does not mean, however, that such complex functions are always affected in the same way. On the contrary, by careful analysis it has been shown that with any particular lesion the disturbance bears certain definite and constant features which clearly distinguish it from lesions in other areas.

Motor disturbances may result from lesions in the posterior or anterior parts of the cerebral cortex. Those which result from posterior lesions involve impairment of afferent integration processes; for instance they are associated with loss of body orientation, objective spatial disorientation, or disturbance of the symbol-object relationships in terms of which patterns of movement are formulated. On the other hand those which result from anterior lesions involve the disruption of temporally ordered processes and are associated with loss of the sequential organization of motor acts. The motor disorders are entirely different. In exactly the same way, there is a difference between the perceptual disturbances observed with anterior and posterior lesions. Whereas lesions of the posterior, afferent areas of the cortex disturb primary recognition, lesions of the anterior areas destroy the purposeful direction of perceptual activity and give rise to perceptual defects of a different type.

The categorization of lesions giving rise to speech disorders is considerably more complicated. Focal damage to different parts of the primary speech zones or bordering areas abolishes different components or basic factors of speech activity. Psychologically, however, speech is such a highly organized and unitary function that partial lesions usually disturb the functional system as a whole.

This does not mean that the syndromes arising as result of a focal brain lesion are due to different degrees of disturbance of a single aspect of speech; speech as a whole is not disturbed in some overall diffuse manner. The "unitary aphasia" hypothesis of P. Marie is not sufficient to account for the multiplicity of syndromes which one observes. The removal of a particular prerequisite for the formulation of speech activity always leads to breakdown of the *system of basic speech processes*.

Thus, a lesion of the left temporal area destroys the secondary part of the central auditory apparatus and leads to the disruption of auditory processes. In particular it abolishes the ability to organize perceptual processes in such a way as to recognize the speech sounds which have become stabilized as phonemes with the historical development of language. The loss of the sound schemata is the underlying cause of the syndrome which arises as a result of lesions in the temporal systems. Lesions of the post-central, kinesthetic cortical areas result in loss of the ability to differentiate the proprioceptive patterns associated with the production of different sounds. With the development of language certain patterns of kinesthetic perception have taken on the character of inner, generalized articulatory schemata, or *articulemes*. The loss of articulemes is the basic defect underlying aphasias resulting from lesions of the afferent systems. Damage to the speech parts of the premotor areas disturbs not only the sequential organization of innervational impulses but also abolishes the *inner speech* which is necessary for the dynamic integration of speech activity. In other words, it destroys the basic mechanism for the transformation of thought into external speech.

From this it is clear that every localized lesion affects the entire system of speech processes. Careful analysis shows that expressive speech, receptive speech, reading, and writing always depend upon a complex constellation of individual functions; thus they all suffer as a result of focal lesions.

Expressive speech can hardly be thought of as a function localizable to some narrowly defined "motor speech zone." In order for expressive speech to be normal phonemic hearing must be intact, kinesthetic schemata must be present to permit the immediate mobilization of articulatory movements, and the capacity to organize the sound-articulatory schemata into sequential patterns must be present. Besides this, the entire apparatus concerned with the external, phasic aspect of speech must act in accordance with the higher level semantic speech patterns which we have discussed in the preceding pages.

Given the complexity of the expressive speech system it is impossible to conceive of its being localized in any "center for the motor images of words". A disturbance of expressive speech by no means always indicates a lesion in Broca's area. Everything that we know about the cerebral organization of speech processes indicates that almost any lesion involving the broad speech area in the left hemisphere may lead to a disturbance of expressive speech and that the particular disturbance may take on any one of a number of forms depending upon precisely what site is involved.

Lesions of the operculum usually lead to loss of the *phasic external organization* of active speech and thus to the type of syndrome which Nielsen (1946) has referred to as "aphasia of a lower level". Articulated speech becomes quite difficult, but the difficulty may take any of several forms depending upon what part of the cerebral cortex is damaged and what type of integration is primarily affected.

It would be incorrect to presume that the loss of any particular psychophysiological prerequisite for speech should affect only the external, phasic aspect of speech. Usually the lesion leads to disintegration of the *semantic aspect* of speech. The semantic disintegration may affect both active, expressive speech and speech comprehension. Thus, a lesion of the secondary or tertiary temporal areas which disturbs primarily the auditory images of words inevitably results in inability to understand the meanings of words and loss of the nominative function of speech. Such a lesion deprives expressive speech of its content and produces a severe disturbance of speech comprehension. A lesion of the parietal, tertiary perceptual system, which is primarily involved in the organization of simultaneous schemata, inevitably deprives both expressive and receptive speech of the continuity which is required if one is to consider a body of material or group of symbols as a whole. Finally, a lesion in the frontal part of the speech area has no effect whatever on the objective, nominative aspect of speech nor on the predicative inner speech which is so important in the transformation of thought into external speech. A frontal lesion affects the dynamics of speech comprehension so that the patient is unable to grasp immediately the meanings of complex statements.

The same can be said for the cortical localization of reading, writing, calculation, and more complex intellectual processes as has been said for expressive speech. It is clear that we cannot talk in terms of the "localization" of such complex processes within particular narrowly defined areas of the cerebral cortex. From this it follows that we cannot attribute damage to a single well-circumscribed area when one of these general "functions" is impaired to give a specific symptom such as alexia or agraphia. What is localized is not a function or a symptom but a *basic component for complex speech activity. Any disturbance of expressive speech, speech comprehension, reading, writing, or computation has localizing significance only after it has been subjected to a careful clinico-psychological analysis.* Such analysis should result in *psychological classification* of the symptom; it should reveal *exactly how* some particular aspect of speech is impaired, and it should show *just which basic factors* have been disturbed in order to give rise to the observed symptoms. Only on the basis of this type of psychological classification is it possible to draw any conclusions as to the site of brain damage from observations of clinical symptoms.

Any attempt to define "centers" for motor or sensory aphasia or "centers" for agraphia, alexia, and acalculia without preliminary analysis of the disturbed functions is just as indefensible as the attempt to establish focal cerebral areas responsible for expressive speech, speech comprehension, reading, writing, and computation. Future clinico-psychological studies must be based upon a proper conception of what roles specific areas play in the various general functions. It is necessary to abandon naive attempts to localize functions; only by careful analysis will it become clear precisely what clinico-psychological changes occur in the different functions with lesions of specific cortical areas.

Thus we return to the position from which we began our investigation. The symptoms which arise as a result of focal brain damage will only become thoroughly clear *in terms of the total syndromes* of which they are a part. The loss of phonemic hearing which results from lesions in the left temporal area affects primarily the recognition of words and the receptive aspect of speech. It inevitably leads also however, to disturbance of the nominative aspect of words and gives rise to important expressive speech defects. By disrupting the ability to recognize the sound pattern of words it gives rise to a writing disorder. In the person for whom reading is not fully automatized and who cannot read at all on the basis of visual ideograms it produces severe reading impairment. Finally, to the extent that verbal habits are necessary for the organization of mathematical operations, it gives rise to substantial difficulty in calculation.

At first glance it may appear that the symptoms resulting from a lesion in a given area are quite hetereogeneous. More careful analysis, however, usually reveals that there are certain *common factors* basic to all of the symptoms and that they all result from the loss of one particular prerequisite. By analyzing for the common feature in what appears to be a heterogeneous group of disturbances one comes to a better understanding of the nature of each particular symptom and why it should result from a given lesion. This has been the primary goal of the psychological investigations carried out in our clinic.

Any psychological analysis of the symptoms which arise as a result of focal brain damage must take into account one other factor of principal significance. Any psychological function of the cerebral cortex is the product of *learning*. In the process of learning all functions undergo important qualitative changes which involve major shifts in psychological structure and basic changes in the organization of brain mechanisms. Perhaps the best example of this is the psychological development of the *reading process*. In its early stages reading is a complex process involving the phonemic analysis of written words. With further development, its psychological structure changes radically; it is gradually transformed into a process involving the direct visual recognition of words as ideograms. The mechanisms involved in phonemic analysis gradually disappear and reading becomes automatic, i.e., those psychophysiological systems which were essential during the first stage of development are no longer required. It is clear that damage to a given cortical system may produce completely different symptoms *depending upon the level of organization of various psychological processes at the time of injury*. Thus, a lesion in the auditory part of the left temporal area completely abolishes the ability to read in patients for whom reading has not become an automatic process. On the other hand, the very same lesion in a patient for whom reading has become automatic may produce a reading defect which is barely detectable. The level of development of psychological functions can influence the syndromes arising from damage to almost any area. The evaluation of this factor is important for the proper evaluation of any given symptom.

PART III

REHABILITATION OF PATIENTS WITH TRAUMATIC APHASIA

INTRODUCTORY REMARKS

The residual speech disturbances following traumatic aphasia are often severe. They result from the functional exclusion of various links in the cerebral systems which are necessary for speech; thus they often fail to remit spontaneously. Patients with central speech disturbances have often been thought of and treated as permanent invalids. Once having done everything possible to insure normal healing of the wound, doctors have often failed to undertake any further therapy.

Brain cells once destroyed do not regenerate. The authors have observed over and over again, however, that residual speech defects in traumatic aphasia may be markedly reduced or overcome to one degree or another by suitable therapy. The same conclusion was reached by K. Goldstein (1942, 1948), an investigator who has contributed perhaps more than any other to our understanding of the restoration of speech functions after focal brain damage. Ombredane (1951) and many others have, likewise, expressed the same opinion. The success or failure of attempts to restore speech functions depends largely upon the ration of the therapeutic measures taken. Appropriate measures can be undertaken only after identification of the basic factors responsible for the various symptoms and with recognition of means whereby the defects may be compensated for.

In some cases functional disturbances arise as a result of temporary loss of activity in certain brain areas. In these cases it is only necessary to alleviate the functional inhibition in order to achieve complete remission of the corresponding speech defects. In other cases functional disturbances result from the destruction of brain tissue. The loss is permanent in these cases, and there is no direct method for reviving the disrupted functional complex. These two types of disturbance are quite different and they should be treated differently.

In order to clarify the problems with which we are dealing, we should pause to mention one other approach to the restoration of cortical functions. We need not consider it in great detail, for while it is quite important for the restoration of motor functions, it has somewhat less significance in the treatment of traumatic aphasia. It has been found that the functional disturbances arising as a result of traumatic brain damage are made up of *two components*. Part of the loss results from damage to particular cortical areas which *destroys* the functional systems to which they contribute. The remainder results from the fact that certain cortical systems not destroyed by the injury are *inhibited*, very likely as the result of loss of the normal conduction of excitation in the areas directly involved. This inhibition differs considerably from the protective type of inhibition. Here the administration of pharmacological agents to act upon intermediate metabolism and to restore the biochemical processes necessary for normal synaptic conduction can restore the disturbed functions.

Among the pharmacological agents shown to be effective in restoring impaired functions are compounds of the anticholinesterase group. The biochemical process of synaptic transmission is dependent upon a certain level of acetylcholine. It is known, however, that acetylcholine is blocked by cholinesterase, and that the level of cholinesterase activity is greatly increased with trauma and other pathological processes. This observation gave rise, during the Second World War, to a series of investigations by Ja. A. Ratner, N. I. Graščenkov, and L. B. Perel'man who administered such anticholinergic agents as eserine and prostigmine, in order to inhibit the cholinesterases and restore the acetylcholine to a level of activity characteristic of the normal nervous system. Much important information was derived from the administration of anticholinergic drugs to trauma patients during wartime (Graščenkov, 1947; Luria, 1948; Perel'man, 1946) and to other types of patients since the war (Ejdinova and Pravdina-Vinarskaja, 1959).

These investigations showed that one or two injections of prostigmine were capable of restoring components of motor activity which were impaired simply by the transient depression resulting from a disturbance of synaptic transmission. Motor defects resulting from the destruction of brain tissue or conduction pathways were not restored. The restoration of depressed motor functions was permanent; thus, the administration of anticholinesterases became a routine part of the therapy in such cases. M. B. Eidinova and E. N. Pravdina-Vinarskaja have shown that the anticholinesterase preparations are useful in the treatment of children with cerebral paralysis, a syndrome which was previously considered irreversible.

These preparations are less effective in the treatment of speech disturbances than in the treatment of more gross motor deficits. In cases where the speech disturbance is only one facet of a more general cerebral paralysis or part of the pseudobulbar syndrome, the anticholinesterases are quite effective; they are capable of relieving the paresis and dystonia characteristic of such disorder (Ejdinova and Pravdina-Vinarskaja, 1959). Attempts to develop modes of pharmalogical therapy useful for aphasias of other types have met with little success; thus we shall not dwell on this approach to the restoration of speech functions.

XV

THE RESTORATION OF SPEECH PROCESSES: DISTURBANCES RESULTING FROM INHIBITION

A. BASIC PRINCIPLES

We have already indicated that any injury which destroys cortical tissue gives rise to a dynamic inhibition or blockade of functional systems as a whole.[1] This phenomenon was originally referred to by Monakow as "diaschisis" and is apparently related to three factors. First, an injury which destroys some cells brings other cells in the same area into a state of *reduced excitability*, or it disrupts *synaptic transmission* in that area. In the acute period after injury this is associated with cerebral edema and changes in cerebral blood flow; it may persist for a long time.

Secondly, a focal injury eliminates one link in a functional system and thus disrupts the system as a whole for a certain length of time. This disturbance is reflected in the apparent loss of normal function in other links of the same system. Monakov studied the disruption of overall functional systems and suggested a three-part classification of "*conductive*", "*associative*" and "*commissural*" *diaschisis*. During the Second World War different forms of inhibition were investigated by a number of Soviet physiologists and clinicians (A. N. Grinštejn, P. K. Anokhin, E. A. Asratjan). These investigators studied primarily peripheral neural phenomena. They found this type of mechanism useful in accounting for the fact that a small lesion of the ulnar nerve, for instance, could produce pathological impulses capable of blocking normal function of the medial and radial nerves, to give a generalized paralysis of the entire forearm, a paralysis which was essentially "*reflex*" in nature.

The third type of functional inhibition is closely related to the second, or reflex type. A person never reacts passively to injury. If a lesion disrupts an entire functional system he naturally reacts by *actively avoiding* use of the affected system. By shifting as much as possible to other systems he may completely dissociate himself from the disturbed system and fail to show any signs of residual capacity whatever. This phenomenon is seen most commonly with peripheral injuries in the skeletal muscular system where a mental "block" or set may suppress the potential restoration of function for a long time.

[1] See A. R. Luria, *The Restoration of Brain Functions After War Trauma* (Press of the Academy of Medical Sciences of the USSR, Moscow, 1948) (English edition, London, Pergamon Press, 1963).

Any rational approach to the rehabilitation of aphasic patients must take into account these dynamic components of functional disturbances. It is essential to free the functional system of inhibition as rapidly as possible. Efforts must be directed toward disinhibiting functions which have been blocked and making use of whatever residual functional capacity exists.

There are different forms of therapy corresponding to the three types of inhibition described above. In the acute phase after injury, when edema is the major cause of functional disturbance pharmacological agents directed against the reduced excitability and faulty synaptic transmission may be of considerable aid.

When a small focal injury leads to inhibition of a whole functional system, i.e., to diaschisis or reflexogenic functional loss pharmacological therapy may fail to yield any noticeable results. In this case attention must be directed toward the removal of pathological impulses arising from the site of injury, e.g., by surgical removal of a foreign body or scar. *The nonfunctional structure must be incorporated into a broader functional system* so as to enhance the chances of its disinhibition. Examples of this approach have been described in the physiological and psychophysiological literature. Early animal experiments by L. A. Orbeli and K. I. Kunstman and later by P. K. Anokhin showed that after deafferentation the restoration of function to an extremity is accelerated if it is kept in its normal working position and if its movements are part of an overall pattern of locomotion involving the four extremities. The restoration of partial functions by incorporating them into general functional systems became one of the fundamental principles of Anokhin's work.

Similar observations were made by A. N. Leont'ev and A. V. Zaporožec.[2] In studying motor disturbances in patients with arm and leg injuries, these authors observed that the ability to move the injured limb varied depending upon the task. An isolated movement such as a shift in position of the affected limb was very difficult for the patient. If the movement was part of a broader functional system such as grasping a fallen object or erasing a blackboard, however, the range of possible movement was greatly extended. This observation gave rise to one of the major therapeutic techniques applied by these authors for the functional rehabilitation of patients during the war. Movements of the injured limb were incorporated into more general functional systems, e.g., into a system of bimanual activity characteristic of wood working. At first the injured arm played only a passive role, as in planing or sawing wood; gradually it was drawn into more active roles. There is now no doubt but that the incorporation of a movement into an active functional system can be considered a general means of disinhibiting functions in the late stages following trauma. This technique is incomparably more effective than passive methods such as massage, physiotherapy, and the like.

This approach is the most appropriate form of therapy in all cases except where

[2] A. N. Leont'ev and A. V. Zaporožec, "The Recovery of Movements", *Soviet Science* (Moscow, 1945).

the major factor is a protective mental set, i.e., a protective personality reaction to the injury. In this case only a *radical change in the patient's surroundings* is likely to reduce the inhibition and to restore the disturbed functional system. The change in the environment must be accompanied by incorporation of the disturbed function into some form of active functional system. Only when the patient becomes confident that he can activate the damaged system does he become capable of creating sufficiently strong intentions to overcome the protective set and to incorporate the injured limb in his motor activity. Thus, basically, the same approach makes it possible to overcome this type of defect.

B. RESTORATION OF SPEECH FUNCTIONS BY DISINHIBITION

In many cases the types of functional disinhibition described above also account for the recovery of speech processes. Speech disorders may appear considerably more extensive than they are as a result of transient reduction of the excitability and conductivity of cerebral cells, by active inhibition of speech as a whole, and by the same protective personality mechanisms which can totally block motor activity. Since the relationships among these three components are extremely variable, the therapeutic approaches vary greatly also.

Focal lesions in the left hemisphere can give rise to temporary suppression of all speech processes (see Chapter I). Thus in the initial period following injury severe speech disorders may arise only to remit spontaneously a few days later. For instance, speech disturbances arising as a result of the inhibition of neuronal elements near the site of injury rapidly disappear. Speech blocks due to inhibition from higher levels may last indefinitely and demand special therapeutic measures. Such blocks are seen most clearly in reactive postcontusional deaf mutism where the functional components play a leading role. The pathogenesis of this wartime disorder was greatly clarified by studies carried out by G. V. Geršuni, V. A. Giljarovskij, L. B. Perel'man, and others during World War II. As a result, the best form of treatment is now fairly well established.

Reactive postcontusional deaf-mutism is produced by the shock waves set up by the explosion of modern weapons. Intense transient changes in air pressure cause contusions and extreme excitation of the auditory nerve which, in turn, produces a temporary form of parabiotic inhibition. The inhibition is accompanied by a general protective personality reaction which Geršuni has shown leads to the cessation of auditory perception. The auditory threshold is elevated so that sounds of normal intensity fall in the "subsensory" range, even though objective recordings indicate that they produce the usual evoked potentials in the temporal cortical area and evoke involuntary reactions such as the cochleo-pupillary reflex. The displacement of auditory reception to the subsensory range, i.e., the cortical block of hearing, can remain for a long time, sometimes for several months.

It is important to note that this long term inhibition of auditory perception is accompanied by a block of the auditory-speech system as a whole. The question arises as to whether this is simply the result of inhibition of the vocal apparatus or the result of inhibition of speech at some higher level. Reactive postcontusional deaf mutism always involves a block of the entire functional system. The immediate cause is presumed to be the contusion produced by the shock wave; this is fixed by an affective personality reaction which creates a set or expectation that the damaged function is permanently lost.

Rehabilitation therapy should obviously be directed toward changing this set. The change can occur only if the inhibited system can be partially incorporated into some functional system involving at a conscious level. Not only must vocal speech be disinhibited, but the disinhibition must occur within the sphere of consciousness. Only if the patient is conscious of the fact that partial disinhibition has been achieved can he gain the confidence necessary for total restoration of function.

The therapeutic techniques are based upon the fact that the more intense the stimulus and the more obvious the expectation that the patient should perceive it, the less likely it is to be perceived. Conversely, the weaker the stimulus and the more peripheral to the sphere of consciousness it appears to be, the greater the chance that it will be perceived. One sees a similar situation to this in cases involving the block of various affective functions. In the first phase of rehabilitation the examiner attempts to clear the way for innocuous auditory stimulation to reach the sphere of consciousness by distracting the patient's attention during presentation of the sound. No further progress can be made until this step has been accomplished.

The following is an example of the use of this technique by L. B. Perel'man in the Rehabilitation Unit of the Clinic for Nervous Diseases.[3]

The patient who complains of total deafness, but who readily answers written questions (usually by written answers) is asked a number of questions. Each question is presented both in written form and orally. Thus, two functional foci are created simultaneously: one central (visual perception of the written question), and the other peripheral to the patient's sphere of consciousness (auditory perception of the oral question does not reach the level of consciousness). Gradually the written questions are presented in less and less legible form and the patient unwittingly begins to respond to the oral questions which he gradually incorporates into the functional system of the written dialogue. Thus the auditory representation of the words gradually enters his consciousness.

An example of such a series of experiments is presented in Figure 78. Once the desired goal has been achieved, i.e., when the patient is able to answer questions written in a totally illegible script, the examiner can point to this as objective evidence of his ability to hear the speech of others. This is a critical moment, for the effectiveness of all subsequent suggestive and psychotherapeutic techniques depends upon the patient's confidence that he retains a residuum of auditory perception, that his hearing will improve, and that he can remaster auditory speech. The major goal is to revise the personality set so as to incorporate the partial function, of which the patient is con-

[3] This work has been described in detail in the small volume by L. B. Perel'man, *Reactive Postcontusional Deaf-Mutism: Diagnosis and Treatment* (Moscow, 1943 [Russian]).

scious, into his overall personality. L. B. Perel'man noted the first signs of disinhibition as early as the second or third day of such therapy. In virtually all cases, full recovery of auditory perception was achieved within two weeks. A spontaneous total recovery was never observed.

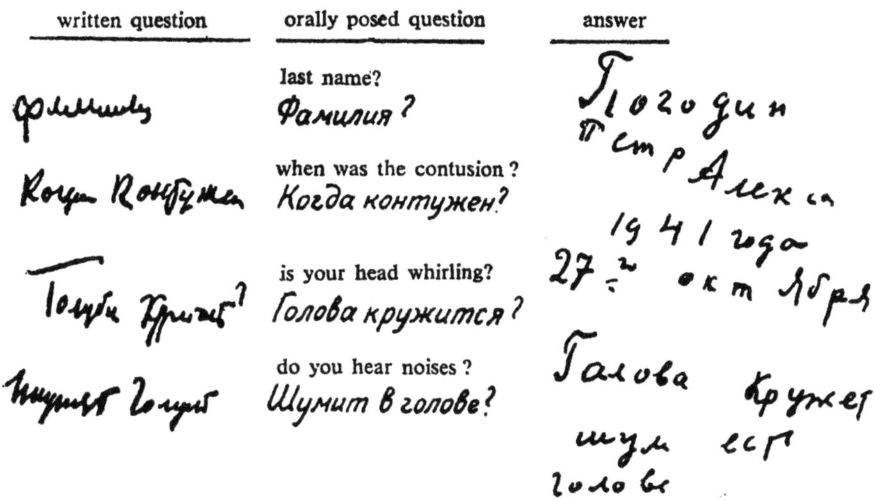

transliteration of Fig. 78.

written questions	orally posed question	answer
Familija (Last Name)	Familija (Last Name)	Pagodin Petr Aleksa
Kogda Kontužen? (When was the Concussion?)	Kogda Kontužen? (When was the Concussion?)	1941 27th of October
Golubi Krichut	Golova Kruzhit? (Is your head whirling?)	head whirls
(The doves are crying) (Illigible)	Šumit v Golove? (Is your head noisy?)	my head is noisy.

FIG. 78. Experiment carried out by L. B. Perelman to test the perception of oral speech in a patient with post-contusional deafness.

(Both written and oral questions are presented simultaneously).

The same type of method is used in cases involving functional speech blocks. Reactive postcontusional mutism is basically an *aphonia* which is due to an articulatory block. By means of various external maneuvers, such as pressing on the chest cavity, applying painful stimulation, etc., the examiner attempts to elicit some form of phonation which he can use as a starting point for reorganizing the basic personality set of the patient. He must do everything possible to incorporate the blocked speech system into the overall behavior of the patient. This is where the disinhibition techniques are useful. Once this first stage is past the patient may go through several stages of dysphonia, stuttering, and the like.

We have intentionally introduced the description of techniques used for the disinhibition of speech functions with a discussion of the restoration of hearing and phonation in cases of reactive postcontusional deaf mutism. The alteration of personality set is especially important in cases where one must overcome the functional dissociation of speech from the main stream of conscious behavior. In traumatic aphasia, especially in the early stages, block, or dissociation, of the impaired function is virtually always present. The picture in traumatic aphasia is more complex than that in postcontusional deaf mutism, however, for it involves permanent destruction of certain cortical areas and the disruption of specific prerequisites with consequent reorganization of the speech function as a whole.

In the early stages the aphasic first discovers that he is unable to speak and he usually abandons the disturbed speech function. He may cease talking altogether or use only very simple forms of speech. If the aphasia is accompanied by general cerebral asthenia, the speech block may be acute. Thus, as M. S. Lebedinski has justifiably pointed out, the initial period of therapy consists of an attempt to alter the protective, inhibitory set of the patient, i.e., to create confidence that he will be able to regain the use of speech. Of course such a set is considerably easier to establish if the patient retains some remnant of speech activity no matter how minor it may appear to be. It is impossible to overestimate the psychotherapeutic value of the slightest success in using whatever remains of his speech, for on this depends all motivation for further retraining. In order to maximize the possibility of utilizing the patient's remaining speech, the therapeutic environment should include the cooperation of nurses and ward mates who can help him to take advantage of every sound he utters.[4]

[4] During the latest period the problems of the restoration of blocked function via disinhibition was specially discussed elsewhere. Cf. A. R. Luria, *Restoration of Function after Brain Injuries* (London, Pergamon Press, 1963). M. B. Eidinova and E. N. Pravdina-Vinarskaya, *Cerebral Palsy in Children and its Treatment* (London, Pergamon Press, 1963).

XVI

THE RESTORATION OF ACTIVITY BY REORGANIZING FUNCTIONAL SYSTEMS

A. GENERAL PRINCIPLES

In the cases considered in the preceding chapter inhibition was responsible for functional impairment. Therapy was directed toward restoring functions in *their original form*. This type of recovery is the exception rather than the rule however, in cases involving the destruction of cortical tissue. Usually the destruction of a mass of nerve cells results in irreversible functional changes, so that recovery of the disturbed functional systems can be achieved only by *major reorganization* of cortical processes.

Early investigators such as Sherrington and, later, Lashley were well aware of the benefit to be gained by reorganizing cortical processes. These authors produced limb paralysis in monkeys by extirpating the appropriate part of the motor cortex. After a period of time the animals regained movement of the paralyzed extremity and the authors carried out numerous experiments to delineate the mechanisms underlying such recovery of function. One hypothesis was that the non-specificity of the cerebral systems was such as to permit the emergence of a new hand "center" or a transfer of function to some other already established "center". Further experiments did not confirm this hypothesis, however. When the animals were subjected to further operations involving extirpation of the adjacent cortex, the corresponding contralateral areas, and related subcortical ganglia, the *original paralysis could not be reproduced. The cortical organization of the restored function proves to be different from that of the original function.*

By observing the recovery of function in patients with traumatic brain injuries it has become possible to describe how the reorganization of function comes about. Damage to the primary projection areas of the cerebral cortex, i.e., to the central parts of the cortical nuclei of the various analyzers, leads *to loss of elementary forms of movement or sensation*. The elementary functions lost as a result of lesions in these areas are not recovered. The only means of compensating for deficits of this type is by transferring the functions to other structures or to other functional systems. Learning to use the other hand when one hand is paralyzed or learning to read Braille when the visual cortex has been destroyed are examples of such "substitutive compensation".

The recovery of function in cases involving the secondary "intrinsic" areas or zones of overlap between the different analyzers is quite different. The injury does not result in loss of an elementary function but in the *disruption of complex functional systems*. The disintegration of such systems is irreversible, but they may be reorganized; the defective link may be replaced by a new link so that the overall function is re-established on a new basis.

In animals, not just any cortical area can substitute for a given functional link to permit reorganization of function. Lashley and Anoxin showed that, "only an area which is already in some way part of the disturbed system is capable of being used in the functional reorganization" (Lashley, 1938). Lashley found that each cortical area is involved in both specific and nonspecific functions. This greatly enhances their capacity to take part in the restoration of disturbed functional systems. His findings were later confirmed by anatomists such as Filimonov (1945). Thus, it became apparent that *not the morphological proximtiy but the participation in common functional systems determines the substitution value of different cerebral areas for one another.*

In animals the functional systems are relatively constant; thus, as Bethe, Asrat'jan, and Anokhin have shown, the reorganization of function within certain systems occurs quite easily. In man, on the other hand, the development of work, the use of instruments, and, most important of all, the presence of speech which underlies the "second signalling system of the brain", permits functional systems of extreme plasticity. In man *almost any cortical area can acquire new functional significance and thus may be incorporated into almost any functional system*. Thus, whatever the human lacks in regenerative potential is made up for by greater functional flexibility. We shall consider a few examples of the ways in which functional systems may be restored by means of reorganization. The first involves the loss of simple motor and sensory functions.

It is well known that in man the act of walking depends largely upon proprioceptive impulses which permit continual check and correction for deviations from the normal walking pattern. Damage to the dorsal spinal columns interrupts the proprioceptive impulses and severely impairs the ability to walk. This disturbance is not irreversible, however, for in a very short time the *visual system* can be incorporated into locomotor system. Sometimes by use of a cane the patient may incorporate *tactile and proprioceptive sensations from the upper extremities* into the system. Eventually walking comes to be accomplished on the basis of a reorganized functional system. Investigations of N. A. Bernštejn in the theory of motor coordination have yielded numerous examples of such types of complex coordinated activities which can be reorganized in this fashion.

Defects in the visual and tactile systems may be compensated for in analogous ways. Sometimes lesions in the occipital lobe result not in an elementary visual defect, but in an overall disruption of complex visual perception. In a classical case described by Gelb and Goldstein the patient was able to identify white and colored spots, but he was unable to recognize objects or letters. He was able to compensate for this defect by substituting *movements of the hand or eyes* for the impaired function of visual integration. By tracing out the contour of an object with a finger or with his eyes he was able to "synthesize" its structure and thus was able to recognize it. Similarly, by outlining letters he developed a new functional system which made it possible for him to read.

The recovery of functions by reorganizing functional systems is probably the major mode of recovery in most cases of focal brain damage. Clinico-psychological analysis has shown the way in which recovery comes about is not the same in all cases. There are at least *two basic types of functional reorganization.* We shall illustrate this by examples drawn from our own previous investigations.

Many years ago we were concerned with developing a means of compensating for the disturbance of motor functions which occurs in parkinsonism. In the cases which were studied, damage to basal ganglia had resulted in the motor disorder characteristic of this disease. The pattern of movement was unaffected, but its automaticity was rapidly exhausted, so that after a few repetitions it became impossible to carry out a given act; a severe increase in muscle tonus would develop and movement would cease.

We were faced with the question of whether or not it was possible to overcome the automaticity defect and the rapid exhaustibility of voluntary movements. It was proposed that the patient's problem might be solved by transferring the act to the cortical level, i.e., by the substitution of a series of individual, conscious impulses for the patterned response cycle. The effect of this reorganization was immediately obvious. When we substituted a series of auditory signals for the single stimulus which had been used to evoke the same complex movement it became considerably more stable and the exhaustibility of the process less sharply (Figure 79). Observation of parkinsonian patients in everyday situations further supported this finding. A patient can take only a few steps along a smooth floor, but he has no difficulty in climbing stairs or walking across a floor which has lines painted at frequent intervals. Thus when reactive movements can take the place of automatic movements the patient has little difficulty in overcoming his motor defect. In order to really compensate for such a defect it is necessary to find the method whereby the patient can himself generate the individual stimuli to which he responds. *If autostimulation can be substituted for environmental stimulation all of the patient's movements can be mediated internally.*

The problem is, of course, that the patient is not in a position to generate the necessary voluntary motor signals himself. Thus it would appear that this method is defeated at the outset. It was thought that this difficulty might be surmounted, however, by using a semi-automatic motor act, such as the blink, as the basis for the voluntary autostimulation system. The patient was instructed to squeeze a rubber ball each time he blinked. He was told to repeat to himself, "Blink and press, blink and press . . ." This degree of reorganization of the motor act was sufficient to

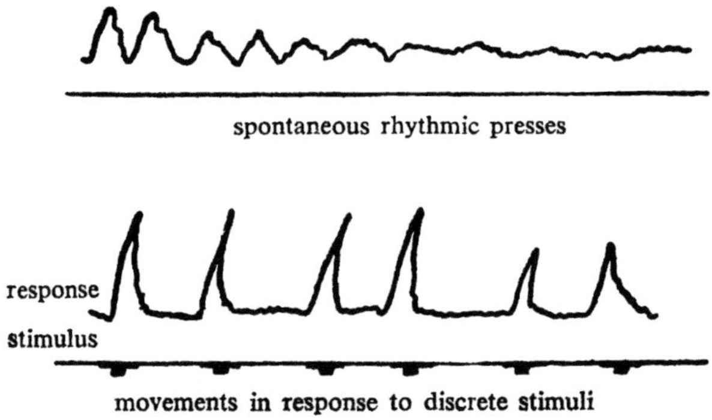

FIG. 79. Spontaneous and responsive movements as performed by a parkinsonian patient.

prevent the onset of muscular rigidity for many repetitions of a given movement and the patient was able to carry out rhythmic movements which had previously been impossible for him (Figure 80). Objectively the movements were the same as those he had performed before, but now they were *carried out on the basis of a new functional system.*

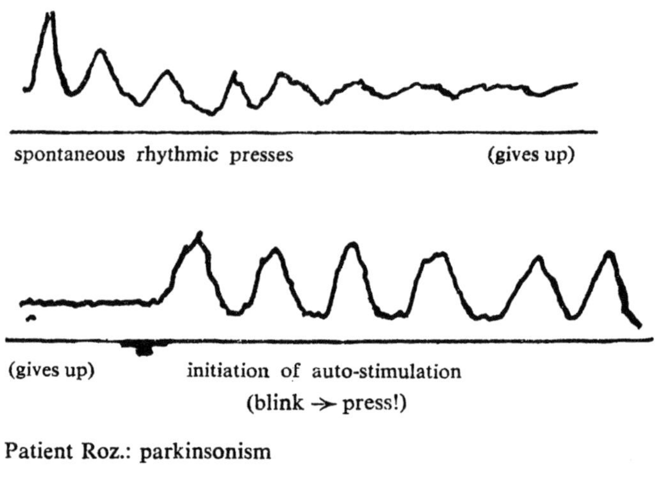

FIG. 80. Reorganization of movement in a parkinsonian patient by means of auto-stimulation.

With this type or reorganization, the major factor on which reorganization is based comes from an entirely different functional system. Ordinarily the eye blink has nothing to do with movement of the hand. In the example above, however, it was incorporated as the initiating stimulus to the act of grasping. We refer to this type of compensation as *intersystemic reorganization.*

The second type of reorganization involves only elements of the disturbed functional system itself. Two possibilities present themselves. One can shift a disturbed function *down* to a lower level, i.e., have it carried out at a more primitive, automatic level, and thus avoid the effects of disorders involving the voluntary execution of the motor acts. The other alternative is to shift the function *up* by giving it new meaning and *transferring its execution to the level of higher cortical processes*. This can be done by employing "second signalling system", speech, to embed the movement in a new meaningful pattern.

This approach was used on the same parkinsonian patient described above. At first he was unable to carry out a series of elementary rhythmic movements of the hand or finger. His attempts to do so rapidly gave way to insuperable rigidity. In this experiment, we attributed a *new meaning* to the movements by incorporating them into more complex patterns of conscious activity. The patient was asked questions to answers to which were numerical in nature and were to be represented by the number of responses. Examples of the effectiveness of this type of reorganization are presented in Figure 81. The patient was unable to press the rubber bulb spontaneously, but when pressing the bulb was made the symbolic response to

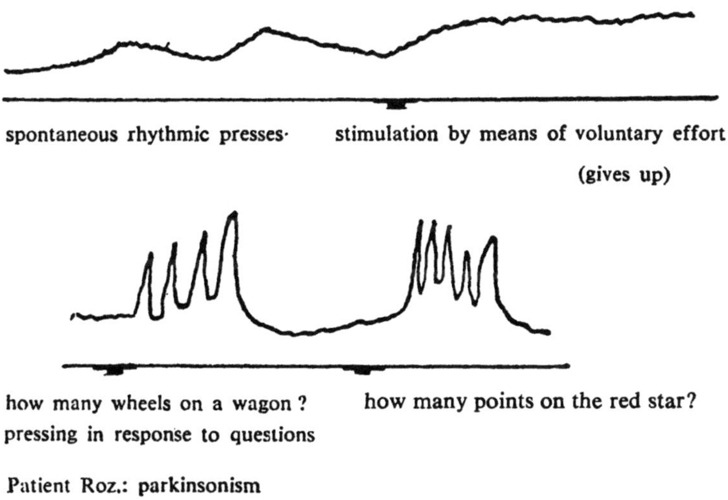

FIG. 81. Reorganization of movement in a parkinsonian patient by the incorporation of a semantic factor.

mental arithmetic problems, e.g., addition, subtraction, counting, etc., it became easy for him to press it. By being incorporated into a new functional system the motor act came to be carried out by a constellation of cortical zones and thus ceased to be subject to such rapid exhaustion as previously. Again, the movements were objectively identical to the ones he was unable to perform before, but they were now being carried out by a new functional system. The difference lay in the fact that reorganization was achieved not by incorporating new links from other functional systems, but by *transferring the same functional system to a new level of organization.* Thus, we can refer to this type of compensation as *intrasystemic reorganization.*

The majority of compensatory mechanisms which develop following focal brain damage belong to one of these two types of functional reorganization. We can summarize both types by the general statement that recovery is brought about by the incorporation of some new type of *afferentation* into the disturbed functional system. This afferentiation may be drawn from another analyzer, in which case it is truly "new" afferentiation, or it may be derived from reorganization of the function at the semantic level so that it comes from a new level of afferent integration. In either case a new functional system takes over an activity which has been disrupted by brain injury.

The reorganization of a functional system usually involves a fundamental change in structure and verbalization of previously nonverbal activity. The restructured activity is incorporated into a system of verbal associations and becomes the object of special consciousness. Before injury, the function is carried out as an unconscious operation, e.g., we are not aware of exactly how we innervate our extremities when we walk, grasp objects, or write. A patient attempting to recover such functions however, must set himself the conscious task of carrying out certain movements such as articulating particular sounds or writing particular letters. What was previously an unconscious operation and part of an on-going process is transformed into an independent movement which must be performed at a conscious level. Consciousness or awareness is a necessary condition for any function which is to acquire a new system of afferentiation. Thus, awareness of an action which was once performed unconsciously characterizes the first step towards the recovery of a disturbed functional system. In succeeding pages we shall come again and again upon the voluntary and conscious execution of movements as the step toward functional reorganization. The following is an example of how one patient recovered motor habits which had been disrupted as the result of lesion in the premotor area.

Patient Čern. suffered a parasagittal shrapnel wound of the premotor area. (This case will be presented in greater detail in Chapter 16.) He lost the ability to carry out complex movements smoothly and skillfully. For instance, he was totally unable to tap out various rhythms. Repeated practice was of little help, but if the function was reorganized so as to involve a new type of afferentation, he recovered the ability to perform such coordinated movements.

The most simple form of reorganization was to *count as he tapped.* When he counted aloud to himself, "1, 2, 3, 1, 2, 3, . . ." he was able to master the rhythm immediately (Figure 82-A). Counting was not the only means by which he was able to master this motor patern, however. The same effect could be achieved by looking at a visual representation of the rhythm as he tapped, e.g., /◡◡/◡◡ . With a diagram of this sort he was able to tap out the rhythm as though he were playing by note. Of course in order to perform such a task he had to be continually conscious of what he was doing. In order for normal rhythmic movements to be produced, the newly reorganized function had to be totally conscious.

At first the mediating activity had to be external in nature. Very quickly, however, it underwent a certain change. The patient ceased to count aloud and began to *count to himself*. He did not have to look at the visual representation of the rhythm, but simply *imagined* it to himself and tapped out the rhythm according to an inner image of the printed diagram. The results were the same as those obtained by using the visual display. The movement was restructured on the basis of internal afferentation. At this point the activity was to all appearances identical to the pretraumatic activity, but the patient was perfectly aware that the underlying mechanism was different. He showed great virtuosity in his ability to devise verbal mediators, e.g., in order to tap out the rhythm //⏑⏑⏑, he pictured to himself two dump trucks and three pickups or two cannons and three machine guns; the force with which he tapped corresponded to the weight of the object which he pictured to himself. If he was forced to give up verbal mediators, his ability to tap rhythmically was immediately disrupted. Genuine automatization did not recur even after numerous practice sessions; the reorganized activity continued to involve an abbreviated form of internal mediation for the entire time that we followed the patient. Figure 82 illustrates his capabilities clearly.

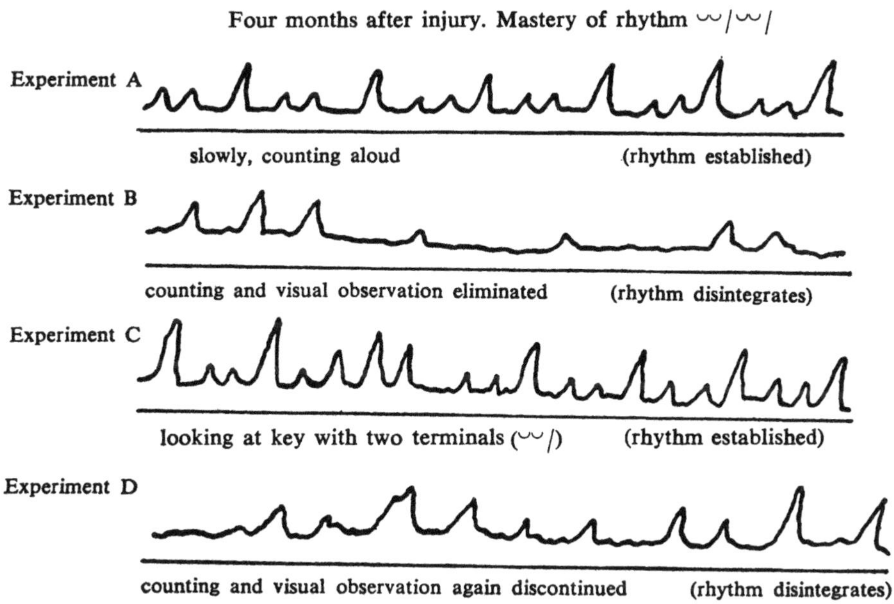

Patient Čern.: lesion in right premotor area.

FIG. 82. Mastery of rhythm in a patient with a lesion in the premotor area.

In many respects this example is the prototype of any attempt to restore a disturbed function. To a certain extent the function may be restored by being incorporated into a new functional system, i.e., by the addition of new afferentation to compensate for the link which has been lost. At first such reorganization requires verbalization; the non-verbal unconscious operation is transformed into a conscious activity. This conscious voluntary aspect is a necessary condition for the reorganization of any functional system. As might be expected, the restored activity requires great effort and is carried out extremely slowly at first. The amount of effort reflects the degree to which the recovered function differs psychologically from the original function.

Gradually the reorganized function becomes more automatic. Essentially the automatization process consists of abbreviation and consolidation of the new processes which can have been incorporated into the disturbed function. These processes are gradually internalized and become less and less dependent upon external stimulation. This facilitates the execution of the reorganized function, but only in very rare cases are all signs of the reorganization so completely lost that the function appears to be exactly the same as before injury.

The major difference between the new function and normal function lies in its mediated character. One can detect signs of such mediation in most cases of restored speech activity. The aid and direction of a therapist is usually necessary during the first stages of recovery. His role is to point out to the patient the methods whereby he can compensate for his defect in mastering specific tasks. The conscious reorganization of disturbed functions is best carried out systematically. Without such training such defects may go unimproved for many months or even years. We have observed many cases in which defects resulting from brain injury remained unimproved for a period of three or four years and then disappeared completely with a few months of retraining. Retraining is necessary if impaired function is to be restored; only in the latest stages of recovery is the patient able to work on his own; it is essential that therapy be initiated under the guidance of a professional therapist (Cf. P. Ja. Gal'perin, 1955, 1957 *et al.*).

The general principles underlying the types of functional recovery we have just described are also important in the recovery of various aspects of speech activity. Next we shall consider their application in the restoration of speech functions functions disturbed as a result of brain damage.

B. THE RESTORATION OF ARTICULATORY SPEECH

The restoration of articulatory movements is one of the major problems in the treatment of traumatic aphasia. Experience has shown that the spontaneous recovery of expressive speech is very limited in patients with motor aphasia. Residual articulatory defects are often quite severe; they seldom undergo total spontaneous recovery and, in the absence of special training, they remain for many months or years. Further, it has been found that patients who began a course of retraining but did not continue showed little spontaneous recovery beyond the point where they left off formal retraining. This reflects the degree to which the recovery of function depends upon radical reorganization of the functional system. The "rebirth" of speech can come about only as a result of special retraining.

The specific approach to restoring expressive speech depends largely upon the nature of the defect responsible for the articulatory difficulty. The various techniques have much in common with one another, however, so that is it possible to describe certain basic characteristics of the techniques employed and then to direct special attention only to those methods which differ significantly from these. A complete description of all the methods used for the restoration of articulate speech after brain trauma would be impossible.[1]

The most clear-cut articulatory defects occur in cases involving apraxia of the speech apparatus. Only rarely are all types of oral movements disturbed equally. Usually it is possible to distinguish levels which suffer different degrees of impairment. As a rule, practical movements which are not a part of the speech system, e.g., chewing, swallowing, pursing of the lips, etc., are better preserved than imitative movements or complex symbolic movements such as the articulatory movements. The practical movements are usually carried out best when the situation is appropriate, e.g., the lips are brought together when the patient takes a bite, blows out a match, or burns his finger. Frequently they cannot be carried out when isolated from such a concrete situation. Preservation of the basic level is most important for the restoration of articulatory movements in severe disturbances of expressive speech.

We shall describe the recovery of speech in several simple cases of apraxia of the speech apparatus. Therapy begins with training in how to utter individual sounds, i.e., with restoration of the articulatory schemata. First one reintroduces the patient to the speech sounds which have the most clear-cut tactile-vibratory characteristics and which are asociated with movements clearly visible to the observer. Thus, the first sounds involve easily observed movements of the articulatory apparatus.

The patient who has completely lost his speech is first taught to produce the sound "p". Usually he retains no trace of the articulatory schema necessary for pronouncing "p". Furthermore he is unable to show how one purses the lips to blow out a burning match. Generally, however, he is able to blow out a match spontaneously if it burns down to his fingers. This involuntary act becomes the starting point for the reestablishment of articulatory movements. From here the problem lies in *fixating* a complex of movement, then in *differentiating* it from other similar complexes, and, finally, in creating the *inner schema* whereby it may be produced voluntarily.

The most difficult task is to fixate the movement pattern as it is elicited unvoluntarily so that it may be produced voluntarily. This involves transfer of the movement from an elementary reflex level to the level of higher cortical activity. Simple repetition is not sufficient. Usually a number of supportive techniques must be

[1] The basic techniques have been presented in the works of Gutzman, E. Fröshels, F. A. Rau, M. E. Xatcev, R. E. Levina, and others.

used to bring the reflex act to a conscious level and, thus, to fixate it. The movement is repeated numerous times in a concrete situation and the patient's attention is directed toward analyzing the component parts and the pattern of the movement. The patient repeats the act of blowing out a match under different conditions so that it becomes less and tied to the concrete situations. The first step may be to blow out the match before it burns his fingers. Next he shows how to blow out a match, blows a bit of fluff from his hand, and, finally, he learns to make only the movements which are associated with blowing. As he goes through this process the therapist continually points out the individual movements involved in the act of blowing. He is instructed to breathe out while the therapist molds his lips with his fingers to form a narrow slit between the lips. He is shown a diagram of the expiratory movements and lip movements which are involved in pronouncing the sound "p". He looks in a mirror in order to follow his own articulatory movements and develop an external aid for reproducing the appropriate articulation.

It will be noted that all these methods combine the principles of intersystemic and intrasystemic reorganization of functions. With time and practice they lead to the fixation of a coordinated pattern of movements, and the patient gains the ability to reproduce the appropriate movement either spontaneously or in response to instructions. Of course, the mediated character of the movement remains for a long time.

The second phase of training is the differentiation of particular components in the overall movement pattern. At this stage the patient shifts *from "practical" movements of the oral apparatus to movements which are specifically articulatory in nature*. This phase is especially important, because it involves learning to differentiate between sounds which are articulated similarly. The phonemes "t", "b", "m", and "f" are all based upon expiratory movements. The patient must learn to recognize the features which distinguish them from one another. Only by identifying the motor distinctions, i.e., the diacritical features, is he able to go from the undifferentiated articulatory pattern to the *articuleme*. In other words, the patient must recognize the distinctive articulatory features of a given sound and be able to compare it with the sounds produced by other articulatory movements. On the basis of this he can recognize the range of sounds which correspond to a given articulatory pattern and which are constant regardless of the intonation or pitch of the voice.

The techniques used at this stage can become quite complicated. Intersystemic functional reorganization plays a large role in many ways, some of which we have already described. First the patient learns to differentiate the phonemes "t" and "m". A number of techniques are used to demonstrate to him that in articulating "p" the air simply passes through the mouth, whereas in articulating "m" the nose and cheeks vibrate. In order to demonstrate this, one may place a small rubber tube in the nostril so that the patient can tell when air is flowing through the nose. In a similar way one can show that in pronouncing "p" the stream of air passes through the mouth. By touching his own nose and cheeks as he pronounces these phonemes he learns to distinguish them on the basis of tactile-vibratory sensation. In addition he is presented a diagram illustrating the coordination of lip, tongue, and expiratory movements appropriate to the two phonemes. His attention is directed specifically to the diacritical features which distinguish one articuleme from the other. Figure 83 is an example of the type of diagram which can be used to aid the patient in recognizing his own articulatory movements.

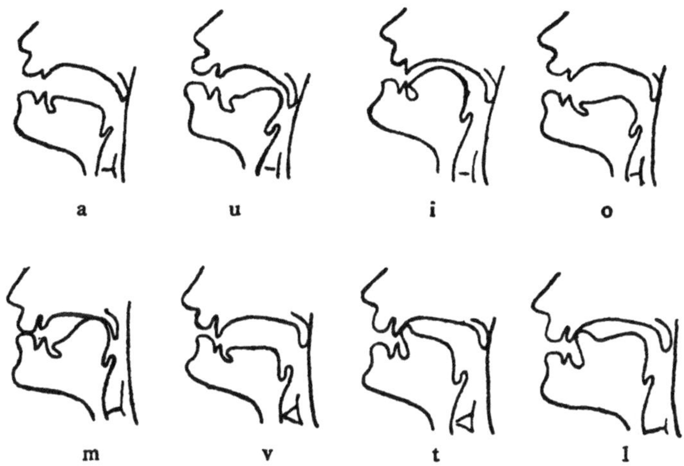

FIG. 83. Articulatory diagrams used for the restoration of expressive speech in cases involving apraxia of the speech apparatus.

Another group of methods are introduced at this stage and quickly come to play a major role in the therapy. The *meanings* of sounds become a part of the articulatory differentiation process. It would be virtually impossible to master the tremendous number of subtle features which distinguish the various articulemes from one another were it not for the fact that they are critical for the differentiation of words having extremely divergent meanings. Only the fact that a very slight change in tactile-vibratory sensation signifies the difference between "papa" and "mama" or "točka" (dot) and "dočka" (daughter) permits a child to master the very fine differences between these two articulemes without recognizing the difference in motor patterns. This is of less absolute significance than certain other factors in the restoration of articulatory movements, but still, it is quite important. Thus in shifting from primary motor patterns to well differentiated articulatory movements, the meaningful aspect of individual articulatory features becomes an important aid to the conscious recovery of function. A patient working on the differentiation of "p" and "m" is greatly aided when it is pointed out to him that this difference defines the auditory distinction between the words "papa" and "mama". Also he is aided by introduction of the *letters* which symbolize the two phonemes and which stand for the ranges of variation which characterize the different phonemes. Written symbols may be used from the beginning as an aid in the recovery of articulated speech.

The introduction of meaning is of further significance in that, in many cases of traumatic aphasia, the loss of articulatory schemata is accompanied by loss of the unity of sound and meaning. There is a disruption of the phonemic organization of speech processes. Thus practice with short meaningful combinations of phonemes is an important step in the recovery of articulatory schemata. At first the patient simply learns to pronounce the sound patterns; later he subjects them to articulatory analysis.

The transformation of a primary motor pattern into an articuleme and the differentiation of correlative articulemes does not occur immediately. For a long time the sounds which a patient produces bear certain traces of their origin in "practical" movements, e.g., the utterance of "p" may be associated with superfluous movements appropriate to blowing out a match. Further, he is often unable to recognize immediately the particular combination of characteristics which distinguish one articuleme from another. He may omit certain diacritical features so as to confuse the articulation of phonemes which are similar but not identical. For instance, he may pronounce "b" as "p" or "m". In the early stages of retraining he may make very gross articulatory errors of this sort. Gradually, however, they decrease in magnitude and in frequency until they occur very rarely. If the auditory recognition of phonemes is intact, the elimination of erroneous articulatory patterns may occur rapidly.

So far we have considered methods used in the first phases of recovery of one particular group of sounds. In principle, the same approach is used in the restoration of the other speech sounds. The major difference derives from the fact that overt oral movements play a lesser role in the production of other groups of phonemes. Still, an important role is played by techniques involving nonsymbolic movements. This is true for instance in relearning the postero-lingual phonemes. On the other hand, sounds whose articulation involves clear-cut overt movements and less complex motor coordination, e.g. the vowels "a", "o", and "u", can be relearned largely on the basis of the visual aid provided by a mirror. A series of examples and diagrams are useful also. One may use a circle to represent "o", a short tube to represent "u", and wide opening of the mouth to represent "a" to a patient with apraxic aphasia. The visual mode is most important for the intersystemic reorganization of the articulatory processes.

The series of techniques has been expanded to include all the speech sounds. It begins with the use of nonsymbolic movements which are modified to represent various groups of sounds, e.g., blowing out a match serves as a basis for the recovery of "p", "b", and "f"; biting the lower lip serves as a basis for the recovery of "v". Imitation of a cow's mooing serves as a basis for the recovery of "m". The fixation and transformation of such movements into symbolic articulemes results eventually in the creation of *generalized articulatory schemata.* This is the major goal in cases of motor aphasia.

The patient is provided a number of aids to help in differentiating the primary articulatory patterns so that he may distinguish the different articulatory groups. This phase is considered completed when the patient is able to recognize articulatory groups under variable conditions of intonation and pitch and when his own articulatory schemata attain adequate degree of constancy. He is aided in reaching this goal by observing the articulatory movements of the therapist, by observing his own movements in a mirror, by studying articulatory diagrams, by attending to the vigration of his nose, mouth, and pharynx, and by relearning the letters which represent the various articulemes. With these aids he becomes able to discriminate specific articulemes.

In the early stages attempts to pronounce any of the antero-lingual sounds give rise only to crude articulatory movements. The patient first learns to distinguish the antero-lingual phonemes, "t", "l", and "n", by the use of special diagrams. This is often the first discrimination he is able to make between different articulatory patterns. At first the antero-lingual sounds are not very well differentiated. At this stage, however, the patient ceases to make such gross errors as substituting the postero-lingual "k" or "x" for the antero-lingual phoneme "t". Still, however, he tends to confuse phonemes within the antero-lingual group. For instance, he may substitute "d" or "t" for "l" or "n". He may shift from one to another in speaking or in writing. Special training is necessary before his ability to differentiate among these sounds becomes permanent. Two important aspects of retraining at this stage are precise explanation of the articulatory positions appropriate to specific sounds (Figure 84) and extensive practice in the recognition of what would appear to be insignificant differences in articulatory positions but which are extremely significant in the extent to which they determine the meanings of words, i.e., they play an important role in the *differentiation of meanings.* Analysis of the articulatory differences between such words as "stol" (table) and "ston" (groan) or "katuška" (spool) and "kaduška" (tub) are often useful in this respect.

Even after a long period of retraining in the articulation of individual sounds the patient may have to expend great effort in order to utter them. They continue to bear traces of their origin in the sphere of voluntary, conscious activity. Self-consciousness and strained pronounciation distinguish the speech of aphasic patients from that of normal subjects in whom speech is generated by completely different mechanisms.

This brings us to the final stage of rehabilitation therapy where the goal is mastery of the articulatory features which vary depending upon context. The patient must complete this phase if he is to make the transition to the pronunciation of syllables in whole words. In Russian the sound "t" in "tip" (type) and "ten'" (shadow) is quite different from the "t" in "Tanja" or "tuflja" (shoe). Whereas in the first two words its articulation is quite similar to that of "c" or "s", in the latter

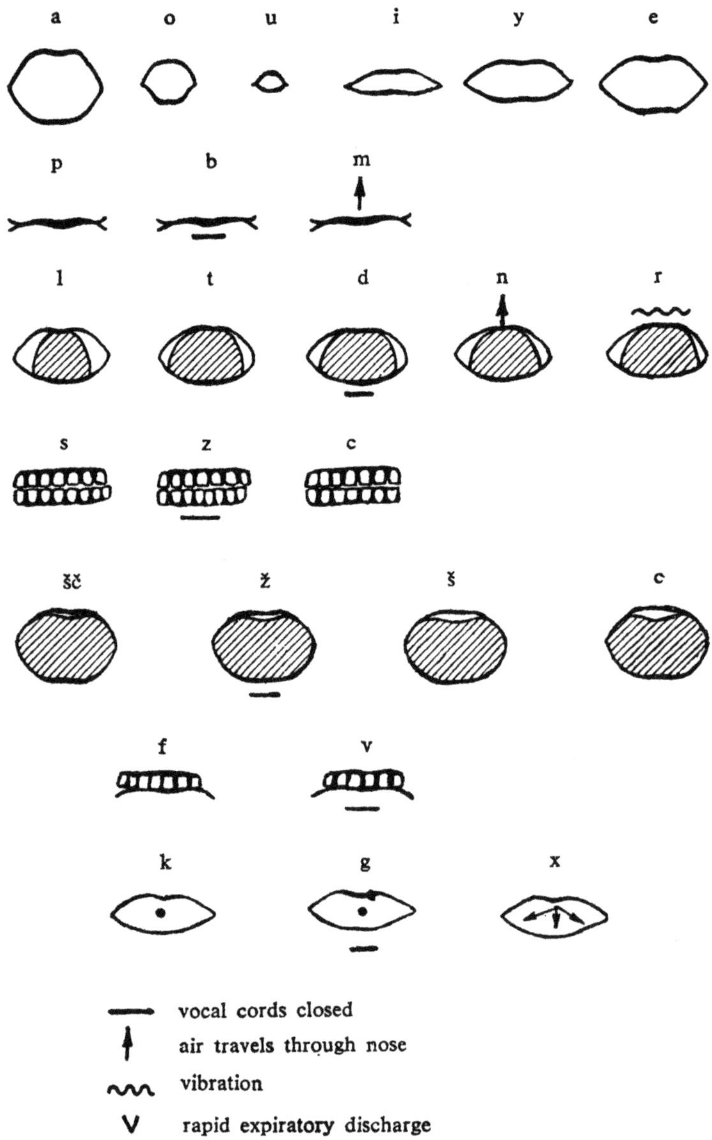

FIG. 84. Articulatory diagram differentiating between sounds similar in pronunciation.

two words it assumes the hard character of the pure "t" sound. The correct pronunciation of "t" depends upon its *transformation into the proper "positional variant."* This problem is not considered in the first two phases of therapy, but in the third phase it is necessary to teach the patient that a sound may be articulated differently depending upon its context.

Here one begins to work with syllables and words. The prototype of this phase of therapy is teaching the difference between *hard and soft consonants*. Experience has shown that a patient who is able to articulate pure sounds with little difficulty is rarely able to make spontaneously the changes in articulatory position which are necessary for pronunciation of the same sounds in soft syllables. The therapist must concentrate on methods of aiding the patient to master such syllables. Here again major benefit is to be gained from careful explanation of the articulatory changes involved and from the incorporation of the different articulatory positions into words having different meanings, e.g., "byl" (was), "bil" (he has beaten), and "pil" (he drank); etc. By working with a large group of such words the patient eventually masters the soft sounds. He must work through numerous exercises which require him to pronounce the some phonemes in different positions, e.g., "lampa" (lamp) – "lipa" (linden) – "Olja" (a name) – "lom" (crowbar).

The following is a case illustrating the sequence of stages through with a patient goes in recovering the speech articulations which are lost as a result of afferent motor aphasia.[2]

Patient Xo. came under our observation in October, 1944, one and a half months after having been injured in the left postcentral area of the cortex. He had a severe apraxia of the speech apparatus, a total loss of writing, and a reading defect so severe that he was only able to recognize familiar ideograms.

At the time therapy was initiated the patient was unable to pronounce a single speech sound. Although he retained some phonation, he was unable to pronounce the sound "a". When he attempted to do so he could only extend his tongue spasmodically and make a hoarse croaking sound. He was unable to vocalize voluntarily on expiration. At the first session he regained the ability to produce the sound "a" by simultaneously palpating for the vibration of his larnyx and pressing on his abdomen. By the second day he had forgotten how to pronounce "a". A mirror was of no help to him, so that, the only way to produce "a" was by the same mechanical means as in the first session. Once he had remastered "a" he was able to go on to learn to produce the sound "o" by rounding his lips and the sound "u" by extending them. He was unable to produce the appropriate lip positions by himself. Then he was given a simple articulatory diagram of the vowels "a", "o", and "u" with the corresponding letters in written form. With several attempts and self-correction by means of a mirror he soon succeeded in pronouncing these vowels correctly.

Once the vowels "a", "o", and "u" were mastered it was possible to go on to the recovery of other phonemes. The first consonant presented was "m". He was shown by means of a diagram and before a mirror what position the lips should assume in the pronunciation of this sound. Further, he palpated the cheeks of the therapist so that he might tactually perceive the phonation. At first the therapist had to hold the patient's lips together so as to fix them in the appropriate position. At the end of the second session the patient was able to pronounce the sounds "a", "o", "u", and "m" by looking at the diagram; if he did not consult the diagram he tended to confuse these sounds and he was not yet able to combine the sound "m" with the vowels to form syllables. The coordinations necessary for shifting from one acticulatory position to another were not yet established. Open or closed syllables were equally impossible for him to pronounce.

[2] The retraining of this patient was carried out by E. N. Hercenštejn. A detailed description of the syndrome has been presented above (Chapter 6).

In order to facilitate the mastery of syllables he was presented a new diagram (Figure 85) which permitted him to anlyze the articulatory positions involved in the pronunciation of the open syllables.

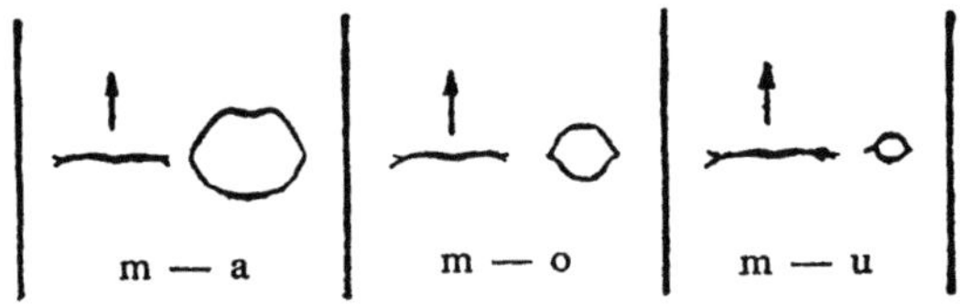

FIG. 85. Schematic diagrams of the articulation of syllables.

After having overcome the initial difficulties it became much easier for the patient to master new sounds, for it was no longer always necessary to resort to mechanical aids. By practicing blowing out matches, blowing bits of cotton or paper from his palm, and other special exercises he was introduced to phonemes "p", "v", "f", "ja", "t", and "l". This was accomplished in eight sessions. By the time these sounds had been mastered he was able to pronounce such words as "Valja" (the name of his sister), "Olja" (a name), "lapa" (paw), etc. These words presented no new difficulties once he could pronounce the component sounds. Recovery of the labial and antero-lingual phonemes of course did not lead automatically to the mastery of other sounds; he was still unable to pronounce the postero-linguals "k" and "x" and the sibilants such as "s" and "š". Recovery of the sound "k" was facilitated by its similarity to "t" which had already been mastered. The tip of the tongue was depressed by a tongue depressor or by the patient's finger as he tried to pronounce the sound "t"; the "k" was established by the end of two sessions of such exercises. Still, however, then the patient had considerable difficulty in pronouncing the syllable "ka". He learned to do so then quickly removing the finger to pronounce "a". After several more sessions he was able to drop this maneuver and pronounce the syllable directly.

Three weeks passed before work was begun on the sibilants. The coordination of tongue position with controlled expiration required the introduction of external aids. A thin rod was used to make a groove in the tongue while the patient blew a rapid stream of air. By this means he rapidly mastered the sibilants. Difficulty arose again, however, when these sounds were incorporated into syllables, e.g., "sa", "so", "as", or "os". He had a tendency to complete a full expiration in pronouncing the first sound and thus was unable to shift to the second. With special practice, however, he succeeded in overcoming this obstacle also.

Although he was able to pronounce the sound "s" he often confused it with "t". In order to correct himself he often resorted to external aids. Thus in reading words which had an "s" at the beginning or in the middle, e.g., "sova" (owl), "suk" (limb), "osa" (wasp), "sup" (soup), or "sam" (himself), he would touch the tip of his tongue with a thin rod as he pronounced the "s". After touching his tongue he would continue to the next syllable. He learned to do this quickly, almost without a pause, and for a long time he refused to give up the rod on the grounds that without it he could not pronounce "s-words" correctly. Eventually it was possible to overcome the need for this maneuver by having him *imagine* that he was pressing the tip of his tongue or blowing on a match when he uttered an "s".

Similar confusion occurred in the pronounciation of "t", "d", and "n". In articulating these sounds the patient always made several incorrect attempts before finding the right sound. Such phonemic searches were gradually overcome by further exercises in which he consulted tongue position diagrams, observed his own articulatory movements in a mirror, and palpated for laryngeal vibration. He was also aided considerably by explanation of the meanings of the different sounds in particular words and by learning to identify them with the corresponding letters.

At first the patient's articulatory movements were very unstable, but with practice this difficulty was overcome. After a certain time he required only the hint of an external aid, e.g., pointing at the tip of his tongue, in order to produce the correct articulatory movements. Eventually, even this became superfluous. The pronunciation of words remained difficult for a long time because of the instability and confusion of articulemes. He would have to search for the proper position of the articulatory apparatus and his attempts at speech were punctuated by substitutions and secondary corrections. Thus in attempting to pronounce the word "polka" (shelf) he would "feel out" the various phonemes, "po-ka ... po-š-ka ... po-d-ka ... po ... l ... ka". Similarly in attempting to pronounce the word "kosa" (braid) he might say, "Kot ... ko ... sa ... ko-ta ..."

With further practice in differentiating the speech sounds and with special readings and writing exercises involving syllables and words his uncertainity gradually disappeared; as the pronunciation of sounds became automatic he came to have no difficulty in pronouncing them as parts of words. By the end of two months of retraining he was able to answer questions in short words using the sounds which he had relearned. He was able to use a few memorized words and phrases in spontaneous speech. The tendency to speak spontaneously grew rapidly, so that within six months he was able to communicate with the hospital personnel and with his friends. Further expansion of the patient's active vocabulary did not require special work. By this time he was able to recognize and use all of the speech sounds and he had little difficulty in recognizing or using new words. The transition from individual phonemes to whole words, from words to short phrases, and from initation to the spontaneous use of words presented no particular difficulty. The only residual signs of speech impairment were the somewhat strained character of his articulation and occasional agrammatisms. He was released after seven months of therapy having recovered his spontaneous speech; reading and writing had been almost fully restored.

In cases where apraxia of the speech apparatus predominates, the major therapeutic effort is directed toward creation of new articulatory schemata of the speech sounds. There is no principal difficulty in the articulation of complex words and sentences. When the major defect is loss of the inner schemata of the sequentiality of sounds in words, however, this stage is reached rather quickly, but more work is required for the restoration of active speech. Here the goal is to create precise, dynamic word schemata and the ability to recognize the sound sequences of which words are composed. Often such patients also have difficulty in overcoming the inertia of articulatory impulses; these two defects often occur together as two aspects of the same disturbance.[3]

In a severe case the patient with an efferent motor aphasia has little difficulty in articulating individual sounds, but he is unable to remember or pronounce com-

[3] Detailed methods of rehabilitation of motor speech are elaborated in the last years in our laboratory by L. S. Cvetkova. Cf. her "Methods of the Rehabilitation of Higher Cortical Functions" (in press) and: A. R. Luria, *et al.*, "Restoration of Higher Cortical Functions after Local Brain Lesions" in: de Bruyn and Vinken, *Handbook of Clinical Neurology* (Amsterdam, North Holland Publishing Co. [in press]).

binations of sounds. This loss of the inner schemata of words is very frequently accompanied by a pathological inertia of articulatory processes, so that it is very difficult to shift from one sound or syllable to another. Initially the problem is to create precise word schemata and to overcome the persistence of established articulatory sets, so that the patient can shift smoothly from one syllable to another.

It is extremely difficult to overcome the pathological inertia of neurodynamic processes. As a rule the usual means of inducing inner inhibition are of little help. The patient is unable to pronounce the word "mukha" (fly) because the inertia or perseveration, of the articulatory set "mu" is so great that he cannot shift to the postero-lingual "xa". As a result he continues to repeat the first syllable, "mu . . . m . . . mu . . . m . . ." as though he is unable to dissociate himself from it.

Usually it does not help to insert long pauses between syllables. There are, however, special techniques which can be used in such a case. These are techniques developed by O. P. Kaufman and ourselves to bring about the speech activity in patients with lesions of the premotor areas.

In devising methods for overcoming the inertia of articulatory patterns we began with the observation that even though a patient was unable to carry out a single complex movement smoothly, he had no difficulty in carrying out two successive acts if they were sufficiently *different* from one another. On the basis of this we tried to find a means of transforming a two-phoneme syllable into two distinct articulatory movements without seriously altering the continuity of pronunciation. It was found that this could be done by relating the individual parts of the word to different affective or semantic contexts. For instance, the patient who has difficulty in pronouncing the word "muxa" (fly) was instructed to think separately of the two syllables as he pronounced them, e.g., "mu" as the lowing of a cow, "xa" as an element of laughter, "ha-ha-ha". Another technique was to have him pronounce the two syllables at different pitches. Usually this type of semantic reorganization of the articulatory process eliminates the difficulty in shifting from one syllable to another. The next step was to equip the patient with enough techniques of this sort to allow him to overcome any difficulties that might arise. Once he was able to talk, the intermediate steps gradually disappeared.

A second common intersystemic method of overcoming the perseveration of articulatory sets is by the use of *auxiliary signalization*. A patient who cannot shift from one syllable to another or pronounce a series of nonsense syllables, such as "ba-bo-bi", smoothly can learn to break down such sequences into individual syllables and accompanying the transition from one syllable to the next with a particular gesture. For instance, "ba" is associated with opening the mouth wide, "bo" is associated with rounding the mouth, and "bi" is associated with flattening the lips horizontally. The same types of gestures may be used when there is difficulty in shifting from one consonant to another. The transformation of a sequential act into several "reactive" articulatory movements each of which depends upon its own auxiliary afferentiation makes it relatively easy to overcome the difficulty in denervating established sets. After a certain amount of practice the patient reaches a point where he needs only to imagine to himself that the auxiliary movements are being carried out. Eventually, he is able to discard them altogether; the reorganized articulatory system is capable of operating independently.

These techniques are most useful in cases involving severe denervational difficulties. In these cases it is necessary to recreate the *acoustic schemata of whole words*. Once such schemata have been established, the majority of denervational difficulties disappear. The restoration of stable acoustic-articulatory schemata is based largely upon reorganization of function about the *meanings of word patterns*. A number of techniques are designed to help the patient recognize the positions of sounds in words and the articulatory differences between similar sounds. It is well known that if a sound sequence is meaningful it is much easier to learn to recognize and remember it than if it is meaningless. One has great difficulty in remembering a sequence of nonsense syllables; whereas one can remember a meaningful sequence, i.e., a word, relatively easily. Often a patient who is unable to repeat such a series of syllables as "bi-ba-bo" has no difficulty whatsoever in repeating the three syllable word "limonad" (lemonade). Moreover, he does not perseverate, omit sounds, or rearrange syllables. The restoration of articulatory processes can often be accomplished by means of exercises which lead to recognition of the meaningful structure of words.

While the semantic analysis of words plays a central role in the retraining of patients with sensory aphasia, it is only one step toward the restoration of word schemata in the motor aphasic. Recognition of the sound sequence of a meaningful word helps to fix its pattern, i.e., gives it a certain constancy on the basis of which the patient can analyze its auditory and articulatory components. A number of teaching techniques have been designed to bring the sequence of sounds to the center of the patient's sphere of consciousness: he writes them, pronounces them aloud before a mirror, analyzes the sequence of articulatory movements by means of diagrams, palpates his throat as he speaks, etc.

If a patient is unable to recognize that the word "lipa" (linden) is articulated differently from "pila" (saw) or that "kto" (who) is pronounced differently from "kot" (cat), the therapist points out to him that the difference in the meanings of the two words depends upon the difference in the order of the letters and sounds. The therapist pronounces them slowly and presents pictures of the letters as he utters them. Visualization of the letters makes it somewhat easier for the patient to analyze the words. An even more effective technique, however, is the presentation of diagrams showing the articulatory positions which correspond to the spoken sounds. The therapist explains for instance, that in the word "pila" (saw) the labial sound appears first and lingual "l" appears in the middle. This sequence is set forth in the diagram indicating the order of articulations in the two words so that the patient comes to think of a given word in terms of its "articulogram." Sometimes the therapist has to explain the articulation of a particular consonant when it precedes different vowels. This is especially true of the hard and soft vowels. Additional exercises are useful in restoring the ability to make smooth transitions from one syllable to another. Supplementary exercises are also frequently necessary for recovery of unaccented vowels at the beginning of words. Otherwise such a patient tends to omit them, e.g., in attempting to pronounce the word "okno" (window) he may say "k . . . ko . . . ko . . ."

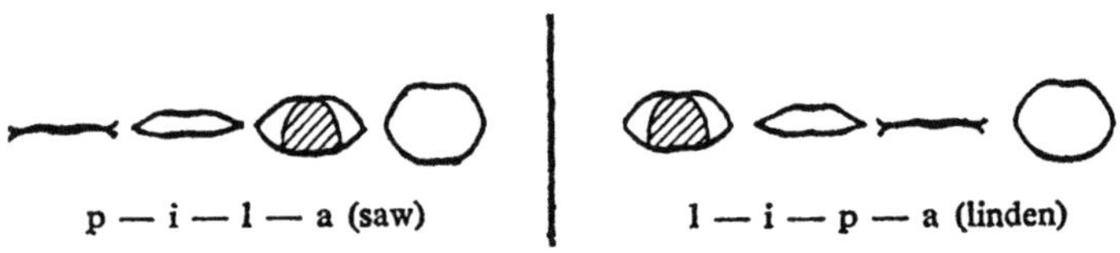

FIG. 86. Schematic diagrams of the articulation of words.

Beyond this restoration of the auditory schemata of words depends upon intensive practice in speaking, reading, and writing. Major effort is directed toward the phonemic analysis and formulation of words, e.g., games with anagrams, filling in the blanks in words where one or more letter has been omitted, and studying words which differ from one another by the order of sounds, such as "kot" (cat), "tok" (current), and "kto" (who). As much attention as possible is given also to the *morphological analysis of words,* i.e., identification of word roots, prefixes, suffixes and inflective endings, for these morphological components determine the range of semantic variability within the patient's speech is formulated.

Since in the motor aphasic the major auditory processes are largely intact, the word schemata become automatic relatively rapidly once they are restored. Soon he can begin to pronounce words correctly again. Often automatization occurs before full recognition of the sound content of the word is attained. As a result, a patient who has regained the ability to speak correctly may continue to experience considerable difficulty in writing. The fact that he is still not always aware of the words he uses is revealed by his tendency to transpose and omit letters as he writes.

C. THE RESTORATION OF THE ABILITY TO RECOGNIZE AND RECALL WORDS

Restoration of the perceptual and memory aspects of speech – the ability to differentiate speech sounds, to recognize word meanings, and to recall verbal images spontaneously is a second important area which often requires treatment in cases of traumatic aphasia. It is very important in most cases in the stage immediately following brain injury and is the central problem in cases of sensory and acoustico-mnestic aphasia.

As we indicated above the first stages of traumatic aphasia are almost always accompanied by impairment of word comprehension. The stable unity of sound and meaning is lost; dissociation between the sound patterns and meanings of words makes it difficult to find the right words or to understand the words of others.

Restoration of the unity of the sound and meaning requires special retraining. Intensive effort must be directed toward this problem in the early stages of traumatic aphasia so as to establish a basis for further recovery of speech. The most common form of therapy consists in the presentation of a series of objects or pictures and naming them as they are presented. At first the patient simply listens to the names of the objects; then he attempts to pronounce the names himself. V. M. Kogan has shown that the number of objects such patients are able to name at first is very small. As the memory expands however, this number increases. If the meanings of words are to be restored to their original flexible and generalized form, their use should not be restricted to the nominative form; they should be included in sentences of variable length depending upon the capacity of the patient's sphere of consciousness, which is often constricted in the initial period following injury. The words should be used in different grammatical forms. By presenting such sentences as "Here is a knife", "cut with the knife", "there is no knife", "here is a pocket knife", "we shall cut with the knife", "there is dirt on the knife", etc. one makes use of concrete surroundings in restoring the meaningful aspect of the word. At the same time one creates for the patient a number of *generalized schemata* of sentences which include a given word in a number of different grammatical contexts. The word retains its constancy, despite the alterations in grammatical construction. This method is quite useful in restoring the unity of sound pattern and meaning.

In cases of motor aphasia where the dissociation of sound and meaning is not the result of a loss of phonemic hearing, the methods just described may be sufficient to restore the word comprehension. On the other hand, if the patient is prevented from recognizing word meanings by a profound *disruption of acoustico-gnostic processes* the problem of rehabilitation is considerably more complex. It is necessary to remove the basic defect, i.e., the phonemic hearing disturbance, for only this will restore the stability of word schemata which are necessary for dependable word comprehension. The therapeutic measures which we have used in cases of sensory aphasia were developed in our laboratory by È. S. Bejn.

Restoration of the precise *phonemic organization of hearing* is by no means a single problem. Patients with sensory aphasia usually hear well enough, but they are unable to pick out the phonemically important cues from a steady flow of speech. For instance, they are unable to recognize the phonemic differences between the words "dočka" (daughter) and "točka" (dot) or between the words "rot" (mouth) and "l̓ot" (lead). The few features which are significant in discriminating the meanings of words are perceived by these patients as no more distinctive than the numerous insignificant features. Thus, the words lose their phonemic constancy and meaning. It is difficult to overcome this loss of phonemic hearing by the usual methods of intersystemic reorganization. A patient who is unable to perceive the differences between the sounds "r" and "l", "b" and "p", "š" and "s", etc., has great difficulty in grasping this difference, even when tactile and visual aids are provided. Palpating the throat, and observing articulatory movements in a mirror are of little help. The absence of adequate auditory feedback prevents him from being able to differentiate or remember the precise pronunciation of sounds. With the incorporation of tactile and visual facors the situation becomes even more complex for the sensory aphasic.

The decisive factor in the recovery of phonemic hearing is use of the *organizing role of meaning*. In numerous observations of sensory aphasics it was found that a patient who was unable to distinguish or remember the difference between the sounds "b" and "p" usually had no difficulty in distinguishing the words "baba" (peasant woman) and "papa" (papa). Apparently the incorporation of a sound into a simple, meaningful sound complex accentuates its meaningful aspect and increases the probability of its being correctly differentiated from other sounds.[4] This observation has been made the basis for a certain therapeutic techniques used to restore phonemic hearing.[5]

If the therapist wishes to teach the patient to recognize the sound "d", he presents a word beginning with "d", e.g., "dom" (house). The word is reinforced by a picture of a house, which fixes its meaning; the word "dom" is written under the picture with the letter "d" standing out from the others. Next a word is given in which the voiced "d" is replaced by the unvoiced "t", so that the meaning of the word is changed to "tom" (book). The second word is also accompanied by a picture under which "tom" is printed with the "t" larger than the other letters (Figure 87). The therapist explains the difference between the sound "d" and "t" and has the patient note visually and by palpation the articulatory differences which distinguish one sound from another and thus determine the meanings of the words.

A second technique supplements the first. It is designed to incorporate the sound into a verbal complex in which its phonemic constancy is maintained. The patient is presented with words which begin with the letters "d" and "t". In the first words these sounds are accented in normal pronunciation, e.g., "bal-byl-bol'-bulka-bočka" (ball-was-pain-roll-barrel). Similar words beginning with "p" are also presented: "pal - pyl - pol - pul'ka - počka" (bollard - ardour - floor - bullet - bud). Each of the words is presented together with a picture. The therapist describes the phonetic differences and similarities between the words. Pairs of words are presented in which the position of a given phoneme determines its sound and

[4] This phenomenon has been reported in the Soviet literature for the somesthatic perceptual system by A. N. Leont'ev and for the visual system by A. I. Bogoslovskij, G. X. Kekčeev and others. More recently the corresponding therapeutic techniques have been studied and given more precision by E. D. Homskaja. See the reports of her work in *Problems of Higher Nervous Activity in the Normal and Abnormal Child*, Vol. I (1956), and Vol. II (1958 [Russian]).

[5] The techniques for restoring speech functions to sensory aphasics were developed by Ė. S. Bejn (1947).

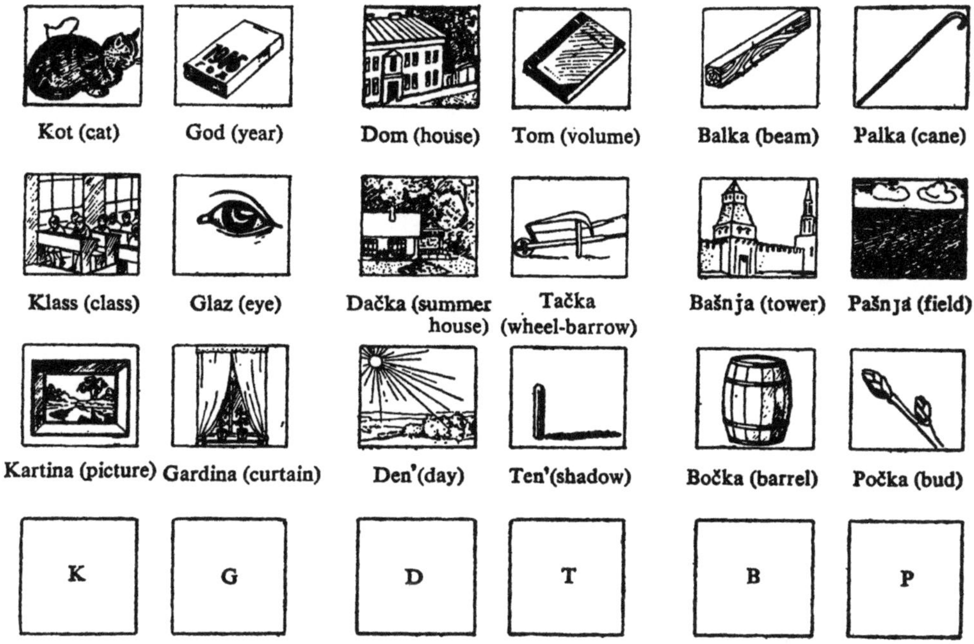

FIG. 87. Drawings with titles used in restoring phonemic hearing to patients with temporal aphasia.

meaning. Words are presented in which the distinguishing characteristic is the hardness or softness of the sound. The sound under study may be combined with another consonant which makes it difficult to recognize, e.g., "brat" (brother) and "bljudo" (dish). It may occur in the middle of the word, e.g., "sbor" (collection) or "vbit' " "to hammer". By working with such words the patient becomes aware of the fact that a given phoneme retains certain constant features even though it seems to change its sound in specific contexts. In working through the variants of a given phoneme it is imperative to represent it always by one and the same letter. The patient does exercises which involve filling in the letters in words printed under the pictures of objects. Exercises of this type re-establish the *phonemic generalizations* which the patient has lost. They reinforce the phonemic organization of hearing, i.e., aid in removing the primary defect in sensory aphasia.

The restoration of precise and stable phonemic hearing contributes also to the *recovery of stable word meanings*. The sound is incorporated into a meaningful word, the word is associated with a picture or an object, and an analysis is made of the phonemic changes which determine the meaning of the word. Other methods may also be used however, to restore the constancy of word meanings regardless their grammatical form.

In Russian a given word appears in a number of different forms, i.e., with different suffixes, depending upon its use. The so-called "null" form or nominative case form or a noun usually serves as the root to which other morphemes are added. It is natural that in the sensory aphasic where the meanings of the words themselves are unstable the meanings of the inflective endings should also be unstable. Thus, a patient may not recognize the common root or different meanings of variants of the word "stol" (table, nominative case) as "stoly" (plural), "stolom" (instrumental case), "stolik" (a small table), "stolovyj" (adjectival form).

Special techniques have been designed for overcoming the lability of word meanings in sensory aphasia. The primary exercise is to analyze the variants of different words by identifying the roots, prefixes, suffixes, and inflective endings. The variants of a given word are compared with the variants of different roots which may be superficially similar but which have entirely different meanings. Simultaneously the patient works on remembering the constant meaning of a word as it appears in different contexts. He is asked to compare such sentences as: "The bread feeds the man", "the bread is eaten by the man", "give me the bread", "tell me about the bread", etc. As the statements are presented the patient's attention is directed to the constant meaning of the word as it appears in different grammatical forms.

	stol		(table)		vod	- a	(water)
	stol	- u	(dative case)		vod	- y	(genetive case)
	stol	- y	(plural)		vod	- janoj	(adjectival form)
	stol	- jar	(joiner)		vod	- orosl	(waterplant)
	stol	- ik	(small table)	za -	vod	- y	(factories)
	stol	- ovaja	(dining room)	pod -	vod	- nyj	(underwater)
za -	stol	- nyj	(adjectival form)	polo -	vod	- ie	(flood)

This work demands a lot of time, because it involves numerous exercises with a large volume of material. Eventually, however, it leads to the development of verbal generalizations which counteract the patient's tendency to dissociate the sound and meanings of words. Words gradually regain their constancy of meaning when used in a variety of different phonemic contexts.

The final problem faced in the restoration of speech to patients with sensory aphasia is to restore the stability of the memory traces of words, i.e., to overcome the amnesic-aphasic disturbances characteristic of such cases. No other task in the treatment of sensory aphasia is so difficult as restoration of the ability to remember words. The patient shows severe impairment of the ability to recall words for a long time even after he has regained the ability to understand the speech of others. His active speech continues to be restricted by an amnesic type of disorder.

It is immediately apparent to anyone talking with a sensory aphasic that he has extreme difficulty in finding words; this is true both in naming objects and in spontaneous speech. It results in numerous literal and verbal paraphasias. The goal of the therapist is to overcome the difficulty in recalling the names of objects and to restore the stability of the memory traces of words.

Restoration of the ability to memorize words and to recall them when appropriate is by no means as easy as one might think. The patient may memorize a word, but it disappears again very quickly, so that within a few hours, or even a few minutes, he will have the same difficulty in recalling it as he had before. Experiments carried out by Franz and, later, Lashley showed that such a patient can repeat a word several hundred times and still be unable to recall it a short time later. Thus, it became apparent that rote memorization is useless in this situation. It was necessary to seek new and more effective ways of helping the patient to recall words. Thus we turned to exercises involving the semantic aspect of speech.

Working with meaningful groups of words leads to the fixation of generalized verbal images. By using a given word root in a variety of combinations the patient learns a whole family of words and thus attains new associations on the basis of which he can produce the word when necessary. The number of memory difficulties is reduced and he can recall words much more dependably then by the rote memorization methods which Franz, Lashley, Goldstein, and others found to help only transiently.

A number of authors have noted the interesting fact that a patient with sensory aphasia who is unable to recognize isolated words is often able to recognize their meaning if they occur in the context of other words. This observation reported by Goldstein (1942), Ombredane (1951), and S. M. Blinkov (unpublished) became the basis for another set of methods useful for the retraining of sensory aphasics.

A patient who is unable to name an object can sometimes recall the name by producing a sentence in which the name appears. For example, if he is unable to remember the word "star", he may be able to recall it by saying, "The sun shines in the daytime, the . . . stars shine at night"; or he may recall the word "comb" by the sentence: "I comb may hair with a . . . comb". This type of compensory mechanism is made possible by the fact that while the sensory aphasic loses the ability to produce isolated words voluntarily, he retains larger, familiar speech patterns. These patterns can be used to advantage by the therapist attempting to restore speech to such a patient.

Experiments have shown that a patient with sensory or acoustico-mnestic aphasia has great difficulty in memorizing the meanings of individual words, but that he has less difficulty in memorizing *lists of related words* or *sentences*. S. M. Blinkov showed that such a patient is able to memorize a list of words such as "bed - blanket - towel - soap - brush" more easily than he can memorize the words individually. Memorizing several sentences each including one of the words also presents less difficulty than memorizing a single such sentence.

Several investigators have attempted to use the memorization of related word lists as a means of restoring speech to patients with acoustico-mnestic aphasia. Sometimes the memorization of lists is facilitated by treating them as rhythmic word patterns. After a great deal of practice the lists are learned; subsequently the patient can use them as a means of recalling individual words. S. M. Blinkov found, for instance, that a patient who wanted to recall the word "soap" would first reproduce the whole list containing the word "soap". From this he selected the proper word. It is interesting to note that the memorized lists gradually lost their rote pattern; they changed spontaneously, were continually reworked and generalized. In time they became quite flexible. After several weeks of use Blinkov observed that the memorized lists "melted away". The patient was able to recall a given word by reciting only a part of the corresponding list. He was able to begin reciting from any one of several words in the list. As the number of words he had to recite became fewer and fewer he was able eventually to recall words without referring to the list at all.

While the value of rote memorization of word lists may be disputed, the value of memorizing sentences and of working through exercises in which a given word appears in a number of different contexts has been well documented.[6] The latter technique is effective both in the amnesic aphasia which accompanies loss of semantic aspect of speech and in cases of verbal amnesia, one of the syndromes of sensory aphasia. Nevertheless amnesic aphasia continues to present some of the most difficult problems faced by doctors and therapists attempting to restore speech to patients with traumatic aphasia. Using these techniques one can expect tangible results only after a great number of sessions.

Patient Zvor.,[7] a trapper, received a penetrating wound in the left temporal area in May, 1942. He entered the rehabilitation hospital three months after injury with a severe sensory aphasia. At the time of admission his comprehension of speech was severely impaired. A few examples drawn from the protocols of his early sessions will suffice to show the inconstancy of perception and vagueness of word meanings at that time.

"When were you wounded?"

"Wounded . . . wounded . . . yes . . . I have a wife . . . Kirova . . . Kirova."

"Where does your wife live?"

"Živet (lives) čived (meaningless) . . . život (abdomen) . . . zovet (he is calling) zovod (factory) . . . zavod (factory)."

"What kind of factory?"

"What kind . . . I don't know. I'm at a factory."

The patient grasped word meanings at random and attempted to continue from whatever word he came up with. For four or five months his speech comprehension was severely disturbed. He attempted to compensate for the disorder by several mechanims; by knowing the situation in which the conversation took place, by guessing from the sounds of words, etc., he attempted to follow the train of thought. Genuine understanding of speech on the basis of discriminative and generalized perception of speech sounds was almost totally lacking, however. He did not differentiate between pairs of sounds. For instance, the pair of syllables "pa-ba" was heard as "ba-da", "ka-ga", or "ga-ga". The word "gora" (mountain) was heard as "kora" (cortex); the word "stena" (wall) as "volna" (wave), etc. The auditory analysis of words was greatly impaired, so

[6] This technique has been greatly elaborated by V. M. Kogan and L. S. Cvetkova.

[7] The examination, therapy, and reporting of this case were carried out by Ė. S. Bejn.

that he was unable to identify or recognize the sounds in a given word, much less recognize their positions within the word.

Retraining was begun by attacking the aphasic defect. The first goal was to restore phonemic hearing, i.e., to restore the ability to differentiate speech sounds spoken aloud. This involved the presentation of similar sounds in meaningful complexes, so that the patient could learn to differentiate them and fix the important phonemic features in his memory. The two most useful aids were visual diagrams of articulatory positions and the remnants of the articulatory processes themselves.

Within a month he was able to recognize letters of the alphabet and single words. He could spell some words, although he occasionally made characteristic errors, e.g., he might spell "okno" (window) as "ogno" (meaningless), or he might read "derevo" (tree) as "terevo" (meaningless). He relied upon a variety of features in relearning to recognize spoken sounds: differences in word meaning depending upon the letters present, differences in the written forms of the letters representing different sounds, etc. During the third week he was able to announce, "I've got it . . . got it . . . I've got it . . . I lay down . . . thought . . . and I've got it . . . here, I'll write it: x . . . x . . . x . . . xata (hut) u . . . u . . . u . . . ulica (street), and the rest the same". Thus, he came to master a series of sounds by using the techniques suggested to him. The role which the visual images of letters played in helping him to remaster the speech sounds is illustrated by the following example. Once during the fifth week he was given the task of selecting a group of several words all beginning with the letter "p". He was unable to do so the basis of the verbal instruction alone, but the moment his eye fell on the letter "p" he exclaimed "Papa! Peter! Paroxod (steamship)!" By this time he was able to analyze the phonemic composition of simple words spoken aloud. Simultaneously, there was a sharp drop in the frequency with which he came upon words, the meaning of which he could not remember. Whereas, initially he failed to recognize 90% of the words he heard, by the third month he rarely had any difficulty in recognizing word meanings. It was now possible to communicate with him verbally. He said, "Now I've begun to understand what it's all about . . . I understand." He actually did begin to understand "what it was all about"; he took an active part in the retraining sessions and sought means of compensating for his defect. He would frequently make auditory and semantic "discoveries" himself, without the aid of the therapist. "Koza (goat) and kosa (braid) . . . s . . . s . . . z . . . s . . . just a minute . . . There's the difference . . . the difference is small . . . but they do sound different . . . amazing!"

As he regained the ability to identify the individual sounds in whole words and to compare them with other sounds he gradually became able to understand the speech of others. At the end of the first stage of retraining, about the third month, he more and more often sought the correct pronunciation of words himself. In the beginning the instability of auditory perception produced a continual feeling of helpless confusion; after three months the inability to grasp the meaning of a word evoked an active response which consisted in his comparing the apparently new sound with sounds already recovered. The following example illustrates this stage of recovery. The patient was asked, "Kakaja segodnja pogoda (How is the weather today)?" "Bagoda (meaningless) . . ." (The patient heard the word "pogoda" in a distorted and, consequently, meaningless form). "Bagoda . . . dagoda . . . bagoda . . . no . . . no . . . (He repeated the word in a pronounceable, but, thus far, meaningless form). "Bagoda . . . bagoda . . . bakota . . . no . . . no . . . then . . . pagoda . . . p . . . b . . . ba . . . no . . . t . . . tagoda." (Recognizing the fact that he was hearing the word incorrectly the patient attempted to figure out its content.) "Pagoda (weather) . . . p . . . p . . . pagoda . . . tagoda (meaningless) . . . bagoda (meaningless) . . . ah, I know, nice weather (pogoda); sunny!"

In the process of searching he tried out the letters "p", "b", and "t" until he discovered which one most nearly matched the original sound and produced a meaningful word. Repeating sounds aloud and comparing them with the sounds he had already remastered reflected a step forward in his capacity to overcome the lack of differentiation of auditory perception. The basis for his progress lay in reduction of the lability of speech sounds, greater ability to retain sounds for a certain length of time, understanding of how to select out the meaningful phonemic units in a verbal sound pattern, and how to represent them by the appropriate letters. Gradually this process of active "search" became shorter and appeared less frequently. He regained the ability to grasp the meanings of words directly.

In the next stage of retraining, part of the time was devoted to reinforcing the constancy of individual words in various grammatical and auditory contexts. The patient analyzed the changes in a word as it was used in singular and plural and in different cases. During the second month, a change in the inflective ending of a word destroyed its meaning for the patient, but by the fourth month this rarely occurred. He was able to understand words and sentences regardless of changes in auditory pattern.

With four months of retraining this patient learned to substitute conscious analysis of speech sounds for the direct perception of word meanings. He learned to rely on several mediating techniques which permitted him to select out important phonemic cues and fix the auditory images of words. As a result, he was able to compensate for a gross disturbance of phonemic hearing; he regained the ability to comprehend the speech of others and succeeded in almost completely overcoming the loss of word meanings. Furthermore, he regained the ability to read and write. Figure 88 shows the changes which occurred in the patient's writing

during retraining and reflects the overall reorganization of his speech activity.

D. THE RESTORATION OF READING AND WRITING

The restoration of reading and writing is an important part of the rehabilitation of patients with traumatic aphasia. Almost every aphasic complains of some degree of difficulty in reading and writing. These functions seldom recover spontaneously, but systematic retraining always leads to improvement and sometimes to full recovery. The appearance of reading and writing disturbances does not depend upon the destruction of any single area, i.e., it does not result from damage to a specific "reading center" or "writing center". Reading and writing are conscious operations which depend upon recognition of the phonemic constituents of words and which are consequently, easily impaired by disturbance of any of the processes underlying the phasic aspect of speech.

Here we shall consider therapeutic techniques appropriate to patients with primary alexia and agraphia. These syndromes usually arise as the result of occipital lesions. They consist in *loss of the meanings of graphemes,* so that the patient fails to recognize letters or forgets how to write them. It may involve *spatial disturbances,* so that the patient writes letters backwards or otherwise incorrectly oriented in space. Finally, it may involve *constriction of the "reading field",* so that the patient is unable to perceive more than one or two letters at a time. Reading is reduced to fruitless attempts to string together a series of letters which can only be perceived one or two at a time. Several investigators have developed effective methods of treating such disorders. The techniques are designed to revive and restore the ability to recognize the range of sounds corresponding to specific graphemes, introduce tactile stimulation to mediate the visual perception of letters, analyze words into their component parts, and, finally, by familiarizing the patient with general groups of letters, to broaden the "reading field". These methods have all been described in detail elsewhere.[8]

Since the reading and writing difficulties resulting from the impairment of auditory speech are so common, they constitute one of the major problems in the rehabilitation of patients with traumatic aphasia. As we pointed out above, reading and writing are based upon different psychological mechanisms depending upon the degree to which they have been mastered previous to injury. The attention of a person who has just learned to read must be directed toward correctly combining the individual letters which he recognizes into syllables and words; a person who has just learned to write must analyze each word into its phonemic components and then write down the letters which represent them. On the other hand, a person for whom reading and writing have become well automatized can skip this step; he is able to write whole words on the basis of established motor engrams[9] and read whole words as visual ideograms. Since the psychological mechanisms are so different, it is not surprising that the reading and writing disorders after brain trauma should be different in skilled and nonskilled readers and writers. There is virtually a total loss of reading and writing in aphasic patients for whom these processes have not become automatic. On the other hand a patient in whom these functions have become highly automatized may show little detectable change in reading and writing, even though his oral speech is severely disturbed. To be sure, in some cases the reading and writing of such patients may undergo peculiar changes. For instance, reading may appear to be largely made up of attempts to guess the identity of verbal ideograms; writing may be reduced to the use of established motor engrams unmediated by sound-letter analysis. Thus, while the

[8] Several valuable investigations have dealt with the restoration of functions in primary alexia and agraphia. See K. Goldstein, *After Effects of Brain Injuires in War,* 1942; B. G. Anan'ev, "The Restoration of Writing and Reading in Agraphia and Alexia", *Works of the Department of Psychology of Moscow University,* 1947; S. M. Blinkov, L. V. Zankov, M. A. Tomilova, Ž. I. Šif, E. N. Zavjalova, and T. A. Moxova in *Proceedings of the Academy of Pedagogical Sciences,* II, 1945; O. P. Kaufman, "On Visual Agraphia", *Works of the Institute of Neurology of the Academy of Medical Sciences of the USSR*; L. S. Tsvetkova (in press) and others.

[9] This process was studied in detail in a series of investigations carried out by E. V. Gurjanov (1940, 1945).

recognition of written words may appear to be intact, the patient is totally unable to read words or syllables which are unfamiliar to him. Similarly, he may be able to write familiar words and sign his name, but not be able to write less familiar words which require the processes of auditory analysis and synthesis.

In every case of traumatic aphasia which we observed the reading and writing disorders resulted from loss of the conscious operations of sound-letter analysis and synthesis which constitute the psychological basis of both processes. There were two ways of compensating for this defect, only one of which is really appropriate. The first, and incorrect, approach maximizes use of the residual automatized reading and writing habits of the patient. This approach is designed to compensate for the reading and writing defects by having the patient memorize whole words presented visually. The words become ideograms and thus permit the patient to compensate for his difficulties. The acquisition of ready-made word images, however, avoids rather than overcomes the basic difficulty. A patient retrained in this manner possesses a relatively limited number of ideograms and his reading remains largely a guessing process whenever he is exposed to unfamiliar words. It is doubtful that any real success results from this approach.

A second, more radical, approach has a greater chance of being effective. This consists of a concerted effort to return the phonemic patterns of speech to the patient's sphere of consciousness, and thus bring it back to a level where reading and writing can be re-established as conscious processes and re-automatized on that basis. Such retraining involves special exercises to strengthen those aspects of auditory function which are disturbed in a particular form of aphasia. In some cases the central problem is to reestablish the constancy of phonemes so that the patient can represent them by the appropriate letters. In other cases one must restore the ability to recognize and remember sound sequences. In still other cases one must contend with denervational difficulties which prevent the patient from reading or writing several words in sequence. This approach often requires a long period of retraining. Sometimes it requires that established ideographic images be broken down and reestablished on the basis of sound-letter analysis. Only this approach can lead to genuine remastery of the reading and writing processes.

1. *The Restoration of Writing*

In many cases the therapist must direct his efforts toward restoring the ability to work with *letters*. The mastery of letters is not difficult in childhood, but it presents great difficulty in certain aphasic disturbances. The major prerequisite for the mastery of letters is an ability to pick out the constant and significant sounds in the flow of speech and to identify them with the basic phonemes of the language. This process is lost in sensory aphasia. Since a patient with sensory aphasia is unable to recognize the sound "ž", he may repeat the word "žar" (heat) as "zar . . .

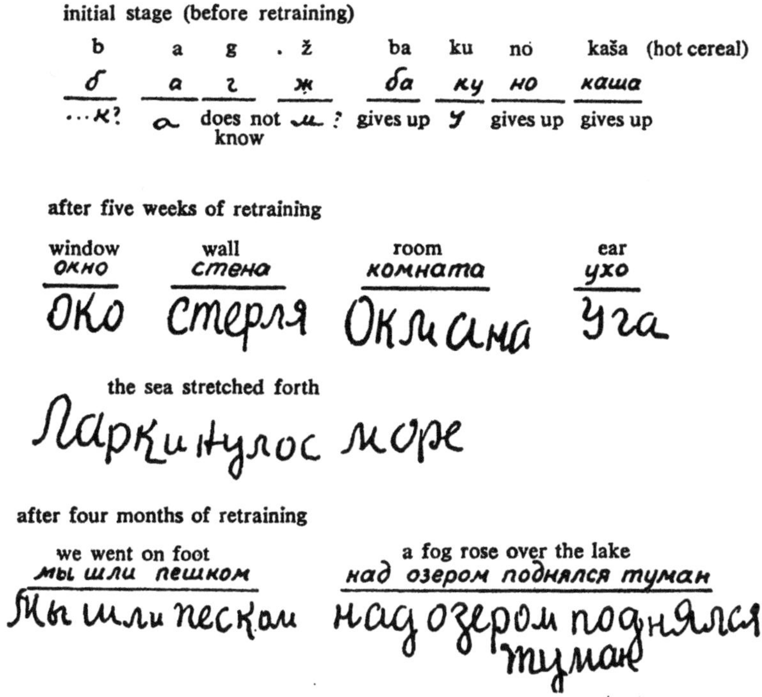

transliteration:

initial stage (before retraining)

b	a	g	ž	ba	ku	no	kaša (hot cereal)
...k?	a		m		u		

after five weeks of retraining

okno	stena	komnata	oxo
oko	sterlja	okmana	uga

raskinulos' more (the sea stretched forth)
Larkinulos' more

after four months of retraining

my šli peshkom	nad ozerom podnjalsja tuman
my šli peshkom	nad ozerom podnjalsja tuman

Patient Zvor.: Lesion in the left temporal area; sensory aphasia.

FIG. 88. Patient Zvor.'s writing before and after retraining.

žar . . . sar . . . šar". Naturally, he is unable to say what letter represents this sound, for he has lost the phoneme itself. A patient with afferent motor aphasia experiences a similar difficulty. The loss of articulemes leads to instability of lines of demarcation between sounds which are similar in articulation, e.g., "l", "m", and "d". As a result, he cannot immediately distinguish the group of auditory cues which represent the grapheme "l". Such a patient may not always recognize the differences between such letters even though he is able to pronounce them in certain words.

The ability to read letters is impaired in either case. The patient with a severe sensory aphasia often reads letters correctly, but he can never be certain that he is pronouncing it correctly, and thus he constantly shifts from one phoneme to another. The patient with afferent motor aphasia complains that letters have lost their precise meanings and he attempts to determine what sounds they stand for by pronouncing the various possible articulations aloud. This does not always help and he too tends to shift from one phoneme to another.

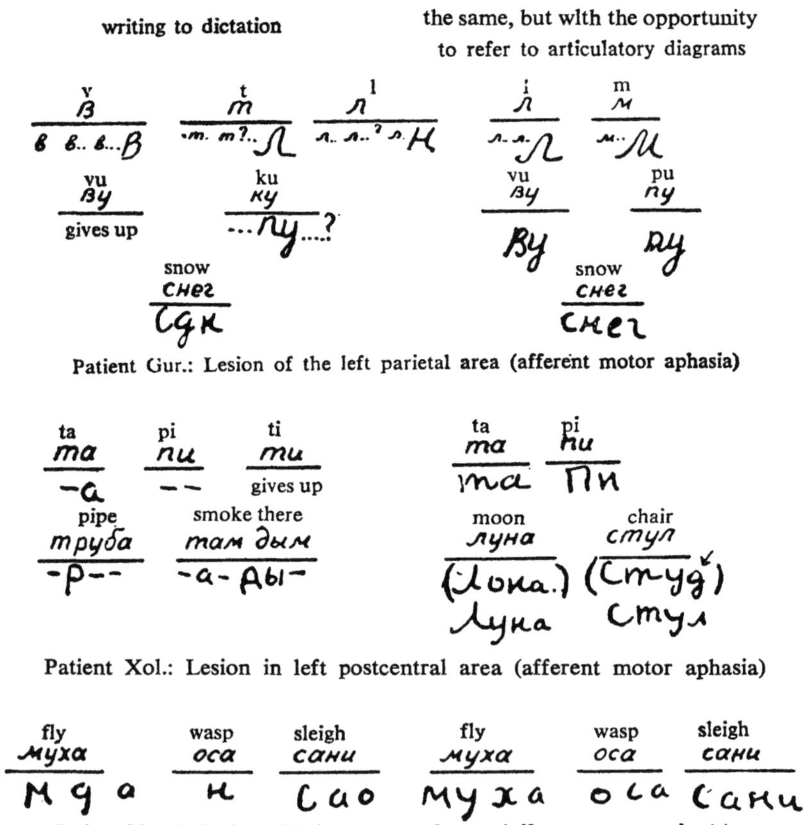

FIG. 89. The role of articulatory diagrams in restoring the ability to write.

In these cases the difficulty in using letters arises not from a visual or motor defect but from *impairment of the auditory or articulatory analysis of sounds necessary for reading or writing.* In both cases the goal of the therapist is to restore the preliminary stage of reading or writing activity. Simply having the patient copy letters is of little help, since it does not involve reorganization of the defective processes responsible for phonemic analysis. Writing individual letters to dictation is of equally little benefit, because the patient is unable to recognize the sounds which he hears. The only thing achieved by dictation is a clear-cut manifestation of the difficulty itself. For the same reason, little benefit is gained from exercises in reading individual letters; here again, the patient is unable to tell what sounds the letters represent.

The patient can make progress only if he acquires means of differentiating one sound from another, recognizing the range of sounds corresponding to given phonemes and representing these generalized phonemes by letters. There are two basic groups of techniques which are useful in this regard. One teaches the patient

transliteration of Fig. 89.

writing to dictation			the same, but with the opportunity to refer to articulatory diagrams	
v / v.. v.. v... V	t / t.. t?.. L	l / l.. l..? l.. N	l / l.. l.. L	m / m.. M
vu / gives up	ku / ... pu..?		vu / Vu	pu / pu
sneg / sdk			sneg / sneg	

Patient Gur.: Lesion in the left parietal area (afferent motor aphasia)

ta / -a	pi / - -	ti / gives up	ta / ta	pi / pi
truba / -r- -	tam dym / -a- dy-		Luna / (Lona) Luna	stul / (stud) stul

Patient Xol.: Lesion in left postcentral area (afferent motor aphasia)

muxa / mda	osa / n	sani / sao	muxa / muxa	osa / osa	sani / sani

Patient Nas.: Lesion in left postcentral area (afferent motor aphasia)

FIG. 89. The role of articulatory diagrams in restoring the ability to write.

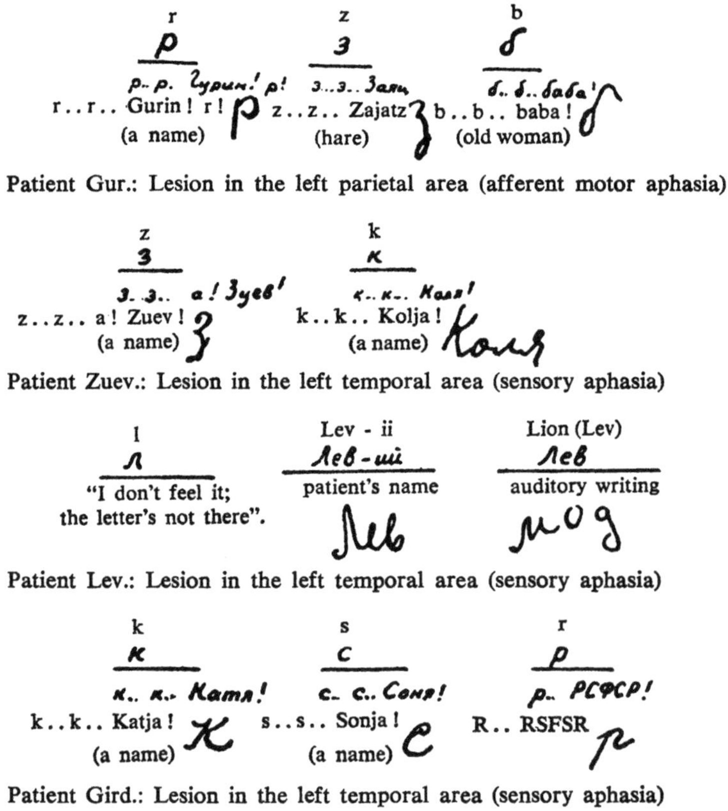

FIG. 90. The role of meaningful ideograms in restoring the ability to write.

to rely on external cues which help to identify sounds as they are uttered; this includes visualization of articulatory movements, palpation of the speech apparatus, etc. The other is designed to make the patient aware of the role played by different sounds in differentiating the meanings of words and thus transforms the physical sounds into true phonemes. Both types of technique are used in cases where the basic defect is a disturbance of the ability to recognize the elements of oral speech.

Retraining begins with the presentation of articulatory diagrams similar to those shown in Fig. 83 and 84. Special attention is given to the articulatory differences between phonemes which sound alike or which are articulated similarly, e.g., "b" and "p", "d" and "t", "l", or "n", etc. Explanations of the differences are reinforced by reference to the diagrams, demonstration of the articulatory positions by the therapist, and tactile impressions which the patient gets by feeling the vibration of his own troat and nose. The phonemic analysis of words requires great precision when the patient begins to work with complex sound sequences, e.g., syllables with two or more consonants in a row. The exercises designed to help

transliteration of Fig. 90.

r.. r.. Gurin! r! r	z.. z.. Zayac z	b.. b.. baba! b
r / (a name)	z / (hare)	b / (old woman)

Patient Gur.: Lesion in the left parietal area (afferent motor aphasia)

z	k
z.. z.. a! Zuev.: z	k.. k.. Kolja! Kolya
(a name)	(a name)

Patient Zuev.: Lesion in the left temporal area (sensory aphasia)

l	Lev - ii	(Lev) Lion
"I don't feel it; the letter's not there".	patient's name Lev	auditory writing mod

Patient Lev.: Lesion in the left temporal area (sensory aphasia)

k	s	r
k.. k.. Katja!	s.. s.. Sonja!	R.. RSFSR
(a name) K	(a name) S	R

Patient Gird.: Lesion in the left temporal area (sensory aphasia)

FIG. 90. The role of meaningful ideograms in restoring the ability to write.

the patient to differentiate and identify sounds are reinforced by having him write down the corresponding letters. This serves as a means of fixing and generalizing phonemes and simultaneously sets the stage for the recovery of writing. Sometimes a patient can learn the distinctive features of speech sounds in a single session. Once this is accomplished he can match the sounds with the corresponding letters and soon begin writing simple syllables. Figure 88 illustrates the degree to which articulatory diagrams can assist in writing letters, syllables, and words.

At first visual and tactile aids play a large role in the patient's writing. The extent to which he relies on them in his attempts to find the sounds is easy to see. He carefully observes his articulatory movements in a mirror and palpates his lips and pharynx until he has established all the features characteristic of the sound he wants. In the early stages he can only write words if simultaneously he pronounces them aloud. The auditory patterns of words must be externalized so that the distinctive features of individual phonemes can become fixed. Gradually these steps become automatized; the conscious determination of phonemic features becomes superfluous, and, within a few weeks, there is a sharp drop in the frequency with which the patient must search for phonemes. He is able to find most sounds directly.

The use of visual and tactile sensations for the recognition of phonemes is not the only method open to a patient wishing to recover the use of letters. A more important method is designed to take advantage of the role which phonemes and letters play in determining the meanings of words. A patient who has already learned to distinguish sounds on the basis of articulatory cues acquires even greater confidence when he recognizes meaningful words in which they appear, e.g., when he becomes aware that the sound "k" is the only factor which distinguishes the word "kora" (cortex) from the word "gora" (mountain). By comparing the meanings of words containing sounds which are similar acoustically or which are articulated similarly helps the patient to differentiate between the sounds themselves. Once he recognizes the sound "k" as part of the sound complex "Katja", he has little difficulty distinguishing it from similar sounds. In cases involving loss of articulemes and in cases of temporal lobe auditory aphasia this is often the most effective method of restoring the ability to write. As a rule the patient has no difficulty in memorizing how to write familiar ideograms such as "Katja", "golub'" (dove), etc.; and he can usually pick out the first letter of the ideogram. He can often use the ideograms he retains for finding the letters he wishes to use. He repeats the sound which is presented to him, listens to it, compares it with the verbal patterns ideograms which he already knows, finds one beginning with that sound. The first letter of the ideogram is the letter he seeks. This method is useful not only for writing individual letters, but also for writing whole words. He simply figures out each letter as he goes. For instance, in spelling the word "kot" (cat) he may say, "kot, kot . . . k . . . k . . . ah, koška! (feminine form of kot) . . . k! . . . kot . . . kot . . . kot . . . o . . . o . . . Olja! (a name) . . . o, – kot . . . t . . . t . . . Tanja! (a name) t!" If such a patient is prevented from speaking aloud he is totally unable to write in this fashion. Figure 90 shows examples of how patients are able to write by the use of auxiliary words. It is important to note that when a patient uses this technique he actually overcomes his defect. This is not merely a means of substituting for the lost auditory analysis but a means of recovering it.

Usually during the first stages of retraining the patient must constantly rely upon intermediate steps in writing to dictation. Gradually, however, the intermediate steps become abbreviated. He begins to try out the various sounds to himself in a way that to the untrained observer is totally undetectable. Eventually this process becomes automatic and writing appears to regain its original direct character. Even in the final stages, however, careful analysis will reveal that the structure of the new process is radically different from the original function.

Difficulties in the recognition of phonemes or letters are not the only reading and writing difficulties with which the speech therapist has to contend. They may account for most afferent motor aphasias, but in cases of efferent motor aphasia and certain disturbances of simultaneous gnostic schemata the major difficulty may be quite different. The patient may have no difficulty in writing individual letters, but when he must write a series of letters in a particular order to form a word he fails. Here the serial organization of sounds or letters is disturbed; the major obstacle lies in the inability to identify the first letter, grasp the word as a whole, and recognize the sequence of phonemes.

The problem of the therapist in a case such as this is to teach the patient to identify the sounds represented by the written symbols and to recognize and to preserve their sequence; in other words his goal is to restore the patient's word schemata. He must help the patient create new word schemata, so that he can recognize the individual phonemes and the ways in which they change their sounds depending upon their position in different syllables. Word schemata are also necessary if the patient is to preserve the correct order of sounds as he writes words. The use of oral and tactile images of individual sounds is not sufficient. These cues contribute nothing to fixing the order of sounds in words; thus they are of little use in cases of this sort. In order to compensate for the basic defect the therapist must find a means of displaying the auditory patterns of words so that the patient can continually refer to it until he is able to recognize the order of sounds himself.

There are several techniques by which one can *externalize the sequential schemata of words*. First one re-establishes the schemata of simple syllables, then of syllables with more than one consonant, and finally of whole words. Experience has shown that patients in this group are not able to grasp the sequential order of sounds. They often omit vowels and anticipate accented consonants, so that they tend to begin words with the accented consonant and rearrange the order of phonemes in complex syllables so as to make for the greatest ease of articulation. Another important difficulty that arises in the absence of stable word schemata is a tendency to repeat the first sounds in words, so that in writing a syllable they are apt to include sounds which were a part of preceding syllables (see Chapter 13).

Exercises in constructing syllables usually begin with the application of several techniques designed to help the patient recognize and remember the sounds of which specific syllables are composed. He is given a diagram showing how to pronounce the vowels; he observes the movements of his own mouth in a mirror as he pronounces the different vowels. In this way he becomes aware of the way the vowels are pronounced. Then he is given exercises in which he writes a series of open and closed syllables, e.g., "pa-ap", "pi-ip", "ma-am", "mi-im", "ka-ak", "ki-ik". Once he is able to write these syllables he learns to pronounce them aloud, again, using all of the aids described above.

The next step is to write complex syllables involving two consonants in a row. Here he is aided by the fact that he can already pronounce simple syllables or words even though he is not conscious of the phonemes of which they are composed. In order to become aware of the phonemes involved, he must learn to pronounce and compare such syllables as "pro-por-rop', 'pru-pur-rup", etc. The difference between these syllables may be emphasized by incorporating them into words having different meanings.

kto	(who)	pri	(attached to)	kru(g)	(circle)
kot	(cat)	pir	(banquet)	ruk(a)	(hand)
tok	(current)				
lipa	(linden)				
pila	(saw)				

The patient is aided by a diagram of the articulatory positions appropriate to the different sounds. He writes them down, pronounces them, and interprets what he says by means of the corresponding diagram (Figure 91).

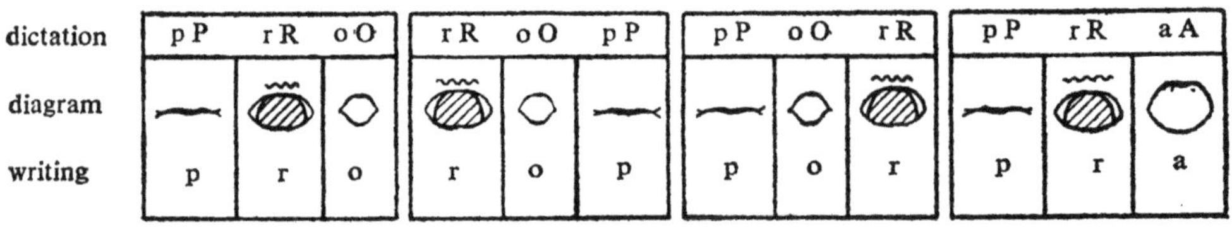

FIG. 91. Sequences of diagrams used in the articulation of complex syllables in response to dictation.

With these techniques the writing process comes to be based upon an awareness of the identity of various articulatory positions; essentially it is transformed into a type of "articulatory dictation". At first the patient analyzes a ready-made diagram. Later he is able to make up his own diagrams corresponding to the schemata of new syllables. He does this by carefully noting the positions of his articulatory apparatus and drawing them in correct sequence on paper. Gradually the intermediate steps become unnecessary and he becomes able to write syllables simply by pronouncing them aloud to himself.

During the first days or weeks the syllables must be spoken loudly and precisely. By multiple repetition, "iteration", of written sounds the patient is able to pick out vowels. Since vowels actually play more of an intermediate role in the transition from one consonant to another than as a part of the word skeleton they are difficult to identify, and thus difficult to bring to the level of consciousness. A typical example of a patients writing at this stage is the following. The therapist dictates the word "rak" (crab). The patient pronounces it, "Rak . . . rak . . . ra . . . ra . . . r . . . r . . . r . . . (he writes "r") r . . . rak . . . raaak . . . raaa . . . aa . . . aaa . . . a (he writes "a") . . . rak . . . raak . . . rak . . . k . . . k . . . k . . . k (he writes "k")."

Sometimes he makes a mistake by writing a given letter twice; but if he is careful in the way he verbalizes, he can maintain the correct sequence of letters. If he is not careful, he makes certain typical errors, e.g., he omits soft sounds or rearranges letters so that the accented consonants come first.

The patient may have considerable difficulty when a given phoneme is articulated differently in different words. He has difficulty both in identifying it and in writing down the proper letter. It is essential that the therapist explain the phonemic equivalence of hard and soft variants of the consonants, e.g., the articulatory difference in Russian between the hard "t" in the syllables "to" and "ta" and the soft "t' " in "te" and "ti".

These techniques not only return writing to a voluntary, conscious level but also radically change the basis of writing by obviating immediate grasp of the sequential schemata of words. Of course, the restoration of writing by these methods depends upon the extent to which external speech is preserved. But it should be noted that external speech itself develops in the course of such retraining.

The first phase of retraining is designed to teach the patient a way of maintaining the order of letters by referring to their order in externalized speech. The second phase consists of a gradual transition to the use of *inner schemata* of syllables and words. There are several ways in which this transition may be brought about. The first is by direct "internalization" based on the vocal repetition of words. Usually the signs of internalization are detectable within two or three months of retraining. A patient who, during the first weeks, can only write by pronouncing words aloud to himself gradually comes to pronounce them in a whisper, and eventually needs only imagine them to himself. In the final stage of recovery there is no overt indication that his writing is directed by such a process. The schemata underlying the overt utterance of words become automatic and gradually give way to the formation of inner schemata which assume full control of the writing process. Figure 92 illustrates the extent to which a patient relies upon speaking words aloud at various stages in recovering the ability to write.

In working with complex words simple automatization of the process of word repetition is often not sufficient. Thus, the therapist should begin as soon as possible to introduce to the patient a second method of developing internal word schemata. He begins by analyzing words into their component syllables and by working through exercises which give him practice in recognizing the most common combinations of phonemes. He learns to break down words into syllables and to transform the syllables into familiar ideograms. The major accomplishment at this phase of retraining is learning to write by syllables rather than by individual letters.

At this stage, one of the important exercises the patient should work with is one in which he compares words with a common root, suffix, or prefix and identifies the common element. He gains practice in the use of frequently occurring letter combinations by reading, copying, and reproducing with anagrams words lists such as the following:

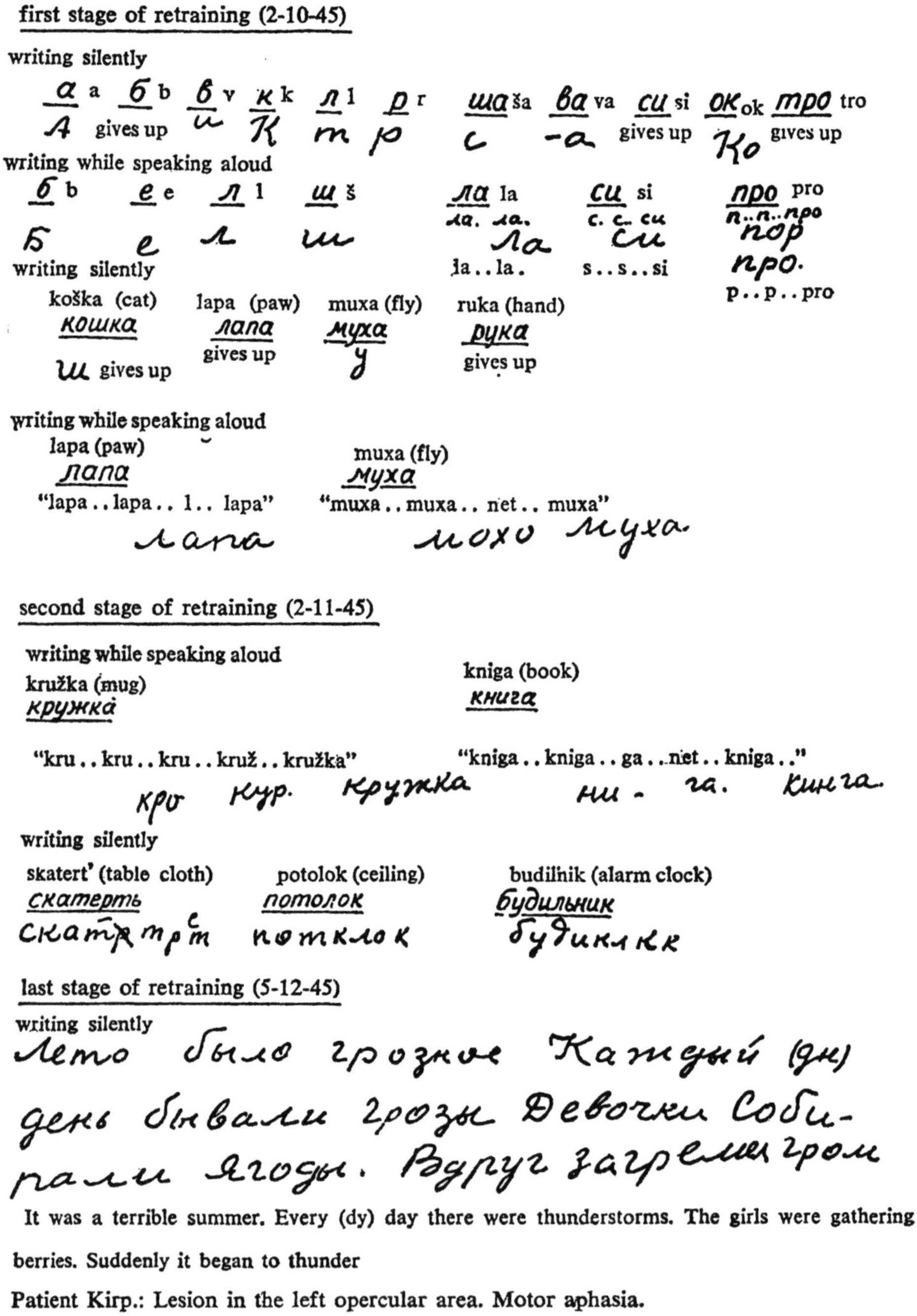

FIG. 92. The role of repeating words aloud in restoring the ability to write in a motor aphasia.

transliteration of Fig. 92.

first stage of retraining (2-10-45)

writing silently

a	b	v	k	l	r	ša	va	si	ok	tro
A	gives up	l	K	t	r	s	-a	gives up	Ko	gives up

writing while speaking aloud

b	e	l	š	la	si	pro
B	e	l	š	la .. la ..	si .. si ..	p .. p .. pro por

writing silently

koška (cat)	lapa (paw)	muxa (fly)	ruka (hand)
š gives up	gives up	u	gives up

writing while speaking aloud

lapa (paw)	muxa (fly)
"lapa .. lapa .. l .. lapa .."	"muxa .. muxa .. net .. muxa"
lapa (paw)	moxo muxa (fly) (meaningless)

second stage of retraining (2-11-45)

writing while speaking aloud

kružka (mug)	kniga (book)
"kru .. kru .. kru .. kruž .. kružka"	"kniga .. kniga .. ga .. net .. kniga .."
kro kur kružka	ni ga kinga

writing silently

skatert' (table cloth)	potolok (ceiling)	budil'nik (alarm clock)
skatrtrt	potklok	budinlkk

last stage of retraining (5-12-45)

writing silently

It was a terrible summer. Every (dy) day there were thunderstorms. The girls were gathering berries. Suddenly it began to thunder

Patient Kirp.: Lesion in the left opercular area. Motor aphasia.

FIG. 92. The role of repeating words aloud in restoring the ability to write in a motor aphasia.

st	ol	(table)	trud		(work)	pis	at' (to write)	po	it'	(to go)
st	ul	(chair)	trud	nyj	(difficult)	čit	at' (to read)	po	smotret'	(to look)
st	oljar	(joiner)	trud	itsja	(to work)	sčit	at' (to count)	po	dymat'	(to think)
st	ojat	(to stand)	trud	ovoj	(working)	kuš	at' (to eat)	po	dat'	(to give)

In another useful type of exercise he fills in the missing letters of words printed under the pictures of various objects.

picture of a kitten (koška)	picture of a fork (vilka)	picture of a window (okno)
ko-ka	vil-a	ok-o
koš-a	vi-ka	o-no
ko-a	vi- -a	o- -o

These methods can greatly enhance the patient's ability to recognize the positions of specific sounds in whole words.

These techniques initially permit the patient to write without the inner schemata of words. Writing is based on the successive recognition of individual sounds as they are spoken aloud. In the early stages of retraining the patient cannot write without simultaneously speaking aloud the sounds he wishes to transcribe. In time, however, these techniques lead to the establishment of new word schemata, and the patient can gradually undertake other modes of writing. He begins to whisper rather than speak aloud as he writes; eventually he may write silently, only resorting to the oral accompaniment when working with difficult words. This last stage comes relatively late, however, and in some cases is never reached. In these cases the loss of inner sound schemata is so great that new schemata cannot be formed and the writing process cannot be reautomatized.

The restoration of writing is brought about by radical reorganization of the process of sound-letter analysis. Sometimes a patient will himself discover techniques which have not been described but which are useful to him. For instance, he may base his writing on the visual images of written words rather than on the phonemic analysis of spoken words. Writing "in whole words" simply avoids the basic impairment of phonemic analysis, however; it should not be encouraged. Seldom can a patient master more than a small group of verbal ideograms, and he can never regain a true mastery of writing.

A number of techniques used in the restoration of writing are similar to those which we have already described as applicable in the restoration of oral speech. Despite their similarity, however, there is one important difference. In the restoration of speech it is possible to make use of anything which the patient remembers about the meanings of words; but in the restoration of writing it is a long time before the patient can go beyond the mastery of simple sounds and sound combinations. Thus, whereas oral speech rapidly becomes a vehicle for the conveyance of thoughts, the act of writing becomes a special conscious process and continues for a long time to require the patient's full attention. The semantic organization of words is important in oral speech, but it is only of minor significance in the recovery of writing.

We shall present two cases involving patients with writing disorders which were overcome by careful retraining. In one case the major defect lay in the identification of sounds and their symbolic representation in letters. In the second case there was a disturbance of the sequential schemata of sounds.[10]

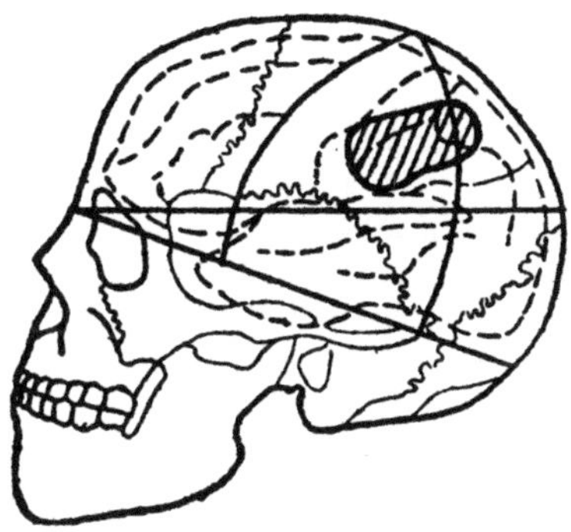

Patient Vas.: Injury diagram.

On March 1, 1945, patient Vas., a 20 year old man with an 8th grade education received a penetrating shrapnel wound in the left opercular area. Bone fragments and necrotic brain tissue were removed from the wound at an operation carried out five days after injury. Local inflammation developed following the operation and there was further extrusion of brain substance. An encephalogram five months after injury revealed an internal hydrocephalus; the ventricular system was drawn toward the site of the lesion.

Immediately following the injury the patient suffered from a right hemiparesis with impairment of all forms of sensation on the right; in time these symptoms diminished, the arm was affected more than the leg. Motor aphasia was also present from the first. Although he was able to comprehend common everyday speech, he did not speak for three months.

The patient came under our observation seven months after injury. At that time the paresis of the upper extremity was still present. There were no signs of apraxia, though there was no severe disturbance of oral movements, a severe speech disorder was noted. The patient could utter only single words. He had difficulty in finding sounds and sometimes omitted sounds from words which were not clear to him, e.g., he said "babu-ka" instead of "babuška" (grandmother). He also had difficulty in making words agree with each other grammatically (this defect will not be considered here). The difficulty in finding particular sounds emerged very clearly when he was asked to repeat

[10] These examples were taken from an investigation of speech therapy carried out by L. K. Nazarova.

words. He had to make several attempts before he was able to repeat individual phonemes and the correct sound was often replaced by another sound similar in articulation. As a rule the sounds substituted were homorgans of the sounds he wished to utter. Acoustically the sounds might differ sharply from one another, but they were similar in articulation, e.g., he might pronounce "n" as "t", or "l", sometimes he even substituted "r". He was able to perceive the difference between oppositional phonemes such as "b" and "p". His attempts to repeat words were marred by the word-searching and substitutions. He tended to omit consonants appearing together and to substitute other sounds. For instance, he pronounced "koška" (kitten) as "ko-ta". He had the same difficulty in naming objects, e.g., instead of "palec" (finger) he said "pa-tit". All of these observations indicated a general *disturbance of the precise structure and differentiation of articulemes.*

The patient showed no signs typical of temporal (acoustico-gnostic) aphasia. He had no difficulty in the auditory differentiation of correlative phonemes nor in remembering word meanings. He often attributed the wrong meanings to words, but this occurred only as the result of substituting similar articulemes. For instance, when instructed to point at his mouth (rot) he pointed at his forehead (lob); he frequently confused numbers involving sounds similar in articulation, e.g., 4 and 6 (četyre and šest') 12 and 18 (dvenadcat' and vosemnadcat) or 6 and 7 (šest' and sem'). His attempts to pronounce or write down these words revealed clearly that the source of his difficulty lay in defective analysis of sounds which were similar in the way they are articulated.

These defects severely affected the patient's writing and somewhat impaired his reading. He had little difficulty in telling how many sounds were present in simple words, and he seldom made an error in reporting their sequence. The identification of the sounds themselves was severely disturbed, however. He identified the first letter of the word "nos" (nose) as "l", "b", or even "r". Even when his answer was correct, he was not confident of it. The same difficulties prevented him from putting together individual sounds to produce whole words. His errors did not result from a difficulty in preserving the order of sounds but in identifying the sounds.

The most direct demonstration of the patient's basic defect was to have him write individual letters to dictation. Here one observed typical substitutions of sounds similar in articulation. He frequently wrote "n" as "d", "l", or "t" and sometimes as "s", or "r", "m" he wrote as "p" or "b." The same defect emerged when he wrote syllables. Occasionally he substituted correlative phonemes such as "k" and "t", but this occurred only if they were parts of syllables in which the vowels were soft and identical, e.g., he might write "ki" for "ti".

In writing syllables with two or more consonants in series the patient had a tendency to alter the phonemes so that the general intonational pattern was retained, but the individual sounds were changed, e.g., "st" was written "nda". His greatest difficulty arose in writing nonsense syllables, though he sometimes had difficulty with meaningful words also, e.g., he wrote "belka" (squirrel) as "betka" (meaningless), "stol" (table) as "slon" (elephant), etc. He made the same types of errors filling in the missing letters of words; e.g., he wrote "obnako" (meaningless) instead of "oblako" (cloud). This type of error occurred even when he wrote names which were quite familiar to him. Figure 93 shows several examples of the types of error he made.

He quickly regained the ability to read to himself, and by the seventh month he had no difficulty in recognizing written words. For the most part, however, his reading was restricted to the recognition of ideograms. When he was unable to grasp a word immediately he attempted to analyze its phonemic composition, but here the defect of sound-letter analysis often prevented him from being able to grasp the word's meaning. Such

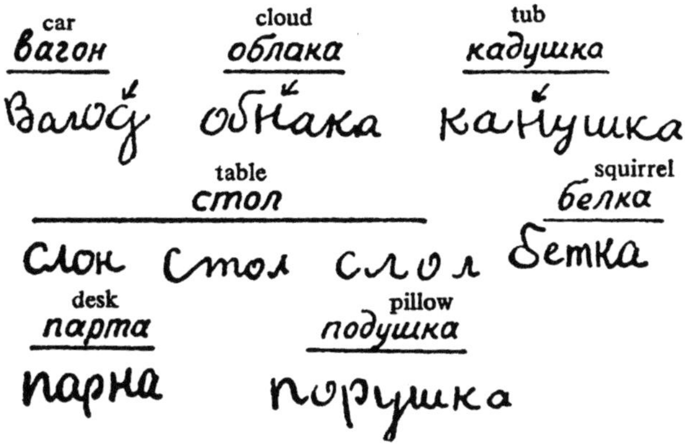

transliteration:

vagon → vagod   oblaka → obnaka   kaduška → kanuška

stol → slon stol slol   belka → betka

parta → parna   poduška → poruška

Patient Vas.: Lesion of the left opercular area (afferent motor aphasia).

FIG. 93. Substitution of letters which are similar in articulation in the writing of Patient Vas.

uncommon words as "pododejal'nik" (quilt cover) and "štepsel'" (electric plug) were impossible for him.

Reading aloud was made difficult for him by his tendency to substitute sounds. Though he made fewer errors than in writing, they were of the same type. His articulatory substitutions often prevented him from understanding the meanings of unfamiliar words. When he read "venki" (wreathes) as "vetki" (twigs) or "sobaki" (dogs) as "somaki" (meaningless) he naturally had difficulty in understanding what he read. Sometimes he had to resort to guessing the meanings of words on the basis of their context.

This patient's basic disturbance was loss of the precise and generalized articulatory groups (articulemes). It became apparent whenever he attempted to articulate a given sound and represent it by a letter. Consequently the major problem for the speech therapist was to help him compensate for this basic defect either by training him to recognize the differences between articulemes or by circumventing the defect and re-

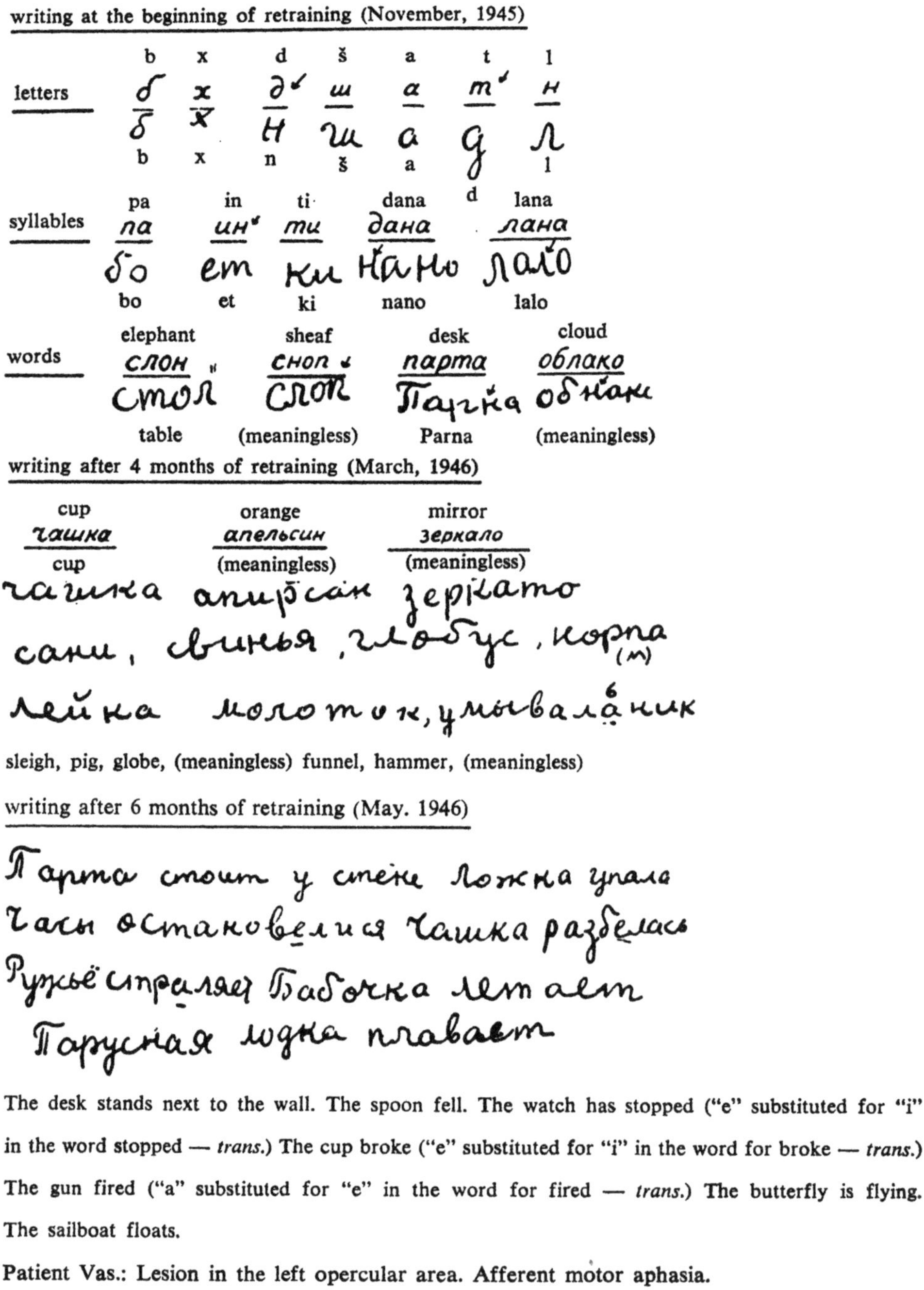

FIG. 94. The development of writing ability in Patient Vas. during six months of retraining.

writing at the beginning of retraining (November, 1945)

letters	b	x	d	š	a	t	n
			↓			↓	
	b	x	n	š	a	d	l

syllables	pa	in	ti	dana	lana
		↓			↓
	bo	et	ki	nano	lalo

words	slon	snop	parta	oblako
	↓ ↓	↓	↓ ↓	↓
	stol	slop	parna	obnako

writing after 4 months of retraining (March, 1946)

čaška	apel'sin	zerkalo
čaška	apirsan	zerkato

sani, svinja, globus, norpa

lejka, molotok, umyvalanik

writing after 6 months of retraining (May, 1946)

sleigh, pig, globe (meaningless), funnel, hammer (meaningless)

Parta stoit u stene. lozhna upala. chasy ostanovelisiaa. chashka razbelas

Ruž'ë stralaet Babočka letaet. Parusnaja lodka plavaet

The desk stands next to the wall. The spoon fell. The watch has stopped ("e" substituted for "i" in the word stopped — *trans.*) The cup broke ("e" substituted for "i" in the word for broke — *irans.*) The gun fired ("a" substituted for "e" in the word for fired — *trans.*) The butterfly is flying. The sailboat floats.

Patient Vas.: Lesion in the left opercular area. Afferent motor aphasia.

FIG. 94. The development of writing ability in Patient Vas. during six months of retraining.

organizing the processes of reading and writing on a new basis. In this case both principles were used.

The first problem was to teach him to differentiate clearly between individual sounds, i.e., to re-establish the constancy of phonemes without relying on his own imprecise articulatory patterns. By overcoming this defect one could immediately alleviate much of his difficulty in writing.

The therapist explained the articulatory patterns which corresponded to different sounds. This was done primarily by comparing the pronunciation of sound patterns all of which had a common articulatory component (Figure 94). The therapist simultaneously pointed out how words assumed different meanings depending upon the distinctive characteristics of the phonemes making them up. The patient practiced pronouncing and writing words in which a change in the first letter altered the meaning of the whole word. At the same time he wrote syllables all of which began with the same letter followed by different letter combinations, e.g., "to-tu" or "te-ti". He also wrote lists of syllables in which the first letter changed while the second letter was constant.

ta-na-la	ba-ma-pa
to-no-lo	bo-mo-po
te-ne-le	bi-mi-pi

The syllables were then incorporated into meaningful contexts. This helped to further fix the distinctiveness of their pronunciation.

Tanja	(girl's name)	Nadja	(girl's name)	Lapa	(paw)
Tolja	(boy's name)	Noga	(leg)	Lošad'	(horse)
Telo	(body)	Net	(no)	Lena	(girl's name)
Tina	(mud)	Nina	(girl's name)	Lipa	(linden)

As a result of such exercises the primary articulatory complexes were re-established on the basis both of articulatory structure and of semantic significance. Gradually they regained their distinctiveness and constancy so that in time the patient had reestablished a whole system of methods which permitted him to escape the defects which made writing difficult for him. In speaking he seldom substituted one sound for another, especially when he restricted himself to simple words. He also ceased to have difficulty in understanding words because he was able to recognize the individual phonemes. He still had a tendency to make substitutions when it was difficult for him to identify the root of a word or when the sound pattern was especially complex. There was a great change in his writing. Whenever a word presented difficulty he read it aloud and listened to his own voice as he isolated each sound or syllable in turn and identified it with one of the mediating words which he had learned. By analyzing the distinctive features of his own articulatory pattern he immediately found the correct letter to represent the component phonemes. At this stage his writing showed errors less frequently than initially, but he was still unable to write without analyzing each word into syllables and reading the syllables aloud. If any step in this process was blocked and a meaningless word was presented the patient was completely unable to write it.

Considerable progress was made in reading; from this stage on he had no difficulty in understanding words of any degree of complexity if he were allowed, to analyze them.

Subsequent retraining was directed toward making these techniques automatic. Continuous practice in the differentiation of meaningful articulatory patterns led to gradual disappearance of the long searches for appropriate articulatory positions. Soon the patient was able to write many words without consciously analyzing their articulatory components. Here an important factor was the accumulation of visual ideograms of words and extensive practice in the recognition of common letter sequences, e.g., prefixes, suffixes, and inflectional endings. Eventually the patient was able to write smoothly and he made fewer and fewer errors. Figure 94 illustrates his progress over a six month period of retraining.

For some time his writing continued to show clear signs that it was mediated by auxiliary process, and it never returned completely to its original functional structure. His reading difficulty disappeared completely as a result of the writing exercises.

The second patient differed considerably from the first in that he had no great difficulty in recognizing and writing individual letters, but het was unable to remember the correct order of letters in syllables and words. The problem in this case was to find a means whereby he could remaster and remember the sequential patterns of letters which make up meaningful words.

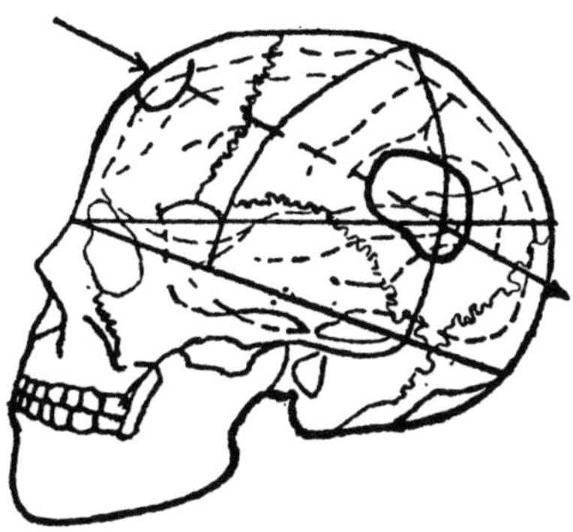

Patient Sux.: Injury diagram.

On April 26, 1945, Major Sux. a 30 year old cadet officer and former instructor in a military school was struck by a bullet which entered the central part of the left frontal area and emerged through the left infero-parietal area. An operation was performed the following day; a hematoma at the site of injury was drained and bone fragments were removed from deep in the parietal wound site; the frontal site was not operated upon. The parietal wound continued to drain for a long time.

A right hemiplegia of the type caused by destruction of their internal capsule was present immediately following the injury. There was no severe sensory deficit; in fact there appeared to be a hyperesthesia in the right extremities. The paresis disappeared from the right leg and, to some extent, from the right arm. No pathological reflexes were present. The visual field on the right was slightly constricted and signs of astereognosis were persistent. Severe motor aphasia was noted immediately following the injury and lasted for about four months. Toward the end of the first month the patient began to pronounce individual sounds and by the end of three months he was able to talk, though still with great difficulty. He had an articulatory disorder and tended to reverse the order of phonemes in certain words. By the end of five months he was able to utter short sentences, but he constantly had to search for the correct articulations of words. In repeating words he still reversed phonemes, e.g., he pronounced "portnoj" (tailor) as "pontroj" (meaningless); only after several attempts was he able to utter the word with the sounds in correct order. His comprehension of logico-grammatical relations was also severely impaired.

During the first month he showed clear signs of the parietal lobe syndrome. He could not identify the right and left sides of an object. He was unable to name fingers; in imitating hand positions he was sometimes correct, but other times he produced a mirror image of the correct position. He was unable to point out countries of the world on a map. Computational operations were severely impaired and showed further signs of the disturbance of complex spatial patterns. Thus, while he had no difficulty in writing down individual digits, he became confused in writing multiple digit numbers. He tended to reverse the order of digits and might write 2,078 as 2,780, or he might read the Roman numeral VI as four and IV as six. He had equally great difficulty in carrying out calculations in his head. In addition, he showed persistent reading and writing disorders.

Tests of the phonemic analysis of words showed that the patient was frequently unable to identify the sounds in words. He was seldom able to tell the number of sounds in a word, and when asked to point out the second or third letter of a simple word he usually failed. He was completely unable to carry out operations of auditory synthesis. Thus he was able to identify the individual sounds "b-r-a-t" (brother) but for him they never combined to form a meaningful word.

These difficulties were reflected in his reading and writing. Five months after injury he was able to write individual letters to dictation without error, but he had great difficulty in writing syllables. He was able to retain and write down short open syllables, but only if he repeated them aloud to himself. In attempting to write closed syllables, such as "or", "as", or "in", he had tendency to confuse the order of letters so as to write the consonant first. When confronted by complex syllables involving two or more consonants in a row, e.g., "kro", "pri", or "tre", or by simple words, such as "kot" (cat), "son" (sleep), or "ris" (rice), his basic disorder emerged very clearly and he tended to write the component sounds in random order. Thus, he might write the syllable "kro" as "kor" or "rko". Even if he wrote the letters in correct order, he was not confident of its accuracy. Similarly the word "okno" (window) might be written "nako", "Moskva" (Moscow) might be written "Mosak". He also tended to reverse letters in exercises which involved filing the letters in more than one blank. The only words he could write easily were such familiar ideograms as "Lenin" or "Petr Sux-n" (his own name).

The inability to maintain the letter sequences of words also complicated the reading process. The patient could read individual letters and open syllables without difficulty. But he had some difficulty in reading closed syllables and great difficulty in reading syllables in which two or more consonants appeared together.

He did not appreciate the sequential pattern of the words which he saw. As a result he sometimes read "op" as "po" or "kru" as "kur". He could avoid this difficulty only by reading slowly and aloud or by recognizing the syllables in new words as part of familiar words, e.g., recognizing "kru" as a letter sequence with which he was familiar as part of the visual ideogram "krug" (circle). Because of the difficulty in recognizing sound sequences he often had to guess at words on the basis of the individual letters and the context of the word as a whole. Thus, he read the word sequence "Šči, kaša, kompanija" (soup, cereal, company) as "šči, kaša, compot" (soup, cereal, compote). Similarly, he read the nonsense sentence "U sobaki jaščiki" (The dog has boxes) as, "U sobaki ščenki" (The dog has puppies).

The reading and writing defects were complex. They were based upon the impairment of the perception of "simultaneous patterns" typical of patients with the parietal syndrome. In addition, however, they were affected by the residue of a motor aphasia which deprived the patient's speech of automaticity. Because of the lack of automaticity he had to constantly correct himself, yet the capacity for self-correction was impaired by inability to perceive sequential patterns.

The goal in retraining this patient was to help him develop a basis for recognizing and remembering the positions of sounds and letters in complex sequential patterns. The first step was to *restore the recognition of individual sounds and awareness of the order of consonants and vowels in simple words.* Since he was still able to pronounce individual sounds and syllables it was necessary to make their pronunciation a *conscious process.* The major difficulty lay in the fact that, while the patient had little difficulty in recognizing consonants, he had great difficulty in recognizing vowels. To him a vowel appeared to be only a part of the preceding consonant. In order to overcome this defect his attention was directed to the articulatory positions appropriate to the consonants. He was shown diagrams of the sequence of sounds in specific words. By bringing the articulation of single sounds to a conscious level the patient acquired a new set of cues by which he could distinguish the sequence of sounds in words which already he was able to pronounce correctly. Using these new cues he could write simple syllables and read simple words. This step was relatively easy for him.

The second step was to develop a means of *organizing the sounds of more complex auditory patterns.* In particular he had to learn to deal with auditory complexes including several consonants. Since he still lacked the differentiated sequential patterns of syllables the basic approaches at this stage were to help him to analyze the letter sequence of syllables and to point out the significance of letter sequence in determining word meanings.

Initially the patient was taught to recognize the *first* sound in a word. This proved to be somewhat difficult in cases where the more distinct phoneme appeared in the middle of the word, for since the general schemata of the word was lost the patient anticipated the most striking phoneme and chose it as the first sound. Exercises in recognizing the consonants and having the patient write words as he spoke them helped him to overcome this difficulty. This constituted a large part of his retraining. The large amount of time was taken up in learning to recognize the pure consonant sounds and combinations of consonants. Such combinations as "t-r", "k-r", "s-t", had to be established on the basis of visual observation of the articulatory movements in a mirror, the use of articulatory diagrams, etc. Here, of course, the goal was not to compensate for articulatory defects but to establish a basis for tracing out the sequential order of sounds in words. Of special help in this regard were exercises involving the comparison of syllables containing the same letters in different sequences, e.g., "bro-bor" or "kro-kor". The distinctions between such syllables were made clearer by incorporating them into meaningful words, e.g., "fro-nt" (front) and "for-ma" (form), "dro-va" (firewood) and "dor-oga" (road).

In order to help overcome the reading difficulty, the method of "cinematic" reading was used. Words were exposed a letter at a time, so that the patient read syllables in the sequence in which they appeared. This protected the patient from the tendency to perceive words as whole letter complexes and thus helped him to pronounce the syllables in the correct order. Furthermore, the therapist insisted that he pronounced words slowly and precisely.

At the end of this stage of retraining the patient was able to write complex syllables and words; he was able to read slowly. In reading he had to pronounce words aloud, for he depended heavily upon auditory cues. The "simultaneous" patterns of words were replaced by sequential patterns. If he was prevented from whispering aloud, his reading and writing were again disrupted and he made the same types of letter reversals as before the *initiation* of therapy. The same degree of disruption of reading was

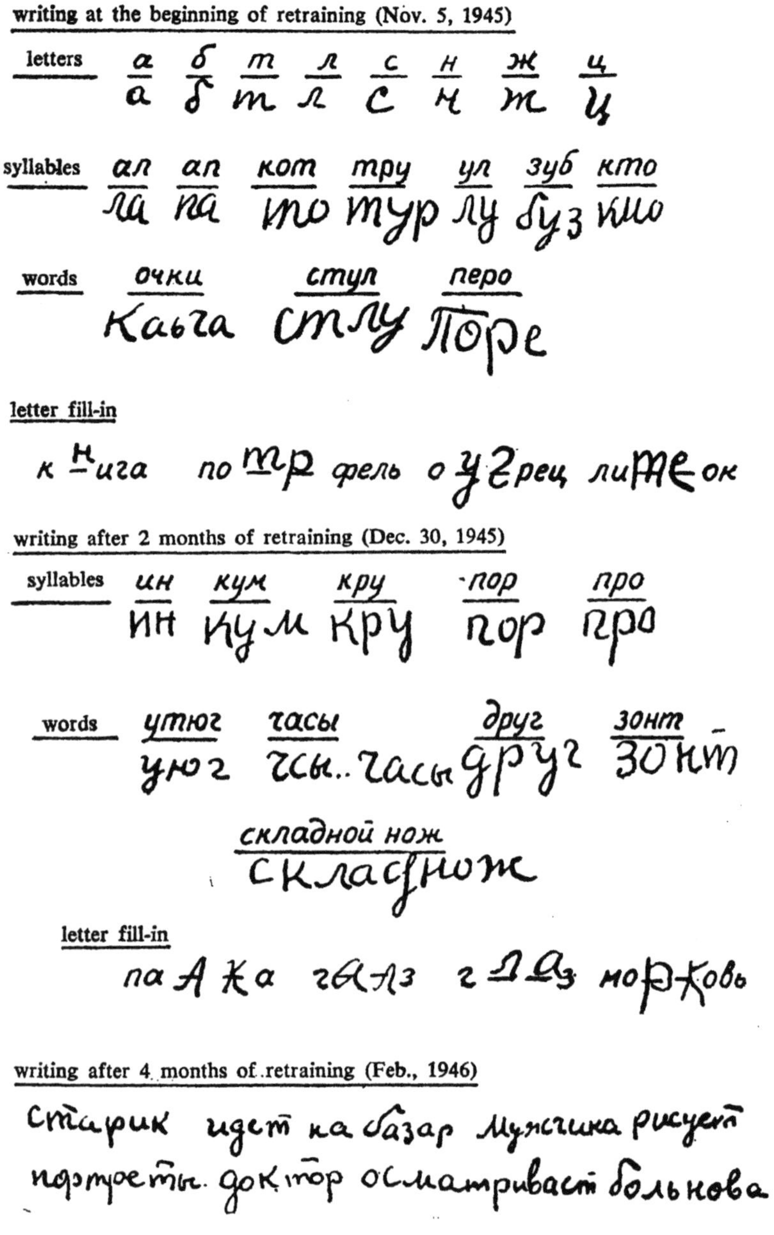

Patient Sux.: Penetrating bullet injury involving left fronto-parietal area. Parietal syndrome. The recovery of writing with retraining.

Fig. 95. The recovery of writing in Patient Sux. with rehabilitation therapy.

transliteration of Fig. 95.

writing at the beginning of retraining (Nov. 5, 1945)

letters	a	b	t	l	s	n	ž	c
	a	b	t	l	s	n	ž	c

syllables	al	ap	kot	tru	ul	zub	kto
	la	pa	to	tur	lu	buz	kio

words	očki	stal	pero
	kacha	stlu	pore

letter fill-in	kniga	portfel'	ogurec	listok
	kniga	potrfel'	ougrec	litsok

writing after 2 months of retraining (Dec. 30, 1945)

syllables	in	kum	kru	por	pro
	in	kum	kru	por	pro

words	utjug	časy	drug	zont
	ujug	čsy časy	drug	zont
		skladnoi nozh		
		sklad nozh		

letter fill-in	palka	galz	___	mozkov
	palka	galz	glaz	morkov

writing after 4 months of retraining (Feb. 1946)

starik idet na bazar Mužčika risuet

portrety. doktor osmatrivaet bolnova

produced if he was presented words tachistoscopically. In either case, exclusion of the opportunity to externalize the sequentiality of phonemes prevented the patient from doing anything other than to guess at the identity of words on the basis of randomly perceived letters.

The third step in retraining was to *transform the externalized sequential schemata established in the second stage into internal schemata.* This step required a lot of time and was by far the most difficult. It involved the simultaneous application of two types of techniques. With extensive practice there was a gradual shift from the utterance of words aloud, to whispering, to internal speech. Thus, after three and a half or four months of retraining the patient was able to write slowly and to read any word without speaking aloud. This internalization of the sequential schemata of words, did not however, restore the simultaneous schemata whereby words are perceived as wholes with letters in their proper sequence. The slowness with which the patient wrote indicated clearly that the writing process was organized differently from before. Thus, a second series of techniques was used. This required that the patient analyze words grammatically. He learned to identify roots, suffixes, inflective changes, etc. This work was based upon the sequential schemata which had just recovered and, in time, provided him with certain generalized sound-letter images. Eventually, he was able to read or write any word without repeating it to himself. At this point, the tendency to guess at word meanings virtually disappeared; even complex words which could not be guessed from the context were read accurately. This process remained unstable, however, so that any alteration in the way words were presented tended to disrupt the reading or writing process and the patient had to resort to the externalized, sequential aids learned earlier. For a long period of time these remained the basic means of compensating for his defect. Figure 95 presents examples of the patient's writing at successive stages of retraining and permit one to trace his progress as he gradually remastered the sequential schemata of words.

2. *The Restoration of Reading*

Reading, like writing, can be disrupted at various stages. Thus, its restoration also requires different techniques depending upon the step disturbed. The same difficulties encountered in teaching schoolchildren to read arise in various forms of aphasia. To these are added other difficulties. As a result, the methods used in restoring the ability to read have both similarities to and differences from those used in elementary education.

In a large number of aphasic disturbances the difficulties arise in the recognition of letters. In such cases the basic therapeutic measures must be directed toward overcoming this defect. In the early stages of traumatic aphasia and especially in cases involving damage to the occipital systems there may be a loss of the ability to recognize graphemes. Such cases are relatively uncommon; the major goal of retraining is to overcome the primary visual disorder. The first step is to have the patient copy letters. He learns to recognize the first letter in a word and write it down. Then he learns to write the letters corresponding to the diagrams of specific articulatory positions. These methods obviate the conceptualization of how the letters are written. The first are methods familiar to instructors who teach reading in grammar school; the latter is a method widely used in schools for deaf mutes. Together they constitute the first step in speech rehabilitation.

Next the patient is presented groups of letters written in different ways, e.g., D, D, d, d, or B, B, b, b. In this way he gradually recovers his generalized concepts of the letters of the alphabet. Also important in cases of alexia are methods which take advantage of the intact kinesthetic schemata of graphemes or which are based upon the visual analysis of printed letters. As pointed out in Chapter 13, a patient suffering from a disturbance of the visuo-gnostic system is unable to recognize letters, but he can often write them to dictation. Conversely, if he simply sees a letter he may be unable to name it, but if he copies it he may recognize it immediately. This phenomenon can be used in reorganizing the reading process as a whole. At first he learns to read letters by copying them or tracing their outlines with a pencil or finger. Eventually, he need only trace their outlines with his eyes in order to recognize them.

Even more important, however, are methods involving analysis of the structure of letters and the creation of letters from their individual elements. These methods were first suggested by B. G. Anan'ev and have been quite successful. A number of investigations, especially those of Ž. I. Šif, have shown that the basic defect preventing the patient from being able to read is that he is unable to differentiate the individual elements of which letters are composed or to recognize their positions relative to one another. It is important to point out to the patient that the individual elements in the letters "H", "K", "b", "r", and "E" differ considerably from those in the letters "A" and "Y" or "P" and "T". Sometimes it takes a little practice in analyzing letters to eliminate the patient's difficulty. The following is a case which illustrates the restoration of function to a patient in this group.

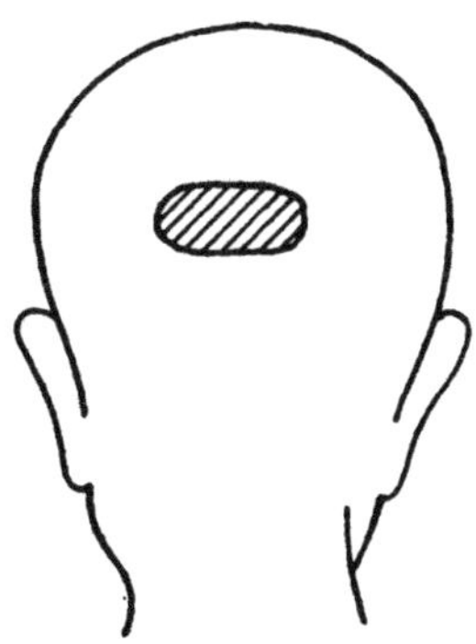

Patient Oz.: Injury diagram.

In December, 1942, patient Oz., a 41 year old draftsman received a direct bullet injury of the left occipital area which resulted in a right hemianopsia and further visual disorders. An abscess developed a year after injury and an operation was performed to drain it. Following the operation his visual defects became considerably more severe. He showed distinct signs of visual agnosia and alexia. In looking at an object or a picture he usually was able to grasp only one or two cues from which he attempted to guess its identity. These visual-gnostic defects emerged especially clearly when he attempted to read. The only letter he could recognize was "O", "Because it's roundish!" Despite the fact that he could not recognize the letters, he was able to write easily, rapidly, and with very few errors. He was unable, however, to read what he had written. This severe reading defect lasted for about two years with no detectable improvement.

The patient came under our observation in January, 1947, and retraining was begun immediately (the therapy was carried out by E. N. Hercenštejn). It became immediately apparent that, whereas the patient was unable to recognize letters visually, he could identify them with little difficulty if he traced them out with a pencil. The image of a letter emerged as he wrote it. This became the basis for retraining. He began by reading letters as he traced them out. A second technique was soon added to the first and consisted in the creation of letters from their basic elements. He learned to recognize the different letters which could be constructed from a common set of elements. These two methods led to very rapid improvement. The patient began to analyze letters by tracing them out with his finger or by mentally analyzing them into their component parts. At first he did this rather slowly but, gradually, the process became more rapid and more abbreviated until after two months the inability to recognize letters was totally abolished and a slow form of reading was restored.

In this case the basic difficulty arose from a visuo-gnostic defect. More frequently, however, the loss of letter meanings results from a different, nonvisual defect. A letter may elicit a sound which is not phonetically precise and which varies from reading to reading. The difficulty in reading letters arises either from the fact that no clear-cut auditory image is evoked or from the patient's shifting back and forth from one phoneme to another. A patient with temporal (acoustic) aphasia may pronounce the letter "ž" as "z", "š", or some other sound. A patient with afferent motor aphasia for whom articulatory schemata have lost their distinctiveness may read the letter "l" as "n" or "d", phonemes which are articulated similarly to "l". A patient with sensory aphasia may read "žar" (heat) as "zar" (meaningless), "zal" (hall), "šar" (sphere), or "sar" (meaningless). Similarly the word "guba" (lip) may be understood by a patient with afferent motor aphasia as "guma" (meaningless). The reading difficulty in a case such as the latter may be so great that the patient reads "stol" (table) as "slon" (elephant); here he has made two substitutions; "l" for "t" and "n" for "l". As we indicated above (Chapter 13) these defects may affect reading whether the patient reads aloud or to himself. The patient who has lost the phonemic articulatory correlates of letters is able to recognize words only if he pronounces them aloud to himself. The only exception occurs in the recognition of ready-made word-idiograms such as "USSR", "Lenin", "Moscow", etc. In some cases the preservation of ideograms may be so great that reading appears to be intact.

The first problem in retraining these patients lies in restoring the precise meanings of letters. This is done, as noted above, by incorporating the letters into meaningful word patterns, e.g., k=Katja (a girl's name), g=gora (mountain), n=Nina (a girl's name), l=Lenin, etc. First the patient works with groups of words all beginning with one letter, e.g., Katja, Kolja, karta (map), kofta (jacket), and kuxnja (kitchen). With each word he differentiates the first letter "k" from letters which sound similar, e.g., "k=kora" (cortex), "g=gora" (mountain), etc. In cases of afferent motor aphasia he also consults diagrams showing the articulatory positions for various letters in order to substitute for the inner articulatory schemata which he lacks and which are also necessary for the correct pronunciation of letters.

Once the recognition of individual letters has been mastered, the patient may or may not have great difficulty in going on to the recognition of whole words. In addition to reading letters as "pure sounds", he must also master the articulatory changes which occur when such sounds are incorporated into syllables. A certain amount of work must be spent on recognizing the differences between hard and soft syllables. The patient reads groups of syllables such as "to-tu-te-ti" or "ba-bo-be-bi" (syllables with "a", "o", or "u" are hard; syllables with "e" or "i" are soft, *trans.*) Soon he is able to recognize the articulatory distinction and certain difficulties in the smooth shift from one sound to another can be overcome.

Once the primary sounds have been mastered and reinforced it is necessary to elaborate the corresponding inner schemata before the patient is able to read to himself. This is the final stage of retraining and is achieved by first learning to read in a whisper, and then to read silently. At all stages the recognition of whole ideograms is understandably attractive to the patient, for it is easier than reading syllable by syllable. He should force himself to use the analytical methods, however, rather than rely upon his ability to guess the meanings of words on the basis of randomly perceived letter patterns.

Sometimes the recognition of visual ideograms may simulate reading in a patient who, previous to injury, was a highly skilled reader. He may read correctly aloud without relying upon the auditory analysis and synthesis of words. M. S. Lebedinskij and later, we ourselves observed a large number of cases in which patients with severe damage to the temporal systems and total loss of the auditory analysis of words able to recognize simple syllables and "read" rather complex words, even though they could not recognize individual letters. On careful analysis, it was found that they simply recognized the words as visual ideograms. Their errors were semantic in character. For instance, one patient read "airplane" as "aircraft", "Kiev" as "Kharkov", and carefully examining the word "Holland" said, "Well, yes . . . I know . . . I know . . . It's a country . . . not Europe . . . no . . . not Germany . . . it's small . . . it was captured . . . Belgium! That's it, Belgium!"

Such reading is obviously not satisfactory. The patient must overcome the tendency to guess at word meanings and reorganize the reading process on the basis of genuine sound-letter analysis. This is often difficult. A patient with severe temporal aphasia who is able to recognize many words may be unable to read a single letter. He is given exercises which force him to relate letters and combinations to letters with sounds rather than with meanings. As he reads his attention is directed toward the phonemic analysis of words. Work carried out by Ė. S. Bejn has shown that he can regain the ability to read letters and syllables on the basis of such exercises. It is interesting to note that once he regains the ability to analyze words there is a complete breakdown in his ability to recognize ideograms. Thus, having remastered letters and syllables the patient, for the first time, is unable to "read". Reading was reestablished by subsequent exercises. It was more difficult than the form of "reading" existing in the early post-traumatic period, but it was more flexible and was based upon genuine analysis of the phonemic composition of words.

The course of retraining is entirely different in cases of efferent motor aphasia. Here the reading of individual letters is usually intact; the primary difficulty lies in combining them into sequential patterns and in maintaining the schemata of the whole words. The difficulty in reading whole words results from inability to shift smoothly from one syllable to another and from inability to preserve the correct sequence of letters. The patient's difficulty is most acute when he attempts to read complex syllables or words. The letters which make up a complex syllable, such as "kru", "kro", or "stro", are read separately and then combined in any order. Some letters may be omitted and the identity of the word guessed at on the basis of the group of letters which remain.

The goals of the therapist in cases of this sort are to facilitate the process of shifting from one syllable to another and to re-establish the schemata of whole words which will permit the patient to retain the correct sequence of letters. In order to solve the first problem the patient must acquire means whereby he can modify the sounds depending upon their position in different syllables. This categorization of the "pure" phonemes to include the variants which occur in different contexts is a prerequisite for the incorporation of individual phonemes into whole words. The appropriate variant of a given phoneme can only be determined, however, if the patient is able to perceive the schemata of whole words. Thus, the first stage in retraining is to restore the schemata of whole words.

The patient first learns to combine individual sounds to form syllables. There are several methods which may be useful in overcoming this difficulty. Some of them are techniques used in teaching children to read; others are not. Some provide external aids in shifting from syllable to syllable; others aid in the establisment of the internal schemata of words. The aids designed to externalize the reading process consist of slow uninterrupted reading of combinations of letters or in writing syllables as a single motor act, i.e., without lifting the pencil from the paper. The second and more important group of techniques involve working with a series of syllables in which one consonant is used in combination with different vowels which alter its sound, e.g., "ta-to-te-tu". The therapist explains the articulatory mechanisms involved in shifting from one sound to another and the patient practices reading the syllables. By using anagrams to build up and break down syllables he acquires further practice in pronouncing words aloud and gradually develops the capacity to grasp whole syllables, recognize the first letter, and smoothly pronounce the whole syllable. Another important exercise involves filling in the blanks in simple syllables from which one or more letters have been omitted, e.g., he may be instructed to fill in "—a—a-" to produce the pair of syllables "pa-pa" or "ba-ba". Exercises of this type lead to the establishment of syllable schemata on the basis of which the patient can perceive and recognize whole syllables.

The next stage of retraining is directed toward restoration of the ability to read whole words. Often when a patient who has recovered the ability to read individual syllables attempts to combine them to form words the syllables themselves break-down so some letters are omitted or their sequence is altered. Again, instability of the inner sound-letter schemata of words forces the patient to resort to guessing and genuine reading is impossible. At this stage the motor aphasic may read "krest" (cross) as "korset" (corset) or "okno" (window) as "kino" (movie).

The methods used to retrain a patient of this sort are designed to help him retain the sequence of letters in words. He identifies the first letter and attempts to suppress the tendency to pronounce the subsequent letters before they actually appear in the word; in other words, his effort is directed toward continuous analytical control of the reading process. This is usually achieved by reinforcing the inner schemata of words. Each word is broken down into its component syllables and the syllables are pronounced slowly and carefully. The method of "cinematic" reading is especially useful in these cases. The patient reads words through a window in a small moving screen. The screen covers the syllables on either side of that which is to be read. This method plays only a secondary role in the restoration of reading, however. The major factors are the inner analysis of words into their component parts and the identification of roots, prefixes, suffixes, and inflective endings. The transition from externalized phonemic analysis of words on the basis of inner schemata is very important, for without this, it is impossible to read rapidly or to overcome the perseverative and random external factors which may interfere with the perception of words (Cf. L. S. Cvetkova [in press]).

Only in the final stage of retraining does the externalization of reading become less important and give way to silent reading. The development of the inner schemata and the transition to silent reading by the inner analysis of the morphological components of words concludes the retraining of patients in this group. It should be noted, however, that the return to automatic reading occurs very slowly. For a long time the patient's reading bears traces of the intermediate processes by which he has regained the ability to read. The recovery of reading is usually associated with the recovery of writing. The two case histories presented in the previous sections illustrate the above principles.

A patient for whom the inner structure of words is unstable easily substitutes guessing for genuine reading. Sometimes such guessing may be based on very fragmentary impressions of words and yet the reading process appears rather well preserved. The tendency to rely on visual ideograms rather than on genuine word analysis is, of course, greater, the more definite the set created by the context. In normal reading, and in the late stages of retraining, context may play a positive role in the reading process. On the other hand, in the early stages of retraining, when the inner schemata of sound sequences and the morphological structure of words are not yet re-established, such contextual reading may be quite hazardous. It can completely supplant the analytical reading process and thus impede restoration of the ability to read accurately. Thus, in retraining patients with efferent motor aphasia, reading by the recognition of words as ideograms should be undertaken very cautiously. It should be introduced only at a stage when the schemata of words have been well enough re-established to serve as a means of self-correction in the reading of ideograms. This is an important part of the reading process and cannot be performed if the patient is unable to analyze the auditory and morphological components of words.

E. THE RESTORATION OF SPEECH COMPREHENSION

The restoration of speech comprehension is one of the most important problems in traumatic aphasia. Yet this is often not adequately recognized and is not given sufficient attention in severe cases of motor, sensory, or amnesic aphasia. Impairment of the comprehension of grammatical speech is encountered in traumatic aphasia much more often than might be supposed on the basis of first impressions gained by talking with aphasic patients. As we have already seen (Chapter 12) it is not limited to cases of sensory aphasia. A large number of patients with motor aphasia, and all patients in whom damage to the occipito-parietal areas is accompanied by semantic aphasia, show defective comprehension of logico-grammatical constructions. While such patients have no difficulty in understanding the primary meanings of words and short statements, they have considerable difficulty in understanding "expansive constructions", in which related parts of the sentence are separated by qualifying phrases. They also have difficulty with "inverted constructions" in which the order of words is different from the logical order of the thoughts expressed, and with logico-grammatical relationships which are symbolized in certain ways, e.g., by inflected endings, prepositions, connectives, or specific word order. These difficulties are rarely brought out in everyday speech, the meaning of which can usually be established by guessing or by context; they emerge quite clearly, however, in the reading of complex material. The patient may complain that the text is incomprehensible, that "It doesn't hang together".

The difficulty in comprehending complex grammatical speech derives from the fact that the patient is unable to grasp the meaning underlying certain grammatical constructions. This is a common defect seen in many forms of traumatic aphasia, but the underlying mechanisms are different in different syndromes; consequently, the methods of retraining patients with comprehension difficulties vary from case to case.

The easiest comprehension defects to overcome are those present in the residual stage of *motor aphasia*. The comprehension difficulties here result from disturbance of the dynamics of verbal thought and the loss of inner speech. The process whereby sequentially perceived words are transformed into meaningful inner schemata is impaired, so that the patient must repeat a grammatical construction several times before he is able to grasp its meaning; external repetition compensates for a function ordinarily accomplished by inner speech. With each repetition the patient can emphasize a different part of the sentence and separate the various thoughts from one another. If he is dealing with an expansive construction he can identify and omit the qualifying phrases long enough to grasp the basic thought. Similarly, he can transform inverted constructions into direct constructions. By repeating the sentence aloud, or in a whisper, the patient can generate a statement, the semantic structure of which he is able to comprehend. The difficulties experienced in comprehending logico-grammatical constructions are nonspicific in these cases and the methods used in retraining are quite simple. The most effective exercise involves reading complex statements over and over in a distinct and expressive voice. Sometimes diagrams aid in comprehending the relationships of different elements within the sentences. Such diagrams differ little from those used in common grammar texts. In extremely severe cases sentences are broken down into their component parts and the parts are considered together in various combinations. The effectiveness of these measures depends upon the severity of the impairment of inner speech and upon the conscientiousness with which the exercises are carried out.

It is more difficult to restore speech comprehension in cases of *semantic aphasia*. Here the basic defect is not a disturbance of inner speech but a primary inability to grasp the entire grammatical structure of a sentence and relate the various details into a simultaneous pattern, i.e., a pattern in which all parts are beheld simultaneously. In this situation, of course, the use of external speech does not help the patient; the more he attempts to grasp the relationships between different phrases, the more confused he becomes. As was pointed out earlier (Chapters 8 and 12), the greatest difficulty of such a patient arises when he is confronted with a sentence in which it is necessary to go beyond the nominative meanings of words and consider them as part of an overall meaningful pattern. Elementary, "inter-systemic" modes of compensation are of little help here. The therapist must take a long roundabout approach which involves major reorganization of the processes whereby the patient grasps logico-grammatical constructions.[11]

Retraining may take either of two forms. The first takes advantage of whatever

[11] The material presented here was gathered in our laboratory by V. K. Bubnova and L. S. Cvetkova. See V. K. Bubnova, *The Comprehension of Grammatical Constructions in Cases of Brain Damage and Recovery with Retraining* (dissertation, 1946) and L. S. Cvetkova, "Methods of Restoration of Higher Cortical Functions after Local Brain Lesions" (in press).

"sense for the language" the patient retains; he is taught to recognize the meanings of certain grammatical constructions on the basis of familiarity with the way they are formulated. The second consists of breaking down complex sentences into their components parts and analyzing the parts one by one. Special investigations have shown that only the second method is capable of producing long term improvement.

We shall describe how these approaches help a patient to comprehend two specific types of grammatical construction, *viz.*, inflective word changes and prepositional phrases. A patient with semantic aphasia is unable to grasp such apparently simple constructions as nouns in instrumental or genitive cases. Since he is unable to grasp the relationships between the objects which are defined by the instrumental or genitive cases, he has great difficulty in carrying out such an instruction as: "Point with the pencil at the comb." Here the information that the pencil is to be used for pointing is carried entirely by the suffix "-om" instrumental case on the word "karandaš" (pencil). Instead of responding as instructed, the patient often points at the two objects in turn saying, "Here is the pencil, and here is the comb". If presented a picture of a mother and daughter he is able to point out the "mother or the daughter" but he is unable to comprehend the terms "daughter's mother", or the "mother's daughter".

Attempts to comprehend such constructions by mastering a number of specific examples are generally unsuccessful. At best they make the patient aware that such constructions refer to a single object rather than two. It does not, however, help him to recognize which object, i.e., it does not help him to grasp the relationship implied by the grammatical construction.

A more rational approach is to break down such constructions into their component parts and to use auxiliary means to help the patient grasp the grammatical relationships involved. He must learn to consciously analyze the rule according to which a given grammatical construction is organized. In considering the instrumental construction in the comb and pencil example described above, the therapist first explains to the patient that the two nouns do not have equal value in the sentence. Only one of the two objects mentioned is to be pointed at. In order to make it easier for him to recognize the relationship between the two objects an etxra preposition may be introduced into the instruction to define the position of the comb (grebešok). "Pokažite karandašom *na* grebešok". Here the preposition "na" (at) appearing after "pencil" and before "comb" in the Russian sentence clarifies at which object the patient is to point. In explaining the relationship the therapist poses a series of questions to further aid the patient. "Karandašom – om – instrumental case; what is used to point? karandašom! Na grebešok (at the comb) – at what? . . . nominative case – at the comb!" The patient is able to understand questions posed in this form despite his semantic aphasia for his "feeling for language" in active speech is relatively intact. While for the normal person such a long complicated approach is more difficult than direct mastery of the instrumental case, it is the only means whereby a patient in this group can master the concept. Once he has mastered this rule he can use the same method to analyze similar constructions by himself.

The same approach is used in helping the patient to remaster constructions involving the genitive case. Here again the process of abstracting the meaning of a word appearing in the genitive case and grasping its attributive or possessive significance must be achieved on the basis of aids provided by the therapist. First the therapist points out to the patient that in constructions of the type "daughter's mother", "mother's daughter", "father's brother", "friend's sister", etc. only one of the two words refers to an object; the meaning of the other is attributive in nature. Pictures may be used in which the two meanings are clearly dissociated so as to show the attributive character of one of the words. For instance, a boy's suit may be used to illustrate "boy's clothing" and a dress used to represent "girl's clothing". These illustrations, however, have only a propaedeutic function. The second step consists in breaking down the expression and using new methods to provide the patient with cues whereby he can analyze its meaning. One technique is to introduce a demonstrative pronoun which goes with and, thus, segregates the noun which has an attributive meaning, e.g., "this mother's daughter" instead of "mother's daughter". This pronoun, which in Russian has a genitive case ending itself, gives the patient one more cue as to the adjectival nature of the accompanying "noun".

In some cases this type of exercise alleviates the difficulty in grasping the meanings of grammatical constructions. In other, more stubborn cases, it is necessary to apply other methods of grammatical analysis to externalize the meaningful relationships implied by the constructions and compensate for the inner schemata which the patient lacks. The therapist can help the patient analyze the term "daughter's mother" by the following type of explanation: "Mother – who – mother – nominative case – the subject; this means you should point at the mother. Daughter's – the ending apostrophe – of whom . . . daughter's – genitive case. This means she is the mother of whom? – daughter's, of this daughter; the word "daughter's" only indicate whose mother." At first this type of analysis must be carried out in great detail so as to provide a concrete external means of substituting for immediate recognition of the meaning of the grammatical construction. Gradually, however, the explanations are shortened; shorter operations provide a sufficient basis for the patient to master such constructions.

It is even easier to show the process of retraining in cases involving the inability to comprehend complex logico-grammatical structures involving pronouns. As a rule the patient with semantic aphasia is totally unable to grasp the meaning of such constructions as "Place the notebook to the right of the book", or "draw a circle under a square". The patient has no difficulty in understanding the individual words, e.g., "circle", "under", "square", etc. But he does not recognize the spatial relationships implied by the construction, i.e., he does not understand which figure is to be placed under the other. If he is presented two constructions for comparison, e.g., "the circle under the square" and "the square under the circle" he is unable to distinguish the meanings of the two; he feels that both constructions refer to the same relationship, and that the only difference lies in the order of the words. He is completely unable to fulfill a three part instruction of the type, "Place the pencil to the right of the notebook and to the left of the book".

Retraining is directed toward overcoming the inability to grasp the semantic schemata underlying such constructions. Again, it involves analyzing the grammatical construction and fulfilling the task in two steps.

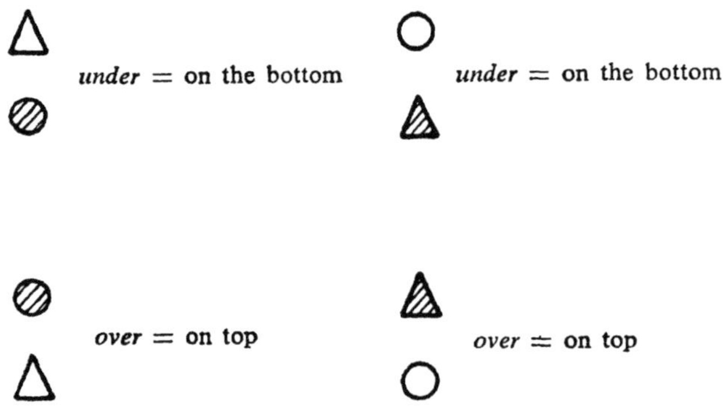

FIG. 96. Diagrams used for the remastery of relationships expressed by prepositions.

The relationship of the two figures is represented diagrammatically by drawing them (Figure 96) and darkening the one which appears in the nominative case in the instruction; (in Russian the object of a preposition "under" or "over" must have a special ending which identifies it as belonging to the instrumental case. *trans.*) Next to these figures is written the preposition "under" or "over" which, in the diagram, is replaced by the adverb "on the bottom" or "on top". The patient with the instruction to draw "a triangle under a circle" looks for that diagram in which a triangle (which occurs first in the construction and in the nominative case) is drawn as a darkened figure and stands next to the preposition "under". Here he sees that the preposition may be replaced by the adverb "on the bottom". Thus, he is able to replace the relative construction, "the triangle under . . ." by the absolute construction "triangle on the bottom". Once this is done he can solve the second part of the construction, ". . . under a circle" by substituting the absolute construction "circle on top". By transforming one relative construction to two absolute constructions he is able to fulfill a task which would otherwise be impossible for him.

A second way of solving this task lies in mastering the rule that a word appearing in the instrumental case, i.e., having an instrumental case ending, is the object with reference to which the other object, that in the nominative case, is to be placed; the preposition tells the position of the second relative to the first. The patient is instructed to draw first he object which appears in the nominative case and then to draw the other object above or below it as indicated by the pronoun. Here again, the direct grasp of a spatial relationship is replaced by a two step operation. It differs from the first approach only in that the patient is able to use the preposition in its original form and yet in terms which are comprehensible to him.

In both cases a short grammatical construction expressing a spatial relationship is replaced by a series of operations. Gradually this series of externalized steps may be shortened, and the patient gains the ability to comprehend such constructions by an abbreviated form of this indirect path. Experience has shown that only in very rare cases does this way of handling instructions become so automatic that the patient is able to grasp the meanings of grammatical constructions as rapidly as before injury. Usually patients who have been through a long period of retraining and who are able to carry out grammatically defined instructions with little difficulty continue to be aware of the fact that their successes are not based upon a genuine "recognition of relationships" of the type they enjoyed before injury. Thus, while the reorganization of logico-grammatical functions leads to a practical mastery of complex constructions, it does not re-establish the function in its original form.

We have presented examples of patients who recovered the ability to understand certain grammatical constructions because these are the defects which are most troublesome in semantic aphasia and for which methods of retraining are best developed. It is important to note that techniques which appear so difficult and artificial to a normal speaker greatly aid the patient in mastering general types of grammatical constructions which occur in many speech situations. At first, of course, he can only apply the methods of grammatical analysis which he learns in exercises whereby he learns them. Eventually however, he is able to generalize to other types of material; the degree of transfer to other situations is greatly expanded. The patient becomes aware of the fact that only by conscious grammatical analysis can he understand constructions which are not immediately comprehensible; consequently, he gradually adopts such analysis as part of his everyday thought.

Only in a few cases have patients succeeded in making the comprehension of grammatical constructions fully automatic, or at least nearly so automatic as to approximate the normal process of grasping grammatical meanings. Usually the retraining only gives the patient a number of rules which he can use to compensate for his comprehension defect. We shall present one example to illustrate the course which one patient followed in recovering the ability to comprehend complex grammatical speech forms.[12]

[12] Speech therapy was conducted in this case by V. K. Bubnova.

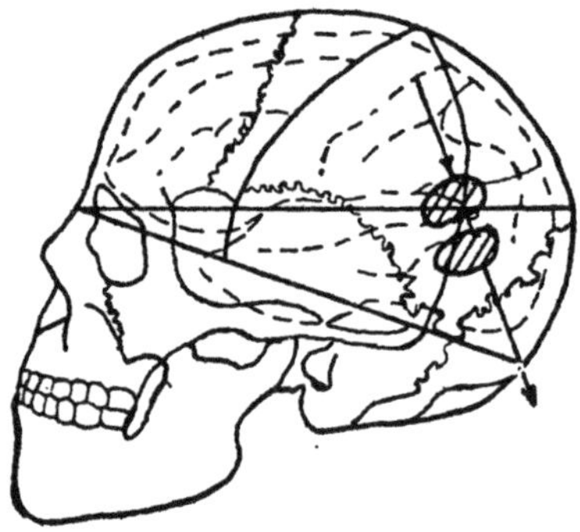

Patient Pryg.: Injury diagram.

In February, 1944, Major Pryg., a 35 year old former engineering student received a penetrating shrapnel wound of the left parieto-temporo-occipital area. At an operation the following day, two skull defects were cleared, bone fragments were removed from the brain substance, and a hematoma was drained. The wound was deep and cerebrospinal fluid drained from the injury for some time. It was finally closed four and a half months later.

The patient was unconscious for 20 to 30 minutes following the injury and them made his own way to the medical post. Paresis was absent; there was a slight sensory deficit on the right which was eliminated by drug treatment. Persistent hemianopsia and astereognosis on the right were noted. Spatial orientation was disturbed in the initial period.

A speech disorder emerged immediately after injury. There was no particular articulatory difficulty, but the patient made many literal and verbal paraphasias without recognizing his errors. He usually understood the speech of others, but he quickly forgot what he heard. His speech gradually returned to normal, but for a long time he showed noticeable signs of a residual amnesic-aphasic-disturbance of connected speech. Severe alexia and agraphia were present for some time; reading was more disturbed than writing. In the residual period of recovery, the patient still had difficulty in reading and writing; if confronted with stylized print, he often had to write down words himself in order to read them. Computation was disturbed but was recovered after extensive practice.

The most persistent disturbance involved the *comprehension of grammatical speech*. The patient was able to understand common everyday speech and easily grasped the meanings of various fables. For instance, when he was told Tolstoj's fable "The Dove and the Pigeons" he had no difficulty in recognizing the moral it illustrated: "Everyone has his own place". He was unable, however, to grasp relationships implied by the grammatical structure of statements. He was unable to understand the relationships implied by such expressions as "mother's daughter, daughter's mother", "father's brother", or "brother's father". He indicated that the change in order of words produced some change of meaning, but he could not say what the change was. He was totally unable to grasp the meaning of the instruction, "Draw a circle under a cross"; his interpretation of the statement was agrammatical as shown by the fact that he produced the symbols as ♀. He was unable to comprehend relative constructions; after a great deal of effort he was unable to solve the problem: "Which of the three circles is larger than the blue one and smaller than the red one?" His comment was, "Somehow it just doesn't hold together". These difficulties naturally hindered him in his work and he felt that it was impossible for him to comprehend complex written material.

The patient came under our observation a year after injury, thus, his retraining was begun in the risidual phase of recovery. In order to restore the comprehension of inflective constructions it was necessary for him to overcome the tendency to recognize only the root or nominative aspect of words. The therapist helped him by directing his attention to the case endings of words and by explaining how changes in suffix affect the meanings of words. The explanations were supplemented by exercises in which words were used in different contexts and he was asked to explain their meanings. This type of grammatical analysis taught him to recognize the common inflective word-endings in statements, the meaning of which he already knew either as a result of immediate recognition or on the basis of newly acquired rules. Eventually he *overcame the tendency to perceive only the meaning implied by the order of words and learned to transform certain constructions into a form comprehensible to him.* Each time he would go through a routine course of reasoning: "Aha! here's the subject ... and this ending '-om' ... means 'with what' or 'by means of what' ... Yes, that's clear ..." or, "the granddaughter's grandmother ... aha! ... there's the subject ... and 'granddaughter's' ... that means 'whose' ... that's whose grandmother ..." This method of analyzing inflective constructions became well established and became a basic method of comprehending grammatical statements. The patient had no difficulty in generalizing this method to any type of grammatical construction. The only types of grammatical constructions he was able to recognize automatically, however, were very simple inflective relationships.

Similar work was carried out in order to restore the comprehension of relationships implied by the grammatical structure of sentences. At first he was unable to comprehend such expressions as "a circle under a cross" or "a cross under a circle". He could not grasp which object was to appear under which. Retraining was carried out as described above. First he was taught to pick out the noun in the instrumental case and then to substitute the absolute abverb "on the bottom" for the relative preposition "under". Having done this, he was able to draw the two figures correctly. Though it appears very complex, this was the only method whereby the patient was able to grasp such a relationship. With a little practice he was able to carry out this type of instruction even though he did not directly recognize the relationship implied by the grammatical construction. Very gradually the intermediate steps became shorter, and the patient was able to reason more rapidly: "A triangle under a cross ... that means the triangle on the bottom with something else on top ... the cross on top ... that's it. But I would have done just the opposite; I would have rotated the thing by exactly 180° ... from my memory I would think "under" means it's on the bottom; but, still, it's on top ... from just reading it I am not sure ... if I say it straight out, I want to do just the opposite. The only way I can do it is to keep in mind the main figure and draw it without paying any attention to the other ..."

With extensive practice the patient was able to carry out this type of construction almost automatically, but by careful observation one could still detect that he was compensating for the initial defect by applying the methods he had learned. While he was able to perform accurately, it was obvious that he had not regained the direct "feeling for relationships" which he had possessed before injury.

F. THE RESTORATION OF GRAMMATICAL SPEECH

In the cases just described the comprehension of complex logico-grammatical relations was severely disturbed, but the expressive speech of the patient remained relatively intact. The preservation of expressive grammatical speech was explained by the fact that these patients retained their "sense for the language" and were, consequently, able to formulate grammatical sentences. Indeed, the preservation of this aspect of speech serves in some cases as a basis for overcoming an impairment of the ability to grasp spatial or grammatical relationships.

In many cases, especially ones involving lesions in the anterior parts of the speech areas, just the reverse situation is observed. As a rule, patients in this group are able to comprehend relatively complex logico-grammatical relationships. In their own speech, however, the predicative function is severely disturbed, so that they can do little more than name individual objects (Chapter 7). The "sense for the language" which is derived from the predicative aspect of inner speech is so disrupted in these cases that patients can no longer make use of the basic parts of speech, e.g., subject, verb, and the subordinate parts of speech. Furthermore, they are unable to create the schema for any type of grammatical statement.

The restoration of expressive speech may be achieved by *substituting external aids for the missing inner dynamic schemata.* A patient who lacks the basis for formulating the predicative aspect of sentences must be provided the external schemata of very simple sentences which he can learn to break down into subject and predicate. He must be taught to feel that any statement involving a single word is incomplete; in addition he must be provided with instructions which force him to attach a verb or adjective to every object mentioned so as to transform the single word into a statement or judgment. Once the basis for predicative statements has been established, he must learn to create sentence patterns. A severe disturbance of the "feeling for language" makes this extremely difficult to achieve. External schemata must be substituted for the missing phraseological schemata. They must represent the relationships between objects and must lead to conscious awareness of the basic grammatical rules adhered to in normal speech. The following is a case illustrating the sequence of stages by which a patient regained the ability to formulate grammatical sentences and thus to recover expressive speech.

Colonel Vin., 37 years of age, came under our observation as a result of a blow to the left hemisphere and hemorrhage of the left middle cerebral artery. He suffered a transient right hemiparesis and a severe motor aphasia. He was able to utter single words either imitatively or spontaneously but he was totally *unable to utter phrases or sentences.* He was even unable to repeat short sentences spoken by the therapist. Thus, while he had no difficulty repeating the word "polden' " (noon), he was unable to repeat the short sentence. "Byl den' " (It was day); he was only able to repeat the word "den' " (day). The patient's spontaneous statements consisted of single words in the nominative case, "... wounded! ... medal ... commission ... overcoat ... boots". By this statement he wished to indicate that he wanted his overcoat and boots brought in order that he might go to the commission which awards military medals. There was no hint whatsoever of sentence structure in his speech. His speech comprehension was better preserved, though signs of a receptive agrammatism were detectable.

The first problem in retraining was to compensate for his expressive speech defect. It was necessary to overcome the purely nominative character of his speech and compensate for the absence of the inner schemata of statements. Attempts to teach the patient the normal predicative structure of a sentence by having him imitate very simple statements were totally unsuccessful. He listened carefully to such examples, but in attempting to repeat them, he immediately reverted to naming single words. Sometimes he was able to repeat only the nouns, sometimes he recalled a verb, but his statements never exhibited any kind of predicative structure. The simple "adaptation" to the speech of others which is so common a factor in the development of speech in children was completely absent.

It was necessary to create external schemata which would force the patient to form elementary, though perhaps agrammatical, combinations of two or more words. These could then serve as a basis for making predicative statements. At first the therapist only indicated the number of words to be used in a simple sentence. The patient was presented a sheet of paper on which there appeared two figures in which he was to write words and, thus, to form a sentence. He was also given sample sentences (Figure 97). With these aids, he was instructed to create other statements having to do with the same objects. This method proved successful in a very short time. Although the patient was not immediately able to produce sentences, he soon began to sense the incompleteness of one-word statements. He began to feel that his own statements were incomplete, and it became clear to him that in order to complete them he must add more words. He was still unable to specify, however, the nature or form of the missing words. The newly established feeling that his sentences were incomplete led him to attempt to add words. These attempts sometimes resulted in agrammatical word patterns and sometimes in nonsense, but they set the stage for the next step in retraining *viz.*, consideration of the relationships among words which constitute the skeleton of a sentence.

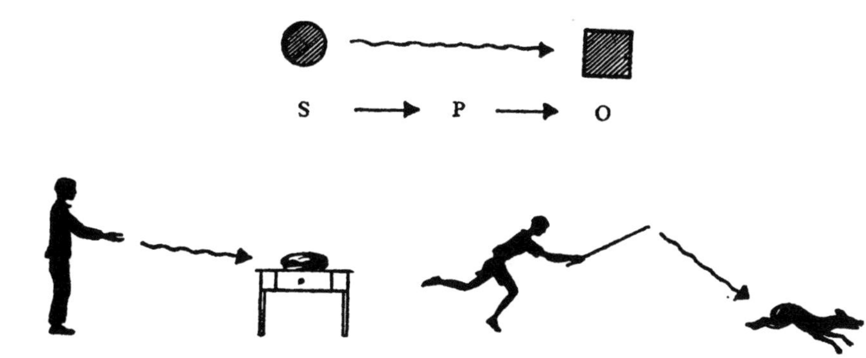

FIG. 97. Diagrams used for constructing sentences.

Since he retained some ability to comprehend abstract categories, it was possible to diagram simple statements for him. For instance, it was possible to symbolize the action in a sentence by an arrow directed toward the direct object. Each component of the diagram was accompanied by a small arrow pointing to a blank space into which he was to write the appropriate word. This technique also produced clear-cut results after a few exercises. By looking at the relationships symbolized in the diagram the patient was able to name them and thus to construct a whole, though still agrammatical, sentence. He was unable to construct such statements in absence of external aids. If the diagram was removed immediately after he completed a statement, he was unable to repeat it.

Thus, it is clear that at this stage retraining the external schemata of statements played a decisive role.

Gradually the external schemata underwent certain changes, so that the patient was able to use them in more generalized forms. It became quite easy for him to use the general sentence pattern involving subject, verb and direct object (Figure 98). By carefully adhering to this pattern he gradually developed the ability to construct similar sentences. At first it was necessary to reinforce this activity by presenting appropriate pictures. Soon, however, he was able to fill in the blanks by referring to a mental image of the relationships between objects.

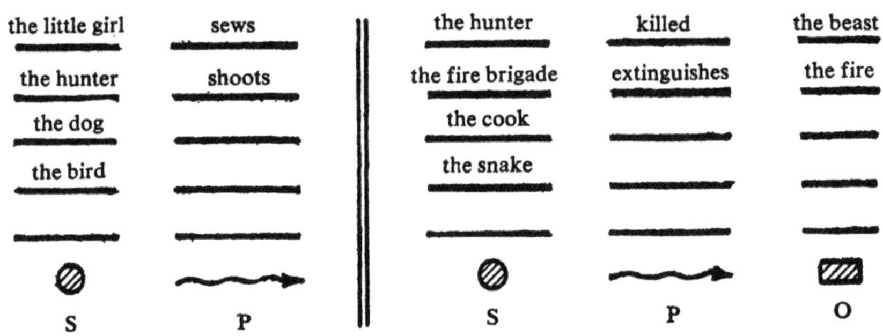

FIG. 98. Generalized diagrams for constructing sentences.

At this stage it became possible for the patient to construct statements of two or three words, but the sentences themselves were agrammatical. The next problem was to provide an external aid for recognizing and using the distinctive characteristics of words with different grammatical significance, Again, the simple repetition of grammatical sentences was of no help. The patient sensed no error whatever in the two or three word agrammatical statements which he was able to construct. If he attempted to reproduce a longer sentence, he often omitted connective elements such as prepositions and conjunctions, and he tended to alter inflected endings at random. He could make such a statement as, "The birds sing . . . the forest" with no sense of error and no attempt at self-correction. It became obvious that we must find some way of representing the grammatical features of inner schemata of sentences in an external form.

We began by working with prepositions. At this stage the patient did not use prepositions; he usually omitted them when reproducing sentences presented to him. The reason for this became clear when we presented sentences with a blank for the appropriate preposition, e.g., "the birds sing ——— the forest". In this particular case he substituted several different prepositions in turn: "The birds sing on the forest . . . in the forest . . . out of the forest . . . about the forest . . ." etc. He was able to insert various prepositions, but he had no feeling for their relative appropriateness. He was provided diagrams symbolizing the meanings of the different prepositions (Figure 99); since he had no difficulty in grasping spatial relationships, this type of diagram was very useful to him. He had a distinct concept of the relationship to be expressed. Thus, with a little practice he could refer to the diagram and construct sentences in which the dynamic relationships were expressed by prepositions. At first he had to refer to the diagram quite frequently, but gradually the intermediate process became more automatic and he was able to dispense with external aids altogether.

Once he was able to use prepositions, we began to work on the inflective aspects of

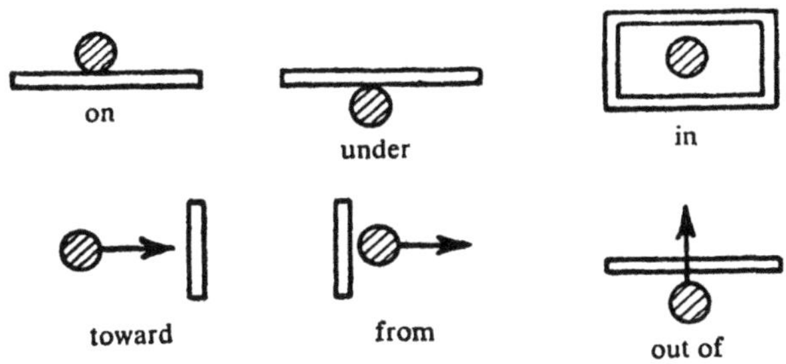

FIG. 99. Diagrams representing the meanings of prepositions.

words. This turned out to be much more difficult than restoring the use of prepositions, for it was impossible to use visual diagrams. The meanings of inflective changes are not generally adaptable to diagrammatic representation. The basic method of restoring the "feeling" for inflective relationships had to involve grammatical analysis of gender, number, and case (when working with nouns and adjectives) or of person and tense (when working with verbs). The patient was given a notebook with examples of how the different cases are formed and how they are used. In order to learn the instrumental case, for instance, he memorized that the endings "-em" or "-om" on a noun imply the question, "By whom?" or "using what?" Next he performed exercises in which he analyzed grammatical constructions involving nouns with instrumental case endings. Each time he saw the suffix "-em" or "-om" he asked himself the questions, "By whom?" or "using what?" Finally, he learned to fill in the blanks in sentences of the type, "A woodcutter chops wood (with what? . . .)" Whereas before he might have written simply, "topor" (axe), he now wrote, "topor*om*" (using an axe).

A long period of practice in recognizing the questions implied by case endings and in using them himself was required before he became able to evaluate different phraseological constructions. After that, he continued to analyze grammatical constructions by a set of intermediate steps. The work was greatly encumbered by the limited degree to which he was able to transfer from one grammatical situation to another. Mastering the instrumental endings "-em" and "-om" which are appropriate to masculine nouns, did not help him to recognize situations calling for the feminine instrumental case ending, "-oj". The work on sentence structure was continued for a long time; the desired results gradually appeared, and eventually he was able to make use of a certain number of the more common grammatical constructions.

The above was a typical case in which speech therapy is directed toward the restoration of grammatical speech. The central problem was to restore the use of predicative statements to a patient who only used words in the nominative case. He was presented a means of substituting external patterns for the inner dynamic schemata of sentences which he lacked. At first he learned to use elementary diagrams specifying only the number of words to be used in a given sentence. Then the diagrams were made more complicated in order to fix the concrete relationships between different words and to help in analyzing their grammatical forms. Further methods were employed to create a feel for the predicative structure of sentences. For instance, the patient was forbidden to begin a two word statement with a noun; thus he was forced to use a construction involving a verb. Gradually the sentences were made more complex. An important aid in this respect was the use of exercises requiring him to supply the missing words in ready-made sentences, or to construct sentences from disordered groups of words using grammatical diagrams. In every exercise, the basic principle was to substitute an external aid for the missing internal schemata and to practice using each aid until it became essentially automatic. By this method it was possible to restore the patient's grammatical speech.

G. THE RESTORATION OF ACTIVE THOUGHT PROCESSES

This is one of the most interesting retraining problems which arises in cases of brain injury. An injury involving the frontal area just anterior to the speech zone usually gives rise to certain changes in active speech. The grammatical structure of speech is relatively well preserved in such a case, but the patient notes that he is unable to initiate a spontaneous narrative. He complains that his thoughts have come to a halt, that he is unable to formulate any particular intention which would help him to generate active speech, and that, while he has no difficulty whatever in comprehending written and spoken material, he is completely lost when confronted with the necessity of thinking productivity.[13]

In order to treat a case of this type the investigator must develop methods of restoring the dynamics of spontaneous thought. The techniques described in the previous section and designed to re-establish grammatical speech give some indication as to how one might approach this complex task. If we were able to teach a patient to go beyond nominative speech by relying on external schemata to aid in the active constructions of sentences, we should be able to apply the same method to encourage the formulation of thoughts and restore the "free flow" of active thought. A psychological analysis of the origin of active thought processes suggests that this problem is by no means unsolvable. Active spontaneous thought is not a primary characteristic of the human mind. The creation of an intension, its expansion into an inner schema for further expression, and its transformation into grammatical speech is a product of long development. This development is closely related to the development of behavior patterns during childhood. It depends upon the child's communication with adults and the mastery of complex grammatical speech. The first factor is responsible for the emergence of problems without which thoughts cannot arise; the second, gives the child a pattern of dialogue which becomes transformed from a means of communication to a means of thought. With final mastery of the grammatical structure of the language, thought processes are executed smoothly and automatically without detectable intermediate mechanisms.[14]

[13] For a more complete description of this syndrome see the works of L. S. Cvetkova in: A. R. Luria and E. D. Homskaja (eds.), *Frontal Lobes and Regulation of Psychological Processes* (Moscow, University Press, 1966 [Russian]) and A. R. Luria and L. S. Cvetkova, *Neuropsychological Analysis of Problem Solving* (Moscow, "Prosvesčenie", 1966 [Russian]) (The French edition: *Troubles de solution des problèmes neuropsychologiques*, Paris, 1968).

The contribution of these factors to what would appear to be the "unitary spontaneity" of thought makes possible several approaches to the restoration of this aspect of intellectual activity. One approach is to substitute a series of external stimuli to elicit successive steps in thought patterns whose inner dynamic schemata have been disrupted. The patient can learn to apply the stimuli which are initially presented by the therapist. Once he can respond to and communicate with other people, corresponding processes can be transformed into inner mental activity. In other words, through the use of special retraining techniques we can give the patient the means whereby he can carry through continuous thought processes. In a sense, these means may be thought of as a "dynamic prostheses". Many studies have demonstrated that such reorganization of mental activity is possible and that the systems which result can compensate for the impaired *dynamics* of mental processes, just as in other cases the reorganization of speech activity compensates for speech defects. The following is a case which illustrates how this type of retraining is carried out.

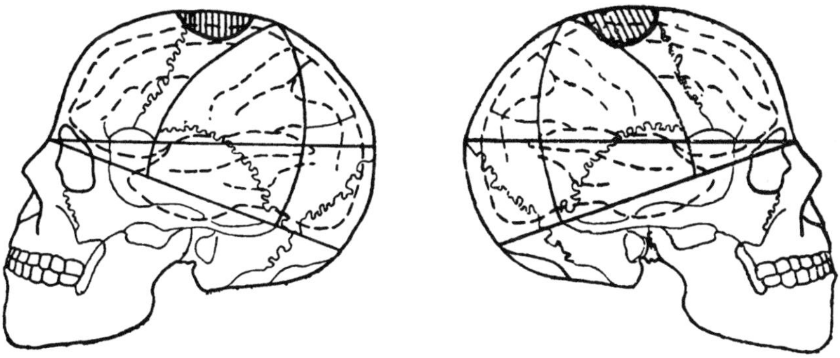

Patient Čern.: Injury diagram.

In early 1943, Lieutenant Čern., 34 years of age, came under our observation as a result of a nonpenetrating parasagittal injury of the premotor area. There was a comminuted fracture of the skull and the inner plate separated from the outer plate to damage the underlying premotor cortex (see injury diagram). There was no severe neurological deficit, i.e., no paresis or sensory loss, and no pathological reflexes. There was, however, a loss of skilled movements and impairment of smooth narrative speech. The patient was able to answer questions, name objects, and explain the contents of a simple picture, but he was totally unable to initiate a spontaneous conversation or narrative. Whenever he attempted to relate any information spontaneously he was unable to do so; "There's no continuity to my speech or to my thoughts . . . there's some kind of block; the words disappear; I don't know where to begin . . . where to go . . . there's some kind of block – and I have to be quiet . . . Sometimes a word which you should say comes out first – and then you just don't know what to do . . . you get embarrased . . . you say a word, or it pops out, but then there's nothing after it – why is it? – I don't know; nothing

[14] The development of intellectual processes has recently been investigated by P. Ja. Gal'perin and his coworkers (P. Ja. Gal'perin, 1956, 1957).

holds together. I used to be able to give whole speeches, but now I can't even say a simple sentence . . ."

These complaints reveal the basic defects of active thought. The patient is unable to formulate an intention on the basis of which to elaborate the schema of a statement. His active thought does not crystallize into a pattern; it does not follow a consistent course. His speech is limited to the enumeration of disordered details. The patient can describe a simple series of pictures and is able to put together a story relating them to one another, but if the pictures are removed before he tells his story, he loses it. In order to tell the story without the picture he must rely upon some kind of inner schema, and the schema is lacking. The absence of an inner plan and the inability to synthesize details according to a spontaneously developing theme make the task impossible.

The only way such a task can be fulfilled is by means of a dialogue, i.e., by the substitution of a series of questions and answers for spontaneous narrative. The fact that this can be done indicates that the disorders is not basically a *memory* defect; it is *dynamic* in character. Taking this into account several methods have been designed to compensate for such defects. In the present case, two types of methods were used. The patient had difficulty in relating thoughts in a connected manner, because, while he could describe a single concrete event, he was unable to associate it with subsequent events to produce a continuous narrative. It was apparent that if he could be provided with a "transitional construction", it would be much easier for him to speak narratively. With this in mind we gave him a sheet of paper on which were printed various words and phrases which might serve as a stimulus for beginning a narrative and other constructions which would aid in the narrative transition from one event to another. This list of "opening and transitional" constructions included such words and phrases as, "however . . .", "when . . .", "while . . .", "after that . . .", "he did not succeed, for . . .", etc. The patient kep this list before him, and when he lost the train of thought he could look at it, select one of the constructions, and continue his account. This "dynamic thought prothesis" helped him considerably. Whereas he had been unable to repeat a simple story on his own, he became capable of reproducing relatively complex narratives. For instance, at first he refused to try to tell Tolstoj's story "The Bear in the Carriage" saying "I remember it all, but I don't know where to begin . . . just the bear is all I can say . . ." Using the list of prepared expressions, he was able to relate one of Tolstoj's simpler stories, "Mad Dog", as follows: (transitional phrases taken from the list are italicized):

"*Once upon a time* there was a rich man who bought a small puppy . . . and *when* the dog grew up, the man took him hunting . . . *one time* a mad dog appeared as though out of nowhere; while there were children playing in the garden . . . the man saw the dog and shouted. The children heard him and began to run toward the rabid dog . . . *at that moment* the young hunting dog attacked, and the two animals fought . . .", etc.

Prepared phrases of this sort can substitute for the questions which would otherwise be necessary to evoke successive statements. At first they were looked upon altogether as external aids or stimuli capable of initiating further statements, but gradually they became a part of the patient's internal repertoire. A number of the expressions were internalized and the patient began to add new phrases himself. The use of "dynamic protheses" provided him with a system of grammatical aids whereby he could make the transitions necessary for the smooth expression of his thoughts. They remained formal in nature, however; he was unable to create an overall, meaningful plan for dealing spontaneously with a whole new topic at once. The formulation of such plans was an extremely difficult problem. Whereas he was able to generate plans for telling short anecdotes, he had difficulty with long stories involving numerous details, and he had even greater difficulty in relating spontaneous thoughts. He was overwhelmed by a mass of confused thought fragments, for he had no feel for their sequential order or order of importance. "I see one part of it, and then another and then a third, but there is no definite pattern or plan to it."

No matter how he tried, the patient was unable to develop the inner plan necessary for narrating a story. In order to help him overcome this defect, the therapist showed him how to break down the formulation of the plan into two steps. The first step consisted in writing down all the component statements in the story without regard to their order; the second was to organize the externalized components into a single plan. It was hoped that in this way he might avoid the difficulties associated with anticipatory impulses and create external conditions whereby the order of thoughts could be restored.

A rather long story was read to him and he was asked to write down on separate cards all of the events in the order in which he recalled them. Having recovered the individual episodes he was allowed to rearrange the cards in correct sequence. Once this was accomplished he had no difficulty in relating the contents of a story by referring to the cards on the table before him.

We shall present only one of many possible examples to demonstrate the effectiveness of reorganizing the narrative process in this way. The patient was read Tolstoj's story "How a Thief Betrayed Himself". When asked to repeat the story directly, he failed, saying, "It all runs together; I can't pick out the main thoughts; for me it's all mixed up . . . first I recall one fact and then another, but I don't know where to begin". Next he was instructed to write down the fragments of the story as he recalled them without regard to their correct order. Once this was done, he was to rearrange the written statements and write his account according to the resulting outline. The patient wrote down the individual episodes (left column) and then rearranged them in the correct order (right column).

Order in Which Plan First Composed

1. He gave himself away by sneezing.
2. Once a thief wanted to rob a merchant's garret.
3. They did not find anyone in the garret.
4. The merchant told the servant that someone had been in the garret.
5. The thief hid in a tobacco bin.

Final Plan

I. Once a thief wanted to rob a merchant's garret.
II. The thief hid in a tobacco bin.
III. The merchant told the servant that someone had been in the garret.
IV. He gave himself away by sneezing.

He was able to tell the story using this method. "Before, all five statements were mixed up; they got in the way of each other, and you didn't know which to throw out and which to keep; but now I think about only one statement at a time, and it goes easily."

The mastery of narrative speech using this "index card plan" not only helped the patient to reproduce the contents of a story read to him but also was a big step towards the recovery of *spontaneous narrative speech*. We asked him to write a description of his experiences from the time of his injury. He wrote three lines and then indicated that he could not go on because he was unable to analyze the mass of minor events which occurred to him whenever he started to write anything down. When it was suggested that he used the method described above he was able to write down the following plan in less than an hour. (The Arabic numerals represent the sequence in which he wrote; the Roman numerals in parentheses indicate the order of statements in the final plan):

1. How I came to the rehabilitation hospital and how I was admitted here. (IX)
2. Leaving City R., I did not know where I was going. I was in the medical car on the train. (VIII)
3. How I arrived in City R. and stayed in the hospital there. (VII)
4. How I started to work with the professor and used different methods. (XIV)
5. How I travelled on a medical train from City V. to City R. (VI)
6. How I was on an operating table in City V. (IV)
7. How I felt in the rehabilitation hospital and what I was able to understand. (X)
8. How they took me from the airport at City V. (III)
9. How they began my treatment at the rehabilitation hospital. (XI)
10. How they took me to the first aid station and what I remembered. (II)
11. How I met the professor with some kind of apparatus and didn't know what it was for. (XIII)
12. The day I was wounded, December 11, and what I remember about it. (I)
13. How I tried to write a letter in Moscow and was unable to. (XII)
14. How I felt after the operation and what I thought. (V)

On the basis of this plan he was able to write a six page description of the history of his illness. The following is taken from his written account:

The Story of my Injury. On December 11, 1942, I was in the front lines. It had been cloudy all morning; it was snowing and there was a slight wind blowing. At that time I was at the command post; with me there was an old political instructor and several soldiers. There was some artillery fire overhead. The soldiers began to ask me whether or not we would soon open fire on the enemy. I answered that it was not time yet. An hour later the command came to open fire. At that time the soldiers were in good spirits; there had been no losses. I could tell from where our shells were falling right over the heads of the enemy.

At sixteen hours I was badly wounded in the head. I remember the words of the old political instructor. He said that the commander had been killed. But I could not tell him that I was alive. At the same time I thought, "How easy it is to die . . ."; I did not remember anything else.

How they got me to the hospital I cannot remember. I remember how they took me to the plane. This was at the airport in City V.; at first I didn't know why they had brought me to City V. but then I found out that the surgical hospital was in that city, and they operated on me. When I entered that hospital the surgeon on duty came to me. He said that the operation would be that evening. That was December 13, 1942. Evening came. The orderlies took me into the operating room and laid me on the table. It was hard for me to lie there, but I only asked whether or not the operation would be over soon. They told me, "Be patient for a little longer". This I, of course, took the wrong way . . . (in Russian the verb "to be patient" also means "to suffer". *Trans.*)

These opening paragraphs show the completeness and continuity with which the patient was able to narrate a series of experiences even though the inner schemata were severely disrupted. This method of externalizing ones thoughts is normally used by writers in organizing long manuscripts. For this patient it became the sole means of formulating a chronological account of familiar experiences. The method underwent certain changes with time as the externalization process became shorter. Even so, it did not become totally automatic during the long period of time in which the patient remained under our observation. He never reverted entirely to the formulation of inner schemata. For a long time after he was released from the hospital and began to work he caried a notebook in which he could jot down a sequence of statements which he could not plan spontaneously.

This example of retraining shows that is is possible to compensate to a certain extent for defects in the dynamics of intellectual processes. As in other cases, the principle underlying the reorganization of function lies in the externalization of a process which has been disrupted. It is broken down into several steps, each of which is performed with the use of external aids. Fundamental changes in the way higher mental processes are generated, and the basis for successful techniques used in the restoration of dynamic psychological processes.[15]

CONCLUSIONS

This concludes our analysis of the methods used in restoring the different aspects of speech activity disturbed by brain trauma. We have shown that in some, though by no means all, cases the function disturbed may be restored in its original form. This may occur either when the injury has given rise to a temporary functional block, in which case recovery follows disinhibition of a functional system, or when the contralateral cortical zone is capable of assuming the function of the damaged area. The latter may ocur with left hemispheric lesions in patients who are slight or latent left-handers.

In the great majority of cases the recovery of disturbed functional systems can be achieved only by a major reorganization of speech processes. It is largely the potential for such functional reorganization that is responsible for the great reputation for "plasticity" possessed by the human brain. The reorganization of functional systems usually involves the incorporation of new afferentation or profound functional reorganization of the overall system. The latter usually involves a semantic reorganization which alters the psychological character of the process and permits the patient to carry out an old process in a new way. Such changes in the way psychological processes are mediated depend upon external aids to create intermediate schemata by means of which the person can carry out the processes consciously and thus compensate for his defect.

The results of functional reorganization which we have described rarely become highly automatic or unconscious. Automaticity is recovered only with the reorganization of purely sensory or purely motor acts, e.g., the reorganization of the visual field with the emergence of "functional maculae" in cases of hemianopsia or the automatic shift to extrapyramidal control of movement in cases of cortical paresis. Usually the reorganization of psychological processes is consciously directed and initially requires the aid of a speech therapist who can prescribe a strict retraining

[15] The detailed technique of the restoration of active thought processes in local brain lesions is elaborated by L. S. Cvetkova. Cf. A. R. Luria, *et al.*, "Restoration of Higher Cortical Functions after Local Brain Lesions" in: de Bruyn and Vinken, *Handbook of Clinical Neurology* (Amsterdam, North Holland Publishing Co. [in print], and L. S. Cvetkova, *Methods of Restoration of Higher Cortical Functions after Local Brain Lesions* (in press).

program. The retraining must be based upon precise knowledge of the nature of the defect and must be directed toward compensation for that defect. The techniques are sometimes directed toward aspects of psychological processes which at first glance, appear to be far removed from the disorder at hand, for in many cases just such factors as these give rise to the major components of the aphasic syndrome. In order to formulate an effective retraining program it is essential that the therapist first performs a painstaking psychological analysis of the inner structure of the defect.

A rehabilitation program grounded in knowledge of the nature of the disturbed function is based largely upon the normal course of development of the function. Auxiliary techniques are often employed which are modifications of the ways in which such functions are normally executed. Never, however, does the retraining of a patient with traumatic aphasia repeat exactly the normal course of development. Usually new processes which previously had no relationship to the disturbed functional system play the major role in reorganization. Sometimes the original function must be broken down into several steps which can be externalized and the psychological process it represents mastered in a new way. This type of retraining rarely culminates in complete automatization of the reorganized function and never results in a function which is identical to that which was lost. A consciously directed, systematic course of retraining is the only method of compensating for a defect arising from primary brain damage. By reorganizing the disturbed function it is possible to restore activities which once appeared hopelessly lost.

BIBLIOGRAPHY

Adrian, E. D., "Afferent areas in the brain of ungulates", *Brain*, vol. 66 (1943), p. 2, LXI.

Ajuriaguerra, J. de, *Langage, geste, attitude motrice* (Cours Internat. de Phonologie et de Phoniatrie, Faculté de médecine de Paris) (Paris, Librairie Malaine, 1953).

—, "Langage et dominance cérébrale", *Journal Français d'Oto-Rhino-Laryngologie*, VI (1957), 3.

Ajuriaguerra, J. de, et Hécaen, H., *Le cortex cérébral*, 2nd ed. (Paris, Masson, 1960).

Alajouanine, Th., "Verbal reaction in Aphasia", *Brain*, 79 (1956), p. 1.

—, et Mozziconacci, P., *L'aphasie et désintégration fonctionnelle du langage* (Paris, 1947).

—, Ombredane, A., et Durand, M., *Le syndrome de désintégration phonétique* (Paris, 1939).

Anan'ev, B. G., "Vosstanovlenie pis'ma i čtenija pri agrafii i aleksii" [The restoration of reading and writing in agraphia and alexia], *Učenye zapiski Moskovskogo Gosud. Universiteta*, III (1947).

Anoxin, P. K., *Problemy centra i periferii v fiziologii nervnoj dejatel'nosti* [Problems of Center and Periphery in the Physiology of Higher Neural Activity] (Gor'kij, 1935).

—, "Problema lokalizacii s točki zrenija sistemnyx predstavlenij o nervnyx funkcijax" [The problem of localization in view of systemic conceptions of neural functions], *Nevropatologija i psixiatrija*, 6 (1940).

—, (ed.), *Problemy vysšej nervnoj dejatel'nosti* [Problems of Higher Neural Activity] (Moscow, Izd-vo Akademii medic. nauk SSSR, 1949).

—, "Novye dannye ob osobennostjax afferentnogo apparata uslovnogo refleksa" [New data regarding the characteristics of the afferent apparatus of the conditioned reflex], *Voprosy psixologii*, 6 (1956).

—, *Vnutrennee tormoženie kak problema fiziologii* [Internal Inhibition as a Problem of Physiology] (Moscow, Gosud. Izd-vo medic. literatury, 1958).

Asrat'jan, È. A., "Kora bol'šogo mozga i plastičnost' nervnoj sistemy" [The cerebral cortex and the plasticity of the nervous system], *Uspexi sovr. biol.*, 1936, 1937.

—, *Fiziologija central'noj nervnoj sistemy* [The Physiology of the Central Nervous System] (Moscow, Izdanie Akademii med. nauk SSSR, 1953).

Astvazaturov, V. W., *Kliničeskie i èksperimental'no – psixologičeskie issledovanija rečevoj funkcii* [Clinical and Experimental Psychological Investigations of Speech Functions], Dissertation (1908).

Babenkova, S. V., "K voprosu ob osobennostjax vzaimodejstvija signal'nyx sistem v processe vosstanovlenija reči pri raznyx formax afazii" [Some characteristics of the interaction of the signal systems during the restoration of speech with different forms of aphasia], *Tezisy VII sessii Instituta Nevrologii Akademii medic. nauk SSSR*, 1954.

Baudouin de Courtenay, J., "Otryvki iz lekcij po fonetike i morfologii" [Selections from lectures on phonetics and morphology], *Akad. ped. nauk RSFSR*, 2.

—, *Ob otnošenii russkogo pis'ma k russkomy jazyku* [On the Relationship of Russian Writing to the Russian Language] (SPB, 1912).

Bay, E., "Untersuchungen zum Aphasieproblem", *Der Nervenartzt*, 28 (1957).

—, "Theorie und Empirie bei der Klassifikation und der Untersuchungsmethoden der Aphasischen Störungen", *Psychiatrie und Neurologie*, Bd. 137 (Basel, 1957).

—, "Die Corticale Dysartrie und ihre Beziehung zur sogenannten motorischen Aphasie", *Deutsche Zeitschrift für Nervenheilkunde*, Bd. 176 (1957), pp. 553-559.

Beck, E., "Das Hörzentrum des Schimpansen", *Journal für Psychologie und Neurologie*, 36 (1928).

—, "Die myeloarchitektonische Felderung des menschlichen Schläferlappens", *Journal für Psychologie und Neurologie*, 36 (1929).

Bejn, È. S., *Psixologičeskij analiz visočnoj afazii (O narušenii myšlenija i reči visočnoj afazii)* [Psychological Analysis of Temporal Aphasia (Concerning the Disturbances of Thought and Speech in Temporal Aphasia)], Dissertation (1947).

—, "Vosstanovlenie rečevyx processov pri senzornoj afazii" [The restoration of speech processes in sensory aphasia], *Učenye zapiski Moskovskogo Gosud. Universiteta*, III (1947).

—, "Osnovnye zakony struktury slova i grammatičeskogo stroenija reči pri afazijax" [Basic laws of word structure and the grammatical structure of speech in aphasias], *Voprosy psixologii*, 4 (1957).

—, *Afazija i ee preodolenije* [Aphasia and its therapy], Medicina (Moscow, Leningrad, 1964).

Bernštejn, N. A., "Problema vzaimootnošenija koordinacii i lokalizacii" [Problems of the interrelationship between coordination and localization], *Arxiv biologičeskix nauk*, XXXVIII (1935).

—, "K voprosu o prirode i dinamike koordinacionnoj funkcii" [The nature and dynamics of the coordinated function], *Učenye zapiski kafedry psixologii MGU*, 90 (1945).

—, *O postroenii dviženij* [The Structure of Movement] (Moscow, Medgiz, 1947).

—, "Nekotorye nazrevajuščie problemy reguljacii dvigatel'nyx aktov" [Certain pressing questions regarding the regulation of motor acts], *Voprosy psixologii*, VI (1957).

Bethe, A., und Fischer, E., "Die Anpassungsfähigkeit (Plastizität des Nervensystems)", Handbuch der norm. und pathol. Physiologie, 15/2 (1931).

Bianchi, L., *The mechanisms of the brain and the functions of the frontal lobes* (Edinburgh, 1922).

Birch, H. G., and Lee, J., "Cortical inhibition in expressive aphasia", *Archives Neurol. Psychiatry*, vol. 75 (1955), p. 5.

Blinkov, S. M., *Variabil'nost' citoarxitektoničeskix polej visočnoj oblasti* [Variability in the Cytoarchitectonic Fields of the Temporal Area], Dissertation (1940).

—, "Materialy po voprosam lečebno-pedagogičeskoj raboty po vosstanovleniju ustnoj reči i pis'ma pri motornyx afazijax" [Materials having to do with questions of therapeutic-pedagogic work in the recovery of oral speech and writing in motor aphasias], *Izvestija Akad. ped. nauk RSFSR*, 2 (1946).

—, *Osobennosti stroenija bol'šogo mozga čeloveka* [Structural Characteristics of the Human Brain] (Moscow, Medgiz, 1955).

Bogorodickij, V. A., *Kurs grammatiki russkogo jazyka. Č. I. Fonetika* [A Course in the Grammar of the Russian Language. Part 1: Phonetics] (1887).

—, *Obščij kurs russkoj grammatiki* [A General Course in Russian Grammar] (Moscow, Socekgiz, 1935).

Bolton, J. Sh., The cortical localisation of cerebral functions (*The Henderson trust lecture*, XII) (Edinburgh, O'liver & Boyd, 1933).

Bonhoeffer, K., "Zur Klinik und Lokalisation des Agrammatismus und der Rechts-Links-Desorientierung", *Mschr. für Psychologie und Neurologie*, 34 (1923).

Bonvicini, G., "Die Störungen der Lautsprache bei Temporallappenläsionen", *Marburg's Handbuch der Neurologie des Ohres*, II, 2 (Wien, 1929).

Boskis, R. M., "Osobennosti rečevogo razvitija u detej pri narušenii sluxovogo analizatora" [Characteristics of speech development in children with disturbance of the auditory analyzer], *Izvestija Akademii pedagogičeskix nauk RSFSR*, vyp. 78 (1953).

Boskis, R. M., and Levina, R. E., "Ob odnoj iz form akustičeskoj agnozii" [On one form of acoustic agnosia], *Nevropatologija i psixiatrija*, 4 (1936).

—, "K probleme ovladenija fonetičeskoj storonoj reči v detskom vozraste" [The problem of mastering the phonetic structure of speech in childhood], *Nevropatologia i psixiatrija*, 6 (1938).

Brain, R., "Visual object-agnosia with special relation to the Gestalt-theory", *Brain*, vol. 64 (1941), p. 1.
—, "Visual desorientation with special reference to the lesions of the right cerebral hemisphaere", *Brain*, vol. 64 (1941), p. 4.
—, *Speech Disorders* (London, Butterworth).
Brickner, R. M., *The Intellectual functions of the Frontal Lobes* (New York, Macmillan, 1936).
—, "A human cortical area producing repetitive phenomena when stimulated", *Journ. Neurophys.*, 3 (1940), pp. 128-130.
Broadbent, D. E., *Perception and Communication* (London, Pergamon Press, 1958).
Brodman, K., *Vergleichende Lokalisationslehre der Grosshirnrinde* (Leipzig, Barth, 1925).
Bruner, J., "On perceptual readiness", *Psychological Review*, vol. 64 (1957), No. 2.
—, Goodnow, J., and Austin, G., *A study of thinking* (New York, J. Wiley, 1957).
Bubnova, V. K., *Narušenie ponimanija grammatičeskix konstrukcij pri mozgovyx poraženijax i ego vosstanovlenie v processe obučenija* [Disturbance of the Comprehension of Grammatical Constructions with Brain Lesions and Recovery in the Process of Retraining], Dissertation (1946).
Bucy, P. (ed.), *The precentral motor cortex* (Chicago, Univ. of Illinois Press, 1944).
Bühler, K., Über das Sprachverständnis vom Standpunkt der Normalpsychologie", in *Berichte des III. Kongresses für exper. Psychologie* (Leipzig, Barth, 1909).
—, *Sprachtheorie* (Jena, Fischer, 1934).
Buscaino, V. M., *Neurobiologia delle Percezioni* (Napoli, 1946).
Buslaev, V. F., *Istoričeskaja grammatika russkogo jazyka* [An Historical Grammar of the Russian Language] (Third Edition, 1868-1869).
Campbell, A. W., *Histological studies on the localisation of cerebral functions* (Cambridge, 1905).
Cassirer, E., *Philosophie der sympolischen Formen*, I-III (1923, 1929).
—, "Le langage et le monde des objects", *Journal de Psychologie*, 30 (1933).
Conrad, K., "Versuch einer psychologischen Analyse des Parietalsyndroms", *Mschr. für Psychologie und Neurologie*, 84 (1932).
—, "New problems of Aphasia", *Brain*, vol. 74 (1956), p. 4.
—, "Aphasie, Agnosie, Apraxie", *Fortschritte der Neurologie*, Nr. 19 (1957).
Critchley, M., *The Parietal Lobes* (London, Arnold, 1953).
—, "Articulatory Defect in Aphasia", *Journal of Laryngology and Othology*, vol. 66, 1 (1952).
Cvetkova, L. S., "Metody vosstanovlenija vysšix korkovyx funkcij posle lokalnix poraženijax mozga" [Methods of Restoration of Higher Cortical Functions after Local Brain Lesions] (in press).
Dandy, W. E., "The effects of the total removal of the left temporal lobe in a right-handed individual", *Journal of nervous mental disasters*, 74 (1931).
Davidenkov, S. N., *Materialy k učeniju ob afazii* [Material for the Study of Aphasia] (Kharkov, 1915).
Dusser de Barennes, J. G., "Experimental researches on sensory localisations in cerebral cortex", *Quarterly Journal of Experimental Physiology*, 9 (1916).
—, "Sensory-motor cortex and Thalamus", *American Journal Psysiology*, 9 (1937).
—, and McCulloch, W. S., "Suppression of motor response obtained from area 4 by stimulation of area 4 s.", *Journal of Neurophysiology*, vol. 4 (1941).
Economo, C., und Koskinas, G. N., *Die Cytoarchitektonik der Hirnrinde des erwachsenen Menschen* (Wien, Springer, 1925).
Ejdinova, M. B., and Pravdina-Vinarskaja, E. N., *Detskie cerebral'nye paraliči i puti ix preodolenija* [Cerebral Palsy in Children and Treament] (1959) (English edition: London, Pergamon Press, 1963).
Èlkonin, D. B., "Konkretnye voprosy psixologii usvoenija gramoty" [Concrete questions concerning the psychological mechanisms involved in mastering reading and writing], *Voprosy psixologii*, 5 (1956).
Ettlinger, B., Jackson, B. V., and Zangwill, O. L., "Dysphasia following right temporal lobotomy in a right-handed man", *Journal of Neurology, Neurosurgery and Psychiatry*, vol. 18 (1955).

Figurin, N. L., and Denisova, M. P., "Opyt refleksologičeskogo izučenija novoroždennogo rebënka" [An experience with the study of reflexes in the newborn child], *Novoe v refleksologii i fiziologii nervnoj sistemy* (Leningrad, 1925).

Filimonov, I. I., "O funkcional'noj mnogoznačnosti arxitektoničeskix formacij kory golovnogo mozga" [On the functional significance of the architectonic formations of the cerebral cortex], *Nevropatologija i psixiatrija*, 1 (1945).

Filippyčeva, N. A., *Inertnost' vysšix korkovyx processov pri lokal'nyx poraženijax bol'šix polušarij mozga* [The inertia of higher cortical processes with focal lesions of the cerebral cortex], Dissertation (1952).

Flechsig, K., *Anatomie des menschlichen Gehirns auf myelogenetischer Grundlage* (Leipzig, 1920).

Foerster, O., *Die Physiologie und Pathologie der Koordination* (Jena, Fischer, 1902).

——, "Restitution der Motilität und Sensibilität", *Deutsche Zeitschrift f. Nervenheilkunde*, 115 (1930).

——, "Die motorischen Felder und Bahnen", in: Bumke-Foerster, *Handbuch der Neurologie*, Bd. VI (1936), pp. 1-357.

Foix, Ch., "Aphasie", *Nouveau traité de Médecine*, t. XVIII (Paris, 1928).

Franz, Sh. I., *Nervous and mental reëducation* (New York, MacMillan, 1924).

——, "Studies in reëducation: the aphasias", *Journal of comparative psychiatry*, vol. 4 (1924).

Froeschels, E., "Zur Behandlung der motorischen Apraxie", *Archiv für Psychologie*, 56 (1925).

Fulton, J. F., "Forced grasping and groping in relation to the syndrome of the premotor area", *Archives of Neurology and Psychiatry*, 31 (1934).

——, "On the function of cerebral cortex", *Journal of Michigan State Medical Society*, 1934.

——, *Physiology of the nervous system*, 2nd ed. (Oxford, 1943).

Gal'perin, P. Ja., "O formirovanii čuvstvennyx obrazov i ponjatij" [On the formation of sensory images and concepts], *Materialy soveščanija po psixologii* (Moscow, Akad. pedag. nauk, 1956).

——, "Umstvennoe dejstvie kak osnova formirovanija mysli" [Intellectual activity as the basis for formulating thoughts and images], *Voprosy psixologii*, VI (1957).

Gal'perin, P. Ja., and Golubova, R. A., "Mexanizmy parafazij kompleksnogo tipa" [The mechanism of complex paraphasia], *Sovetskaja psixonevrologija*, 6 (1933).

Gelb, A., "Medizinische Psychologie", *Acta psychologica* (Stockholm, 1937).

——, "Remarques générales sur l'utilisation des données pathologiques pour la psychologie et la philosophie du langage", *Journal de psychologie*, volume spécial: *Psychologie du langage*, 1933.

——, und Goldstein, K., *Psychologische Analysen hirnpathologischen Fälle* (Berlin, Springer, 1920).

Gerstmann, J., "Fingeragnosie", *Klin. Wschr.*, 37 (Wien, 1924).

Geršuni, G. V., "Ob izučenii oščuščaemyx (senzornyx) i neoščuščaemyx (subsenzornyx) reakcij pri dejstvii vnešnix razdražitelej na organy čuvstv čeloveka" [On the study of sensory and subsensory reactions on the action of external stimuli on human sensory organs], *Izvestija Akad. nauk SSSR*, 2 (1945).

——, "Reflektornye reakcii pri vozdejstvii vnešnix razdražitelej" [Reflex reactions to external stimuli], *Fiziol. žurnal SSSR*, XXXV (1949), 5.

——, "Izučenie dejatel'nosti zvukovogo analizatora čeloveka na osnove ispol'zovanija raznyx reakcij" [Study of the function of the auditory analyzer of man based upon the use of different reactions], *Problemy fiziol. akustiki*, 3 (1955).

——, "Obščie rezultaty issledovanija dejatel'nosti zvukovogo analizatora čeloveka pri pomošči raznyx reakcij" [The general results of an investigation of the function of the auditory analyzer in man with the help of different reactions], *Žurnal vysšej nervnoj dejatel'nosti*, 7 (1957), 1.

——. et al., *Narušenie dejatel'nosti organov čuvstv i nekotoryx drugix nervnyx funkcij pri vozdušnoj kontuzii* [Disturbance of the Function of the Sense Organs and Certain Other Neural Functions with Blast Contusions] (Moscow, Akad. nauk SSSR, 1945).

Giljarovskij, V. A., "O lečenii isteričeskix rasstrojstv u kontužennyx" [On the treatment of hysterical disturbances in blast injured patients], *Nevropatologija i psixiatrija, XII* (1943).

—, *Starye i novye problemy psixiatrii* [Old and New Problems of Psychiatry] (Moscow, Medgiz, 1946).
Goldstein, K., "Über die Störungen der Grammatik bei Hirnkrankheiten", *Mschr. für Psychologie und Neurologie*, 34 (1913).
—, "Das Symptom, seine Entstehung etc.", *Archiv für Psychiatrie und Neurologie*, Bd. 76 (1925).
—, "Über Aphasie", *Schweiz. Archiv für Neurologie und Psychiatrie*, 19 (1926).
—, "Die Lokalisation in der Grosshirnrinde", *Bethe's Handbuch der normalen und pathologischen Physiologie*, Bd. X (1927).
—, "L'analyse de l'aphasie et l'étude de l'essence du langage", *Journal de psychologie*, volume spécial: *Psychologie du langage* (1933).
—, *Der Aufbau des Organismus* (Haag, Nijhoff, 1934).
—, *After-effects of brain injuries in war* (New York, Grune & Stratton, 1942).
—, *Language and Language Disorders* (New York, Grune & Stratton, 1948).
Goodglass, H., and Quadfasel, "Language Laterality in Left Handed Aphasics", *Brain*, vol. 77 (1954).
Granit, R., *Receptors and Sensory Perception* (New Haven, 1956).
Graščenkov, N. I., "O probleme funkcional'noj asinapsii" [On the problem of functional asynapsia], *Nevropatologija i psixiatrija*, VII (1946).
—, *Čerepno-mozgovye ranenija i metody ix lečenija* [Skull-brain Injuries and Methods of Treatment] (Moscow, Gosud. Izd. medic. literatury, 1947).
—, (ed.), *Nevrologija voennogo vremeni* [Neurology in Wartime] (Moscow, Izd. Akad. medic. nauk, 1948).
—, and Luria, A. R., "O sistemnom principe lokalizacii funkcii v kore golovnogo mozga" [On the systemic principle of the localization of function in the cerebral cortex], *Nevropatologija i psixiatrija*, I (1945).
Grünbaum, A. S. T., and Sherrington, C. S., "Observations on the physiology of the cerebral cortex of some of the higher apes", *Proceedings Royal Society*, vol. 69 (1901).
Gurevič, M. O., *Psixomotorika* [Psychomotor Functions] (Moscow, Gosizdat, 1928).
—, "K teorii lokalizacii psixičeskix rasstrojstv" [On a theory of the localization of mental disturbances], *Nevropatologija i psixiatrija*, 1 (1935).
Gurianov, E. V., *Razvitie navyka pis'ma u škol'nika* [The Development of Writing Habits in School-Children] (Moscow, Učebno-pedagog. Izdvo, 1940).
—, "Navyki i dejstvija" [Habits and Actions], *Učenye zapiski Mosk. Universiteta*, 90 (1945).
Gurova, E. V., "Rol' levšestva v semiotike mozgovyx poraženij" [The role of left-handedness in the diagnosis of brain-lesions], *Trudy Instituta Nevrologii Akad. med. nauk SSSR*, 1947.
Hartmann, F., "Beiträge zur Aphasie", *Mschr. Psychiatrie und Neurologie*, XXI (1907).
Head, H., *Aphasia and kindred disorders of speech*, I-II (Cambridge, 1926).
Hécaen, H., David, M., Van Reeth, P., and Clément, J., "Über parietale Tumoren", *Wiener Zeitschrift für Nerven Heilkunde*, VIII, 1-2.
—, Dell, M. B., and Roger, A., "L'aphasie de conduction", *L'encéphale*, 2 (1955).
—, and Piercy, H., "Paroxismal Dysphasia and Problem of Cerebral Dominance", *Journal of Neurology, Neurosurgery, Psychiatry*, vol. 19 (1956).
Hécaen, H., and Angelergues, R., *Pathologie du Langage* (Paris, Librairie Larousse).
Henschen, S. E., "Über die Hörsphäre", *Journal für Psychologie und Neurologie*, 22 (1917).
—, *Klinische und anatomische Beiträge zur Pathologie des Gehirns* (Stockholm, 1920-1922).
—, "Aphasiesysteme", *Mschr. für Psychiatrie und Neurologie*, 65 (1927).
Hermann, H., und Pötze, O., *Über die Agraphie* (Berlin, 1927).
Holmes, G., "Disturbances of vision by cerebral Lesions", *British Journal of Ophtalm.*, 1 (1928).
—, "Cerebral integration of ocular movement", *British Medical Journal*, 2 (1938).
—, and Horrax, G., "Disturbances in special orientation and visual attention", *Archives of Neurology and Psychiatry*, 1 (1919).
Humphrey, M. E., and Zangwill, O. L., "Dysphasia in left-handed patients with unilateral brain lesion", *Journal of Neurology, Neurosurgery and Psychiatry*, XV (1952), p. 184.
Isserlin, M., "Über Agrammatismus", *Zschr. für den ges. Neur. und Psych.*, 75 (1922).

—, "Die pathologische Physiologie der Sprache", *Ergebnisse der Physiologie*, 29 (1929), 33 (1931), 34 (1932).

Ivanova, M. P., *Narušenie vzaimodejstvija dvux signal'nyx sistem v formirovanii složnyx dvigatel'nyx reakcij pri poraženii mozga* [Disturbance of the Two Signal Systems in the Formulation of Complex Motor Reactions with Brain Damage], Dissertation (1953).

Ivanov-Smolenskij, A. G., "O vzaimodejstvie pervoj i vtoroj signal'nyx sistem pri nekotoryx fiziologičeskix i patologičeskix uslovijax" [On the interaction of the first and second signal systems under certain physiological and pathological conditions], *Fiziol. žurnal SSSR*, XXXV (1949), 5.

—, *Očerki patofiziologii vysšej nervnoj dejatel'nosti* [Notes on the Pathophysiology of Higher Neural Activity] (Moscow, Gos. izdat. med. literatury, 1949).

—, "Ob izučenii sovmestnoj raboty pervoj i vtoroj signal'nyx sistem mozgovoj kory" [On the study of the coordinated functions of the first and second systems of the cerebral cortex], *Žurnal vysšej nervnoj dejatel'nosti*, I (1951), 1.

Jackson, H., *Selected papers*, I-II (London, 1932).

Jacobson, C. F., "Function of frontal association areas in primates", *Archives Neurology and Psychiatry*, 33 (1935).

Jacobson, F., "Electrophysiology of mental activity", *American journal of Psychology*, vol. 44 (1932).

Jakobson, R., "Le développement phonologique du langage enfantine etc.", in *Ve Congrès International de Linguistes, Bruges* (1939).

—, *Kindersprache, Aphasie und allgemeine Lautgesetze* (Uppsala, Universitets Arsskrift, 1942).

—, and Halle, M., *Fundamentals of Language* (The Hague, Mouton & Co. 1956).

Jarbuss, A. L., *Rol' dviženija glaz v processe vosprijatija izobraženij* [The Role of Eye Movements in Perception of Images] (Moscow, Nauka).

Jasper, H. H., "Diffuse projective System", *Electroencephalography and clinical Neurophysiology*, no. 1 (1949).

—, and Ajmon-Marsan, C., "Thalcemocortical and integrating mechanism", *A. Kes. Nerv. Ment. Dis. Proc.*, vol. 30 (1952).

—, Ajmon-Marsan, C., and Stroll, I., "Cortico-fugal projections to the brain stem", *Archives Neurology, Psychiatry*, v. 67 (1952).

Kabeljanskaja, L. G., *Sostojanie sluxovogo analizatora pri senzornoj afazii* [The State of the Auditory Analyzer in Sensory Aphasia], Dissertation (1955).

—, "Sostojanie sluxovogo analizatora pri senzornoj afazii" [The state of the auditory analyzer in sensory aphasia], *Žurnal nevrol. i psixiatrii*, LVII (1957), 6.

—, and Viting, A. I., "K voprosu o tak naz. transkortikal'noj senzornoj afazii" [On the question of so-called transcortical sensory aphasia], *Žurnal nevropatologii i psixiatrii*, LVIII (1958), 1.

Kaufman, O. P., "Ob optičeskoj agrafii" [On optical agraphia], *Trudy Instituta nevrologii Akad. med. nauk SSSR*, 1947.

Klein, R., "Über d. Wortgestalt u. ihren Bedeutungsinhalt bei Aphasiker", *Zschr. für den ges. Neurologie und Psychiatrie*, 129 (1930).

—, "Zur Symptomatologie der Parietallappens", *Zschr. für den ges. Neurologie und Psychologie*, 135 (1931).

Kleist, K., "Über Leitungsaphasie", *Mschr. für Psychiatrie*, 17, 6 (1905).

—, "Kortikale (innervatorische) Apraxie", *Jahrbuch der Psychiatrie*, 28 (1907).

—, "Der Gang und der gegenwärtige Stand der Apraxieforschung", *Ergebnisse der Neurologie* (1911).

—, "Über Leitungsaphasie und grammatische Störungen", *Mschr. für Psychiatrie*, 40 (1916).

—, "Die Gehirnverletzung und ihre Bedeutung für die Gehirnlokalisation", *Allg. Zeitschrift für Psychiatrie*, 1918.

—, "Die psychomotorischen Störungen und ihre Verhältniss zu den Motilitätsstörungen", *Mschr. für Psychiatrie*, 52 (1922).

—, "Die alogischen Denkstörung", *Archiv für Psychiatrie*, 90 (1930).

—, *Gehirnpathologie* (Leipzig, Barth).

Kogan, V. M., "Vosstanovlenie smyslovoj storony reči pri afazii" [Restoration of the semantic aspect of speech in aphasia], *Učenye zapiski Mosk. Gos. Univers.*, III (1947).
Kogan, V. M., *Vosstanovleni Reči Pri Afazii* [Recovery of Speech in Aphasia] (Dissertation, Moscow, 1963).
Kol'cova, M. M., *O formirovanii vysšej nervnoj dejatel'nosti rebënka* [On the Formation of Higher Neural Activity of the Child] (Leningrad, Gos. Izdat. medic. literatury, 1958).
Konorski, J. M., and Miller, O. M., "Uslovnye refleksy s dvigatel'nogo analizatora" [Conditioned reflexes of the motor analyzer], *Trudy fiziol. laboratorii I. P. Pavlova*, VI (1936).
Kramer, V. V., *Učenie o lokalizacii v golovnom mozgu* [Study of Localization in the Brain] (Moscow, Gosizdat, 1928).
Krasnogorskij, N. I., *O processe soderživanija i lokalizacii kožnogo i dvigatel'nogo analizatora v kore bol'šix polušarij* [On the Process of Delay and the Localization of the Somesthetic and Motor Analyzers in the Cerebral Cortex], Dissertation (1911).
Krol', M. B., "K klinike i topičeskoj diagnostike afazičeskix i apraktičeskix rasstrojstv" [On clinics and the topological diagnosis of aphasic and apraxic disturbances], *Žurnal nevropatologii i psixiatrii im. Korsakova*, 1911.
—, *Novoe v učenii ob afazii, agnozii, apraksii* [New Findings in Aphasia, Agnosia, Apraxia] (Moscow, Gosizdat, 1934).
—, *Nevrologičeskie sindromy* [Neurological Syndromes] (Moscow, OGIZ, 1936).
Kryšova, N. A., Kok, E. P., and Smirnov, V. D., "Kliniko-fiziologičeskoe issledovanie bol'nyx s afaziej" [A clinico-physiological investigation of patients with aphasia], *Žurnal nevropatologii i psixiatrii*, LIV (1954), 12.
Kvassov, D. G., "Sobstvennyj myšečnyj apparat analizatorov" [The motor apparatus of the analyzers], *Fiziol. žurnal SSSR, XLII* (1950), 8.
—, "Reflektornaja organizacija recepcii i propriomuskuljarnyj apparat analizatorov (organov čuvstv)" [The reflex organization of reception and the propriomuscular apparatus of the analyzers (Sensory organs)], *Orientirovočnyj refleks i orientirovočno-issledovatel'skaja dejatel'nost'* (Moscow, Izd. Akad. pedag. nauk RSFSR, 1958).
Lashley, K. S., *Brain mechanisms and intelligence* (Univ. of Chicago Press, 1931).
—, "Functional determinants of cerebral localisation", *Arch. of neurology and Psychiatry*, vol. 38 (1937).
Lashley, R. S., *The Neuropsychology of Lashley* (N.Y., McGraw-Hill, 1960).
Lassek, A. M., "The human Pyramid tract", *Archives of Neurol. and Psychiatry*, vol. 42, 44, 45. *Journal Comparative Neurology*, 76, 83 etc. (1939-1948).
Lebedinskij, M. S., *Afazija, agnozija, apraksija* [Aphasia, Agnosia, Apraxia] (Kharkov, 1941).
Leonhardt, K., "Apraktische Formen vom Aphasie", *Neurol. u. Mediz. Psychologie*, Bd. 9 (Leipzig), p. 151.
Leont'ev, A. N., *Razvitie pamjati* [The Development of the Memory] (Moscow, Izd-vo Akad. komm. vosp., 1930).
—, *Problemy Razvitija Psixiki* [Problems of Mental Development] (Moscow, Acad. Pedag. nauk, 1959).
—, and Zaporožec, A., *Vosstanovlenie dviženij* [The Restoration of Movement] (Moscow, Izd-vo Sovetskaja Nauka, 1945).
Levina, R. E., *O nedostatkax čtenija i pis'ma v detskom vozraste* [Reading and Writing Defects in Childhood] (Moscow, Učpedgiz, 1933).
Lewis, M., *Infant speech* (London, 1936).
Liepmann, H., *Der Krankheitsbild der Apraxie* (Berlin, Karger, 1900).
Lorente, de Nó, "Analysis of the activities of the chains of internuncial neurones", *Journal of Neurophysiol.*, 1 (1938).
Lotmar, F., "Zur Kenntnis der erschwerten Wortfindung und ihre Bedeutung für das Denken der Aphasischen", *Schw. Arch. f. Neur. u. Psych.*, 5 (1919).
—, "Zur Pathophysiologie der erschwerten Wortfindung bei Aphasischen", *Schw. Arch. für Neurologie und Psychiatrie*, 30 (1933).
Luria, A. R., *Učenie ob afazii v svete mozgovoj patologii*, č. I: *Visočnaja (akustičeskaja) afazija*. č. II: *Temennaja (semantičeskaja) afazija* [The Study of Aphasia from the Point

of View of Brain Pathology, Part I: Temporal (acoustic) Aphasia]. Dissertation. [Part II: Parietal (semantic) Aphasia], Manuscript, 1940.

—, "Problema afazii v svete mozgovoj patologii" [The problem of aphasia in view of brain pathology], *Sbornik v česť V. P. Osipova* (Leningrad, 1941).

—, "Narušenie dviženij pri poraženii promotornyx sistem" [The disturbance of movements with damage to the premotor systems], *Učenye zapiski kafedry psixologii MGU*, 90 (1945).

—, "Narušenie ustanovki i dejstvija pri mozgovyx poraženijax" [The disturbance of set and action with brain lesions], *Trudy Instituta psixologii Akad. nauk gruzinskoj SSR*, 1945.

—, "O narušenii grammatičeskix operacij pri mozgovyx poraženijax" [On the disturbances of grammatical operations with brain lesions], *Izvestija Akad. ped. nauk RSFSR*, III (1946).

—, "O patologii čisla i sčeta" [On the pathology of computation and numbers], *Izvestija Akad. ped. nauk RSFSR*, III (1946).

—, "Vosstanovlenie funkcij mozga posle voennoj travmy" [The restoration of the brain function after war trauma] (Moscow, Izd-vo Akad. medic. nauk SSSR, 1948) (English Edition: Restoration of Function after Brain Trauma, London, Pergamon Press, 1963).

—, *Očerki psixofiziologii pis'ma* [Essays on the Psychophysiology of Writing] (Moscow, Izd-vo Akad. ped. nauk RSFSR, 1950).

—, "Osnovnye problemy kliniki očagovyx poraženij golovnogo mozga v svete idej I. P. Pavlova" [Basic clinical problems relating to focal brain lesions in the light of the theories of I. P. Pavlov], *Žurnal vysšej nervnoj dejatel'nosti*, II (1952), 5.

—, "Rol' slova v formirovanii vremennyx svjazej u čeloveka" [The role of words in the formation of temporary connections in man], *Voprosy psixologii*, 1 (1955).

—, "O regulirujuščej roli reči v formirovanii proizvol'nyx dviženij" [On the regulatory role of speech in the formation of voluntary movements], *Žurnal vysšej nervoj dejatel'nosti*, VI (1956), 5.

—, "Dvigatel'nyj analizator i problema korkovoj organizacii dviženija" [The motor analyzer and the problem of the cortical organization of movement], *Voprosy psixologii*, 2 (1957).

—, *Problemy vysšej nervnoj dejatel'nosti normal'nogo i anomal'nogo rebënka* [Problems of Higher Neural Activity in the Normal and Abnormal Child], vol. I and vol. II (Moscow, Izd-vo Akad. ped. nauk RSFSR, 1956, 1958).

—, *The Role of Speech in the Regulation of Normal and Abnormal Behavior* (London, Pergamon Press, 1961).

—, *Vysšije Korkovye Funkcii Čeloveka* [Higher Cortical Functions in Man] (Moscow University Press, 1962) (English edition: N.Y., Basic Books).

—, *Mozg Čeloveka i psixičeskie Processy* [Human Brain and Psychological Processes] (Moscow, Acad. Ped. nauk, 1963) (English edition: N.Y., Harper and Row, 1966).

—, "Factors and Forms in Aphasia" in: *Disorders of Language* (CIBA Foundation Symposium, London, 1966).

—, "Brain Disorders and Language Analysis", *Language and Speech*, I (1958).

—, and Leont'ev, A. N., "Psixofiziologičeskie problemy vosstanovlenija funkcij posle travm mozga" [Psychophysiological problems in the restoration of function after brain trauma], *Učenye zapiski MGU*, III (1947).

—, and Judovič, F. J., *Reč' i razvitie psixičeskix processov rebënka* [Speech and the Development of Mental Processes of the Child] (Moscow, Izd-vo Akad. ped. nauk RSFSR, 1956; also transl.: *Speech and the Development of Mental Processes*, London, Staples Press, 1959).

—, "Two Kinds of Motor Perseveration in Massive Injury of the Frontal Lobes", *Brain*, Vol. 88 (1965), pp. 1-10.

—, and Homskaja, E. D. (eds.), *Lobnye doli i regulacija psixičeskix processov* [Frontal Lobes and Regulation of Psychological Processes] (Moscow University Press, 1966).

—, and Cvetkova, L. S., *Nevropsixologičeskij analiz rešenija zadač* [Neuropsychological Analysis of Problem Solving] (Moscow, Prosveščenije, 1966).

—, Naidin, V. L., Vinarskaja, H. N., and Cvetkova, L. S., "The Restoration of Higher Cortical Functions in Local Brain Lesions", in: de Bruyn and Vinken (eds.), *Handbook of Cortical Neurology* (Amsterdam, The North Holland Publishing Co. [in press]).

Magoun, H. W., "The ascending reticular activating system", *A. Res. Nerv. Meul. Dis. Proc.*, v. 30 (1952).
Malinowsky, B., "The Problem of meaning in primitive languages", in Ogden's *Meaning of meaning* (London, 1930).
Marie, P. et Foix, Ch., "Les aphasies de la guerre", *Revue neurologique*, 31 (1917).
Markova, E. A., "Osobennosti narušenija nevrodinamiki pri amnestičeskoj afazii" [Characteristics of the disturbance of neurodynamics in amnesic aphasia], *Žurnal vysš. nerv. dejat.*, VII (1957), 3.
Marr, N. J., *Izbrannye raboty* [Collected Works], vol. 1-5 (Moscow, Socekgiz, 1933-1937).
Mayer, A., "The relation of the auditory center to aphasia", *Journal for Psychology and Neurology*, 13 (1908).
McCulloch, "The functional organisation of the cerebral cortex", *Physiological Review*, 3 (1944).
Meščaninov, I. I., *Problema klassifikacii jazykov v svete novogo učenija o jazyke* [Problems in the Classification of Languages in the Light of New Studies of Language]. Moscow, Izd-vo Akad. nauk SSSR, 1935.
—, *Novoe učenie o jazyke* [New Studies of Language] (Moscow, Socekgiz, 1930).
—, *Členy predloženija i časti reči* [The Components of Sentences and Parts of Speech] (Moscow, Izd-vo Akad. nauk SSSR, 1945).
Meščerjakov, A. I., *Narušenie dvux signal'nyx sistem s formirovaniem prostyx dvigatel'nyx reakcij pri lokal'nyx poraženijax golovnogo mozga* [Disturbance of the Two Signal Systems in the Formulation of Simple Motor Reactions with Focal Lesions of the Brain], Dissertation (1953).
Mettler, F. A., "Extracortical connection of the primate frontal cerebral cortex", *Journal Comparative Neurology*, v. 86, pp. 95-117 (1947).
Miller, G., *Language and Communication* (N.Y., McGraw-Hill, 1951).
Monakow, C., *Die Lokalisation im Grosshirn* (Wiesbaden, Bergmann, 1914).
Morel, F., *Introduction à la psychiatrie neurologique* (Paris, Masson, 1947).
Nazarova, L. K., "O roli rečevyx kinèstezij v pis'me" [On the role of verbal kinesthesia in writing], *Sovetskaja pedagogika*, 6 (1952).
Needles, W., "The problem of crossed aphasia", *Journal of Nervous and Mental Disorders*, 1942.
Nielsen, J. M., "Function of the minor cerebral hemisphere in language", *Bulletin Los Angeles Neurological Society*, 3 (1944).
—, *Agnosia, apraxia, aphasia* (Los Angeles, 1946).
Nissl v. Mayendorf, E., *Die aphasische Symptome und ihre kortikale Lokalisation* (Leipzig, Engelmann, 1911).
—, *Vom Lokalisationsproblem der artikulierten Sprache* (Leipzig, Barth, 1930).
Ombredane, A., *L'aphasie et l'élaboration de la pensée explicite* (Paris, Presses Universitaires, 1951).
Orbeli, L. A., *Lekcii po fiziologii nervnoj dejatel'nosti* [Lectures on the Physiology of Neural Activity], Second Edition (Moscow, Gosizdat, 1935).
—, *Voprosy vysšej nervnoj dejatel'nosti* [Questions of Higher Neural Activity] (Moscow-Leningrad, Izd-vo Akad. nauk SSSR, 1949).
Orton, S., *Reading, writing and speech problems in children* (New York, 1937).
Pavlov, I. P., *Dvadcatiletnij opyt ob"ektivnogo izučenija vysšej nervnoj dejatel'nosti životnyx* [Twenty years of Experience in the Objective Study of Higher Neural Activity of Animals] (= *Polnoe sobranie sočinenij*, III, Izd-vo Akad. nauk SSSR, 1951).
—, *Lekcii o rabote bol'six polušarij golovnogo mozga* [Lectures on the Function of Cerebral Cortex] (= *Polnoe sobraine sočinenij*, IV, Moscow, Izd-vo Akad. nauk, 1951).
Penfield, W., "Memory mechanisms", *Archives Neurology and Psychiatry*, 67 (1952).
—, "A consideration of the neurophysiological mechanisms of speech", *Proceedings American Academy of Arts & Sciences*, vol. 82, No. 5 (1953).
—, and Boldrey, F., "Somatic motor and sensory representation in the cerebral cortex of man", *Brain*, vol. 60 (1937).
—, and Erickson, T. C., *Epilepsy and cerebral localisation* (Springfield, Illinois, 1941).

——, and Rasmussen, T., *The Cerebral Cortex of Man* (New York, Macmillan, 1950).

——, and Jasper, H., *Epilepsy and the functional anatomy of Human Brain* (Boston, Little, Brown & Co., 1954).

Penfield, W. and Roberts, L., *Speech and Brain Mechanisms* (Princeton University Press, 1959).

Perel'man, L. B., *Postkontuzionnaja (reaktivnaja) gluxonemota, ee raspoznavanie i lečenie* [Postcontusional (Reactive) Deafmutism: Evaluation and Treatment] (Moscow, Medgiz, 1943).

——, "Farmakologičeskaja terapija dvigatel'nyx i čuvstvitel'nyx narušenij pri travme central'noj nervnoj sistemy" [Pharmacological therapy of the motor and sensory disorders resulting from trauma to the central nervous system], *Sovetskaja medicina*, 8-9 (1946).

Pfeiffer, R. A., "Pathologie der Höhrstrahlung und der orticalen Höhrsphäre", im Bumke-Foerster, *Handbuch der Neurologie*, Bd. 6 (1936).

Phillips, C. G., "Precentral motor area", in: J. Eccles (ed.), *Brain and Conscious Experience* (Berlin, Springer 1966).

Pick, A., "Über Sprachverständnis", *Ber. des III. Kongr. für exper. Psychologie* (Leipzig, 1909).

——, *Die agrammatischen Sprachstörungen* (Berlin, Springer, 1913).

——, "Aphasie", in Bethe's *Handbuch der norm. und pathol. Physiologie*, Bd. XV (1931).

Poliak, S., *The main afferent fiber systems of the cerebral cortex in Primates* (Univ. of Calif. Press, Berkeley, 1932).

Polivanov, E. D., "La perception des sons d'une langue étrangère", *Travaux de Cercle Lingutstique de Prague*, VI (1931).

Poljakov, G. I., *O rannem ontogeneze kory bol'šix polušarij* [The Early Ontogenesis of the Cerebral Cortex], Diss. (1939).

——, "O sootnošenijax osnovnyx tipov nejronov v kore mozga čeloveka" [The correlations of the basic types of neurons in the cortex of man], *Žurnal vysšej nervnoj dejat.*, 1 (1956), 3.

Poppelreuter, W., *Die psychischen Schädigungen durch Kopfschuss*, Bd. I-II (Leipzig, Voss, 1917-1918).

Potebnja, A. A., *Mysl' i jazyk* [Thought and Language] (SPB, 1862, Fifth Edition, Kharkov, 1926).

——, *Iz zapisok po russkoj grammatike* [Essays on Russian Grammar], vol. I and II (Kharkov, 1888).

Pötzl, O., "Die Aphasielehre vom Standpunkt der klinischen Psychiatrie. Die optisch-agnostischen Störungen", in Aschaffenburg's *Handbuch der Psychiatrie*, Spez. Teil, Abt. 3, H. 2 (Leipzig, Deutike, 1928).

——, *Zur Klinik und Anatomie der reinen Worttaubheit* (Berlin, Karger, 1919).

Pribram, K., *Neocortical functions in behavior. Symposium on interdiscriptionary research in the behaviore etc. Sciences* (Madison, University of Wisconsin Press, 1957).

——, *Comparative Neurology and the evolution of behavior. Behavior and evolution* (Yale University Press, 1958).

——, "Intercorrelation of Psychology and Neurological disciplines", *Files* (1957).

——, "On the Neurology of Thinking", *Behavioral Sciences*, 4.

Quensel, P., "Erkrankungen der höheren optischen Zentren", *Handbuch der Ophtalmologie*, 6 (1931).

Ratner, J. A., "Doklad na zasedanii Moskovskogo Obščestva Nevropatologov i Psixiatrov" [Report on sessions of the Moscow Society of Neuropathologists and Psychiatrists], *Žurnal nevropatologii i psixiatrii*, 1942.

Rose, J. E., "Cortical connexions of the reticular complex of the thalamus", *A. Res. Nerv. Ment. Dis. Proc.*, vol. 30 (1950).

Rosengardt-Pupko, G. L., *Reč' i rasvitije vosprijatija* [Speech and the Development of Perception] (Moscow, 1947).

Rossi, G. F., and Zanghetti, A., "The Brain stem reticular formation. Anatomy and Physiology", *Archives italiennes de biologie*, tome 95, fasc. 3-4 (1957), p. 199-435.

Rudenko, Z. Ja., *Narušenie sčeta pri mozgovyx poraženijax* [The Disturbance of Calculation with Brain Lesions], Dissertation (1953).

Salomon, E., "Motorische Aphasie mit Agrammatismus und sensorisch-agrammatische Sprachstörungen", *Mschr. für Psychiatrie*, 35 (1914).

Sapir, E., *Language* (1934).

Sapir, I. D., "Die Neurodynamik des Sprachartes bei Aphatiker", *Journal für Psychologie und Neurologie*, XXXVIII (1929).

—, "Afazija, reč', myšlenie" [Aphasia, speech and thought], *Žurnal nevropatologii i psixiatrii*, III (1934).

Saussure, F. de, *Cours de Linguistique générale* (Paris, 1922).

Šaxmatov, A. A., *K istorii zvukov russkogo jazyka* [The History of Sounds of the Russian Language] (Izd-vo Akad. nauk SSSR, 1900).

Ščelovanov, N. M., "Opyt refleksologičeskogo izučenija novoroždennogo" [Experiences in the study of reflexes of the newborn], *Novoe v refleksologii i fiziologii nervnoj sistemy* (Leningrad, 1926).

Ščerba, L. J., *Russkie glasnye v kačestvennom i količestvennom otnošenii* [Russian Vowels: Qualitative and Quantitative Relations] (1912).

—, *Fonetika francuzskogo jazyka* [Phonetics of the French Language] (Moscow, OGIZ, 1943).

Schaeffer, P., "Die kindliche Entwicklungsperiode des reinen Sprachverstehens, *Schr. Päd. Psych.*, 22 (1921).

Schell, H., "Diagnosis and Prognosis in Aphasia", *Archives of Neurology Psychiatry*, vol. 74 (1955).

—, "Auditory impairment in Aphasia", *Journal of Speech and Hearing Disorders*, vol. 18 (1953).

—, Jenkins, J. and Jimenez-Pabon, E., *Aphasia in Adults* (N.Y., Harper and Row, 1965).

Sečenov, I. M., *Èlementy mysli* [The Elements of Thought] (= *Izbrannye trudy*, I) (Moscow, Izd. Akad. nauk SSSR, 1947).

Semernickaja, F. M., *Ritm i ego narušenie pri različnyx mozgovyx poraženijax* [Rhythm and Its Disturbances with Different Brain Lesions], Dissertation (1945).

Sepp, E. K., "Osnovnye principy lokalizacii funkcij v mozgovoj kore" [Basic principles of the localization of function in the cerebral cortex], *Žurnal nevropatologii i psixiatrii*, 1 (1945).

Sherrington, Ch., *The Brain and its mechanisms* (Cambridge, University Press, 1934).

—, *Man on his Nature* (London, Macmillan, 1941).

Šif, Ž. I., "O narušenijax sravenenija pri čtenii" [Disturbances of comparison in reading], *Izvestija Akad. ped. nauk RSFSR*, 2 (1945).

Skipin, G. V., "K izučeniju fiziologičeskogo mexanizma tak naz. proizvol'nyx dviženij" [On an investigation of the physiological mechanism of so-called voluntary movements], *Žurnal vysš. nerv. dejat.*, I (1951), 6.

Škol'nik-Jarros, E. G., *Narušenie dviženij pri poraženii premotornoj zony* [The Disturbance of Movements with Lesions of the Premotor Zones], Dissertation (1945).

Šmidt, E. V., and Suxovskaja, I. A., "K patofiziologii senzornoj afazii" [The pathophysiology of sensory aphasia], *Žurnal nevropatologii i psixiatrii*, LIV (1954), 12.

Smirnov, L. I., *Patologičeskaja anatomija i patogenez travmatičeskoj bolezni golovnogo mozga* [Pathological Anatomy and Pathogenesis of Traumatic Disorders of the Brain] (Moscow, Izd-vo Akad. med. nauk SSSR, 1946).

Sokolov, A. N., "Vnutrennaja reč' i ponimanie" [Inner speech and Comprehension], *Učenye zapiski instituta psixologii*, 2 (1941).

—, "O rečevyx mexanizmax umstvennoj dejatel'nosti" [On the speech mechanisms of intellectual activity], *Izvestija Akad. pedag. nauk RSFSR*, 81 (1956).

—, "K voprosu o rečevyx mexanizmax umstvennoj dejatel'nosti" [On the question of speech mechanisms of intellectual activity], *Materialy soveščanija po psixologii* (Moscow, Izd-vo Akad. ped. nauk RSFSR, 1956).

Sokolov, E. N., *Vosprijatie i uslovnyj refleks* [Perception and the Conditioned Reflex] (Moscow, Izd-vo Mosk. Gos. Universiteta, 1958).

Spirin, B. G., *Narušenie podvižnosti nervnyx processov posle operacij na golovnom mozge* [Disturbance of the Flexibility of Neural Processes After Brain Operations], Dissertation (1958).

Stengel, E., and Lodge Patch, I. C., "Central Aphasia associated with parietal symptoms", *Brain*, vol. 78 (1955), p. 3.
Stern, W., *Kindersprache* (Leipzig, Barth, 1927).
Stier, E., *Die Linkschhändigkeit* (Jena, Fischer, 1911).
Stockert, F .G., "Werkzeugstörung und Aphasie", *Der Nervenartzt*, 29 (1958).
Subirana, A., "The prognosis in Aphasia in relation to the factor of cerebral dominance and handedness", *Brain*, vol. 81 (1958), p. 3.
Suxovskaja, N. A., *Izučenie reflektornyx reakcij čeloveka v norme i patologii po pokazatelja funkcional'noj mobil'nosti* [The Study of Reflex Reactions in Man: Functional Mobility as an Indicator under Normal and Pathological Conditoins], Dissertation (1958).
Šumilina, A. I., "Funkcional'noe značenie lobnyx oblastej kory golovnogo mozga v uslovno-reflektornoj dejatel'nosti sobaki" [The functional significance of the frontal areas of the cerebral cortex in conditioned reflex activity of the dog], *Problemy vysšej nervnoj dejatel'nosti* (Moscow, Izd-vo Akad. medic. nauk SSSR, 1949).
Šustin, N. A., *Narušenie nervnoj dejatel'nosti posle udalenija lobnyx dolej bol'six polušarij u sobak* [The Disturbance of Neural Activity after Extirpation of the Frontal Lobes of the Cerebral Cortex in the Dog], Dissertation (1955).
—, "O patologičeskoj inertnosti processa vozbuždenija v dvigatel'nom analizatore posle udalenija lobnyx dolej bol'šix polušarij" [The pathological inertia of the excitatory process in the motor analyzer after extirpation of the frontal lobes], *Žurnal vysšej nervn. dejatel'nosti*, VIII (1958), 2.
Švackin, N., *Fonetičeskoe razvitie detskoj reči* [The Phonetic Development of Children's Speech], Dissertation (1940).
Svedelius, C., *L'analyse du langage* (Uppsala, 1897).
Tapolet, "Die Sprache des Kindes", *Dtsch. Rundschau*, 131 (1907), 49.
Thorson, A. M., "The relation of tongue to internal speech", *Journal experimental psychiatry*, vol. 8 (1925).
Tixomirov, O. K., "Rečevaja reguljacija dviženij umstvenno-otstalogo rebënka v uslovijax konflikta neposredstvennyx i slovesnyx signalov" [Speech regulation of movements in the mentally retarded child given a conflict between direct and verbal signals], *Problemy vysšej nervnoj dejatel'nosti normal'nogo i anomal'nogo rebënka*, Vol. II (Moscow, Izd-vo Akad. pedag. nauk RSFSR, 1956).
—, "O formirovanii proizvol'nyx dviženij u detej doškol'nogo vozrasta" [On the formulation of voluntary movements in children of pre-school age], *Problemy vysšej nervnoj dejatel'nosti normal'nogo i anomal'nogo rebënka*, vol. II (Moscow, Izd-vo Akad. pedag. nauk RSFSR, 1958).
Traugott, N. N., "O senzornoj alalii i afazii v detskom vozraste" [On sensory alalia and aphasia in childhood], *Referaty naučno-issledov. rabot, Mediko-biol. nauki*, 1 (Moscow, Izd-vo medic, literatury, 1947).
—, Balonov, L. J., Ličko, L. E., *Očerki fiziologii vysšej nervnoj dejatel'nosti čeloveka* [Notes on the Physiology of Higher Neural Activity of Man] (Moscow, Gos. Izd-vo medic. literatury, 1957).
Travaux du cercle linguistique de Prague, vol. IV, VI (Prague, 1934, 1936).
Troubetzkoy, N., *Grundzüge der phonologie* (Prague, 1939).
Tsang, Y. Ch., "The functions of the visual areas of the cerebral cortex", *Comp. psych. Monogr.*, 50 (1936).
Vygotskij, L. S., *Myšlenie i reč'* [Thought and Speech] (Moscow, Gosizdat, 1934) (English edition: MIT Press, 1947).
—, "Psixoligija i učenie o lokalizacii" [Psychology and the study of localization], *Tezisy 1-j Vseukrainskoj psixonevrologičeskoj konferencii* (Kharkov, 1934).
—, *Izbrannye psixologičeskie issledovanija* [Collected Psychological Investigations] (Moscow, Akad. pedag. nauk PSFSR, 1956).
—, *Razvitie Vysšyx Psixičeskix Funkcij* [Development of the Higher Mental Functions] (Moscow, Akad. Pedag. Nauk RSFSR, 1960).
Wada, J., "New method of the determination of the side of Cerebral speech dominance", *Acta Medica Hokkajdo*, vol. 24 (1949), p. 1-10.

Walker, A. E., *The primate thalamus* (Chicago, Univ. of Chicago Press, 1938).
Walshe, F. M. R., "On the syndrome of the premotor cortex", *Brain*, 58 (1935).
Warrington, E., and Zangwill, O. L., "A study of dyslexia", *Journal of Neurol. Neurosurgery and Psychiatry*, XX (1957), p. 208.
—, "On the mode of representation of movements in the motor cortex", *Brain*, 66 (1943).
Weisenburg, Th., and McBride, K., *Aphasia, A clinical and psychological study* (New York, 1935).
Wernicke, S., *Der Aphasische Symptomenkomplex* (Breslau, 1874).
Woerkom, W. van, "Über Störungen im Denken bei aphasischen Patienten", *Mschr. für Psychiatrie und Neurologie*, 59 (1925).
Woolsey, L. N., *Organization of Somatic Sensory and Motor Areas of the Celebral Cortex, Biological and Biochemical Bases of Behavior* (Madison, University Wisconsin Press, 1958).
Xoroško, V. K., *Ob otnošenii lobnyx dolej mozga k psixologii i psixopatologii* [The Relation of Frontal Lobes to Psychology and Psychopathology] (Moscow, 1912).
Zambran, I. I., *Rol' afferentnyx sistem v organizacii dvigatel'nogo akta* [The Role of the Afferent Systems in the Organization of the Motor Act] (Diplomnaja rabota biolog. fakul'teta Moskovskogo Universiteta, 1948).
Zankov, L. V. (ed.), "Psixologo-pedagogičeskie problemy vosstanovlenija reči pri čerepno-mozgovix ranenijax" [Psychological-pedagogical problems in the restoration of speech with skull-brain injuries], *Izvestija Akad. ped. nauk*, II (1945).
Zaporožec, A. V., *Razvitie proizvol'nyx dviženij* [The Development of Voluntary Movements] (Moscow, Izd-vo akad. ped. nauk RSFSR, 1959).
Zavarzin, A. A., *Očerki po èvoljucionnoj gistologii nervnoj sistemy* [Notes on the Evolutional Histology of the Nervous System] (= *Izbrannye trudy*, t. III, Moscow, Izd. Akad. nauk SSSR, 1955).
Žinkin, N. I., *Mexanizm reči* [Speech Mechanisms] (Moscow, Akad. pedag. nauk RSFSR, 1959).

INDEX OF AUTHORS

INDEX OF MATTERS

Bei Fragen zur Produktsicherheit wenden Sie sich bitte an:
If you have any questions regarding product safety,
please contact:

Walter de Gruyter GmbH
Genthiner Straße 13
10785 Berlin
productsafety@degruyterbrill.com